Preface

The aims and objectives outlined in the preface to the first edition remain the same, together with the general format, but the text has been revised and expanded to take into account developments during the 7 years since the preparation of the first edition.

The chapter on Automated Blood Cell Analysis has been completely rewritten and significant additions include sections on the myelodysplastic syndromes and cell markers. The rate of progress in certain areas is exemplified by the increase in the number of interleukins from 6 to 9 since the manuscript was submitted! Although increased understanding of the mechanisms of thrombosis, the introduction of new methods of investigation, together with changes in monitoring anticoagulant therapy, have justified the restructuring of the chapters dealing with disorders of haemostasis and their investigation, I have been conscious throughout of the desirability of limiting the inevitable increase in text to a reasonable level.

Once again I am grateful to colleagues in many laboratories for their encouragement and help. Particular thanks are due to the staff of Butterworth–Heinemann for their encouragement, patience and expertise. It is hoped that this second edition will continue to contribute to the high standard of laboratory haematology and be as well received as the first.

Roger Hall
December 1990

Preface to the First Edition

Many years involvement in teaching, in examining and in the practice of laboratory haematology, together with frequent requests to recommend suitable books, have indicated a need for a single volume that combines physiology, pathophysiology and the practical aspects. The aim has been to produce a textbook that is more than adequate for first qualifications and a sound basis for further study, which will also serve as a bench-book in the haematology department of a general hospital. We have therefore attempted to maintain a balance between the haematological disorders and the methods used in investigation, but in certain areas where technology is advancing rapidly, e.g. instrumentation or immunoassays using radioisotope or enzyme labels, we have confined the text to general principles and avoided recommending particular instruments and methods (or test kits!). This book is primarily for technologists, scientists and medical colleagues involved in laboratory haematology; and although inevitably the content is related to laboratories and examinations in the United Kingdom, we are confident that much of the content is relevant to laboratory haematology in other countries.

The photomicrographs have been restricted to those capable of illustrating morphological appearances in monochrome; those features that can be appreciated only by colour reproduction have been deliberately, though regrettably, omitted to maintain the book at a reasonable price. Clinical aspects and therapeutic considerations are included only when the laboratory is involved in monitoring treatment or when symptoms or physical examination indicate a particular line of laboratory investigation.

We are grateful to the many colleagues who knowingly or unknowingly have contributed in any way to the preparation of this book. Particular acknowledgement is made to the assistance of David Howard and the Department of Medical Illustration, St James's University Hospital for preparing the photomicrographs and to Alan Tunstill and the Department of Medical Illustration, Royal Hallamshire Hospital for the figures illustrating aspects of haemostasis. *Figure 13.1* is based on a scheme devised by Mr C. S. Scott. Mrs Wendy Mitchell and Mrs Eileen Murat skilfully transformed the draft into presentable form. To Butterworths for their patience, tolerance and encouragement, we extend our thanks.

Roger Hall
Robert G. Malia

Contents

Chapter 1

Haemopoiesis

The blood volume of the normal adult accounts for approximately 7% of body weight or about 70 ml/kg, of which 30 ml (45%) is occupied by the cellular elements and 40 ml (55%) is plasma. The cells are heterogeneous. They consist of erythrocytes, which are disc shaped, non-nucleated, non-motile and contain haemoglobin; the nucleated, motile leucocytes and the platelets. The leucocytes are further divided into granulocytes (neutrophils, eosinophils and basophils), lymphocytes and monocytes. Plasma contains many organic and inorganic compounds, notably proteins, electrolytes, substances absorbed from the gastrointestinal tract, hormones and products of metabolism.

All blood cells have a finite life span which may be shortened in disease. Plasma components, particularly proteins, have a determined rate of turnover which is often expressed as T_{50} – the time during which half the substance is removed from the circulation and, in health, renewed. The 'turnover times' may be altered by disease.

The loss of cells through the normal processes of ageing, physiological consumption, and, in certain circumstances, by loss from the body, is normally compensated by the process of renewal by the proliferation, maturation and release of new cells from the haemopoietic system – a process referred to as *haemopoiesis*. The haemopoietic system in the adult consists of the bone marrow and the lymphatic system. Other sites of haemopoiesis are active in the embryo and fetus.

Blood formation in the embryo and fetus

Haemopoiesis in the embryo and fetus takes place in three overlapping phases – the extraembryonic (in the yolk sac), the hepatic (and to some extent the spleen) and the bone-marrow phase. The yolk sac is the principal site in the early embryo and declines rapidly to be entirely replaced by the liver at about 2.5 months' gestation. The hepatic phase is maximal between 4 and 5 months' gestation and then gradually declines towards term though some activity is still present at birth. The contribution of the spleen is maximal at the same time as the liver but starts at about 2.5 months with a contribution that lasts until about 6.5 months. The hepatic and splenic contribution is gradually taken over by that of the bone marrow which begins at 4 months and replaces the liver at term.

Erythropoiesis

Recognizable erythropoietic cells are found in the mesoderm of the yolk sac as early as the 14th day of development and produce erythrocytes for about 10 weeks. Initially morphology is similar to the megaloblasts associated with vitamin B_{12} and folate deficiencies. Normoblastic appearances are seen at 6 weeks. Mesodermal erythropoiesis is transferred to the liver which becomes the principal source of red cells during the second trimester of development. Hepatic erythropoiesis is macronormoblastic resulting in the production of macrocytic red cells. At 12 weeks' gestation circulating normoblasts are in the order of 50×10^9/l with the red cells having an MCV of 180 fl. By 20 weeks the normoblast numbers have fallen to 1.0×10^9/l and the MCV at 28 weeks is about 120 fl falling to a range of 100–120 fl at term. Maximum response to erythropoietin is demonstrable between 14 and 18 weeks.

The bone marrow contains recognizable erythroblasts at about 10 weeks, foci of development at 4 months, and by the 6th month has become the major site of erythropoiesis.

The transfer of erythropoiesis to different sites is associated with changes in the polypeptide chains of the globin molecule of haemoglobin. The production of α chains commences at about the 5th week and continues into and throughout adult life and is preceded by the formation of ζ chains. The precursors of the β and δ chains of adult haemoglobin are designated, in order of appearance, ε and γ chains. The normal haemoglobins found during erythropoiesis in the embryo and fetus are therefore:

$\zeta_2\varepsilon_2$	Gower I	Extraembryonic source detectable up to 12 weeks?
$\zeta_2\gamma_2$	Portland I	
$\alpha_2\varepsilon_2$	Gower II	
$\alpha_2\gamma_2$	Hb F (fetal Hb)	– hepatic phase
$\alpha_2\beta_2$	Hb A	Bone-marrow phase
$\alpha_2\delta_2$	Hb A_2	

Hb F is detectable very early in embryonic life and at the 34th week constitutes about 90% of the circulating haemoglobin falling to between 50 and 85% at term. Hb F has a higher oxygen affinity than Hb A which would facilitate transport of oxygen across the placental membrane. Hb A is detectable in small amounts as early as 8 weeks of gestation but remains the minor haemoglobin component during fetal life. Hb A_2 appears at about 7 months' development as a minor Hb component.

Granulopoiesis

Though granulocyte formation can be observed in various embryonic and fetal tissues from about 7 weeks, the developing bone marrow is the major source of granulocytes starting at about 10 weeks. Relatively little activity is found until after 4–5 months' gestation. At 20 weeks circulating granulocytes number fewer than 1×10^9/l but thereafter rise rapidly towards term.

Thrombopoiesis

A few megakaryocytes are found in the yolk sac at 6–7 weeks. They then develop in the liver and spleen and eventually the bone marrow at 13 weeks. Little is known of the production and numbers of platelets in the fetal circulation though at term the number is similar to that of the adult.

Lymphopoiesis

Lymphocytes have not been identified in the yolk sac. Formation commences in lymph plexuses at about 8 weeks and then the thymus, lymph glands, spleen and in the bone marrow. About 2% of marrow cells are lymphocytes at 26 weeks rising to 8% at 30 weeks. Lymphocytes are found in the circulation as early as the 8th week reaching a maximum of 4–10 × 10^9/l at 6 months and falling to 3 × 10^9/l at term.

Bone-marrow structure and function

At term all the bone marrow apart from perhaps the terminal phalanges of the fingers and toes is active or 'red', and has a volume of about 1.4% of fetal weight.

The totally haemopoietic marrow of the new-born is gradually replaced with fat cells until adult development is attained when about half the marrow is fatty. The bone marrow is one of the largest organs of the body, having a volume of 30–50 ml/kg body weight. Thus in a 70 kg adult the active marrow has a volume of about 1000–1750 ml. The gradual replacement of haemopoietic marrow by fat commences at the periphery of the skeleton and proceeds in the limb bones until, in the adult, active marrow is confined to the central skeleton.

The blood supply to the bone marrow is provided from a central artery which leads to branching arterioles and capillaries which open into sinusoids. The walls of the sinusoids consist of a single layer of cells without a basement membrane. The lining cells simply touch or overlap each other. This loose arrangement of sinusoidal endothelium separates the haemopoietic and fat cells of the extravascular tissue from the intravascular system and forms the marrow–blood barrier (MBB) [1]. The sinusoids are drained by a system of venules leading to the central vein.

The MBB controls the migration of formed blood cells from the extravascular haemopoietic compartment into the circulation and conversely probably influences the passage of essential nutrients, humoral stimulators and inhibitors of haemopoiesis, and possibly the selective trapping of circulating cells. In normal marrow the release of cells from the extravascular space is determined by the deformability of the cells. Thus segmented neutrophils can be aligned to squeeze between or through the endothelial cells [2]. The release of erythrocytes is associated with removal of the nucleus (the so-called 'pitting' function). In certain abnormal states such as haemopoietic hyperplasia or when the architecture is altered by the presence of non-marrow elements the MBB is unable to control cell release effectively and immature cells can reach the circulation.

A similar situation arises when haemopoiesis occurs in tissues other than the bone marrow (extramedullary haemopoiesis) where an effective barrier does not exist. The effectiveness of the MBB is shown by its ability to control the release of about 6 × 10^{11} mature cells daily (about 6 × 10^6 cells every second!) into the circulation while retaining the immature cells and maintaining the proliferative capacity of the marrow. The ability of the bone marrow to provide prompt delivery of cells to the circulation suggests that the MBB responds to humoral signals. Not only is there a prompt response but it is also selective in that erythrocytes are delivered when needed or granulocytes are released if required though some non-specific release of other cell lines may occur.

It has been suggested that the PCV is an important determinant of red-cell release into the sinusoids independent of erythropoietin levels[3, 4]. *In vitro* studies support the hypothesis that red-cell egress may be driven by a hydrostatic pressure difference across endothelial 'pores'[5]. Platelet release is an exception in that there is little marrow reserve, as indicated by the delay in recovery of circulating platelet numbers in individuals made thrombocytopenic. The megakaryocytes are located close to the sinusoidal endothelium and extend projections into the lumen and thus the circulation. A high proportion of megakaryocytes enter the sinusoids intact and migrate to the lungs, where platelet formation takes place[6–8].

The extravascular space of the marrow consists of haemopoietic cells and non-haemopoietic elements or stromal cells. The stromal elements of the marrow include fat cells, mononuclear phagocytes and connective tissue cells capable of synthesizing collagen and to form reticulin fibres. It is recognized that the non-haemopoietic connective tissue provides a micro-environment which is essential for the proliferative and self-renewal capacities of normal haemopoiesis and is an example of cell–cell interaction in haemopoiesis[9, 10]. To a great extent this concept is based on observations of long-term bone marrow cultures[11].

Yellow marrow is predominantly fat and even red active marrow contains fat, particularly towards the centre of the marrow cavity. The degree of haemopoietic activity varies considerably, not only between different bones but between adjacent sites within the same bone. The lymphocytes of the adult bone marrow are distributed in nodules either as lymphoid follicles or lymphoid infiltrates. Follicles account for about 80% of the nodules with a reticulin framework, some having germinal centres[12].

In addition to its haemopoietic function the bone marrow, as part of the reticuloendothelial system, contains many macrophages which ingest particulate material, micro-organisms, extruded nuclei and in certain circumstances intact erythrocytes. The role of the marrow in removing effete red cells in normal subjects is not clear.

Cell proliferation

Proliferating cell systems vary in their growth characteristics in that the total number of cells may increase, remain constant or diminish. Haemopoiesis during intrauterine life is an example of an increasing cell population while haemopoiesis in the adult is normally in a steady state: production equals loss or destruction. Within a steady-state population, different cell types can vary greatly in the frequency of cell division; the relatively rapid turnover of erythrocytes requires that the earlier erythroblasts are in the cell cycle leading to mitosis, while others – e.g. the lymphocytes – divide only rarely and are not in cell cycle.

The cell cycle (*Figure 1.1*) is the period between the formation of a cell and the completion of mitosis in the newly formed cells and is known as the interphase. The development of techniques of microspectrophotometry for quantitation of DNA and autoradiography using radioactive DNA precursors has enabled the cell cycle to be divided in relation to the period of interphase when DNA synthesis occurs, the 'S' phase. Cells in the S phase are recognized by their uptake of radioactive thymidine as shown by autoradiography. The S phase is preceded by a postmitotic,

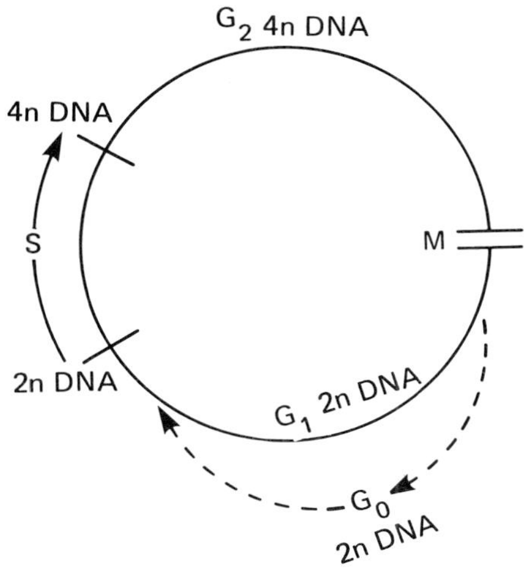

Figure 1.1 The cell cycle. The stages of cells in interphase are shown by: G_0 = cells not engaged in proliferation; G_1 = 'gap 1', the presynthesis phase of cells with a 2n DNA content; S = phase of DNA synthesis; G_2 = the post-synthesis/premitotic phase, the cells having replicated their DNA content though still having a diploid number of chromosomes; M = mitosis

pre-synthesis phase known as G_1 (or gap 1) in which the cells have a diploid (2n) DNA content. The post-synthesis, premitotic phase in which the cells have a 'tetraploid' (4n) DNA content is known as G_2 (or gap 2). Cells in S phase have a DNA content between 2n and 4n. Cells with a 2n DNA content that do not enter S phase are thought to have an extremely prolonged G_1 or are in a 'resting phase' designated G_0. However, G_0 cells may be stimulated to enter the cycle. The combined techniques of DNA quantitation and autoradiography following thymidine labelling, allow determination of the proportion of each cell type in G_1 (and G_0), S and G_2 phases. Further, the duration of G_1, S and G_2 phases can be measured and the 'labelling-index' of mitoses calculated.

Rates of cell proliferation may be adjusted by several mechanisms. Cells in G_0 may be stimulated to commence DNA synthesis, the period of G_1 may be shortened or prolonged as may S and G_2, and the duration of mitosis may vary. In certain disorders of haemopoiesis, cell development may be arrested in G_2 with resulting cell death. Therapeutic drug regimens designed to reduce a cell population are often based on the stages of the cell cycle.

Haemopoietic development

In 1961 Till and McCullough[13] observed that cells that form colonies in the spleens (colony forming units–spleen, CFU–S) of irradiated syngeneic recipient mice are able to self-renew and differentiate into granulocyte, erythrocyte, macrophage and megakarocyte cell lines. Subsequent developments in *in vitro* techniques of cell culture in semi-solid medium have established many of the processes by which pluripotent stem cells (PSCs) give rise to the mature or end-cells of the blood.

Most models of haemopoiesis have four compartments:

1. Pluripotent stem cells with the capacity for self-renewal.
2. Committed pluripotent stem cells.
3. Committed unipotent progenitor cells.
4. Mature end-cell compartment.

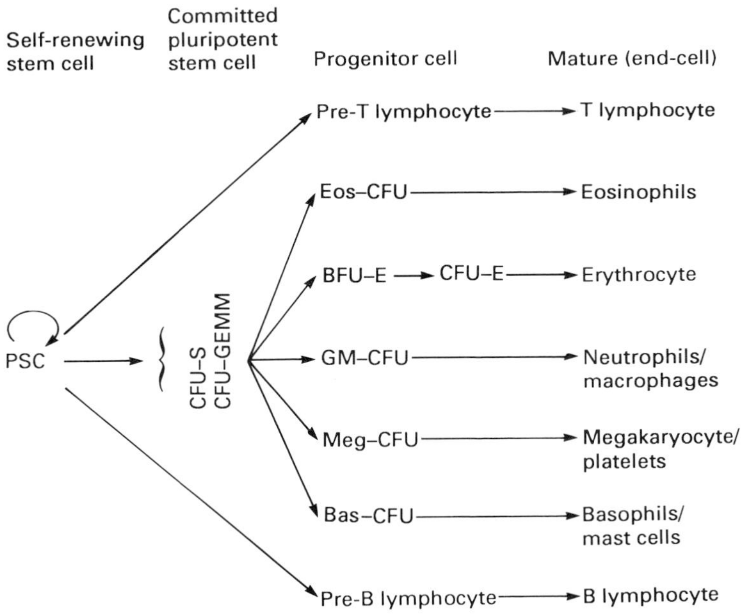

Figure 1.2 A model of haemopoiesis based on observations in irradiated mice and in clonal cell culture. PSC = self-renewing pluripotent stem cell; CFU–S = colony forming unit–spleen; CFU–GEMM = colony forming unit–granulocyte, erythroid, macrophage, megakaryocyte; Eos–CFU = eosinophil colony forming unit; BFU–E = burst forming unit–erythroid: CFU–E = colony forming unit–erythroid; Meg–CFU = megakaryocyte colony forming unit; Bas–CFU = basophil colony forming unit

A model is shown in *Figure 1.2*. All models are based on culture studies and therefore represent the 'state of the art' of cell cloning and are almost certainly an oversimplified diagrammatic representation of a more complex process. Variation to this model could be to include a compartment of oligopotent progenitors which have mixed potential in culture but are not pluripotent.

Self-renewal is the process of cell division in which one of the daughter cells proceeds to differentiation while the other retains the properties of the parent stem cell. Most authorities appear to prefer a stochastic model of self-renewal expressed as the probability (P) that a daughter cell will retain the characteristics of the parent stem cell. In the steady state $P = 0.5$.

There is evidence from recloning studies that human, committed, pluripotent cells (CFU–GEMM), like the CFU–S in the mouse, have limited self-renewal capacity.

By conventional methods of study the earliest identifiable precursors seen in the bone marrow are already committed 'blast' cells with morphological, biochemical, cytochemical or immunological characteristics that identify their lineage. The production of monoclonal antibodies against determinants on pluripotent and differentiated precursors together with the use of fluorescence-activated cell sorters, has permitted immunological identification and separation of progenitor cells[14, 15].

Haemopoietic growth regulators

Growth inducers

The early work on *in vitro* cell culture demonstrated that, in addition to the micro-anatomical contribution of the other cells and structures of the marrow, soluble cell products are essential for colony growth and are collectively termed 'colony stimulating factors' or CSFs. Some CSFs have wide activity and encourage growth of multilineage colonies while others are restricted or even specific for a single cell line. For example, CSF–GEMM supports colonies containing cells of granulocyte, erythroid, macrophage and megakaryocyte series, while CSF–GM supports only granulocyte and macrophage proliferation and CSF–G only granulocytes. The earliest defined specific growth factor is erythropoietin (Epo) which influences the growth of erythroid burst forming units (BFU–E) and further differentiation.

Assays based on *in vitro* colony formation have allowed purification and characterization of several growth factors. They are all glycoproteins and, by recombinant DNA technology, some have been cloned and can be produced in either mammalian or bacterial systems[16].

The current terminology reflects the role of cell–cell interactions by the use of the term 'interleukin' (IL) for soluble cell products which influence the proliferation or maturation of other cell lines. The ILs either act directly or stimulate the release of growth factors from other cell types. *Table 1.1* summarizes the characteristics of certain growth factors.

Growth inhibitors

Most biological systems have inhibitory or negative feedback mechanisms. These processes may simply reduce the level of growth factor, e.g. tissue oxygenation on Epo production. Others are, again, examples of cell–cell interactions. Acidic isoferritins (AIFs) are found in granulocytes, monocytes, lymphocytes, erythrocytes and in erythroblasts. Not all AIFs have inhibitory activity though it has been suggested that AIF from macrophages or monocytes contribute to a normal inhibitory feedback mechanism affecting CFU–GEMM, CFU–GM and BFU–E progenitor cells[17].

The iron-binding protein lactoferrin present in neutrophils has been suggested as a negative feedback mechanism for control of granulopoiesis by suppressing GM–CSF from mononuclear cells, and that decreased release from neutrophils can result in increased granulopoiesis[18].

Interferons (IFNs) are a group of naturally occurring inducible proteins with several biological activities including, *in vitro*, inhibitory effects on the growth of progenitor cells from normal bone marrow, including CFU–GEMM, CFU–GM, BFU–E, CFU–E and CFU–Mk. Both alpha and gamma IFN have been cloned and

Table 1.1 Characteristics of haemopoietic growth factors

Growth factor	*Synonym*	*Source*	*Activity*
IL-1		'All' cells	Synergistic with other growth factors G–CSF; GM–CSF; IL-2; IL-3
IL-2		Activated T lymphocytes	Proliferation of activated T lymphocytes
IL-3	Multi-CSF	Activated T lymphocytes, myeloid cells	Proliferation and maturation of 'all' cell lines including erythroid
IL-4	BSF-1	Activated T lymphocytes	Activation of B lymphocytes, T-helper cells, mast cell/basophils in synergy with IL-3
IL-5	(a) BCGF-II (b) mEDF	Activated T lymphocytes Activated T lymphocytes	Growth of B lymphocytes Eosinophil differentiation
IL-6	BSF-2	Activated T lymphocytes	Ig secretion by B lymphocytes
Epo	Erythropoietin	Renal activator	BFU–E and subsequent stages of proliferation and maturation
Insulin		Pancreatic hormone	CFU–E in absence of Epo
BPA	Burst promoting activity	Activated T cells and other cells	Induces differentiation of BFU–E
MkPA	Megakaryocyte potentiating activity	T lymphocytes	Synergistic with IL-3
EPA	Erythroid potentiating activity	T lymphocytes	Synergistic with Epo
IL for DA lymphs	HILDA	Activated human T lymphocytes	Eosinophils

BSF, B cell stimulating factor; BCGF, B lymphocyte colony growth factor; mEDF, murine eosinophil differentiating factor.

Note: Many growth factors have been derived from murine cell lines. Although human equivalents have been isolated and purified, this may not always be the case

in vitro studies indicate that recombinant alpha and gamma IFN have inhibitory activity, although the effect of gamma IFN is mediated by other cell populations, notably T lymphocytes [19].

Leucotrienes (LTs) are products derived from the arachidonic acid 5-lipo-oxygenase pathways originating in cell membranes and certain LTs influence prostaglandin PGE_2 and thromboxane B_2 production. LTs are produced by human granulocytes, monocytes, macrophages and T lymphocytes and appear to have both inhibitory and stimulatory effects on normal marrow haemopoiesis [20].

Erythropoiesis

Figure 1.3 shows the concept of orderly development of the erythroid series from stem cell to mature red cell and the role played by erythropoietin.

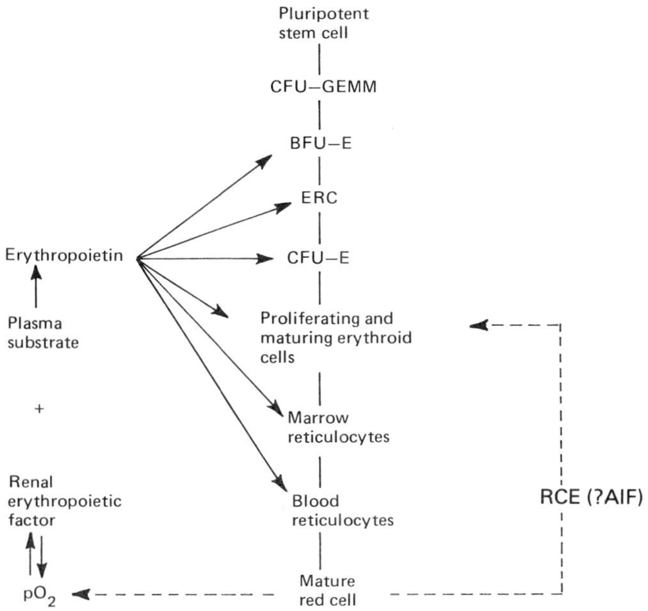

Figure 1.3 Schematic representation of erythropoiesis. CFU–GEMM = Colony forming unit–granulocyte, erythrocyte, macrophage, megakaryocyte; BFU–E = burst forming unit–erythroid; ERC = erythropoietin-responsive cells; CFU–E = colony forming unit–erythroid; RCE = red cell extract; AIF = acidic isoferritins. ——— = stimulatory pathways; ---- = inhibitory pathways

The burst forming unit–erythroid (BFU–E)

This cell is so called because of its ability to promote a number of erythroid clusters or 'bursts' after 5–6 days' culture and is the earliest cell committed to erythroid development. The number of BFU–Es is not influenced by erythropoietin though the number of 'bursts' shows a dose-related response to erythropoietin.

Erythropoietin-responsive cells (ERCs)

These are later stages of committed cells than BFU–Es and their number and differentiation is controlled by erythropoietin to give rise to small colonies of erythroid cells which have been shown to be derived from single cells.

The colony forming units–erythroid (CFU–E)

When cultured from human marrow these reach size in 10–20 days with maturation and the synthesis of haemoglobin. CFU–E are probably a few cell divisions earlier than the first recognizable erythroid precursor – the pronormoblast.

Subsequent development is through the basophilic, early polychromatic and late polychromatic stages to the non-nucleated reticulocyte and finally to the mature erythrocyte. Of these recognizable cells only the pronormoblast and the basophilic and early polychromatic cells are in cell cycle and normally four cell divisions transform one pronormoblast into 16 erythrocytes with a small loss of proliferating cells (ineffective erythropoiesis). Maturation occurs both in the proliferating and in the non-proliferating pools. There is evidence that DNA synthesis, and consequently cell division, is inhibited at a critical intracellular haemoglobin concentration.

Normally the nucleus of the normoblast is lost by extrusion rather than fragmentation (karyorrhexis), and the cell enters the circulation through gaps in the walls of the marrow sinusoids (diapedesis). The newly formed reticulocytes are apparently motile. ^{59}Fe studies have indicated that the time of development from pronormoblast to reticulocyte in the circulation is about 7 days, of which 3 days is the transit time in the marrow reticulocyte pool.

Erythropoietin [21, 22]

The suggestion that the rate of erythropoiesis is regulated by a humoral factor rather than a direct action of hypoxia was made over 80 years ago and was confirmed by inducing reticulocyte responses in normal animals by the injection of plasma from anaemic animals. The plasma factor was termed erythropoietin (Epo). Erythropoietin is a heat-stable, sialic-acid-containing glycoprotein present in very small amounts in normal plasma but excreted in higher concentration in urine. The molecular weight of human Epo is about 34 000 daltons.

The kidney is the major site of Epo production in the adult with a small percentage (5–15%) produced by other organs or tissues. The major source of extrarenal Epo is the liver. The physiological production of Epo is regulated by oxygen delivery to the tissues. Thus the presence of anaemia produces tissue hypoxia in the kidney resulting in increased Epo production and consequent increase in erythropoiesis. Conversely, in hypertransfused subjects or when oxygen affinity of haemoglobin is reduced, Epo is reduced and erythropoiesis suppressed.

The effects of erythropoietin on red-cell kinetics may be summarized as follows:

1. Stimulation of erythropoietin-sensitive cells to differentiate into pronormoblasts.
2. Shortening of cell-cycle times or increase of the proportion of dividing cells among the unrecognized erythroid precursors.
3. Shortening the cell-cycle times of proliferating erythroblasts.
4. Shortening the total maturation time in the recognizable red-cell precursor pool.
5. Causing the production of macrocytes.
6. Promoting reticulocyte release from the marrow.

Erythropoietin also influences RNA and DNA synthesis, the transfer of iron from transferrin to erythroblast, the rate of haem synthesis and the rate of glycolysis via the pentose phosphate pathway. In other balanced biological processes there are usually inhibitory mechanisms, and inhibitors to erythropoietin have been isolated from tissue extracts and urine. Their precise role is not clear. Of particular relevance may be negative feedback influences of extracts from mature red cells and normal bone marrow. Of particular importance is the observation that extracts of mature red cells (RCE) inhibit the incorporation of tritiated thymidine by marrow cells *in vitro*. RCE may affect the recognizable proliferating cells by prolonging cell-cycle times and thus acts as a fine control on cell production.

Influence of other hormones on erythropoiesis

There is good evidence that hormones other than erythropoietin influence erythropoiesis in that endocrine deficiency is often associated with an anaemia that responds to replacement therapy. Furthermore the administration of the male hormone testosterone can induce erythrocytosis and conversely oestrogen administration depresses erythropoiesis. The mechanisms by which these hormones influence erythropoiesis is not entirely clear but there is evidence that much of their effect is achieved by influencing erythropoietin production by modifying either REF production or the plasma substrate, or even by influencing the effect of erythropoietin on the ERC compartment. *In vivo* studies in mice have shown the influence of testosterone in inducing CFU–S to enter the cell cycle.

Granulopoiesis

The earliest cell committed to granulocyte production is the granulocyte-macrophage colony forming unit GM–CFU, growth of which *in vitro* is stimulated by its specific growth factor GM–CSF or in synergism with other factors. In practice, GM–CFU refers to neutrophil lineage and the other granulocyte cell lines can be stimulated by appropriate growth factors, e.g. eosinophils by Eo–CSF or IL-2 with activated T lymphocytes, and basophil/mast cell lines by IL-3/IL-4.

Differentiation and maturation of granulocytes

The recognition of the myeloblast as the precursor of granulocytes is based on subtle morphological appearances supplemented by cytochemistry, electron microscopy and immunological characteristics. The long-held view that neutrophils, eosinophils and basophils are derived from a common myeloblast is not justified and each may well have a distinct myeloblast precursor.

Neutrophil proliferation and maturation is a good model for the concept of proliferating and non-proliferating compartments and subsequent release into marginating (MGP) and circulating pools (CGP) (*Figure 1.4*).

Transfer of neutrophils from the MGP to the CGP without an increase in the total blood granulocyte pool (TBGP) can be caused by physiological influences such as exercise or release of adrenaline which cause increased blood flow through the microcirculation. In such circumstances the increase in circulating neutrophils is not associated with release of neutrophils from the marrow. The injection of bacterial endotoxin results in a shift of neutrophils from the MGP to the CGP and also an increase in TBGP by an influx of cells.

The TBGP must be regarded as a transit population between the bone marrow and the tissues and body secretions, in which the neutrophils normally perform their phagocytic function. The transfer of neutrophils from blood to tissue is considered to be ‘one-way only’.

Regulation of granulopoiesis

The regulation of granulopoiesis is by a homeostatic balance between stimulatory and inhibitory humoral factors. Although CSF activity derived from macrophages may represent the major ‘granulopoietin’ which is influenced by endotoxin stimulation of macrophages, there is evidence of oestrogen control of the proliferating pool possibly by increasing CSF activity, by modifying cell-cycle times or by influencing the rate of release from the marrow. There is evidence that there is a long-cycle periodicity of the CGP in normal humans and this is supported by the disorder of ‘cyclical neutropenia’ which occurs at intervals of about 21 days and is associated with a reduction in the proliferating neutrophil pool.

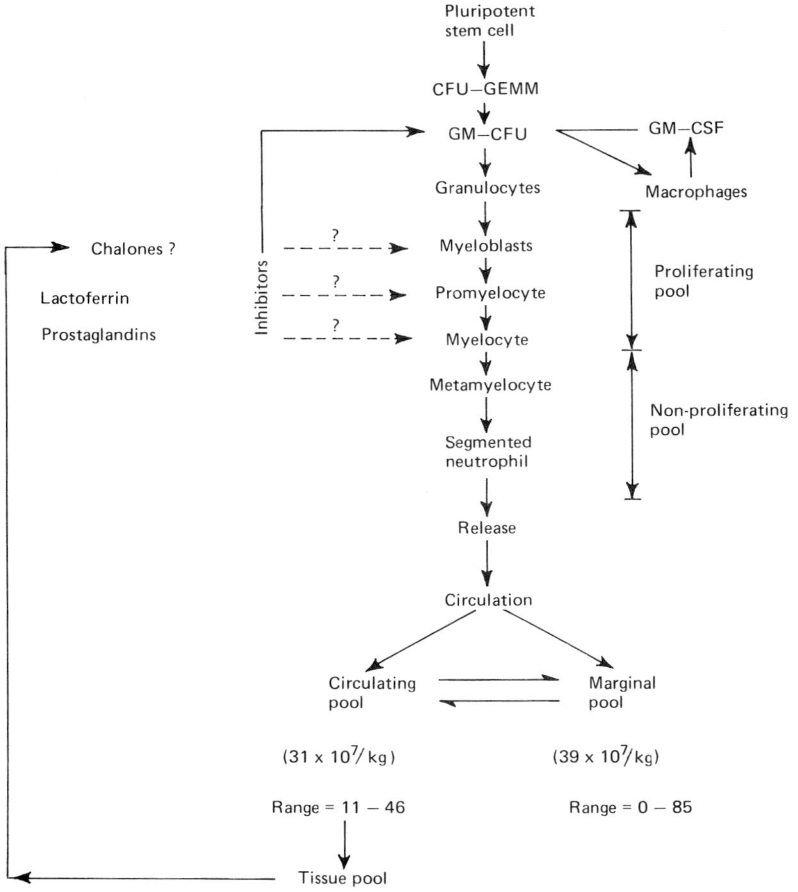

Figure 1.4 Schematic representation of granulocytopoiesis. CFU–GEMM = Colony forming unit–granulocyte, erythrocyte, macrophage, megakaryocyte; GM–CFU = granulocyte–macrophage colony forming unit; GM–CSF = granulocyte–macrophage colony stimulating factor. The numbers of granulocytes in the circulating and marginal pools refer to neutrophils. ——— = stimulatory pathways; ---- = inhibitory pathways

Studies of granulopoiesis *in vitro* have shown that prostaglandins of the E series (PGE), notably PGE_2, have a marked inhibitory activity. PGE_2 can be produced by the stimulation of blood monocytes and thus the monocyte–granulocyte system has a dualistic role in producing both stimulatory and inhibitory factors.

The role of granulocytes in providing a negative feedback control can be shown by *in vitro* studies. Colony inhibiting activity (CIA) has been ascribed to lactoferrin (normally present in the secondary granules of mature neutrophils) apparently by inhibition of CSF. However, it does not inhibit CSF produced by endotoxin-stimulated macrophages which suggests that its role is to regulate normal granulopoiesis while allowing the neutrophil response to bacterial infection to be sustained. A second negative feedback loop is provided by an inhibitor of thymidine incorporation obtained from mature granulocytes and therefore analogous to RCE associated with the control of erythropoiesis.

The release of granulocytes from the bone marrow is probably determined mainly by cell maturity. However, some evidence suggests that when plasma from leucocyte-depleted humans is injected into normal subjects it is followed in only a few hours by a several-fold increase in circulating neutrophils, including metamyelocytes.

Most of the information on the origin and formation of granulocytes has been derived from studies of the neutrophil series, and the production of eosinophils and basophils probably follows the same pathway. Less is known of the regulation of basophil production but the regulation of eosinopoiesis and eosinophil release has been studied in animals. Experiments analogous to the demonstration of the 'plasma-release-factor' for neutrophils have shown that humoral factors are involved. The ability of helminths to stimulate eosinophils has been used in rats to show that T lymphocytes are apparently involved in promoting the eosinophilic response. Antigen-antibody complexes have been shown to provoke a tissue or blood eosinophilia and blood histamine levels may regulate release from the bone marrow.

Monocytopoiesis

That the origins of monocytes and granulocytes are closely associated has been shown by the characteristics of the GM–CFU. Evidence that the bone marrow is the only source of blood monocytes is that in bone-marrow failure monocytes are depleted with the other cell lines and that in healthy subjects and in pregnancy there is a linear relationship between the concentration of neutrophils and monocytes in the blood[12, 23].

The transition from the granulocyte–monocyte precursors to the circulating monocyte and then to the tissue macrophage is generally accepted. There are fewer morphological stages than for the granulocyte and a hypothetical model is shown in *Figure 1.5*.

The regulation of monocyte production is undoubtedly closely linked to that of the neutrophil granulocyte.

Thrombopoiesis[24]

Thrombocytes or platelets are produced by fragmentation of the cytoplasm of megakaryocytes. Though megakaryocyte production is normally confined to the bone marrow it has been known for many years that megakaryocytes are present in large numbers in the lungs. The evidence is that the pulmonary megakaryocytes originate from the bone marrow and are carried to and retained in the lungs via the venous return. The contribution of the pulmonary megakaryocytes to the body platelet pool has been calculated to be from 7% to almost 100%[25].

Megakaryocytes originate in the bone marrow from the pluripotent stem cell as evidenced by the formation of megakaryocyte clones by CFU–GEMM and CFU–M (colony forming units in culture–megakaryocyte) with IL-3 as growth factor. The megakaryocytes are unique in that during maturation they develop a highly polyploid DNA content which is associated with giant multi-lobed nuclei. As the earliest recognizable megakaryocyte precursors already have 4–16 times (8n–32n) the normal diploid (2n) DNA content, it follows that the unrecognized

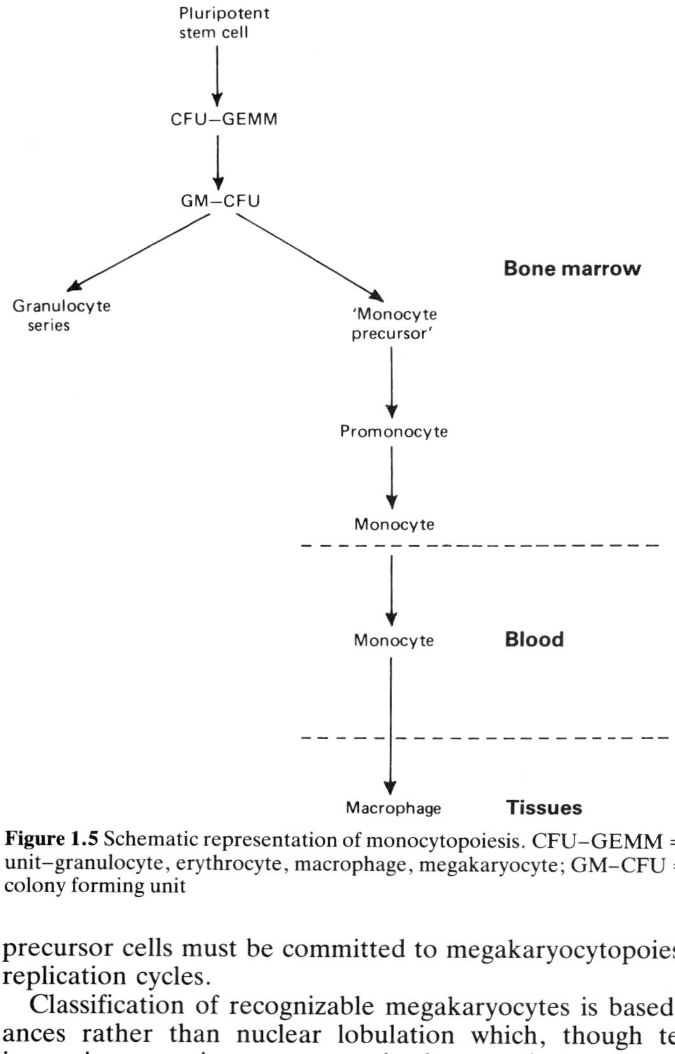

Figure 1.5 Schematic representation of monocytopoiesis. CFU–GEMM = Colony forming unit–granulocyte, erythrocyte, macrophage, megakaryocyte; GM–CFU = granulocyte–macrophage colony forming unit

precursor cells must be committed to megakaryocytopoiesis for at least two DNA replication cycles.

Classification of recognizable megakaryocytes is based on cytoplasmic appearances rather than nuclear lobulation which, though tending to develop with increasing maturity, may occur in the most immature cells. The classification of human megakaryocytes into stages I, II and III[26] correspond to the megakaryoblast, promegakaryocyte and granular-megakaryocyte terminology. These stages of cell maturation are non-proliferative in that neither DNA synthesis nor cell division occurs though there is production of cytoplasmic contents and demarcation membranes, by which future platelets are delineated.

Formation of platelets in the marrow does not appear to be by a simple shedding or disintegration but rather by projection of megakaryocyte cytoplasm through the sinusoidal endothelium though further division presumably follows. It has been suggested that newly produced platelets are larger and more dense than those that have aged in the circulation but most of the evidence supports the view that platelet size and density are independent of age and are determined by the state of megakaryocyte development.

Regulation of megakaryocyte proliferation and platelet production

The level of circulating platelets mediates a feedback regulation by a humoral factor, thrombopoietin. Normal plasma will stimulate thrombocyte formation, plasma from thrombocytopenic donors is a more potent stimulus and plasma from donors with transfusion-induced thrombocytosis is not stimulatory. The induced positive feedback changes include changes in size, DNA content, endomitotic index and number, and more rapid maturation. Negative feedback loops induce the converse changes.

A 'tissue sensor' analogous to the renal control of erythropoietin has not been identified, and why the abnormal platelet count induced by altered splenic function is not normalized by regulation of platelet production is not known. The rate of platelet destruction may influence the level of thrombopoietin.

The role of the spleen as an inhibitory regulator of thrombopoiesis has been suggested by the increased platelet mass after splenectomy which is not accounted for by the removal of the splenic pool. A negative feedback analogous to RCE and CIA in erythrocytes and neutrophils respectively has not been substantiated.

A schematic model of thrombopoiesis is shown in *Figure 1.6* and further expanded in *Table 2.4*.

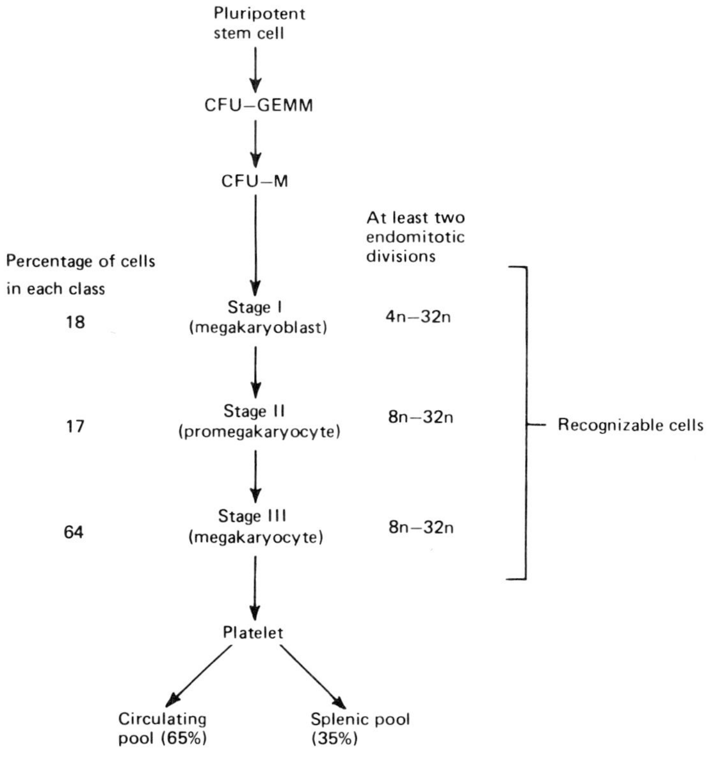

Figure 1.6 Schematic model of platelet production. CFU–GEMM = Colony forming unit–granulocyte, erythrocyte, macrophage, megakaryocyte; CFU–M = colony forming unit–megakaryocyte

Lymphopoiesis

The blood lymphocytes are divided into two main classes, designated 'T cells' and 'B cells'. The terms 'T' and 'B' refer to the tissue sites to which the precursor cells migrate and differentiate: T cells are derived from the thymus and B cells from the bone marrow.

The repopulation experiment of Till and McCullough[13], resulting in the recognition of the CFU–S, also results in the reconstitution of the lymphoid tissues of irradiated mice. In addition to the PSC restricted to the myeloid lineages (CFU–GEMM), stem cells restricted to T lymphocyte generation and with both myeloid and lymphoid lineage are found. Long-term bone marrow cultures (LTMC) are capable of repopulating the B and T cells of irradiated mice. Additional evidence of pluripotent origins of lymphocytes is found in studies of blast-cell transformation in chronic granulocytic leukaemia and adult acute lymphoblastic leukaemia (*see* Chapter 13).

The importance of activated T cells in the production of growth factors such as the interleukins and other lymphokines is evident, not only by their influence on myeloid and erythroid cell lines but also by their activity on the maturation and functional differentiation of T cells themselves and of B cells[27].

T and B lymphocytes are differentiated by membrane 'markers' and the T cells are further divided into sub-populations with differing membrane characteristics

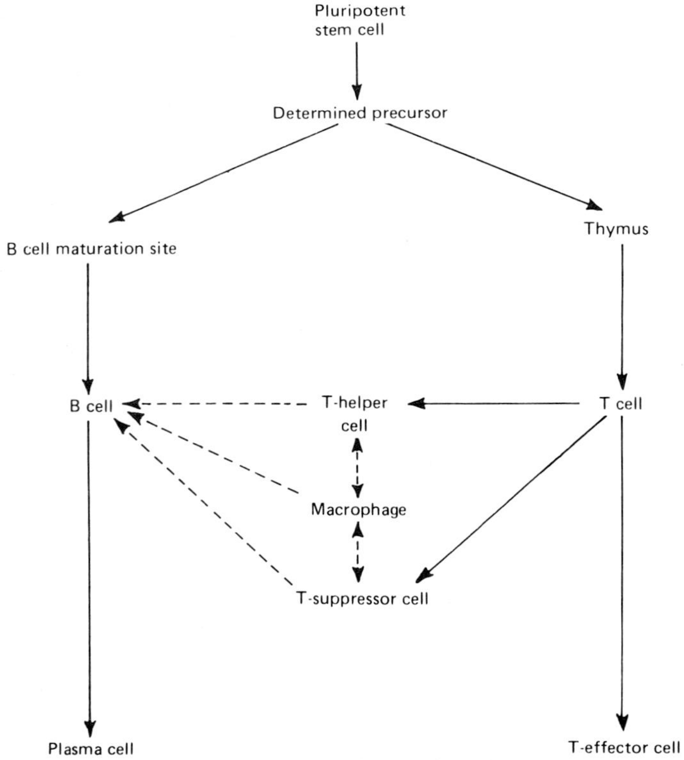

Figure 1.7 Lymphocyte production and interaction of sub-populations. ——— = Cell differentiation; ---- = cell effectors

and functional activities and are designated as 'helper', 'suppressor' or 'effector' cells (*see* Chapter 2).

It is emphasized that the differentiation of B and T cells is based on functional, immunological and biological reactivity rather than morphological appearances. A scheme of lymphocyte production and interaction is shown in *Figure 1.7*.

Cell culture – an overview [28]

The development of techniques of cell culture has clarified the processes involved in normal haemopoiesis, particularly in the stages of development prior to the recognition of precursors by morphological, cytochemical or immunological methods. The importance of cell–cell interaction at the anatomical level in long-term marrow culture and the recognition and isolation of specific or multilineage growth factors and inhibitors have opened the way to therapeutic applications.

Colony culture in semi-solid media has helped to understand the aetiology of haematological malignancies and the role of viral oncogenes. An early application of the technique was in the assessment of the storage of harvested bone marrow cells for transplantation and the viability of manipulated cells. The recognition, using colony culture, that pluripotent stem cells are present in the circulation has opened a further therapeutic approach.

The production and assessment of recombinant growth factors and inhibitors are now being applied to clinical situations, e.g. recombinant erythropoietin (rEpo) in the treatment of the anaemia of chronic renal failure and the use of recombinant interleukins (rIL) and interferons (rIF) in the treatment of malignant disease.

Colony culture

The general requirements for the culture of colonies from single cells are: tissue culture medium conditioned by growth factors from other cells or by isolated growth factors, human or animal serum or plasma, and semi-solid support provided by methyl cellulose, agar or even fibrin clot. The cultures are incubated for 12–28 days in an atmosphere containing 5% CO_2 and controlled humidity. The colonies are counted and examined by low power microscopy and by additional techniques to identify cell lineage and stages of development. What appears to be a reasonably straightforward technique is, in fact, extremely sensitive to variations in procedure, reagents and culture conditions. Certain batches of plastic containers can be inhibitory to growth as can different batches of plasma or serum and the atmospheric condition must be free of traces of volatile substances.

Long-term marrow culture (LTMC)

The essential difference from colony culture is that LTMC is performed in fluid medium and that it requires the growth of an adherent layer of stromal cells on the interior of the culture flask. Again, tissue culture medium with added serum is necessary and hydrocortisone is added unless the growth of B lymphocytes is being studied. The temperature is generally 33°C to increase stromal cell growth which is three-dimensional rather than in a monolayer. Growth represents a balance between stimulatory and inhibitory factors. Additional stimulatory or growth factors may be added to study the proliferation of particular cell lines.

Cell markers in cell culture

The gross appearances of the colonies can reflect their nature, e.g. the characteristic appearance of colonies arising from BFU–Es. Similarly, the synthesis of haemoglobin in erythroid colonies can be readily seen. However, for the identification of other cell lines and to determine the level of differentiation more precise methods are required.

Conventional morphological recognition of myeloid precursors can be made from imprint preparations and Romanowsky staining. Cytochemical demonstration of esterase activity is useful for studying mixed granulocyte-monocyte colonies. Determination of G6PD iso-enzyme type has been much used to demonstrate the clonal origin of proliferative disorders.

More recently monoclonal antibodies (MoAbs) have become available which recognize antigens on granulocytes, monocytes/macrophages, erythroid cells, the megakaryocyte series, stem cells and committed progenitor cells [29]. Lymphocytes in culture can also be monitored by MoAbs. They may be directed against membrane or cytoplasmic antigens and their interaction recognized by fluoresence microscopy, immuno-enzyme techniques, autoradiography and flow cytometry.

Receptors for interleukins, complement and for the Fc fragments of immunoglobulins are also markers of differentiation and maturation. For many diagnostic applications of colony culture, however, simply identifying and counting colonies provides informative data.

References

1. Tavassoli, M. (1979) The marrow–blood barrier. *Br. J. Haematol.*, **41**, 297–302
2. Tavassoli, M. and Yoffey, J. M. (1983) *Bone Marrow: Structure and Function,* p. 17. New York: Liss
3. Chamberlain, J. K., Weiss, L. and Weed, R. I. (1975) Bone marrow sinus cell packing: a determinant of cell release. *Blood*, **46**, 91–102
4. Aoki, M. and Tavassoli, M. (1981) Dynamics of red-cell egress from bone marrow after blood letting. *Br. J. Haematol.*, **49**, 337–47
5. Waugh, R. E. and Sassi, M. (1986) An *in vitro* model of erythroid egress from bone marrow. *Blood*, **68**, 250–7
6. Crosby, W. H. (1977) Delivery of megakaryocytes by the bone marrow, the derivation of platelets. In *Topics in Haematology* (eds S. Seno, F. Takako and S. Irino), p. 538. Amsterdam: Excerpta Medica
7. Tavassoli, M. (1980) Megakaryocyte–platelet axis and the process of platelet formation and release. *Blood*, **55**, 537–45
8. Tavassoli, M. and Aoki, M. (1981) Migration of entire megakaryocyte through the marrow–blood barrier. *Br. J. Haematol.*, **48**, 25–9
9. Bentley, S. A. (1982) Bone marrow connective tissue and the haemopoietic microenvironment. *Br. J. Haematol.*, **50**, 1–6
10. Singer, J. W., Keating, A. and Wight, T. N. (1985) The human haemopoietic environment. In *Recent Advances in Haematology,* No. 4 (ed. A. V. Hoffbrand), pp. 1–24. Edinburgh: Churchill Livingstone
11. Boettiger, D. and Dexter, T. M. (1984) Long term marrow cultures in the analysis of viral leukaemogenesis. *Clin. Haematol.*, **13**, 349–70
12. Wickramasinghe, S. M. (1986) *Blood and Bone Marrow.* Edinburgh: Churchill Livingstone
13. Till, J. E. and McCullough, E. A. (1961) A direct measurement of the radiation sensitivity of normal bone marrow cells. *Radiat. Res.*, **14**, 213–22

14. Bodger, M. P., Izaquirre, C. A., Blacklock, H. A. and Hoffbrand, A. V. (1983) Surface antigenic determinants on human pluripotent and unipotent haemopoietic progenitor cells. *Blood*, **61**, 1006–10
15. Falkenburg, J. H. F., Fibbe, W. E., van der Vaart-Duinkeken, N. *et al.* (1985) Human erythroid progenitor cells express rhesus antigens. *Blood*, **66**, 660–3
16. Metcalf, D. (1986) Haemopoietic growth factors now cloned. *Br. J. Haematol.*, **62**, 409–12
17. Jacobs, A. (1983) Do acidic isoferritins regulate haemopoiesis? *Br. J. Haematol.*, **55**, 199–202
18. Brown, R. D., Rickard, K. A. and Kronenburg, H. (1985) Lactoferrin in the myeloproliferative disorders: a search for granulopoietic regulatory defects. *Br. J. Haematol.*, **59**, 617–26
19. Ganser, A., Carlo-Stenna, C., Greher, J. *et al.* (1985) Effect of recombinant interferons alpha and gamma on human bone marrow-derived megakaryocytic progenitor cells. *Blood*, **70**, 1173–9
20. Estrov, Z., Halperin, D. S., Coceani, F. and Freedman, M. H. (1988) Modulation of human marrow haematopoiesis by leucotrienes *in vitro*. *Br. J. Haematol.*, **69**, 321–7
21. Zanjani, E. D. and Ascensao, J. L. (1989) Erythropoietin. *Transfusion*, **29**, 46–57
22. Spivak, J. L. (1989) Erythropoietin. *Blood Rev.*, **3**, 130–5
23. Twomey, J. J., Douglas, C. C. and Sharkey, O. Jr. (1973) The monocytopenia of aplastic anaemia. *Blood*, **41**, 187–95
24. Hoffman, R. (1989) Regulation of megakaryocytopoiesis. *Blood*, **74**, 1196–212
25. Martin, J. F., Slater, D. N. and Trowbridge, E. A. (1983) Abnormal intrapulmonary platelet production: a possible cause of vascular lung disease. *Lancet*, **i**, 793–96
26. Williams, N. and Levine, R. F. (1982) The origin, development and regulation of megakaryocytes. *Br. J. Haematol.*, **52**, 173–80
27. Izaguirre, C. A. (1984) Colony formation by lymphoid cells. *Clin. Haematol.*, **13**, 405–46
28. McCullough, E. A. (ed.) (1984) Cell culture techniques. *Clin. Haematol.*, **13**, (2)
29. Robak, T. and Goldman, J. M. (1985) Monoclonal antibodies reacting with myeloid cells. *Br. J. Haematol.*, **61**, 1–9

Chapter 2

Physiology of the blood

Blood is composed of *cellular elements* (erythrocytes, leucocytes and platelets) and *plasma* which consists mainly of water and contains electrolytes and proteins. The overall function of the blood is to transport nutrients, exchange gases, remove waste products, provide an efficient defence against infection and maintain the integrity of the circulatory system.

The blood constitutes approximately 8% of total body mass and the total blood volume is about 70 ml/kg body weight, of which 40 ml is plasma. It has physicochemical properties such as isotonicity, colloid osmotic pressure, viscosity and characteristic rheological properties all of which collectively permit efficient circulation and function of the blood constituents. The constituents of the blood are in a state of balance between loss, or escape, from the circulation and regeneration or replacement; this balance is referred to as *homeostasis*.

Erythrocytes

The mean cell life of red cells is 120 days, during which they will travel about 175 miles. On average slightly less than 1% of red cells are the newly formed reticulocytes released from the bone marrow, which take 1–2 days to develop into mature red cells. It is a simple calculation that in a 70 kg subject approximately 2×10^{11} red cells are destroyed and replaced each day or an incredible 2.3×10^{6} cells per *second*.

The mature red cell is circular, biconcave and discoid, with an average diameter of 8.4 μm in 'wet preparations'. (This is considerably greater than the 7.2–7.4 μm diameter in fixed, dried, blood films.) It measures 2.4 μm at its thickest point and 1 μm at the biconcavity and has an approximate surface area of 140 μm^2. The total surface area of the circulating red cells is variously quoted as being between 1500 and 2000 times that of the surface area of the body. The average (±2 SD) red-cell volume (MCV) is 88 ± 6 fl.

Red cells are readily deformable which enables them to pass through the smallest blood capillaries and between cell junctions. *In vitro* they can be drawn through capillaries or micropore filters 3 μm in diameter and still regain normal shape. The deformability of the red cell is not matched by an ability to withstand swelling which can only increase cell volume by about 10% before the membrane loses its integrity and releases the cell contents.

A biconcave shape is the maximum surface area for a given volume and is therefore suited to the major function of taking oxygen from the lungs and delivering it to the tissues. To fulfil this role the red cell requires an organized structure and active energy source and phosphorylated intermediates. The red cell is clearly a complex structure and consists of lipids, proteins, carbohydrates, anions and cations.

Red-cell membrane [1, 2]

Chemical composition

The dry weight of 10^{10} red-cell ghosts is about 15 mg which is composed of approximately 50% protein, 40% lipid and 8% carbohydrate.

Membrane proteins
Membrane proteins have been characterized by polyacrylamide gel electrophoresis (PAGE), conventional amino-acid analysis, isotopic protein labelling and immunological techniques. By conventional PAGE up to 15 bands can be demonstrated which correspond to molecular weights of $30–240 \times 10^3$ daltons. The proteins are numbered in order of decreasing molecular weight and can be divided into three groups: (1) the proteins of the internal aspect of the membrane; (2) the integral proteins which span the membrane; and (3) proteins on the external aspect. The internal proteins comprise alpha and beta spectrins (bands 1 and 2), ankyrin or syndein (band 2.1), bands 4.2, 4.9, band 5 (actin), band 6 and several band 7 subclasses. The integral proteins are represented by band 3, band 4.5, the adenosine triphosphatases (ATPases) and a group of sialoglycopeptides known as glycophorins A, B, C and D. Glycophorin A carries most of the negative surface charge. External protein is represented by acetyl cholinesterase (AChE). The classification, position and function of membrane proteins are summarized in *Table 2.1*.

Lipids
By weight the membrane lipid is 70% phospholipid and 30% free (unesterified) cholesterol. Membrane lipids can be completely extracted by solvents and studied by simple quantification of the lipid classes and by chromatographic procedures for the quantitation of the phospholipid classes and analysis of the associated long-chain fatty acids. The total phospholipid is composed of approximately 33% phosphatidyl choline (lecithin), 30% phosphatidyl ethanolamine, 8% phosphatidyl serine, 28% sphingomyelin and 1% lysolecithin. The polar phosphoric acid esters are hydrophilic and the fatty acid tails hydrophobic which in part determine the arrangement of the phospholipids in the membrane. Red cells cannot synthesize lipid therefore any change in phospholipid composition is by incorporation of different free fatty acids (FFA), lipid exchange between membrane and plasma, and conversion of phosphatidyl ethanolamine to phosphatidyl choline. These changes are slow and are influenced by the phospholipids and FFAs of the plasma. The FFA composition of the red-cell membrane can be altered by changes in dietary FFA.

In contrast to the phospholipids, cholesterol in the membrane is in free exchange with the free cholesterol of the plasma and studies with labelled cholesterol show that equilibrium between membrane and plasma is completed in 8 hours. Esterification of plasma cholesterol is controlled by the enzyme lecithin cholesterol acyl transferase (LCAT). A reduction in LCAT activity results in increased plasma

Table 2.1 Red-cell membrane proteins classified by separation on PAGE–SDS, structural type and function

Protein (band)	*Synonym*	*Position*	*Function*
1	Spectrin	Internal	Form tetramers and cytoskeleton
2	Spectrin	Internal	
2.1	Ankyrin (syndein)	Internal	Links spectrin to protein 3
3	–	Integral	Anion transport, binding of GAPD, aldolase, ankyrin, haemoglobin, Ii blood groups
4.1	Phosphoproteins	Internal	Cytoskeleton, binds to protein 3
4.2	–	Internal	
4.5	–	Integral	Glucose transport
4.9	–	Internal	Actin bundling
5	Actin	Internal	Spectrin cross-linking
6	GAPD	Internal	Protein 3 binding
7	a,b,c,d,+	Internal	?Actin stabilization
Hb	–	Internal	Binds to protein 3
ATPases	–	Integral	Na^+, K^+ transport
AChE	–	External	
Glycophorins	A,B,C,D, sialoglycopeptides	Integral	MNS blood groups

free cholesterol and consequently an increase in membrane cholesterol which increases the surface area of the membrane. The composition, structure and conformation of red-cell membranes can therefore be influenced by changes in the plasma environment.

Carbohydrates

The 8% of carbohydrate is found in glycoproteins and glycolipids and is predominantly on the outer surface of the membrane.

Structure

The lipids of the red-cell membrane may be extracted without disruption or loss of shape of the cell. It can therefore be inferred that the proteins control the structure or cytoskeleton of the cell and underlie the 'plasma membrane'. The skeleton is a lattice of spectrin, band 4.1 and actin. Spectrin accounts for 75% of the protein and consists of heterodimers of an α and β chain, which can combine to form heterotetramers cross-linked by actin with attachment of band 4.1. Ankyrin (band 2.1) links the integral protein 3 to the cytoskeleton via β spectrin (*Figure 2.1*). Band 3 and the glycophorins A and B span the lipid bilayer. Haemoglobin and the glycolytic enzyme glyceraldehyde-3-phosphate dehydrogenase are bound to protein 3. The binding of Hb can be important in determining red-cell shape and function. The lipids are arranged on the protein framework in an asymmetrical bilayer with the hydrophilic polar heads of the phospholipid at the outer and inner surfaces and the fatty acid tails pointing to the interior. The aminophospholipids are located on

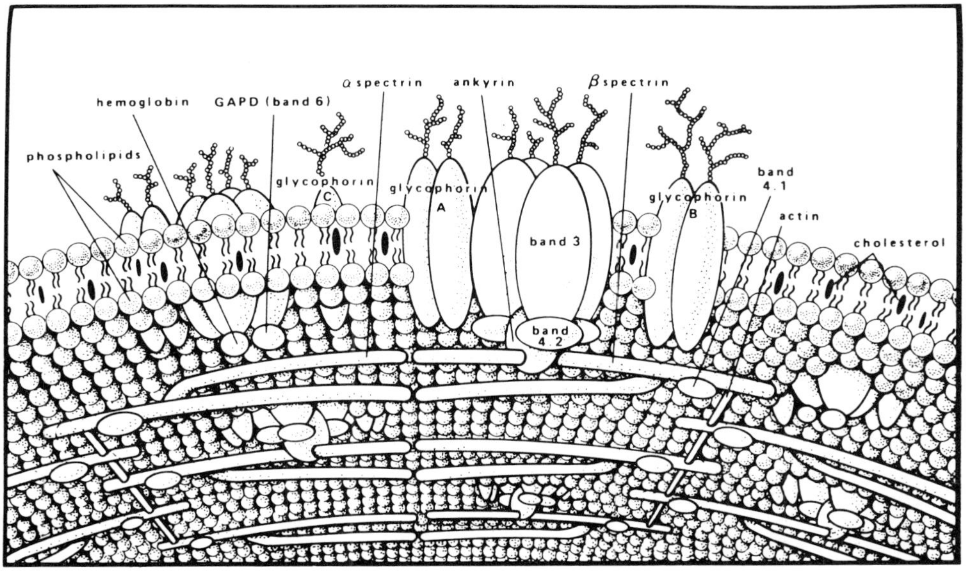

Figure 2.1 The structure of the human red-cell membrane. For description see text. Reprinted from *Scientific American. Medicine*, Vol. VII, No. 5 IV-5

the inner leaflet of the bilayer and most of the phosphatidyl choline and sphingomyelin is present in the outer leaflet. The asymmetry within the bilayer and the incorporation of the planar cholesterol molecule inserted between the fatty acid chains has been likened to a lipid mosaic or film, within which globular proteins not connected to the cytoskeleton may be free to move laterally. The combined lipid–protein arrangement confers the discoid shape of the cell yet allows molecular re-arrangement and flexibility under stress from one direction.

Membrane function

The principal functions of the red-cell membrane are:

1. To separate cell contents from the plasma yet allow the cell to function.
2. To maintain cell shape and deformability.
3. To maintain intracellular concentration and electrochemical gradients, i.e. osmotic equivalence between red cell and plasma.
4. To facilitate transport of cell requirements.
5. To act as support for surface antigens.

The principal content of the red cell is haemoglobin and the membrane effectively contains the haemoglobin yet allows diffusion of gases across the membrane at a rate measured in milliseconds.

The maintenance of normal red-cell shape is a function of the cytoskeleton. Abnormalities of cell shape can generally be ascribed to altered cytoskeletal protein assembly. Membrane stability appears to be a function of the assembly and maintenance of spectrin tetramers which requires ATP as an energy source. Depletion of ATP leads to spectrin aggregation and loss of membrane material in the form of vesicles depleted in spectrin. Deformability of the membrane is dependent on the two-dimensional cytoskeletal network; additional membrane protein cross-linking or disulphide couplings are associated with a marked decrease in deformability and the fixation of cells in abnormal shapes.

The maintenance of cell concentrations and electrochemical gradients and the transport of essential cell requirements depend on transport across the cell membrane. Transport processes can be divided into: (1) *passive*, by simple diffusion through pores or lipid domains and does not require energy; and (2) *active* transport against a gradient which requires energy, which in the case of the red cell is supplied by ATP. Active transport is mediated by proteins acting as carriers which bind to the substrate and translocate it to the other side of the membrane. Carrier transport depends on substrate concentration, exhibits substrate specificity and can be competitively or non-competitively inhibited. Various models of carrier transport systems have been formulated and have in common recognition of the substrate, binding to the carrier, translocation and release. Examples of passive transport are oxygen and glucose diffusion; active transport is necessary for the passage of potassium, sodium and calcium ions.

Haemoglobin structure, synthesis and function

Haemoglobin is a globular chromoprotein consisting of four *globin* (polypeptide) chains each containing a prosthetic *haem* group. The synthesis of the haem and globin moieties proceeds separately, though not entirely independently, being controlled by feedback mechanisms. The haem is inserted into a globin subunit followed by final assembly of the whole molecule.

Haem synthesis

The haem molecule is a porphyrin ring with an iron atom at its centre. Porphyrins are tetrapyrroles (the four pyrroles being linked by methane bridges), are widely distributed in nature and can be synthesized. Different porphyrins are characterized by the pyrrole side groups – methyl, vinyl, acetic or propionic acid, the last two containing carboxyl groups. Four isomeric porphyrins have been synthesized and designated types I, II, III and IV. Only types I and III occur naturally. The porphyrin in haem is a protoporphyrin type III having four methyl, two vinyl and two propionic acid groups; these three groups can be arranged into 15 possible isomers. The protoporphyrin of haemoglobin is asymmetrical and designated protoporphyrin 9. The type I protoporphyrins have two types of side chain, the substituted groups alternating regularly, i.e. in uroporphyrin I acetic and propionic acid and in coproporphyin I methyl and propionic acid.

Biosynthesis of haem

Succinyl CoA combines with glycine, with pyridoxal-5-phosphate as coenzyme, to form δ-aminolaevulinic acid (δ-ALA) – a reaction catalysed by the enzyme ALA-synthetase (ALA-S). This is the major rate-limiting step in haem synthesis. Two molecules of δ-ALA condense to form the monopyrrole porphobilinogen (PBG) in the presence of δ-ALA dehydrase (ALA-D) and glutathione. Four molecules of PBG condense to form the tetrapyrrole uroporphyrinogen III (UPG III), a reaction catalysed by PBG-deaminase and UPG-isomerase (UI). PBG-deaminase alone converts PBG to uroporphyrinogen I. The conversion of UPG III to coproporphyrinogen III and subsequently to protoporphyrin 9 is by a series of decarboxylations and one oxidation step. Uroporphyrin III and coproporphyrin III are by-products of protoporphyrin 9 synthesis. The insertion of iron into haem is catalysed by the enzyme ferrochelatase (haem synthetase) and occurs in the mitochondria.

The synthesis of haem is co-ordinated with that of globin synthesis and requires control of protoporphyrin and globin synthesis and control of the entry of iron into the cell. As previously stated the major rate-limiting enzyme is ALA-S which has high activity in the early erythroblast and gradually diminishes until the mature red cell has no activity. Haem depresses the formation of ALA-S and also inhibits its activity. Low concentrations of iron activate ALA-S while high concentrations are inhibitory. The formation of haem increases globin synthesis and lack of haem reduces globin synthesis, the effect being greater on the α chain than the β chain. Whether globin synthesis stimulates haem formation is uncertain. The pathway of haem synthesis is shown in *Figure 2.2*.

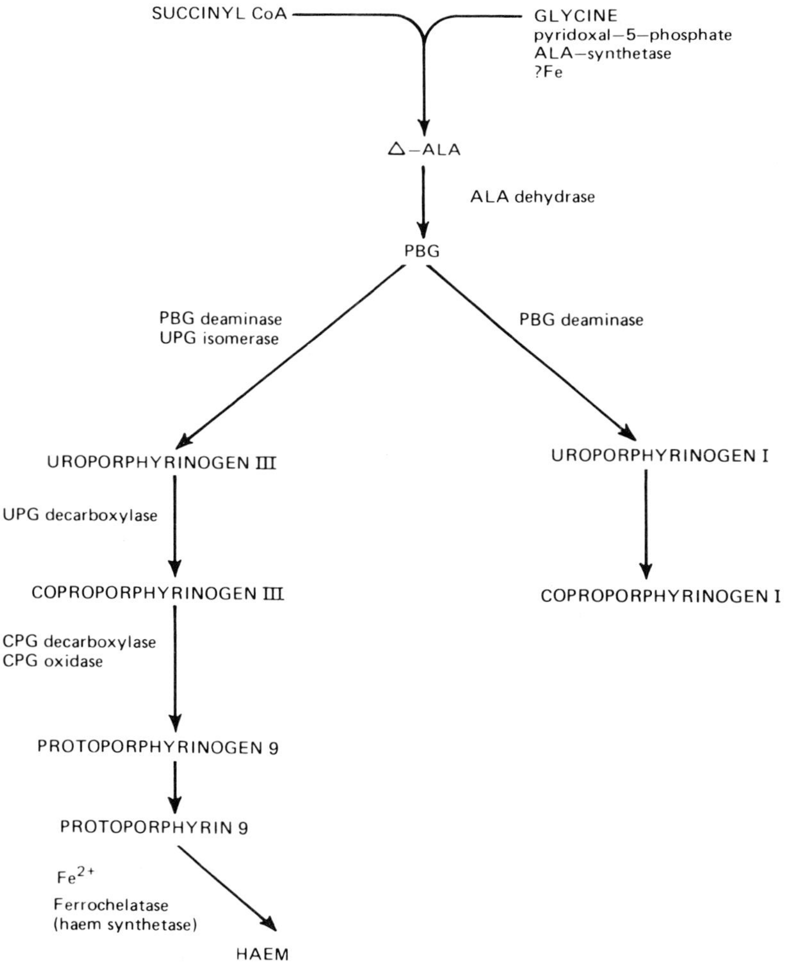

Figure 2.2 The mitochondrial biosynthesis of haem

Globin synthesis and structure

The genes controlling the synthesis of the globin chains are located on two chromosomes. The embryonic ξ globin chain, a pseudo ξ gene (ψ ξ), pseudo α genes (ψα) and the two adult α globin genes are closely linked on chromosome 16 in the order 5 – ξ_2–$\psi\xi_1$–$\psi\alpha_2$–$\psi\alpha_1$–α_2–α_1–3′. The α-chain genes are therefore duplicated in most or all human populations and in normal subjects chain synthesis is therefore controlled by four α-chain genes.

The γ-, δ-, and β-globin genes are closely linked on chromosome 11 in the order γ^G, γ^A, δ, β. The ε gene is on the same chromosome but is not closely linked. The synthesis of the δ and β chains is therefore controlled by two δ and two β chain genes and γ-chain synthesis is controlled by four γ chain genes the products of which differ slightly in that either glycine (γ^G) or alanine (γ^A) is found at position 136. Hb F is therefore a mixture of two molecular forms in normal individuals and at birth the $\gamma^G\gamma^A$ ratio is usually 3:1.

The complete globin structure consists of four polypeptide chains formed by two dissimilar pairs. Apart from the embryonic haemoglobins (Gower 1, Gower II and Portland (*see* page 2)), normal globin consists of two α chains and two β, γ, or δ chains.

The α chains are therefore common to all the normal haemoglobins. Each α chain consists of a chain of 141 amino acids; the β, γ and δ chains have 146 amino acids. The normal haemoglobins are Hb A (adult $\alpha_2\beta_2$) which comprises 96–98% of total haemoglobin, Hb F (fetal $\alpha_2\gamma_2$) normally less than 1% and Hb A_2 ($\alpha_2\delta_2$) 2–3.5%.

Primary structure A single globin chain is a sequence of polar and non-polar amino acids which are conventionally numbered from the N-terminus of the chain.

Secondary structure About 80% of the amino acids form a right-handed spiral, an α-helix, with 3.6 amino acids in each complete turn. The helix is stabilized by hydrogen bonding between amino acids above or below each other in adjacent turns. Each globin chain consists of eight helical segments designated A–H, joined by short non-helical sections designated AB, BC, CD etc. Using this nomenclature the position of an amino acid is identified by its position in the segment which is more meaningful in terms of its contribution to the function and stability of the molecule. The non-helical sections are often, but not always, associated with the presence of a proline residue which cannot be incorporated into the α-helix because of its pyrrolidone ring.

Tertiary structure The non-helical sections result in the chain bending back on itself and its structure is determined mainly by the siting of the polar and non-polar amino acids. The polar, or charged, side-chains are on the exterior surface of the molecule and the non-polar (non-charged) side-chains on the inner aspect of the helix, with the hydrophobic chains forming intramolecular bonds which impart stability to the molecule. The haem molecule fits into a non-polar, and consequently hydrophobic, pocket and is held in position by amino acids bonding with its methyl, vinyl and propionic groups. The iron molecule is hexacovalent and links with the four nitrogen atoms of the pyrrol rings, the fifth bond attaches to the imidazole ring of a histidine residue (proximal histidine) and the remaining bond can attach reversibly to oxygen. Haem imparts stability to the tertiary structure and loss of the haem moiety is associated with unfolding the chain and loss of helical content.

Quaternary structure The complete haemoglobin molecule or tetramer normally consists of the two pairs of dissimilar chains. Hb A has a pair of symmetrically arranged α chains on top of a symmetrical pair of β chains, though the arrangement should be regarded as the association of two $\alpha\beta$ dimers. The arrangement results in four areas of contact between dissimilar chains. There are two large, firm contact areas between dissimilar chains designated $\alpha_1\beta_1$ (or $\alpha_2\beta_2$) which stabilize the formed $\alpha\beta$ dimers. The other areas of contact designated $\alpha_1\beta_2$ (or $\alpha_2\beta_1$) are not rigid and allow movement during oxygenation and deoxygenation. The $\alpha_1\beta_1$ contact consists of 34 amino acids, 16 in the α chain and 18 in the β chain. The $\alpha_1\beta_2$ contact, consisting of 19 amino acids, allows sliding rotation and is influenced by movement of the proximal histidine on oxygenation and deoxygenation. The movement of the $\alpha_1\beta_2$ contact is a major influence on the oxygen dissociation curve of human haemoglobin. The assembly of $\alpha\beta$ dimers is by electrostatic attraction of a positively charged α subunit to a negatively charged β or γ subunit and dissociation is extremely slow. The difference between the rate of dissociation of $\alpha\beta$ dimers and $\alpha\gamma$ with increasing pH explains the alkali resistance of Hb F. The sulphydryl group of the cysteine at β_{112} is ionized at high pH and contributes to dissociation. In the γ subunit, 112-Cys is replaced by threonine [3, 4].

Haemoglobin function

The position of the haem group in the polypeptide chains imparts the property of reversible oxygenation without oxidative damage to the haemoglobin molecule. Oxygen uptake, transport and delivery to the tissues is a complicated process involving interaction of the haem group (haem–haem interaction), configurational changes in the tertiary and quaternary structures, binding of 2,3 diphosphoglycerate (2,3-DPG) and is influenced by pH (Bohr effect). These factors collectively confer and influence oxygen affinity and the characteristic sigmoid shape of the oxygen dissociation curve (*Figure 2.3*).

The reaction of oxygen with haem depends on the hydrophobic haem pocket maintaining the iron molecule in the ferrous state (Fe^{2+}). When oxygen enters the haem pocket it shares the 'spare' electron of Fe^{2+}, forming a weak ionic link which is readily broken by lowering the oxygen concentration (pO_2).

Haem–haem interaction confers the sigmoid shape to the oxygen dissociation curve and is dependent on the presence of four closely associated haem molecules (the haem protein myoglobin is a haem–globin monomer and has a hyperbolic dissociation curve). When one haem molecule is oxygenated there is a conformational change at the $\alpha_1\beta_2$ contact which permits a stepwise oxygenation of the other haem groups. The interaction of the haem groups is measured as Hill's constant n; the tetramer of human haemoglobin has an n value of 3 and myoglobin a value of 1. The value of $n = 3$ applies only to tetramers of two dissimilar pairs of globin chains and therefore the tetramers γ_4 and β_4 have n values of 1.

Oxygen affinity is the amount of oxygen the molecule takes up at a given oxygen tension and is usually expressed as P_{50}, i.e. the pO_2 required to half-saturate the molecule. The terms 'shift to the right' and 'shift to the left' are used to describe changes in the position of the oxygen dissociation curve. A 'shift to the left' indicates that the haemoglobin has a higher affinity and will give up its oxygen only

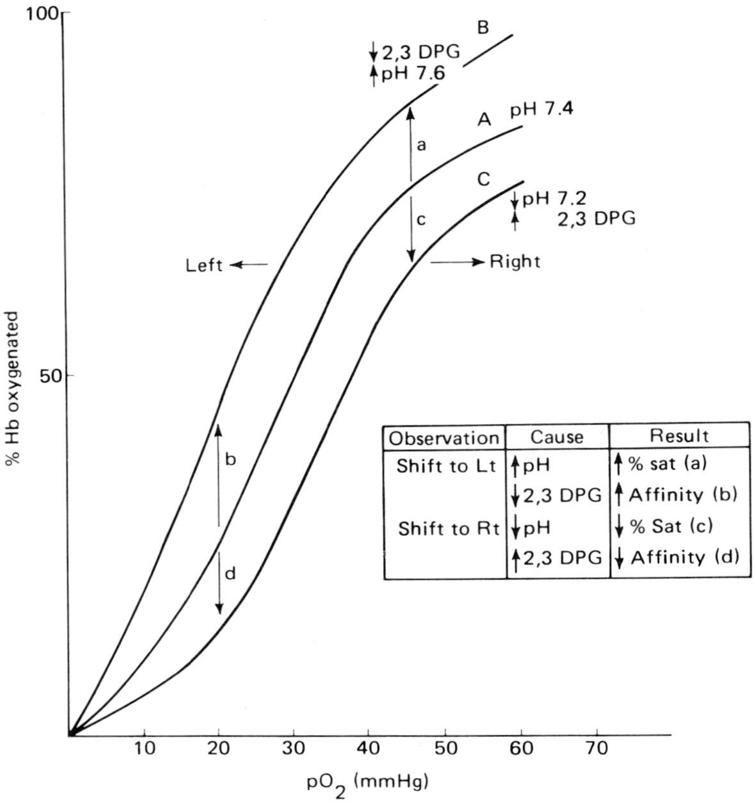

Observation	Cause	Result
Shift to Lt	↑pH	↑% sat (a)
	↓2,3 DPG	↑Affinity (b)
Shift to Rt	↓pH	↓% Sat (c)
	↑2,3 DPG	↓Affinity (d)

Figure 2.3 Effect of pH and 2,3 diphosphoglycerate (2,3-DPG) concentration on the oxygen dissociation curve of Hb A

at a lower pO_2 than normal. Conversely a 'shift to the right' indicates a lower oxygen affinity with greater release of oxygen at any pO_2.

Oxygen affinity is affected by pH (Bohr effect); a lower pH will reduce affinity (shift to right). Physiologically, the Bohr effect operates only in the alkaline range; the alkaline Bohr effect.

The organic phosphate 2,3-diphosphoglycerate (2,3-DPG) is an intermediate in the pathway of anaerobic glycolysis (*see* page 29) and is held between two β chains, thus keeping the chains apart and in the deoxygenated conformation, i.e. it reduces oxygen affinity with a shift of the curve to the right. Depletion or impaired binding of 2,3-DPG by the β chain results in increased oxygen affinity (shift to left). The increased oxygen affinity of Hb F is accounted for by its amino-acid structure which binds 2,3-DPG less well than Hb A.

Transport of carbon dioxide

An additional function of haemoglobin is the binding of CO_2 to form carbamate complexes, thus influencing the formation of carbonic acid and consequently blood pH. Carbamate formation occurs on the amino groups at the commencement of the α and β chains. Deoxygenated haemoglobin is able to bind more CO_2 than the oxygenated form and tends to fix the molecule in the deoxy form with release of further oxygen. The N-terminal valine of the α chain also binds hydrogen ions as well as CO_2 and there is therefore competition for these sites. Similarly, there is competition between CO_2 and 2,3-DPG for the terminal binding sites of the β chains.

Metabolic pathways of the mature red cell

The maturation of polychromatic erythroblast to reticulocyte and then to mature red cell is associated with loss of metabolic function (*Table 2.2*). The loss of the

Table 2.2 Metabolic capabilities of the erythrocytes and precursor cells

	Erythroblast	*Reticulocyte*	*Erythrocyte*
DNA synthesis	+	0	0
RNA synthesis	+	+	0
Krebs cycle	+	+	0
Haem synthesis	+	+	0
Protein synthesis	+	+	0
Lipid synthesis	+	+	0
Cytochrome activity	+	+	0
Glycolysis	+	+	+
Hexose monophosphate pathway	+	+	+

nucleus obviously precludes *initiation* of further protein synthesis but reticulocytes retain the remaining capabilities until mitochondria and ribosomes are lost. The mature erythrocyte retains anaerobic glycolysis (the Embden–Myerhof (EM) pathway) and the hexose monophosphate pathway (HMP) as the only source of energy and reducing power. As the red cell ages, enzyme activities decrease, with the conversion of glucose to glucose-6-phosphate by hexokinase being the rate-limiting step for both anaerobic glycolysis and the pentose phosphate pathway. The metabolism of glucose and glutathione is shown in *Figure 2.4*.

Embden–Myerhof pathway

The conversion of glucose to lactate by anaerobic glycolysis results in (1) a net gain of up to 2 moles of ATP for each mole of glucose metabolized; (2) the formation of NADH; and (3) the formation of 2,3-DPG. ATP is required as the source of energy for the membrane cation pump, the preservation of membrane flexibility, glutathione synthesis, nucleotide salvage and further glucose metabolism. Under normal conditions NADH is the co-factor for methaemoglobin reductase which catalyses the reduction of methaemoglobin to functional haemoglobin. The role of 2,3-DPG in haemoglobin function has been described (*see* page 28).

Hexose monophosphate pathway (HMP)

The HMP is the sole source of NADPH which is essential in maintaining levels of reduced glutathione, which is the main antioxidant of the red cell, and in the formation of 5-carbon sugars which eventually return to the anaerobic pathway for

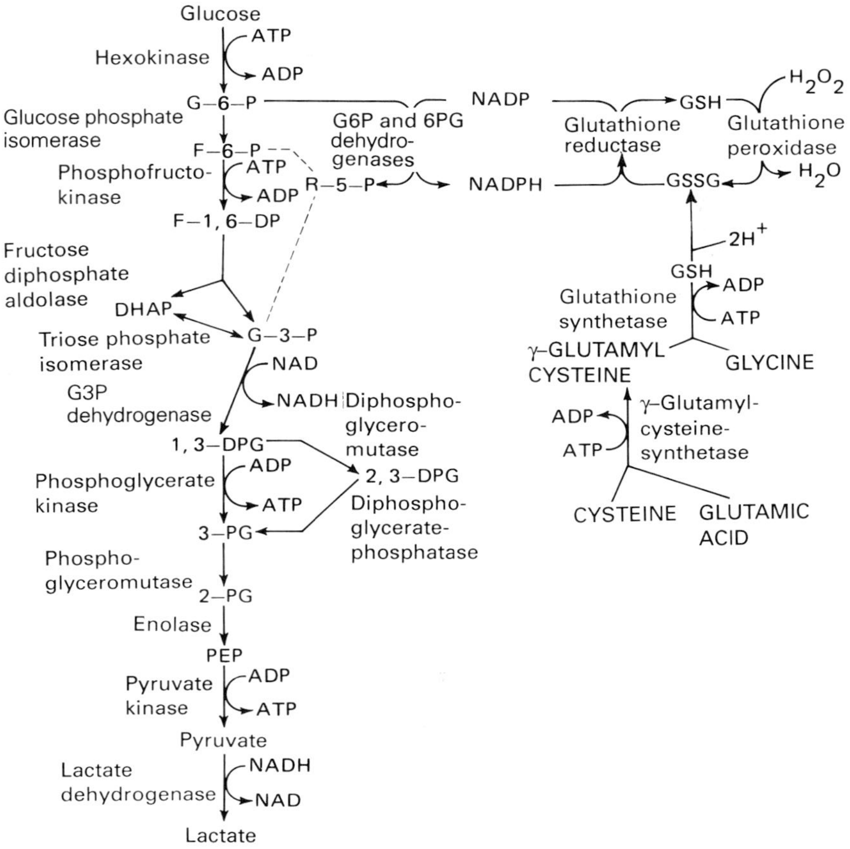

Figure 2.4 Glycolytic pathways and glutathione metabolism in the red cell

conversion to lactate. The rate-limiting enzyme of the HMP is glucose-6-phosphate dehydrogenase which, with 6-phosphogluconate dehydrogenase, converts glucose-6-phosphate to ribulose-5-phosphate with the generation of NADPH from NADP. NADPH in turn converts glutathione (GSSG) to reduced glutathione (GSH). NADPH also acts as co-factor for NADPH-methaemoglobin reductase (diaphorase) which can be stimulated by linking with methylene blue which also increases the activity of the HMP by increasing the supply of NADP in the first reaction (*Figure 2.5*).

Red-cell ageing and destruction

Red cells have a finite life span within a relatively narrow range of about 120 days. Hence a specific factor or factors determine the survival time. Isotopic labelling of a red-cell population of similar age (cohort labelling) followed by centrifugation and/or density gradient separation show that young red cells (reticulocytes) are the least dense and that density increases as the red-cell population ages. Separation and analysis of red-cell populations of increasing age shows alterations in metabolic

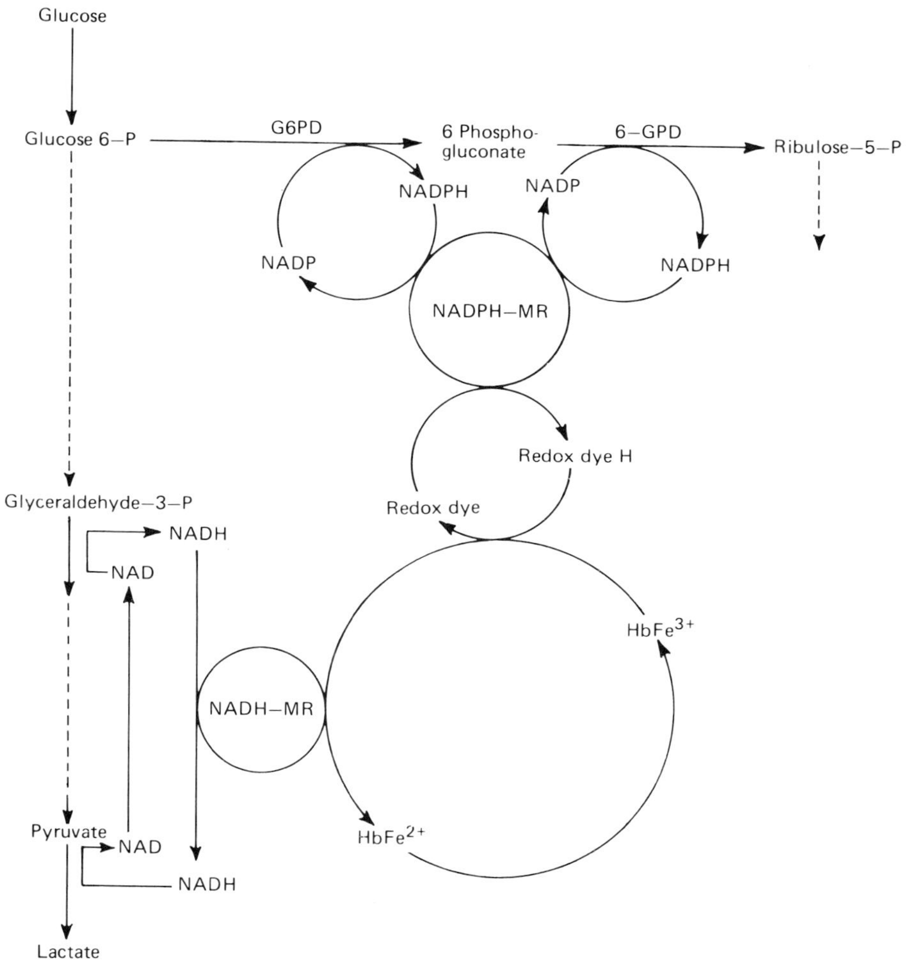

Figure 2.5 Pathways of methaemoglobin reduction. NADH–MR = NADH-methaemoglobin reductase; NADPH–MR = NADPH-methaemoglobin reductase (or diaphorase)

activity and composition and change in the composition of the red-cell membrane and in biophysical properties.

The activity of red-cell enzymes decreases with increasing age of the red cell. The decrease in hexokinase activity, the rate-limiting enzyme in glycolysis, was considered to be of particular importance because a reduction in glycolysis inevitably results in reduced levels of ATP and the intermediate 2,3-DPG. ATP depletion affects active cation transport with loss of intracellular potassium and accumulation of sodium and calcium. Lower levels of 2,3-DPG are reflected by a left shift of the oxygen dissociation curve. However, the concept of enzyme decay in a single first-order (exponential) manner no longer seems tenable. The decay of most enzymes occurs in at least two components – a rapid loss of activity during reticulocyte maturation followed by only slight loss of activity during the remaining life span of the red cell [5, 6]. It follows that red-cell enzyme activity may have only a minor or negligible role in the ageing of red cells.

Oxidative cross-linking of haemoglobin and spectrin is greater in the oldest, dehydrated and most dense fraction of circulating red cells [7–9]. Haemoglobin/spectrin complexes are associated with alteration of the surface of the red-cell membrane and binding of IgG and IgM immunoglobulins [10, 11]. Furthermore, it has been suggested that naturally occurring anti-galactosyl IgG antibodies bind to α-galactosyl residues exposed in the course of red-cell ageing [12]. The presence of immunoglobulins on the red-cell membrane predisposes to recognition by the Fc receptors of macrophages.

Ageing is associated with increasing membrane rigidity and consequent loss of deformability which implies alteration to the structure of the protein cytoskeleton. ATP depletion *in vitro* results in polymerization of spectrin and Ca^{2+}-dependent cross-linking. There is a symmetrical loss of cholesterol and total phospholipid which indicates loss of membrane. Changes in physical properties other than increasing density are reduced resistance to osmotic and mechanical lysis. Although the reductive potential via GSH is not greatly diminished, old red cells are more susceptible to auto-oxidation by free radicals.

Mechanically produced red-cell fragments visible by light microscopy can survive in the circulation for some days and if this were a major mechanism of red-cell destruction in health, the loss of 1% of red cells each day would surely result in recognizable changes in the blood film of normal blood. A possible process of normal red-cell fragmentation is the formation of microvesicles, containing haemoglobin but lacking spectrin, formed from spinous processes of the red-cell membrane. Such projections can be induced by ADP depletion and are irreversible in the presence of increased membrane calcium concentration. Ultracentrifugation (about 100 000 *g*) of blood that has aged *in vitro* reveals the presence of microvesicles 100–150 nm in diameter and is a possible model for normal *in vivo* red-cell fragmentation.

Possibly more than one mechanism of red-cell destruction exists [13]. Clearly, changes occur during red-cell ageing that collectively, or even singly, result in loss of red-cell integrity. Most, if not all, of the suggested mechanisms are extrapolations of the processes associated with reduced red-cell survival in haematological disorders – phagocytosis by macrophages of the reticuloendothelial system (RES), selective removal of membrane by macrophages, trapping in the microcirculation due to loss of deformability and mechanical fragmentation. The role of the spleen in removing pathological red cells has received particular attention because of its macrophage content and the 'trapping' capability of the splenic microcirculation, but splenectomy is not associated with prolongation of normal red-cell life span. Destruction is generally accepted to be mainly extravascular in the RES with only minor intravascular haemolysis. However, the distinction between extravascular and intravascular destruction is not a clear one. Destruction may occur predominantly within an organ of the RES, e.g. the spleen, yet haemolysis may still take place within the vascular system of that organ. Extravascular destruction should be interpreted as removal and destruction of red cells by phagocytosis.

Haemoglobin catabolism

Approximately 6 g of haemoglobin is released from effete red cells each day. Free haemoglobin can be broken down within macrophages or transported, in complex with plasma haptoglobin, to the liver where it is further degraded. Irrespective of whether haemoglobin is broken down at the site of red-cell destruction or in the liver, the catabolic sequence of haem is probably the same: haem→biliverdin→free bilirubin→conjugated bilirubin→urobilinogen→urobilin.

Oxidation of the α-methene bridge of haem opens the porphyrin ring with degradation of the molecule into iron, protein and the straight-chain tetrapyrrole derivative, biliverdin. Whether intermediate steps involve oxidation of the iron, loss of globin and formation of haematin, or alternatively the formation of choleglobin, is not clear. Biliverdin is reduced to free (prehepatic) bilirubin by NADH-biliverdin reductase. Bilirubin is transported to the liver bound to albumin as it is virtually water insoluble. In the liver bilirubin is conjugated with glucuronic acid at each of the propionic acid residues of the central pyrrole rings, which renders the pigment water soluble. It is transported in the bile to the small bowel where it is further transformed by reduction to urobilinogen and oxidized to urobilin. Some urobilinogen is reabsorbed in the intestine and returned to the liver via the portal circulation and re-excreted in the urine. The normal breakdown products of haemoglobin are therefore: iron which is returned to the body iron pool, globin which is broken down to amino acids and reutilized, free and conjugated bilirubin, urobilinogen and urobilin. The binding of free haemoglobin to plasma haptoglobin prevents excretion of haemoglobin in the urine which would result in loss of iron, and is therefore an important mechanism for iron salvage. Free haem binds to plasma haemopexin and is cleared from the circulation by the liver. It should be remembered that haemoglobin is not the sole source of bilirubin; myoglobin, cytochromes and catalase are all degraded to bilirubin.

Requirements for red-cell production

Cell proliferation and maturation require a wide variety of materials. There is nothing to suggest that any substance is unique in being required for red-cell production alone, or that a deficiency of an essential requirement only affects the red cells. Nevertheless the complex and specialized composition, structure and function of red cells described in the preceding sections make the red cell a sensitive 'target' for deficiency states. The large volume of erythropoietic cells and mature erythrocytes, coupled with their rapid turnover, results in deficiencies becoming manifest in red cells by the development of anaemia before measurably affecting other tissues. Of particular importance are iron and the B-group of vitamins, B_{12} (cobalamin), B_6 (pyridoxine) and 'folic acid'. Other trace elements that influence erythropoiesis are copper and cobalt while the B vitamins riboflavin, nicotinic and pantothenic acids, thiamine and vitamin C have all been ascribed a role. Hormonal influences will not be considered in this section.

Iron and iron metabolism

The tissues of a 70 kg adult male contain between 3 and 4 g of iron which is distributed in various compartments (*Table 2.3*) of which haemoglobin is the largest and therefore has the greatest influence on iron kinetics by virtue of its continual turnover. The iron compartments of the body and data on the movement of iron between compartments are shown in *Figure 2.6*. Iron metabolism involves absorption, transportation, utilization, storage and excretion.

Table 2.3 Iron distribution in a 70 kg male

	Total amount (g)	*Iron content* (g)	*% of total iron*
Haem compounds:			
Haemoglobin	750	2.6	65
Myoglobin	40	0.4	10
Enzymes	5.8	0.008	0.2
Transferrin	7	0.004	0.09
Storage iron	–	1.00	25
Total iron	–	4.1	100

Requirements

The average daily loss of iron in urine, faeces and sweat, mainly by cell desquamation, is 1–2 mg and although the normal daily diet contains about 15 mg of iron, only 1–2 mg are absorbed. Additional iron is required for body growth, pregnancy and to compensate for blood lost by menstruation (50 ml of blood contains approximately 25 mg of iron). Blood loss of 2 ml daily is on the brink of a negative iron balance. Pregnancy creates an iron requirement of about 700 mg (fetus, placenta, blood loss and lactation) but is partly offset by the absence of menstruation.

Nutrition

The 10–20 mg of iron per day in a normal Western diet is contained in meats, vegetables and fish. Iron is in organic and inorganic forms with a higher proportion of organic iron being absorbed. In some countries iron supplements are added to white flour. The iron in the diet is mainly in the ferric (Fe^{3+}) form.

Absorption

Iron is released from food complexes by digestive enzymes and is partially reduced to the ferrous form (Fe^{2+}) by the low pH and ascorbic acid. Iron chelated to low molecular weight compounds is more readily absorbed. Organic iron is more readily absorbed than inorganic forms which are inhibited by phosphates and phthylates. The intestinal mucosa controls iron absorption from food sources by an energy-dependent process but high iron content in the gut may result in absorption by passive diffusion, though free iron is unstable and toxic due to free radical membrane damage. The manner by which iron is absorbed from the gut remains controversial and, in particular, the roles of mucosal ferritin and mucosal transferrin, or indeed, whether transferrin has any role in the transfer from the lumen to the mucosal cell [14]. It is likely that the level of mucosal ferritin controls iron absorption – high levels inhibit and low levels enhance absorption. The process is undoubtedly complex with absorption also influenced by anaemia, hypoxia and level of erythropoiesis, though a humoral influence appears unlikely.

Transport

Iron absorbed from the gut or released by haemoglobin catabolism is transported by the plasma protein, transferrin. One molecule of transferrin may bind one or two molecules of ferric iron, the diferric form having a greater ability to transfer iron to tissue cells possibly due to more spheroidal diferric transferrin [15]. Most of the iron bound to transferrin is recycled rapidly (half-life 90 minutes) and mainly to

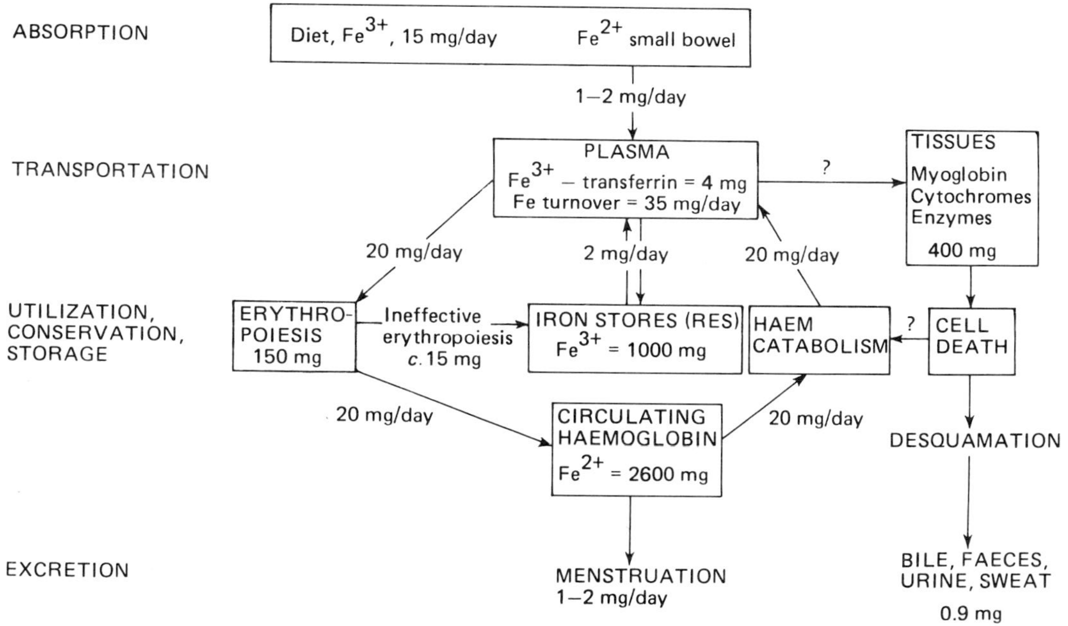

Figure 2.6 Iron metabolism in a 70 kg subject

the erythroblasts and reticulocytes. Plasma transferrin concentration is about 1.8–2.6 g/l but its level is usually expressed as iron-binding capacity. Total iron-binding capacity is 47–72 μmol/l, mean 54 μmol/l (260–400 μg/l, mean 300 μg/l). Normally about one third of the transferrin (18 μmol/l, 100 μg/l) is saturated with iron, giving in total about 3–4 mg of iron.

Transferrin releases iron to erythroblasts and reticulocytes. The cellular uptake is initiated by the binding of the transferrin–iron complex (Tf–Fe) to specific membrane receptors. A group of Tf–Fe complexes produce an invagination of the cell membrane leading to a vacuole or endosome within the cell membrane, release of the iron, and return of the apotransferrin to the outer membrane and dissociation into the plasma to resume iron transport. Free or non-transferrin plasma iron would be toxic due its catalytic activity in the formation of free hydroxyl radicals.

Utilization

Iron within the cell is found in the mitochondria, or in the cytosol in the form of ferritin which may represent iron surplus to requirement or an intermediate in the transfer of iron to the mitochondria. The mitochondrial iron is incorporated rapidly into protoporphyrin to form haem. The ferritin iron is eventually released from the cell at the reticulocyte stage. The concept of erythroblasts acquiring iron from iron-laden macrophages by 'rhopheocytosis' should be considered doubtful.

Iron storage

Iron is stored in the tissues in two forms: as a soluble form, ferritin, and as insoluble iron or haemosiderin.

Ferritin [16] This consists of a protein termed apoferritin with a molecular weight of 500 000 daltons and made up to 24 subunits to form a hollow shell which can contain up to 4500 atoms of iron in the form of ferrihydroxyphosphate. The stimulus for apoferritin synthesis is iron. Iron readily enters and leaves ferritin and mobilization is associated with reduction to the ferrous form. Ferritin is found in all tissues and in high concentration in liver, spleen and bone marrow. These isoferritins have different subunits. Three subunit types have been described: L (light, molecular weight 19 000), H (heavy, molecular weight 21 000) and G (glycosylated, molecular weight 23 000). H subunit isoferritins are acidic, L subunit isoferritins are more basic. The H and L subunits can be differentiated immunologically. Plasma ferritin contains almost only L and G subunits whereas tissue ferritins have variable proportions of H and L subunit types. The virtual absence of H subunits in plasma has been attributed to their binding or complexing with a ferritin-binding β_2-glycoprotein followed by rapid clearance [17]. About 70% of storage iron is present as ferritin, and the remainder as haemosiderin. Ferritin is present in plasma in amounts related to available storage iron and a normal concentration of 12–250 μg/l. It is accepted that plasma ferritin is normally derived from cells of the RES; any movement of iron from red cells to the storage compartment is reflected by a corresponding change in plasma ferritin concentration. Ferritin may also be released from the cytoplasm of damaged tissue cells.

Haemosiderin This is a non-crystalline, insoluble, protein–iron complex with a higher iron content than ferritin (37% by weight). Haemosiderin is generally amorphous – though aggregates of ferritin can be seen by electron microscopy – and may be a degraded form of ferritin. Haemosiderin is stainable by the Prussian Blue reaction and is visible by light microscopy.

Vitamin B_{12} (cobalamin)

Vitamin B_{12} or cobalamin has a similar structure to haem in having four pyrrole rings; but these are linked to a cobalt atom, with a nucleotide at right angles and a cyano, methyl, hydroxyl or deoxyadenosyl group. The major form in tissues is deoxyadenosyl cobalamin (co-enzyme B_{12}). Methylcobalamin is the major component in plasma together with hydroxycobalamin, to which methyl and deoxyadenosyl forms are converted by exposure to light. Cyanocobalamin is a stable synthetic form which can be converted to hydroxycobalamin. Vitamin B_{12} is formed primarily by bacterial synthesis and the only source available to man is dietary and mainly in foods of animal origin.

Requirements
Between 1 and 4 µg are required daily to replace that lost by the body. Total body B_{12} is about 3000 µg (2–4 years' supply) and is stored mainly in the liver. A normal diet contains over 5 µg daily; the 1 µg/day content of a strictly vegetarian diet reflects the absence of the vitamin in fruit and vegetables; the small amount of B_{12} present is due to water and bacterial contamination.

Absorption
Dietary B_{12} is released from its avid binding to proteins by gastric and intestinal enzymes. Passive absorption does occur but very inefficiently (1% of oral dose) and is ineffective unless there is a very high B_{12} intake. The alternative, and physiologically effective, mechanism is by binding to gastric 'intrinsic factor'.

Intrinsic factor (IF)
This glycoprotein is secreted by the parietal cells of the stomach. Free IF is destroyed by proteolytic enzymes in the stomach or gut, but when complexed with vitamin B_{12} the molecule is resistant to digestion. One molecule of IF binds one molecule of B_{12}. The IF–B_{12} complex traverses the small bowel and attaches to specific mucosal receptors in the terminal ileum (the last 2 m). The attachment requires a neutral pH and Ca^{2+}. The number of receptors is limited and about 2 µg can be absorbed from one meal. Vitamin B_{12} separates from IF in, or on, the ileal cell and appears in the blood of the portal vein 3–6 hours later. The fate of the IF is not known.

Transport [18]
Vitamin B_{12} binding proteins are found in plasma and are known as transcobalamins (TC). Three binding proteins, TCI, TCII and TCIII, have been identified. TCI and TCIII are known as 'R-proteins' or 'R-binders' due to their more rapid migration on electrophoresis. TCI is an alpha-glycoprotein and carries the great proportion of circulating B_{12} which is not given up to tissue cells. TCIII in plasma is mainly derived from leucocytes. Physiological roles for TCI and TCIII have not been identified.

The physiologically active transcobalamin TCII is a β globulin (molecular weight 35 000), produced by the liver, macrophages and the ileal enterocytes. B_{12}

absorbed in the ileum is bound to TCII. Tissue cells have receptors for TCII and the TCII with attached B_{12} is internalized by endocytosis.

Folates

'Folates' are a group of compounds with a parent compound, folic acid (pterylglutamic acid), consisting of pteridine, para-amino-benzoic acid and glutamic acid. Folic acid can be considered a synthetic substance; the naturally occurring compounds are in the form of reduced polyglutamates with an additional methyl or formyl group.

Dietary sources

Most foods contain folate, the highest content being found in liver, yeast, green foods and nuts. A normal daily mixed diet contains 200–600 μg of folate, about 75% being polyglutamates. Unlike B_{12}, it is labile and as much as 90% may be lost during cooking, by exposure to light, and by oxidation.

Requirements

Body folate totals 10–20 mg and is stored mainly in the liver. The daily requirement is 100–200 μg which is increased in pregnancy. In contrast to B_{12}, the body stores may only be sufficient for 50–100 days.

Absorption

Folate polyglutamates are hydrolysed to monoglutamates by a folate conjugase within the intestinal epithelial cells and reduced by dihydrofolate reductase to 5-methyl tetrahydrofolate which is the main transport form of folate. Folate is absorbed in the upper small intestine very rapidly.

Transport

Folate in plasma appears to be free, or weakly and non-specifically bound to a variety of protein fractions.

Leucocytes

The leucocytes in blood are of three major classes: granulocytes, monocytes and lymphocytes. Using morphological criteria three types of granulocytes are identified: neutrophils, eosinophils and basophils. By immunological and functional criteria the lymphocytes of the normal adult are of two types, B cells and T cells; a distinction that is not apparent from their morphology. The monocytes are regarded as a single cell line.

Granulocytes [19]

Development and structure

The transformation of myeloblast to mature granulocyte takes 10–15 days. The greater part of this period is within the bone marrow and is accompanied by an eight-fold increase in cell numbers. The mitotic compartment extends to the myelocyte stage, followed by maturation to metamyelocyte, 'band' and mature segmented forms.

The nucleus of the *myeloblast* contains 1–5 nucleoli in a fine chromatin network. The cytoplasm is scanty and in the more mature myeloblast contains a few 'azurophilic' or 'primary' granules, which contain myeloperoxidase (MPO) and other enzymes. The *promyelocyte* nucleus still has nucleoli, the primary granules are numerous and additional granules known as 'secondary' or 'specific' granules are formed but are not readily seen by light microscopy. The *myelocyte* nucleus shows aggregation of the chromatin and a nucleolus is no longer visible; this indicates the loss of ribosomal RNA synthesis and consequent reduction in major biosynthetic processes. The cytoplasm contains fewer primary granules and an increasing number of secondary granules. The type of secondary granule determines the classification and functional characteristics of the granulocytes.

Neutrophils

The secondary granules of the neutrophil series do not have clear basophilic or eosinophilic staining properties, and stain pale pink to lilac, depending on the properties of the stain. The granules do not show myeloperoxidase activity but contain alkaline phosphatase (AP), lysozyme and lactoferrin. The transition from myelocyte to segmented neutrophil mainly involves changes in nuclear shape and structure, though the number of primary granules further decreases and secondary granules fill the cytoplasm. *Metamyelocytes* show further condensation of the chromatin and nuclear indentation to form a horseshoe, or band form, and eventual segmentation into two, three or four lobes connected by fine chromatin strands. The number of lobes is not an indication of cell age and can be modified *in vitro*. Maturation of neutrophils is associated with functional differentiation beginning with the appearance of Fc receptors and terminating with chemotaxis[20]. Advances in fractionation methodology have shown that the simple differentiation of neutrophil granules into primary (MPO-rich) and secondary (AP-rich) granules is insufficient to explain experimental observations. Of particular significance in neutrophil function is the recognition of several naturally-occurring polypeptides from neutrophil granules which have antibiotic properties and have been termed 'defensins'[21].

Mature neutrophils are active in terms of metabolism and movement and require an active energy source. As mitochondria are relatively scanty, oxidative phosphorylation as a source of energy is limited, and there is therefore great dependence on glycolysis.

Neutrophil kinetics

Neutrophils are the most common leucocyte of the circulating blood (about 4.0×10^9/l) yet only about half the total blood granulocyte pool are in the circulating granulocyte pool (CGP); the remainder – or marginal pool (MGP) – are associated with a loose adherence to the vascular endothelium. Nevertheless the exchange between the CGP and the MGP is very rapid. Neutrophils spend on average only about 10 hours in the blood before passing into the tissues. There is no evidence that tissue neutrophils re-appear in the blood. Migration of the marginating neutrophils to the extravascular or tissue space is greatly accelerated by damage to the vessel or local inflammation.

Neutrophil function

The prime function of neutrophils is bacterial killing which involves four stages – chemotaxis, opsonization, ingestion and killing.

Chemotaxis Neutrophils are motile but do not depend on random movement. They react by accelerated mobility (chemokinesis) to specific chemical stimuli (chemotaxins). Most (or possibly all) of the chemotaxins are protein derived from activation of plasma protein pathways such as the complement, fibrinolytic, coagulation and kinin systems. The complement system has been the most intensively studied and the major chemotactic factor is a cleavage product of the fifth component of complement designated C5a. C3 and $\overline{C567}$ also have chemotactic activity. Kallikrein, plasminogen activator and fibrinopeptides are stated to be chemotaxins. Low molecular weight bacterial products are chemotactic but this may be due to their ability to activate complement. As with other biological pathways, homeostatic control mechanisms are present which act as inhibitors of chemotaxins or by immobilizing the neutrophils.

Opsonization This is a process by which the surface of the bacteria is modified to allow phagocytosis. Opsonins differ in heat stability. The heat-labile opsonins are from the complement pathway and have been identified as C3b or related fragments. Heat-stable opsonins are IgG immunoglobulins of the IgG_3 subclass.

Opsonization is associated with immune adherence, by which the opsonized bacterium is bound to the neutrophil membrane by specific receptors for the Fc fragment of IgG, or for C3b.

Ingestion The adherence of the bacterium to the neutrophil membrane is followed by ingestion (phagocytosis). The particle is enclosed in a phagocytic vacuole (phagosome) into which is discharged the contents of the primary and secondary granules (lysosomes) to form a phagolysosome. Discharge of the lysosome contents is associated with degranulation.

Bacterial killing This final stage of neutrophil function involves a number of mechanisms that can be divided into oxygen-dependent and oxygen-independent systems. Oxygen-dependent systems are mediated by myeloperoxidase, hydrogen peroxide formation with a halide as co-factor, and with the formation of superoxide and hydroxyl radicals. Myeloperoxidase is derived from the primary granules and hydrogen peroxide is generated from a burst of activity of the pentose phosphate pathway. The oxygen-independent factors are – a low pH of the phagolysosome, binding of iron by lactoferrin, the direct action of lysozyme on the bacterial cell wall and the bactericidal property of cationic protein from the primary granules.

Each of the stages of neutrophil function may be abnormal and can be studied by *in vitro* tests.

Eosinophils [22]

The secondary granules of eosinophils are large and refractile and are stained bright orange-pink by eosin. Eosinophils are clearly recognizable at the myelocyte stage and further nuclear maturation follows that of the neutrophil series, but segmentation is limited to two or occasionally three lobes. Ultrastrucural studies of the secondary granules show a double-layer membrane and an electron-dense crystalline core. The granules contain peroxidase activity which is distinct from that of myleperoxidase in its resistance to methanol and cyanide, and its inability to decarboxylate amino acids, notably L-alanine. The lysosomes have many enzymes in common with the neutrophils, but have no lysozyme. Aryl sulphatase is 10–20 times more active than in the neutrophil. The granules are rich in protein, notably a zinc-rich major basic protein (MBP), and a cationic protein (ECP).

Eosinophils have a half-life of 4–5 hours in the circulation and a tissue life span of 8–12 days, with some evidence of re-circulation between tissues and blood.

Eosinophil function

Eosinophils respond to chemotactic stimuli and immune complexes (antibody and antigen), complement, and agents released from mast cells have been identified. Phagocytic activity is less than that of the neutrophils and although more hydrogen peroxide is produced, the overall bactericidal activity is less than that of neutrophils. Phagocytosis is associated with degranulation.

Apart from bacterial killing two specific roles have been suggested for eosinophils:

1. Inactivation of mediators released by tissue mast-cell degranulation and consequent reduction of the body's response to IgE-mediated reactions. A role for the high aryl sulphatase activity is the inactivation of substances released in hypersensitivity reactions.
2. The associate between parasitic infection and eosinophilia in blood and tissue is well established. A possible role of the eosinophil is in destroying the larval stages of parasites by eosinophil attachment via receptors of the cell membrane to antibody-sensitized larvae, followed by release of the major basic protein and eosinophil cationic protein which damages or destroys the larvae.

Basophils [23]

Basophils are the least numerous of the circulating leucocytes. They are readily identified by the coarse blue-black staining of the secondary granules, which can be seen at the myelocyte stage of development by light microscopy. Nuclear maturation proceeds to band and bilobed stages. Electron microscopy shows that basophil granules have a substructure consisting of electron-dense particles.

Biochemistry

Histamine is synthesized by basophils, is present in the granules and released during degranulation. The demonstration that basophil granules have an acid pH and stain by metachromatic dyes such as toluidine blue indicate the presence of acid mucopolysaccharides which, coupled with the demonstration of an ability to inhibit blood coagulation that is neutralized by protamine sulphate, has led to the conclusion that basophils are a source of heparin.

Basophil enzymes are quite dissimilar from those of the other granulocytes. Hydrolytic enzymes such as alkaline phosphatase, non-specific esterase etc. are not demonstrable by cytochemistry, but peroxidase activity is present. Basophils have been identified as a source of a platelet-activating factor which is released during degranulation. IgE binds to basophil but not to other leucocytes. IgE binding is associated with degranulation and histamine and heparin release.

Function

Basophils are motile and are attracted by chemotaxins such as complement components and products of activated lymphocytes (lymphokines). The phagocytic power of basophils is weak but they have considerable pinocytic capability in transporting exogenous compounds to cytoplasmic granules. The histamine and heparin content, IgE binding and degranulation point to a role in anaphylaxis, cell-mediated hypersensitivity reactions and local inflammatory responses.

Blood basophils and tissue mast cells
Basophils and mast cells have features in common but almost certainly arise from distinct progenitor cells. Mast cells are virtually confined to the tissues and are readily recognized by the abundant, densely packed and deeply stained basophilic granules, an appearance that is partly due to the insolubility of the granules in water, in contrast to the properties of the basophil granules. The mast-cell nucleus is usually round rather than lobed. The heparin content of the mast cell is much greater than that of the basophil. Both types of cell bind IgE.

Monocytes [24]

The blood monocyte is an intermediate stage in the development of the tissue macrophage, the series being referred to as 'mononuclear phagocytes'. Monocytes originate in the bone marrow from a progenitor cell which is probably similar to, or even identical with, the myeloblast. Cytochemical and tissue culture studies support the concept of a common progenitor cell, with differentiation occurring after the blast-cell stage.

The monocyte is a large cell with a copious cytoplasm, fine azurophil granules and an indented, or even folded, nucleus. The cell is sluggishly motile and is phagocytic. Myeloperoxidase activity is weak but there is strong non-specific esterase activity. It has characteristics that differentiate it from mononuclear cells such as large lymphocytes, e.g. specific receptors for the Fc fragment of IgG and for C3.

Monocyte kinetics

The blood monocyte pool consists of circulating and marginal pools with about 75% of cells in the marginal pool. The mean circulation time in the blood is 10–12 hours before the cell migrates to the tissues. After leaving the circulation, further development as a tissue macrophage is associated with increased enzyme activity and increase in the number of mitochondria. It is important to recognize that the tissue macrophage is capable of further proliferation, and in certain circumstances can give rise to multinucleated giant cells. The survival of the tissue macrophage pool is probably in the order of several months and the tissue macrophage pool is some 400 times the size of the blood monocyte population.

Function

As the blood monocyte is an intermediate stage of development, the full range of functions refers to the tissue macrophage.

Microbial killings To some extent the mechanisms are those of the neutrophil: chemotaxis, phagocytosis and killing by an oxygen-dependent, hydrogen peroxide system.

Removal of debris Damaged or dying cells, antibody-sensitized red cells, haemosiderin and other particulate materials such as coal-dust, silica and carbon, are phagocytosed by macrophages.

Immune response There is ample evidence that macrophages contribute to the immune response by 'processing' antigens to facilitate recognition by lymphocytes and the consequent humoral response. Macrophages are also part of the cellular immune response in that 'antigen-activated' macrophages are more phagocytic and have increased metabolic and mitotic rates. Tissue macrophages are involved in delayed hypersensitivity reactions.

Lymphocytes

Lymphocytes are the second most frequent leucocyte type in the blood. They are small cells (about 10–12 μm diameter) with a small amount of cytoplasm surrounding a dense, round nucleus. Cells with more copious cytoplasm or 'large lymphocytes' are more common in children. Until relatively recently the lymphocyte was regarded as an end-stage of development with no known function, although it was realized that in certain infections morphological changes occur, and the number of lymphocytes might increase. The discoveries that lymphocytes could be stimulated to divide, and that they produce antibodies (immunoglobulins) led to the recognition of two separate lymphocyte populations: one having the ability to produce immunoglobulins (B lymphocytes) and the other being responsible for cell-mediated immunity (T lymphocytes). These observations form the basis of the modern concepts of immunity.

Morphology

The typical small lymphocyte is remarkably featureless by conventional Romanowsky staining. The thin rim of cytoplasm is pale blue and contains a few azurophil granules; the nucleus is dense and featureless but nucleoli are always present and can be demonstrated by special stains. The two classes of lymphocyte cannot be distinguished by light microscopy of Romanowsky-stained preparations, or with certainty by either scanning or transmission electron microscopy, and are differentiated mainly by immunological characteristics though cytochemical techniques also reveal differences between T and B lymphocytes (*see* Chapter 13).

Lymphocyte kinetics

The committed T and B cells cannot function as progenitor cells but populate the blood, lymphatics and secondary lymphoid organs such as the lymph nodes, spleen and alimentary canal. The distribution of T and B cells in these organs is organized into compartments, with B cells predominating in the cortex and germinal centres and T cells in the inner cortex and follicular mantle.

In the blood 70–80% of 'small lymphocytes' are T cells and 15–20% are B cells with a small proportion of cells lacking the characteristics of either mature T or B cells and designated 'null' cells. Whether the null-cell population represent a distinct class or represent the limitations of the methodologies and techniques for identifying T and B cells is debatable; certainly, different workers using different techniques report variable numbers of null cells in healthy persons.

The majority of small lymphocytes have a long survival and unlike other blood cells are extensively recirculated through the lymphoid tissues, lymphatics and blood. T and B cells appear to have short- and long-lived populations with a mean survival time estimated to be from 4 to 10 years.

Functional differentiation of B lymphocytes

The function of B cells is the formation of specific immunoglobulins. Surface-membrane immunoglobulin (smIg) receptors specific for an antigenic determinant are expressed on the membrane and if the cell encounters a complementary antigen binding occurs which can stimulate proliferation of the cell to form a 'clone', with differentiation to plasmacytes which are not often found in the blood. Plasmacytes have a characteristic morphology with an eccentrically placed nucleus and deeply basophilic cytoplasm which indicates the presence of large amounts of RNA associated with immunoglobulin synthesis. Immunoglobulin synthesis and secretion of IgG and IgA is associated with the production of 'memory cells' with long survival which can promptly differentiate to plasmacytes upon re-exposure to the antigen.

Early B cells are recognized by the presence of intracellular or cytoplasmic immunoglobulin (cIg) of IgM type. These cells represent about 1% of the total nucleated bone-marrow cells. The presence of cIgM is followed by smIgM or smIgD which is replaced by IgG and IgA molecules. Other developmental markers are the presence of Fc receptors (*see* below) and, later, C3 receptors and Ia antigens. A further characteristic of B cells is the formation of rosettes with mouse red cells.

Functional differentiation of T lymphocytes

Unlike B cells, T cells do not produce immunoglobulins or differentiate to plasmacytes. They do not therefore express cytoplasmic or surface immunoglobulins but are characterized (in mice) by the presence of a membrane antigen designated Thy 1.

The T cells are made up of a number of subpopulations or subsets which can be identified by membrane antigens or receptors for the portion of the heavy chain of IgG or IgM which have a constant amino-acid sequence or 'constant fragment', designated the Fc fragment. The presence of receptors for the Fc fragment of IgG or IgM correlates with functional activity; T cells having Fc receptors of IgG are desinated Tγ and have a suppressor function while cells with receptors for IgM are designated Tμ and are 'helper' or 'inducer' cells. The ratio of helper to suppressor cells is about 2:1.

A further functional T-cell subpopulation are the effector cells associated with cytotoxicity, delayed hypersensitivity, and graft-versus-host disease. The introduction and use of monoclonal antibodies against T-cell membrane antigens has allowed further identification of T cells and the subpopulations. Monoclonal antibodies with identical or very similar specificities prepared by different workers or available from commercial sources have different designations, e.g. OKT8, leu 2. To clarify the nomenclature, antibodies with similar determinants have been 'clustered' and allocated a 'cluster determinant' or CD number. Thus CD3 has pan-T cell specificity, CD4 reacts with the helper/inducer subset and CD8 the suppressor/cytotoxic cells.

Natural killer cells [25]

Cell-mediated cytotoxicity independent of antibody suggested the existence of a 'natural killer cell' (NK) population. NK cells do not have phagocytic or adherent properties, lack demonstrable surface-membrane immunoglobulin (smIg) and lack the pan-T antigen recognized by CD3 monoclonal antibodies, i.e. are null cells. Separation techniques suggest that NK cells are large, granular lymphocytes with a proportion having reactivity with certain monoclonal antibodies which are reactive with T-cell subsets.

In addition to cytotoxicity, NK cells probably modulate haemopoiesis, a role in common with activated T cells (*see* Chapter 1).

Interaction between T and B cells

The differentiation of resting B cells to plasmacytes with antibody production may be independent or dependent on T cells, depending upon the antigen involved.

Differentiation independent of T cells can be stimulated by antigens of high molecular weight which are often polymers, e.g. polysaccharides, which primarily stimulate IgM antibody with no memory-cell formation.

T-dependent B-cell differentiation is associated with antigens such as proteins, glycoproteins and haptens and therefore encompasses the majority of antigens, and induces IgM, IgG and IgA antibodies and the formation of memory cells. The role of the T cell is to produce *non-specific* B-cell activators which, in the presence of an antigen, stimulate B cells and formation of specific antibody. Alternatively in the presence of an antigen, T cells produce a *specific* activator which in the presence of the antigen stimulates *only* those B cells capable of forming the specific antibody. These mechanisms are clearly examples of T-helper-cell function.

Other functions of T cells in the immune response

The activation of T cells results in the production of soluble substances other than the B-cell activators, which have been termed 'lymphokines'. Lymphokines have a variety of actions and include chemotactic factors which attract phagocytic cells, mitogenic factor which stimulates non-activated T cells, and lymphotoxin with direct cytotoxic action. By enhancing antibody production against an antigen, T cells indirectly increase the activation of the complement system.

Platelets and platelet function

Following the first description of the platelet in 1842 by Donne, it was not until 1886 that Booth and Himmelburgh introduced the concept that platelets played an important primary role in the formation of haemostatic plug. They showed in experiments on cut carotid arteries of the dog that platelets plugged the gap in the vessel wall, formed aggregates and fused into one another. In the early part of this century, the first report on the production of platelets from megakaryocytes was published[26]; but interest turned from the platelet to other components of blood coagulation, in particular, those related to the formation of fibrin. During the last 20 years, however, extensive advances have been made in our understanding of the role of platelets in vessel-wall injury, arterial and venous thrombosis, atherosclerosis and of antiplatelet therapy.

Before turning to the relationship between platelets and haemostasis, it is necessary to review the cellular basis of platelet production and the biochemistry and structure of the circulating platelet.

Platelet production [27, 28]

Platelets are formed in the cytoplasm of megakaryocytes, which are found mainly in the bone marrow. The megakaryocyte shares with the myeloid and erythroid series a common precursor, the pluripotent marrow stem cell (*see* page 6). Megakaryocytes have a unique pattern of cellular maturation in that, although DNA synthesis is completed at an early stage (2n), the cells undergo a series of nuclear divisions with a progressive increase in the volume of the cytoplasm, but without cell division (*Table 2.4*). The earliest recognizable type of megakaryocyte found in the marrow has a nucleus that has undergone three divisions (8n cell). The nuclei of the megakaryocyte divide again several times to form a 16n, 32n and then 64n cell with all the nuclei in a single megakaryocyte dividing synchronously. Each successive nuclear division results in an increase in cytoplasmic volume which in turn increases the number of platelets that are formed. A single megakaryocyte is calculated to produce 2000 platelets.

Table 2.4 Megakaryocytopoiesis

Stage	*Approximate maturation* (h)	*Cell classification*	*Minimum ploidy number*	*Recognizable features*
		Pluripotent stem cell	2n	No characteristic morphology
I	9.5	Committed precursor (megakaryoblast)	4n	First recognizable stage with deeply basophilic cytoplasm, 2–8 nucleoli. Specific membrane and cytoplasmic markers
II	9.5	Promegakaryocyte	8n	Larger, less basophilic. Nuclear polyploidy
IIIa	9.5	Immature megakaryocyte	16n	Granular cytoplasm, first platelets formed in cytoplasm. Increase in size
IIIb	8.0	Mature megakaryocyte	32n	Further increase in size. Separation of cytoplasm into platelet subunits
IIIc	32.0	Mature megakaryocyte Mature megakaryocyte	32n 64n	Further increase in size PAS positive

Daily platelet formation = 1.41×10^4

Regulation of platelet production

There appears to be a regulatory mechanism that keeps the circulating platelet population to precise circulating levels. In situations where there is a fall in or transfusion of platelets, the rate of platelet production adjusts very rapidly, suggesting a feedback effect via the circulating platelet mass. A regulatory hormone analogous to erythropoietin termed 'thrombopoietin' [29] is responsible, directing its effect by (1) increasing the number of megakaryocytes formed from precursor cells and (2) increasing the rate both of cytoplasmic maturation and of platelet release. Problems with bioassy and purification have limited identification of the site of synthesis of thrombopoietin; two main organs involved appear to be the kidney and the liver.

Platelet kinetics [28]

Following their release from the bone marrow, the life span of the platelet is regulated by a finite internal metabolism and its dynamic interaction with the vascular endothelium, inflammatory response and the coagulation system. The total population is split between the spleen (30%) and the circulation (70%). Platelet survival studies using [^{51}Cr]chromate, [^{14}C]serotonin, or DF^{32}P indicate a survival time of 10 days with a half-life of about 70 hours, whilst those using non-isotope techniques such as aspirin acetylation of the platelet enzyme cyclo-oxygenase give a figure of 8–11 days.

The spleen has an effect on the distribution of platelets in that it sequesters approximately 30% of labelled platelets into the splenic cords of the red pulp: these can be exchanged freely with the circulating platelets. In splenomegaly a larger proportion of platelets sequester in the spleen (up to 80%) and in some cases, one of the benefits of splenectomy is seen by a postoperative rise in platelet levels due to removal of the splenic pool.

Platelet structure

Circulating platelets are anucleate bodies of discoid shape. Sectioned platelets show the cell as circular or ellipsoid depending on the plane of the section and having a mean long axis of 2.9 μm and a short axis of 1.4 μm. Volume is 5–8 fl. By transmission electron microscopy the platelet is shown to be a complex structure with membrane, microtubules, microfilaments and organelles (*Figure 2.7*).

Plasma membrane

The basic structure and composition is similar to that of membranes of other cells. The membrane bilayer is composed of proteins, phospholipids and cholesterol with the proteins being integral to the lipid matrix or more loosely associated surface structures. The phospholipids provide the source of fatty acids which are of fundamental importance in platelet metabolism, notably arachidonic acid; phosphatidyl ethanolamine and phosphatidyl serine have a direct role in the coagulation process. The most important functional membrane proteins are glycoproteins (GP), seven having been shown to have specific properties (*Table 2.5*).

Other cell-surface receptors act as transducers in the formation of signal-generating enzymes both for activating and inhibitory pathways [30]. In addition to

Table 2.5 Platelet membrane glycoproteins

Glycoprotein	*Function*
Ia	Adhesion to collagen
Ib	von Willebrand factor (vWf) binding, adhesion to vascular subendothelium
IIb–IIIa	Fibrinogen binding, aggregation
IV	Thrombospondin binding
V	Thrombin binding, aggregation
IX	Adhesion, associated with Ib complex

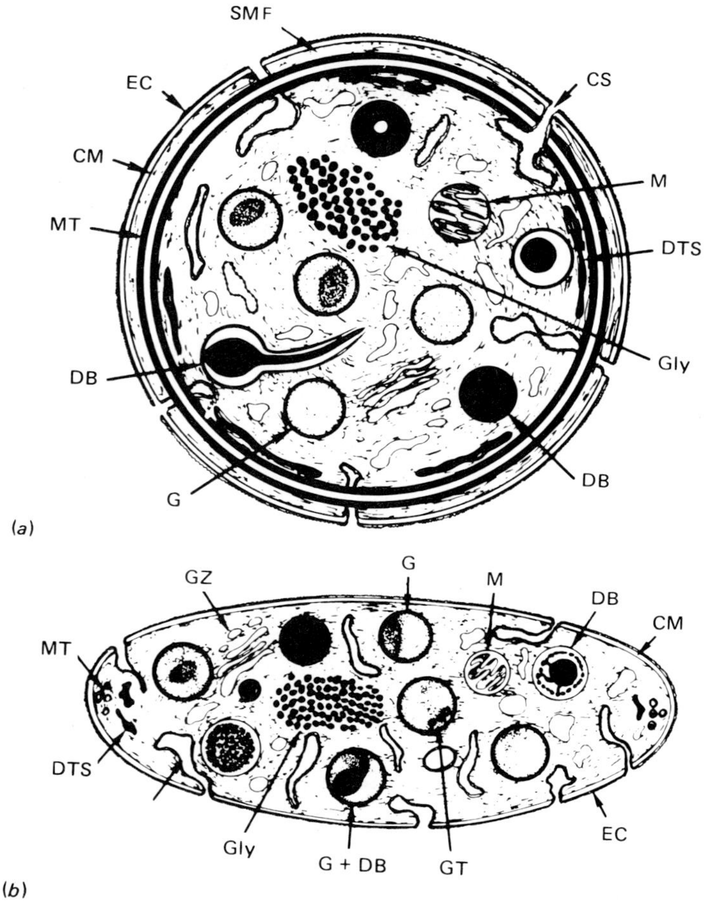

Figure 2.7 Platelet ultrastructure. (*a*) Equatorial plane. (*b*) Cross-section. Peripheral zone: EC = exterior coat; CM = trilaminar membrane. Matrix/sol–gel zone: SMF = submembrane filaments; MT = microtubules; Gly = glycogen. Organelle zone: M = mitochondria; G = granules; DB = dense bodies; DTS = dense tubular system

the structural proteins of the membrane and the binding of vWf and fibrinogen, the external surface of the membrane absorbs several protein factors of the coagulation mechanism including factors V, X, XI and XIII.

Cytoskeleton

Immediately underneath the membrane are microtubules and microfilaments which maintain the shape of the non-activated platelet. They consist of contractile proteins, some attached to integral proteins of the membrane. Following stimulation or activation of the platelet, the proteins contract centrally and are associated with pseudopodia formation and with the release or expulsion of cytoplasmic granules from the platelet.

Cytoplasmic components

The platelet cytoplasm contains several organized structures – mitochondria, numerous 'alpha-granules', less frequent 'dense' granules as defined by electron microscopy, lysosomes and the 'dense tubular system' or endoplasmic reticulum.

The alpha-granules are protein-storage sites, the dense granules contain adenine nucleotides (ADP and ATP), 5-hydroxytryptamine (5-HT, serotonin) and calcium ions, and the lysosomes store acid hydrolases. The components of the cytoplasmic granules are shown in *Table 2.6*. The dense tubular system is associated with prostaglandin synthesis and calcium flux, both involved in the platelet 'release reaction' and aggregation.

Table 2.6 Cytoplasmic platelet structures, content and function

Structure	*Content*	*Function*
Alpha-granules	Platelet factor 4	Heparinoid neutralization
	Beta-thromboglobulin	? Chemotaxis
	Thrombospondin	Thrombin binding, protein C activation
	Platelet-derived growth factor (PDGF)	Mitogenesis, fibroblast stimulation, vessel repair
	von Willebrand's factor	Adhesion
	Fibrinogen	Aggregation, coagulation
	Factor V	Factor X activation
	Fibronectin	Fibroblast and platelet adhesion
	Plasminogen activator inhibitor 1	Inhibition of fibrinolysis
	Factor XIII	Fibrin cross-linking
Dense bodies	ADP	Aggregation, vasoconstriction
	ATP	Degrades to ADP
	5-HT	Vasoconstriction, aggregation
	Calcium	Shape change, aggregation
Lysosomes	N-acetylglucosamidase	
	N-glucuronidase	
	N-galactosidase	

Modified from reference [31].

Haemostasis

Normal haemostasis is a balance between maintaining the fluidity of the blood in normal intact vasculature and the restriction of blood loss from damaged blood vessels. This equilibrium is dependent on the presence of activating and inhibiting processes with regulatory positive and negative feedback pathways. The requirement to prevent excessive blood loss is dependent on the complex interaction between the vessel wall, platelet function and the formation of thrombin and fibrin via the coagulation factors of the plasma. On the other hand, the prevention of thrombus formation is primarily due to inhibitory influence of the vascular endothelium and its capability to initiate dissolution of formed fibrin by fibrinolysis. The haemostatic processes are also linked to complement activation and generation of kinins.

Haemostasis can be considered under five headings:

1. The vessel wall, blood flow and response to injury or damage.
2. Platelets, the vessel wall and coagulation.
3. Fibrin formation via the plasma coagulation factors.
4. The regulatory role of the natural inhibitors of coagulation.
5. The removal of fibrin by activation of the fibrinolytic system.

Vessel wall, blood flow and response to injury

All blood vessels are lined by cells which form a single continuous layer of endothelium. The cells are flat, of varying thickness and have a positive charge due to the presence of glycoproteins and glycosoaminoglycans which repel platelet adhesion. The capillary walls consist of endothelial cells covering a basement membrane of collagen microfibrils. Arterioles are supported by collagen and smooth muscle which constricts in response to humoral or local controls. Under normal physiological conditions leucocytes, nutrients and water pass through the capillary wall while the red cells and platelets are retained. In the intact capillary, platelets circulate in proximity to the vessel wall without adhering to each other or the endothelium. Following injury there is a transient vascular constriction reducing blood flow which aids platelet adherence. The release of vasoactive amines (5-HT) from activated platelets enhances vasoconstriction. Changes in blood rheology, and consequently blood flow, can also influence platelet–vessel wall interaction due to increased aggregation of red cells (rouleaux formation) and displacement of platelets to the vessel wall.

Platelets and the vessel wall

Damage to the endothelium and exposure of subendothelial structures promote platelet adhesion with resulting platelet activation. Adhesion results from the interaction of platelets with collagen and other subendothelial macromolecules and, in particular, von Willebrand factor (vWf) via the high affinity glycoprotein Ib (GPIb) platelet membrane receptor. The activated platelet undergoes major structural changes by transformation from discoid shape to spiny sphere with multiple pseudopodia. The shape change is mediated by changes in the cytoskeleton and accompanied by release of the contents of the platelet granules.

Activation and shape change results in ‘exposure’ of the GPIIb–IIIa complex which allows binding of dimeric fibrinogen to adjacent platelets, resulting in aggregation which is stabilized by the presence of calcium. ADP from damaged cells or platelets binds to a specific receptor and further facilitates exposure of the IIb–IIIa complex.

In addition to aggregation due to shape change and membrane binding of activators, chemical pathways are activated which result in the formation of powerful aggregation-promoting compounds and further release reaction. Arachidonic acid, generated from membrane phospholipid by phospholipase A_2, is converted to the prostaglandin thromboxane A_2 (TXA_2) by cytoplasmic enzymes including cyclo-oxygenase and thromboxane synthetase. TXA_2 is inactivated to form the stable metabolite thromboxane B_2 (TXB_2).

A second pathway is the action of phospholipase C on phosphatidyl inositol 5-diphosphate (PIP_2) to form diacylglycerol (DG) and inositol triphosphate (IP_3).

IP_3 is a calcium ionophore which transfers calcium from the dense tubular system to the cytoplasm resulting in activation of a kinase which phosphorylates the light chain of myosin and induces shape change, contraction, release and aggregation. Diacylglycerol is a cofactor for protein kinase C which phosphorylates a protein of uncertain function. Platelet activation is modulated by cAMP which promotes calcium uptake by the dense tubular system, thus reducing cytoplasmic calcium and inhibiting those reactions which are calcium-dependent. The biochemical pathways of platelet activation are summarized in *Figure 2.8*.

In addition to the formation of TXA_2, the arachidonic acid pathway can also result in the formation of prostaglandin I_2 (PGI_2, prostacyclin, epoprostenol). PGI_2 is the major prostaglandin produced by endothelial cells and inhibits platelet adhesion and aggregation and has antithrombotic and vasodilatory action. PGI_2 stimulates adenylate cyclase which leads to an increase in cAMP levels in the platelets. Under normal physiological conditions there is a dynamic balance between production and interaction of PGI_2 and TXA_2 mediated through cAMP

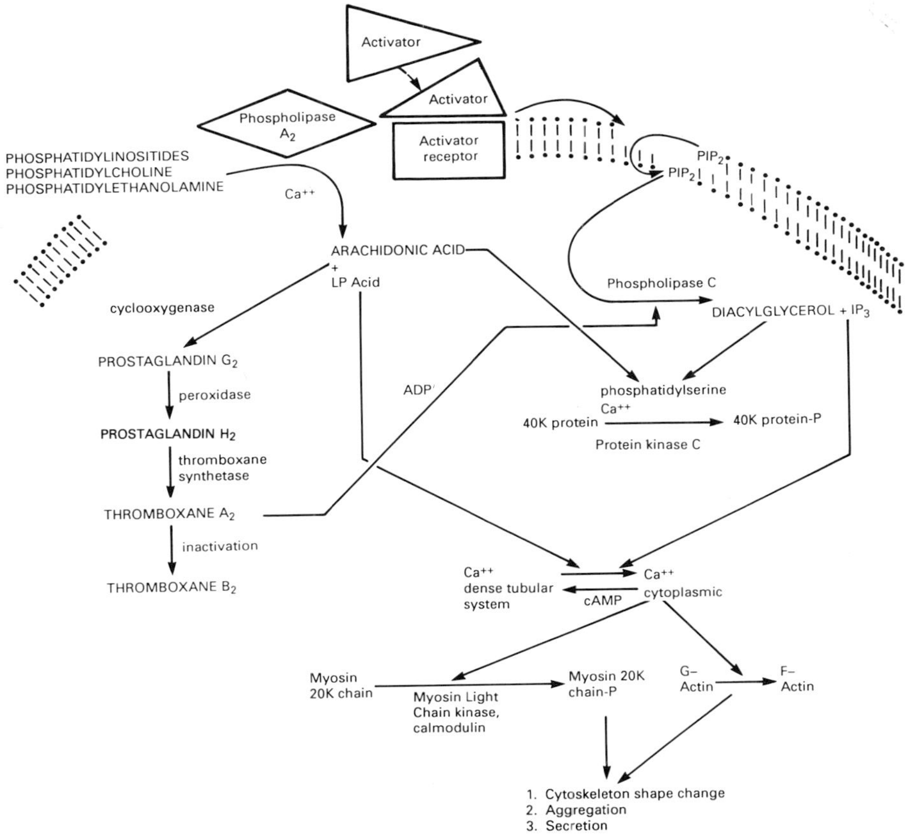

Figure 2.8 Chemical pathways resulting in platelet activation. Abbreviations used are: IP_3, inositol-1,4,5-triphosphate; LP Acid, lysophosphatidic acid; PIP_2, phosphatidyl inositol 4,5-biphosphate. Reproduced from reference [32] with permission

concentration within the platelets (*Figure 2.9*). The consequences of vascular damage are the exposure of subendothelial collagen and loss of PGI_2 release, thus enabling platelet adherence and aggregation (*Figure 2.10*).

Platelet adhesion and aggregation is followed by local fibrin formation which stabilizes the platelet 'plug'. This process is facilitated by the coagulation factors absorbed onto platelets (particularly factor XI), those made available by the release reaction, together with phospholipid contributed by platelet membranes and 'tissue factor' at the site of damage (*Figure 2.11*).

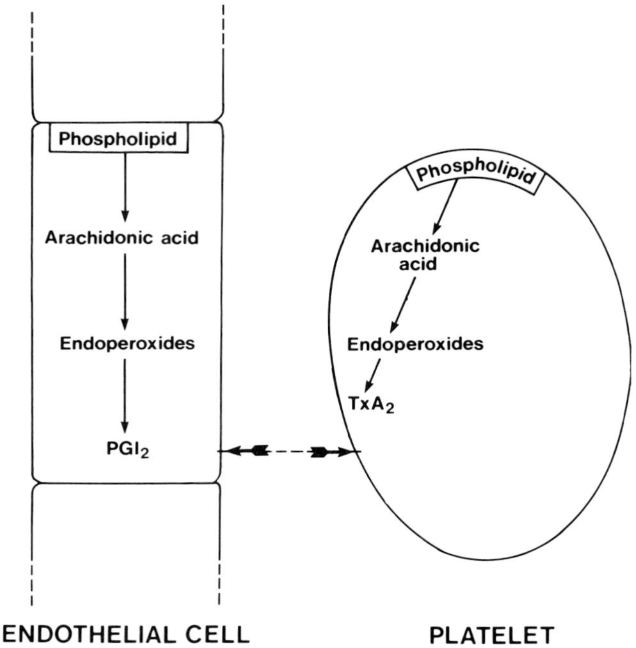

Figure 2.9 Interaction between anti-aggregating activity of vessel-wall prostacyclin and pro-aggregating production of platelet thromboxane A_2

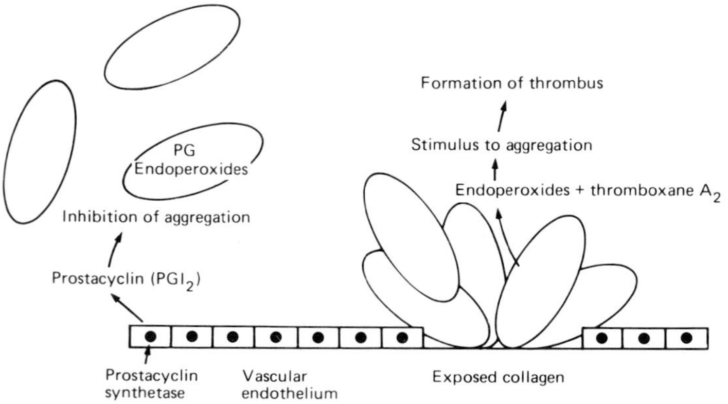

Figure 2.10 Proposed mechanism of platelet aggregation caused by lack of prostacyclin production

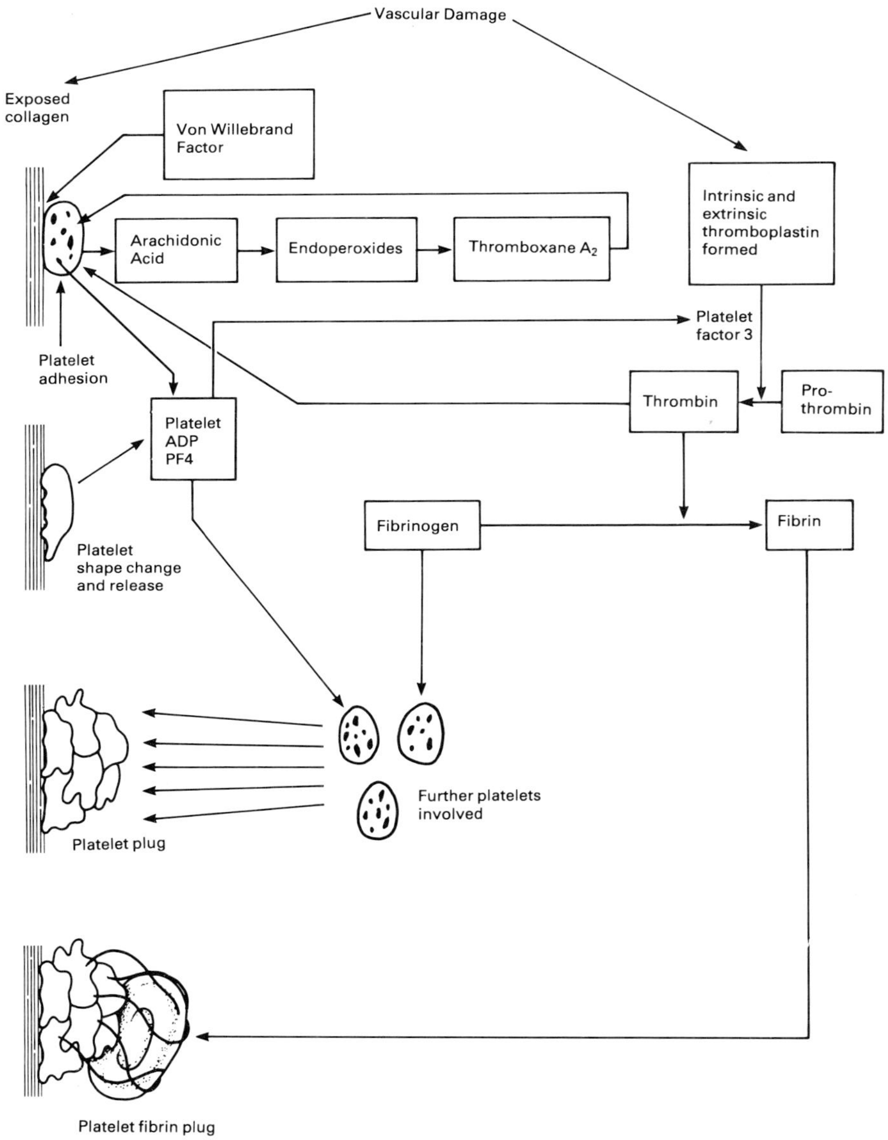

Figure 2.11 Interaction between platelets, plasma factors and vessel wall in haemostasis

The interaction of platelets with the coagulation process

In addition to the role of platelets in primary haemostasis after vascular damage, platelets have procoagulant activity by:

1. Platelet-associated coagulation factors.
2. Providing membrane phospholipids to allow assembly of coagulation factor complexes.
3. Activation of the 'contact system' of the coagulation pathway.

A number of coagulation factors are associated with platelets either bound to the membrane or within the alpha-granules. Certain factors, plasma fibrinogen, factors II, VII, IX, X and vWf are loosely bound and can be removed by washing the platelets. Tightly bound proteins and those associated with alpha-granules include platelet fibrinogen, factors V, XI, platelet factor XIII and vWf. Following platelet activation these platelet-associated proteins are made rapidly available and procoagulant activities develop on the platelet membrane. This localization of procoagulant activity allows fibrin formation at the site of the platelet plug with consequent stabilization.

Shape change and aggregation results in reorganization of negatively-charged membrane phospholipids, notably phosphatidyl serine, phosphatidyl choline and possibly phosphatidyl inositol. This provides the phospholipid interface onto which coagulation factors can bind via specific receptors or calcium bridges. Two complexes are specifically identified, that resulting in the activation of factor X in association with activated factors IX and VIII, and that resulting in the activation of factor II to IIa in the presence of factor Xa and factor Va (*Figures 2.12* and *2.13*).

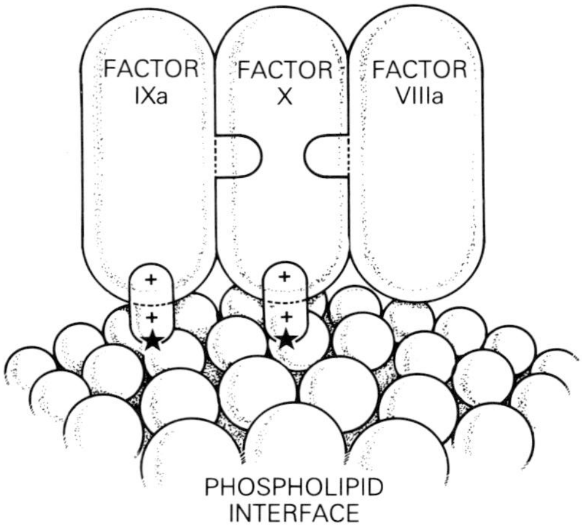

Figure 2.12 Formation of factor Xa-forming coagulation complex. ★ = Calcium-binding site

Platelets can contribute to the contact-activation of coagulation[33]. In the presence of ADP, intact platelets promote the activation of factor XII in association with prekallikrein and high molecular weight kininogen. Collagen-stimulated platelets promote the proteolytic activation of factor XI in the presence of prekallikrein but not requiring factor XII.

Role of coagulation in haemostasis

Thirteen plasma proteins or coagulation factors have been identified as contributing to the sequence of events leading to the formation of fibrin. Most of the coagulation factors have been identified by investigation of subjects with inherited haemorrhagic disorders or abnormalities in *in vitro* experiments, due to deficiency of a single factor. Subsequent isolation, purification, determination of amino-acid sequence and structure, and preparation of specific antibodies have provided a fuller understanding of the complex interactions in the coagulation process.

Excluding fibrinogen (factor I) and factor XIII, the clotting factors can be divided into different types. Factors II, IX, X, XI, XII and prekallikrein circulate as inactive precursors or zymogens which, by limited proteolysis or activation, are converted to active enzymes which possess a serine residue at their 'active site' and are termed serine proteases. The activated forms are designated as IIa, IXa etc. (strictly the nomenclature uses a subscript – II_a, IX_a etc.). Factor VII zymogen also has weak enzyme activity and when both zymogen and enzyme are referred to, the designation VII(a) is used. A further group of proteins, factors V and VIII, high

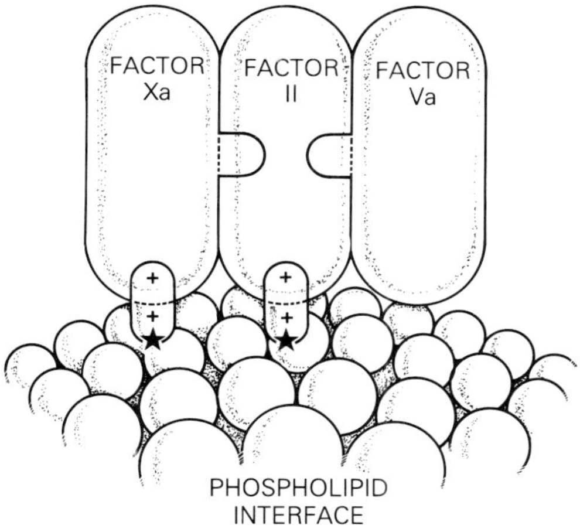

Figure 2.13 Formation of factor IIa-forming (prothrombinase) coagulation complex. ★ = Calcium-binding site

molecular weight kininogen (HMWK), and 'tissue factor', act as co-factors which may be modified during the coagulation process and greatly accelerate the reaction rates of the serine proteases, possibly by as much as 300 000 times! Fibrinogen is the substrate for factor IIa (thrombin) and factor XIII is activated by thrombin to reveal an active cysteine site and transamidase activity.

Calcium ions are required at most stages of the coagulation cascade with the notable exceptions of the 'contact system' and the conversion of fibrinogen to fibrin monomer.

As with other plasma proteins the major site of synthesis is the liver hepatocyte, though smaller amounts of some factors are produced by platelets and endothelial cells. *Table 2.7* summarizes characteristics of the coagulation factors.

Factors II, VII, IX and X, together with the anticoagulant proteins C and S, require carboxylation of γ-glutamic acid residues (glu) to form γ-carboxyglutamic acid residues (gla), a process dependent on vitamin K. This group of factors is referred to as 'vitamin K-dependent factors'. Dietary vitamin K absorbed from the

Table 2.7 Nomenclature and characteristics of clotting factors

Factor	*Common synonym*	*Molecular weight*	*Plasma concentration* (μg/ml)	*Half-life* (h)	*Storage stability*
I	Fibrinogen	340 000	2–4 × 10^3	90	Stable
II	Prothrombin	72 000	120	65	Stable
III	Tissue factor	29 593	0	–	–
IV	Calcium	40	100	–	–
V	Pro-accelerin	330 000	10	15	Labile
VII	Proconvertin	48 000	1	5	Stable
VIII	Antihaemophilic factor (AHF)	360 000	0.05	10	Labile
IX	Christmas factor	57 500	4	24	Stable
X	Stuart–Prower factor	55 000	12	40	Stable
XI	Plasma thromboplastin antecedent	160 000	6	45	Activated
XII	Hageman factor	85 000	40	50	Activated
XIII	Fibrin stabilizing factor	320 000	20	200	Stable
–	Prekallikrein (Fletcher factor)	90 000	40	35	Activated
–	High molecular weight kininogen (Fitzgerald, Reid, Williams, Flaujeac factors)	120 000	70	150	Stable

small intestine is reduced (K_1) in the liver and in the presence of CO_2, O_2 and ATP converts glu- to gla-residues (*Figure 2.14*). During the glu–gla carboxylation, a vitamin $K_{2,3}$ epoxide is produced which is reduced to the active form via the enzyme DT-diaphorase. If the vitamin K-dependent mechanism is blocked, the precursor is released into the plasma in a functionally inactive form or 'protein induced by vitamin K absence (or antagonist)' or PIVKA protein (*Figure 2.15*).

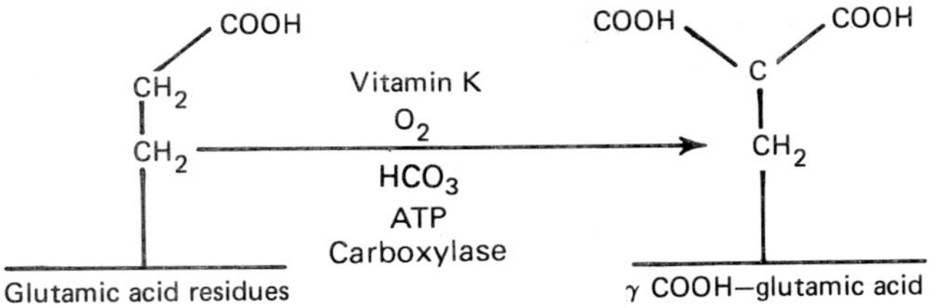

Figure 2.14 Carboxylation of glutamic acid residues

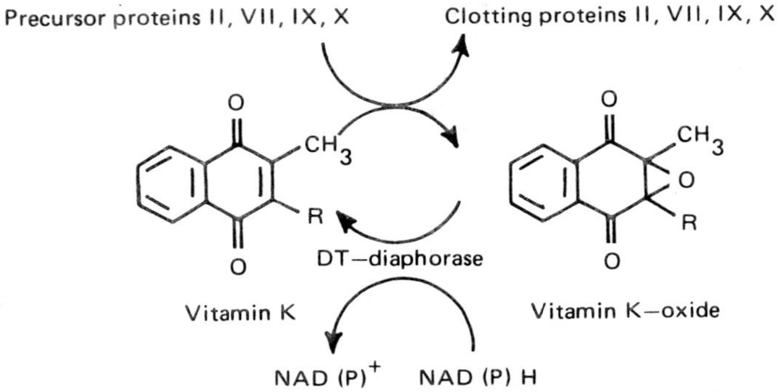

Figure 2.15 Production of the vitamin K-dependent clotting factors incorporating the vitamin K-dependent step

Activation of coagulation, the coagulation pathways and fibrin formation

Description and discussion of the processes leading to the formation of stable fibrin is confused by failure to differentiate between the physiological mechanisms and those taking place when blood is allowed to coagulate *in vitro*. Although it is essential to understand the mechanisms of coagulation in the laboratory, there are clear distinctions from the *in vivo* processes.

As a result of laboratory experiments, tests and findings, coagulation has been separated into an *intrinsic pathway* initiated by plasma contact with negatively-charged molecules such as glass, kaolin, celite, collagen, dextran sulphate, ellagic acid [34], and an *extrinsic pathway* activated by the addition of concentrated 'tissue extract' or 'thromboplastin'. The intrinsic and extrinsic pathways each result in the formation of activated factor X (Xa or 'intrinsic thromboplastin') which activates a 'common pathway' leading to thrombin formation and the conversion of fibrinogen to stable fibrin.

In vitro contact activation of coagulation

The 'contact system' is comprised of factor XII, HMWK, prekallikrein (PK) and factor XI. The primary role of the contact system is the activation of factor IX. Exposure of plasma to negatively-charged surfaces or molecules results in binding of factor XII with change in molecular configuration (XII′) which is more susceptible to proteolytic cleavage to form activated factor XII (αXIIa). Prekallikrein and factor XI are also bound via the co-factor HMWK which facilitates the interaction of the proteins. Factor XIIa activates PK to kallikrein (KK) which in turn converts XII to XIIa, a reciprocal activation mechanism. Factor XIIa is responsible for the activation of HMWK-bound factor XI to XIa which activates factor IX to IXa. The events leading to XIa formation are independent of calcium ions. The sequence is illustrated by *Figure 2.16*.

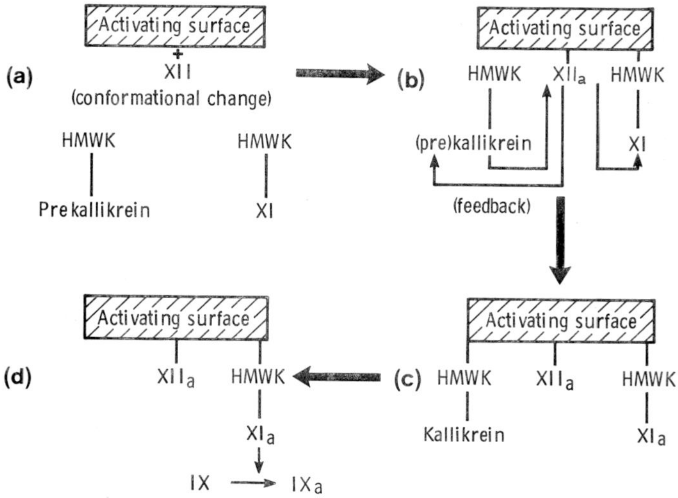

Figure 2.16 Surface-dependent activation of coagulation via factor XII. (*a*) Factor XII is attached to an activating surface and undergoes a conformational change. (b) 'Reciprocal' activation of factor XII occurs in the presence of a high molecular weight kininogen (HMWK). (*c*) Factor XIIa activates surface-bound (via HMWK) factor XI. (*d*) Activated XIa then activates the intrinsic coagulation pathway via factor IX

An alternative stimulus of factor XIa formation is via activated platelets[33]. Factors XIa and XIIa also activate factor VII to VIIa. Naturally occurring inhibitors are found at all stages of the haemostatic process and using purified systems *in vitro* inhibition of XIIa and kallikrein is effected by C1-inhibitor, while α_1-antitrypsin has the reactivity with factor XIa.

In addition to its role in the activation of the coagulation cascade, the formation of βXIIa (the activation fragment of XII to XIIa) and kallikrein from prekallikrein can be shown to result in the activation of the fibrinolytic, complement, kinin-generation and renin-angiotensin pathways and is also associated with bacterial chemotaxis. It is emphasized that these activation processes are *in vitro* observations and are of doubtful physiological significance because severe deficiencies of factor XII, prekallikrein or HMWK are not usually associated with clinical symptoms, though in a minority of cases minor bleeding tendencies have been reported and a tendency to thrombosis suggested[35]. Factor XI deficiency is associated with a bleeding tendency of variable severity which does not, however, correlate with factor XI level. Alternative physiological route(s) of coagulation activation must be present.

'Intrinsic' factor Xa generation

The conversion of factor X to Xa involves the formation of a protein–lipid complex comprising factor IXa, factor VIIa, Factor X, phospholipid and the presence of calcium ions.

Factor IX[36] is activated by specific proteolytic cleavage in the presence of Ca^{2+} to form a light and heavy chain held together by a disulphide bridge. Factor IXa cleaves factor X at a specific site to form the active serine protease factor Xa. Factor IXa alone has a low but measurable capacity to activate factor X; addition of Ca^{2+} results in modest stimulation and added phospholipid has an additional effect. The presence of activated factor VIII (VIIIa) in the complex increases the velocity of the reaction manyfold. This is achieved by binding of the factor VIII to the phospholipid surface to act as receptor for the IXa and X which are stabilized by calcium binding to the phospholipid. *In vivo* the phospholipid surface is provided by platelets and endothelial cell membranes after activation or damage.

Factor VIII[37] is tightly but non-covalently bound to the vWf molecule in molar ratio of vWf:VIII of 36:1. Factor VIIIa is formed by the proteolytic action of trace amounts of thrombin to form several peptides, two of which enhance the velocity of factor X activation. Activated factor VIII is labile and is degraded by excess thrombin, activated protein C and plasmin.

Factor X[38] is a vitamin K-dependent glycoprotein consisting of a light and heavy chain with a total molecular weight of 59 500 which is a structure unique among the serine proteases. Factor X is converted to factor Xa by cleavage of a single peptide bond of the heavy chain. The primary enzymatic function of factor Xa is the conversion of prothrombin (factor II) to thrombin (factor IIa) in the presence of calcium, phospholipid and activated factor V (Va), the so-called 'common pathway' of the coagulation cascade. In addition to the proteolysis of prothrombin, factor Xa significantly activates factor VII which in turn results in further X to Xa conversion, a positive feedback loop. Factor Xa can also be demonstrated to activate factor V and VIII *in vitro*. Factor X can also be activated by other proteolytic enzymes, notably the protease in Russell's viper venom.

'Extrinsic' factor Xa generation

In addition to the 'intrinsic' formation of factor Xa by factor IXa, the same peptide bond is cleaved by activated factor VII (VIIa) in the presence of 'tissue factor', Ca^{2+} and phospholipid.

Factor VII is a single-chain, vitamin K-dependent glycoprotein which is converted to VIIa by cleavage of a single peptide bond resulting in a light chain and a heavy chain which contains the active serine site. Uniquely, however, the intact molecule or zymogen has weak enzyme activity. When referring to both the zymogen and the activated form the abbreviation VII(a) can be used.

Tissue factor (TF) [39, 40]
The action of tissue damage on the coagulation process has been known for many years. Early studies showed that 'tissue factor' was a lipoprotein which could be separated into its protein and lipid components. The lipid components are phosphatidyl choline and phosphatidyl serine. The term 'tissue factor' (TF) is now properly reserved for the protein moiety which has been characterized as a single chain protein with a molecular weight of 29 593. TF is found on the surface of many cells that are not normally in contact with the blood. Tissue damage will therefore allow interaction of TF with the coagulation system. Furthermore, TF expression on cell membranes may be initiated by a variety of agonists.

Activation of factor VII
Factor VII(a) binds to TF in the presence of Ca^{2+}. This active complex generates factor Xa which in the presence of phospholipid rapidly converts factor VII to its two-chain derivative factor, VIIa, with a resulting 100-fold increase in coagulant activity.

The role of TF: factor VII(a) in haemostasis
The observations that deficiencies of the contact factors XII, HMWK and PK are not associated with a bleeding diathesis and that factor XI deficiency has a very variable effect on *in vivo* coagulation, indicate that the activation of factor IX is the first critical reaction in the coagulation cascade.

TF:factor VII(a) complex activates factor IX to factor IXa. This explains why factor VII deficiency results in a bleeding disorder in the presence of an intact 'intrinsic' pathway. The apparent normality of the TF:VII-mediated *in vitro* coagulation tests in the presence of factor IX or VIII deficiency can be explained by artefactual excess of TF in test systems [41]. A possible model of the initiation of the *in vivo* coagulation cascade is shown in *Figure 2.17*.

The 'common' coagulation pathway – prothrombin activation and fibrin formation

The activation of factor X results in the formation of a Xa–Va–II–phospholipid–calcium complex and the rapid conversion of prothrombin to thrombin.

Prothrombin is a 72 000 d, vitamin K-dependent, single-chain glycoprotein. The molecule is split by factor Xa into two almost identically sized fragments. The carboxy-terminal section, prethrombin 2, is further hydrolysed to produce active α-thrombin consisting of a small fragment A linked to a larger B chain which contains the active serine site. The amino-terminal portion, fragment 1.2, is subsequently cleaved by thrombin into fragments 1 and 2 (F1, F2) (*Figure 2.18*). Fragment 2 is involved in binding to the heavy chain of factor Va.

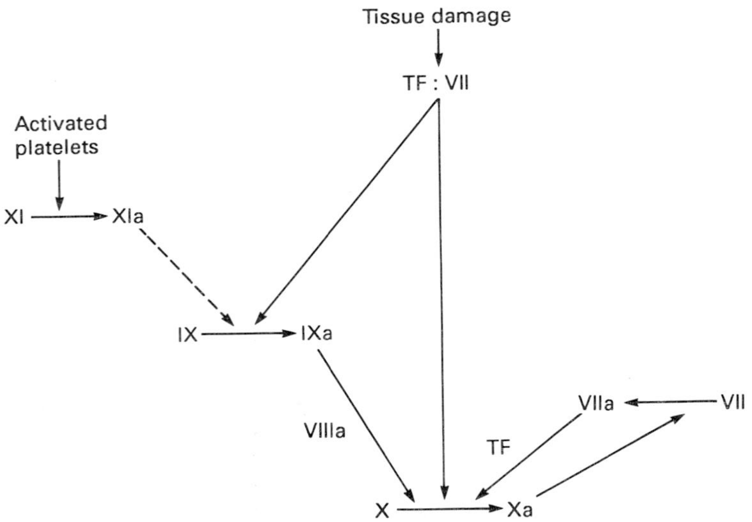

Figure 2.17 Possible model representing the initiation of *in vivo* activation of coagulation. The interrupted line represents a pathway of doubtful importance

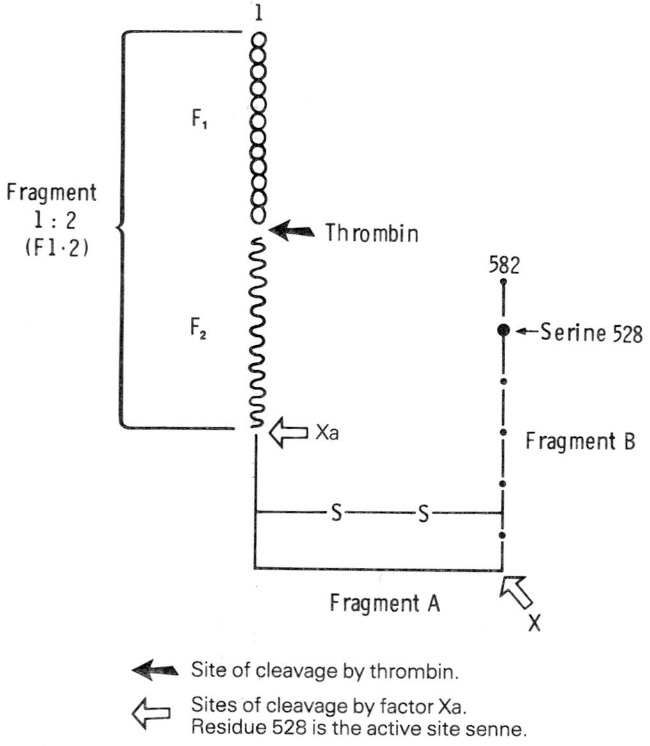

Figure 2.18 Activation of the prothrombin molecule

Factor V is a single-chain glycoprotein with a molecular weight of 330 000 and has physical and chemical properties remarkably similar to factor VIII [42]. Each acts as a co-factor by providing receptors for their respective enzymes, Xa and IXa, to provide the linkage to the phospholipid bilayer. Factor V is converted to Va, first by factor Xa and then more rapidly by thrombin, thus providing a positive feedback mechanism.

Thrombin produced by proteolysis of prothrombin has various substrates other than fibrinogen. Factor V, VIII and XIII are converted to active co-factors and therefore trace formation of thrombin results in positive amplification of the coagulation process. Additionally, thrombin is an agonist in platelet activation via a specific receptor site.

Fibrinogen, fibrin formation and stabilization

The final stages of blood coagulation are the transformation of soluble fibrinogen into stable fibrin polymer which *in vivo* reinforces and stabilizes the primary platelet plug at the site of vessel damage and by the enmeshment of red cells forms blood clot. This is followed by tissue repair and healing and the eventual removal of fibrin by the fibrinolytic mechanism.

Fibrinogen [43]

Fibrinogen is synthesized by the hepatocyte of the liver and has a plasma concentration of between 1.5 and 4.0 g/l. Fibrinogen is also located within the alpha-granules of the platelet which accounts for about 3% of total blood fibrinogen. Native fibrinogen has a molecular weight of 340 000 and comprises about 70% of circulating fibrinogen; the remaining 30% consists of slightly lower molecular weight forms thought to be due to partial degradation by plasmin. All forms of fibrinogen are thrombin-clottable.

A physiological fibrinogen variant is found in newborn and premature infants. The amino-acid composition is identical to that of adult fibrinogen though the sialic acid content is higher and results in delayed fibrin monomer polymerization.

Fibrinogen has a dimeric structure, each dimer containing three dissimilar polypeptide chains (Aα, Bβ and γ). The dimers are linked by disulphide bridges between the two α chains and the two γ chains close to the N-terminus. Intradimer bonds link the three chains (*Figure 2.19*). The terminal segments of the two longer, α and β, chains consist of fibrinopeptides A and B respectively.

Fibrin formation

Thrombin transforms fibrinogen to soluble fibrin monomer by splitting off fibrinopeptides A and B by hydrolysis of specific arginyl–glycine bonds. Fibrinopeptide A (FPA), consisting of 16 amino acids, is first produced and then fibrinopeptide B (FPB) is generated from the initial 14 amino acids of the Bβ chain. The loss of the fibrinopeptides exposes polymerization sites in the central domain of the molecule which react with complementary structures in the carboxy-terminal region of adjacent molecules to form overlapping fibrillar aggregates of unstable or 'soluble' fibrin (Ia^s).

Fibrin cross-linking and factor XIII [44]

The final stage of the coagulation pathway is the formation of an insoluble fibrin polymer. The insoluble fibrin network results from the action of an enzyme, factor

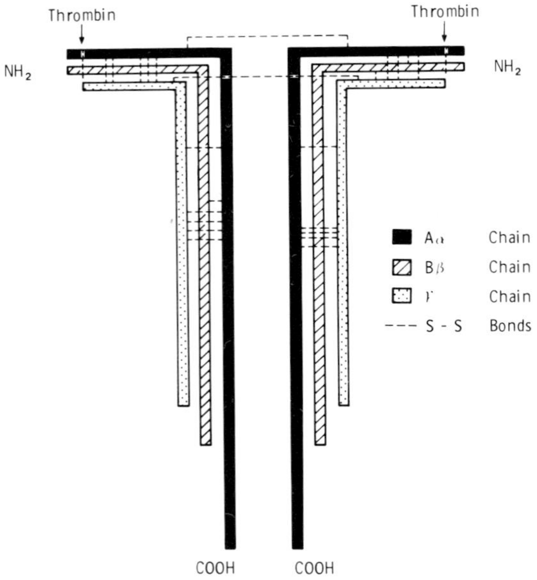

Figure 2.19 Structure of fibrinogen

XIIIa (molecular weight 28 000). Its precursor, plasma factor XIII, has a molecular weight of 320 000 and is made up of two pairs of dissociable subunits (a_2b_2), whereas intracellular factor XIII only has two 'a' subunits. To activate the precursor factor XIII, a thrombin-catalysed reaction removes a peptide from the NH_2 terminus of the 'a' chain by breaking an arginyl–glycine bond. The result is a calcium-dependent transglutaminase. During physiological fibrin formation in the presence of factor XIIIa (*Figure 2.20*), the ε-amino group of lysine from one fibrin monomer forms a peptide bond with a glutamyl residue of an adjacent fibrin monomer. This reaction (ε-(γ-glutamyl) lysine cross-linkage) occurs quickly between the γ-chains of the two different fibrin molecules (*Figure 2.21*). A slower cross-linkage may take place between the α chains of different fibrin monomers. The covalently stabilized and cross-linked fibrin is not only mechanically stronger, it is also more resistant to plasmin digestion.

Calcium is not needed for cleavage of factor XIII subunit 'a' by thrombin. Once this occurs, however, calcium is needed to dissociate subunit 'a' from 'b' and expose the active site of factor XIIIa (on subunit 'a').

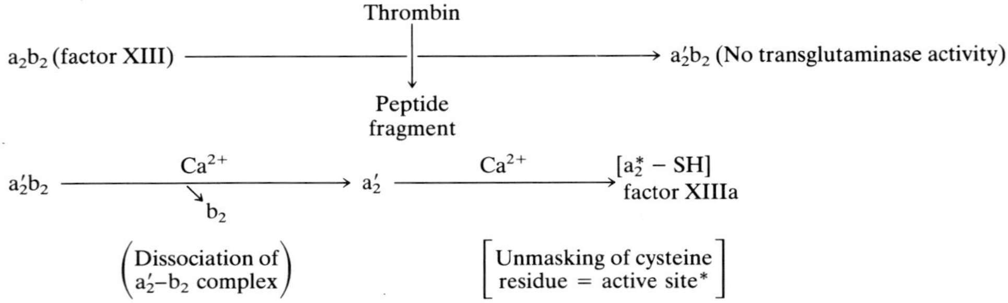

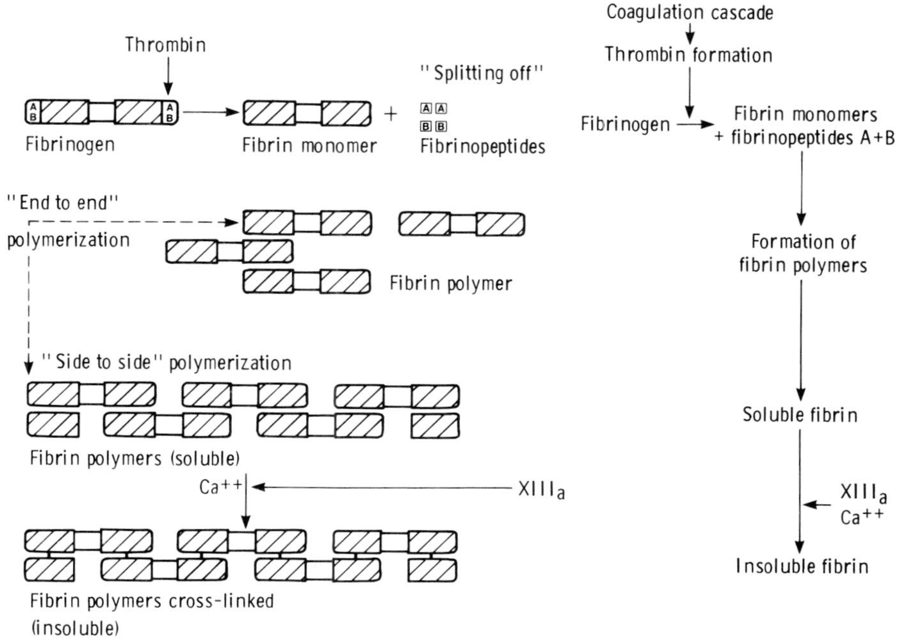

Figure 2.20 Fibrin formation and stabilization

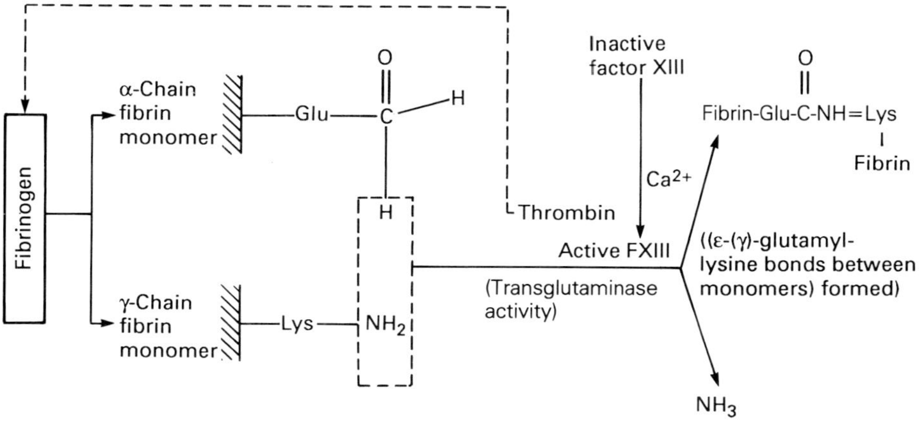

Figure 2.21 Fibrin cross-linking and factor XIII

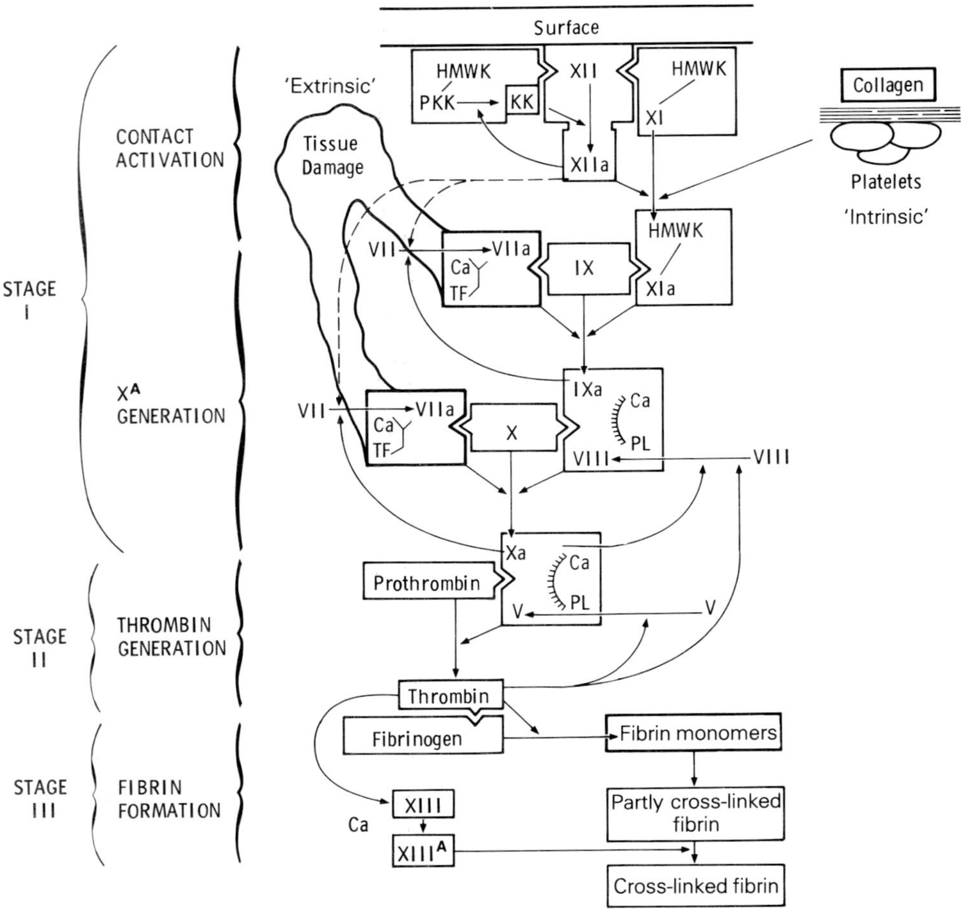

Figure 2.22 Activation of plasma coagulation mechanism via extrinsic and intrinsic systems. HMWK = high molecular weight kininogen; PKK = prekallikrein; KK = kallikrein; TF = tissue factor; PL = phospholipid

The entire coagulation process from activation to stable fibrin formation is shown by *Figure 2.22*.

Naturally occurring inhibitors of coagulation

The rapid response of the coagulation mechanism to tissue damage is normally confined to the site of the platelet plug and the vicinity of the damage. Localization and limitation is achieved by the presence of naturally occurring inhibitors/anticoagulants of serine proteases and activated co-factors. In addition, free or excess thrombin is absorbed by fibrin or fibrin degradation products, and inhibitor–protease complexes are removed by the liver.

Serine protease inhibitors (serpins)

At least six inhibitors of serine protease coagulation factors are found in plasma, though only two – antithrombin III and heparin co-factor II – act by inhibition of active serine sites. Inhibition is achieved by progressive formation of stoichiometric complexes.

Antithrombin III (ATIII) [45]
ATIII is a single-chain, 61 000 d glycoprotein, synthesized in the liver and by endothelial cells. The mean level in plasma is 0.25 g/l and has a half-life of 2.8 ± 0.3 days. It forms a stable 1:1 complex with all serine protease coagulation factors except factor VII, by the formation of a covalent bond between an arginine residue of ATIII and the active serine site which, together with steric hindrance, results in protease inhibition.

The rate of inhibition of different serine proteases varies. The major affinities of ATIII are with thrombin and factor Xa, *in vitro* inactivation half-life being 35 s and 90 s respectively, compared with 10 minutes and longer for factors XIIa, XIa and IXa.

Heparin, heparin-like substances and ATIII
Heparins are sulphated mucopolysaccharides (glycosaminoglycans) which carry a strong positive charge. Heparin has a marked accelerating effect on the formation of ATIII–protease complexes. ATIII–thrombin complex formation is accelerated at least 2000-fold.

Heparin binds to aminolysyl sites of ATIII resulting in conformational change which exposes the reactive arginine site and increases binding with the active serine of thrombin and other proteases. It is emphasized that heparin used for therapeutic purposes is not found in plasma and is not therefore of physiological significance. However, heparan sulphate proteoglycans are present in the surface membranes of endothelial cells and have a similar ability to accelerate ATIII–protease reactions.

Heparin co-factor II
Heparin co-factor II (HCII) is a single-chain 66 000 d glycoprotein. Like ATIII, HCII forms a 1:1 complex with thrombin but appears to have little or no activity against factor Xa or other serine proteases. Again, like ATIII, the presence of heparin or naturally occurring heparin-like substances markedly enhances thrombin neutralization. A difference between ATIII and HCII is that dermatan sulphate enhances HCII activity but has no effect on ATIII.

Other serine protease inhibitors
Several other inhibitors of serine protease coagulation factors have been identified in plasma though their physiological role is questionable because natural deficiencies do not appear to result in thrombotic disorders.

Alpha-2 macroglobulin reacts with a variety of proteases in addition to serine proteases. Binding to thrombin results in steric hindrance due to the large size of the molecule (725 000 d) rather than by inhibition of the active serine site.

C1 esterase inhibitor is primarily an inhibitor of the first component of complement but also reacts with kallikrein, XIIa and XIa by binding to the active serine sites.

Alpha-1 antitrypsin has a wide range of substrate proteases but a significant physiological role in the control of the serine protease coagulation factors has not been established.

Inhibition of coagulation co-factors

Activated coagulation co-factors are VIIIa and Va. As these factors have such a significant effect on the rate of coagulation activation, it is to be expected that they must be subject to control if the equilibrium of haemostasis is to be maintained.

The inhibitory mechanism is complex and several factors have been shown to be involved in the process – thrombomodulin, protein C, protein S, C4B-binding protein, phospholipids, calcium and activated protein C inhibitor.

Thrombomodulin [46]
In addition to prostacyclin, plasminogen activator and glycosoaminoglycans, vascular endothelial cells exhibit a cell surface glycoprotein termed thrombomodulin. Thrombin forms a 1:1 complex with thrombomodulin, a process which results in loss of coagulant function and platelet activation capability but results in a 1000-fold greater efficiency in activating the anticoagulant protein C (APC).

Protein C [47]
An anticoagulant activity in thrombin-treated plasma was described in 1960, and later shown to be a phospholipid-binding serine esterase precursor which in the activated form causes limited degradation of factors Va and VIIIa. The factor was termed protein C as it was the third component to be separated by ion exchange chromatography of barium citrate eluates of bovine plasma. Importantly, protein C is a vitamin K-dependent factor.

The APC degradation of Va and VIIIa is further enhanced by the presence of a co-factor in normal plasma termed protein S. APC has also been shown to enhance fibrinolysis by blocking tissue plasminogen activator inhibitor.

Protein S [47]
This vitamin K-dependent factor isolated in Seattle (hence the term protein S) is not a serine protease inhibitor. It is found in free (40%) and bound (60%) form in plasma. The bound form is a 1:1 stoichiometric complex with C4b-binding protein and does not react with protein C. Changes in C4b-binding protein may therefore influence the amount of available free protein S. Free protein S forms a calcium-dependent complex with protein C in the presence of phospholipids exposed on activated platelets.

Activated protein C inhibitor (APCI)
This single-chain polypeptide maintains the haemostatic equilibrium by controlling APC. In addition to its action on APC it has similar properties to ATIII. The interaction of thrombomodulin, protein C, protein S and APCI is shown in *Figure 2.23*.

Tissue factor pathway inhibitor [48]

An inhibitor of the 'extrinsic pathway' which requires the presence of clotting factors present in serum has been demonstrated *in vivo*. It is suggested that in the

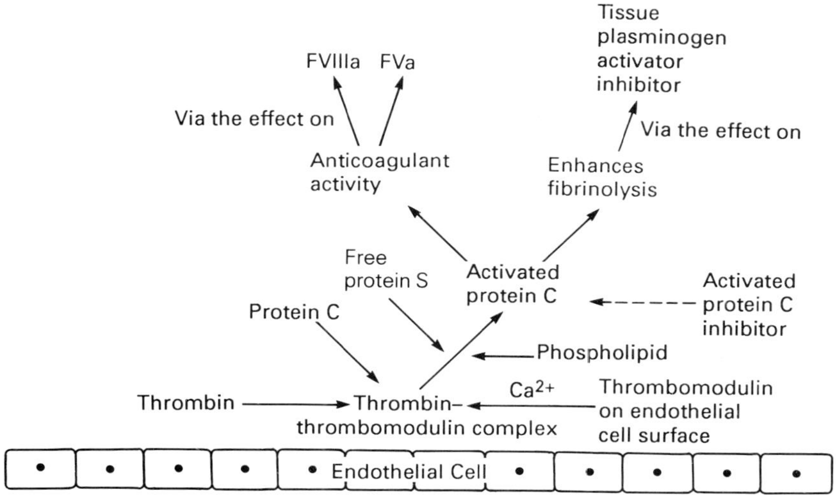

Figure 2.23 Protein C pathways

presence of Ca^{2+} an inert TF:VII(a):Xa:inhibitor complex is formed. The inhibitor has been identified as a 35 000 d protein found in the lipoprotein-rich fraction of plasma. Physiological significance has not been demonstrated as no patient lacking the inhibitor has been identified.

The role of fibrinolysis in haemostasis

The degradation of fibrin (fibrinolysis) by enzymatic proteolysis is generally accepted as the principal defence mechanism against vascular occlusion. The fibrinolytic mechanism, like the coagulation system, is a multi-component system consisting of inactive zymogen precursors, activators, proteinases, co-factors and inhibitors [49]. Although the main role of fibrinolysis is the removal of intravascular fibrin or thrombolysis, it is also involved in controlling fibrin deposited during tissue repair, inflammation and by immune response.

Components of the fibrinolytic system

The key enzyme in fibrinolysis is the serine protease *plasmin* formed by limited proteolysis of the inactive zymogen precursor *plasminogen* by one of several possible activators and controlled by a series of inhibitors.

Plasminogen and plasmin

Plasminogen is a single-chain glycoprotein (92 000 d) with an amino-terminal glutamic acid residue referred to as glu-plasminogen. The single plasminogen chain has 790 residues containing five looped structures or 'kringles' which contain 'lysine-binding sites' by which the molecule interacts with the lysine residues of substrates particularly fibrin, fibrinogen and certain inhibitors. Activation of glu-plasminogen to the active serine protease lys-plasmin, requires two enzyme cleavages. Plasminogen activators hydrolyse the arginine 560–valine 561 peptide bond to form a heavy (A) chain and a light (B) chain linked by a single disulphide bridge. The A-chain contains the kringles and lysine binding sites and the B-chain the active serine site. This structure is referred to as two-chain glu-plasmin. Glu-plasmin converts further glu-plasminogen molecules to a higher affinity single-chain lys-plasminogen by removal of an 8000 d terminal peptide from the A-chain. Lys-plasminogen is then activated to form lys-plasmin. Lys-plasmin may then generate further active enzyme by converting glu-plasmin to the lys-plasmin form. Both glu-plasmin and lys-plasmin convert glu-plasminogen to lys-plasminogen which binds more effectively to fibrin before developing protease activity.

Plasmin hydrolyses a range of substrates by cleaving lys–arg bonds. Its main substrates are fibrin and fibrinogen but it can also hydrolyse factor V and factor VIII, and activate factor VII and the complement system.

Tissue-type plasminogen activators (extrinsic pathway)
Plasminogen activator activity has been demonstrated in a variety of tissues, secretions, and in urine. Two biochemically and immunologically distinct types are recognized: tissue-type (t-PA) which is enhanced by the presence of fibrin, and the urinary or urokinase-type (u-PA), the activity of which is not affected by fibrin. Each type occurs as single- and two-chain forms designated sct-PA and scu-PA for the single-chain forms and tct-PA and tcu-PA for the two-chain types.

Although u-PA is synthesized predominantly by the kidney it is produced in small amounts in other organs and cells, but the physiological role is clearly to prevent occlusion of the renal tract by fibrin. Similarly, secretions of the ducted glands such as the salivary and lachrymal glands contain t-PA to maintain duct patency. Of particular relevance to haemostasis and physiological fibrinolysis is the presence of t-PA in vascular endothelial cells.

Plasma has a very low level of t-PA (5 ng/ml) which is increased by exercise, venous occlusion stress, diet and the environment. Following release from the vascular endothelium, t-PA is in the sct-PA form with a half-life of 2–5 minutes. The physiological activity of the t-PA is minimal until it is bound to fibrin where its activity on plasminogen is markedly enhanced. Plasmin converts sct-PA to tct-PA which enhances the formation of t-PA:fibrin:plasminogen complexes. In contrast to the avidity of t-PA for fibrin-bound plasminogen, t-PA has minimal affinity for plasma fibrinogen which allows localization of *fibrin*olysis without the potential for widespread *fibrinogen*olysis.

Inhibitors of tissue plasminogen activators
Several inhibitors of PA have been identified. In addition to the ability to synthesize and release t-PA, endothelial cells also produce a specific PA inhibitor termed PAI-1. This glycoprotein is also produced by hepatocytes and fibroblasts and is also found in the alpha-granules of platelets. PAI-1 is a fast-acting inhibitor which eventually forms an irreversible complex with t-PA. PAI-1 reacts equally well with single-chain and two-chain t-PA and with tcu-PA. PAI-1 is decreased by activated protein C and therefore effectively promotes fibrinolysis. Thus lowered levels of protein C and protein S not only result in decreased inhibition of coagulation co-factors but also reduce fibrinolytic potential.

Placenta contains another form of inhibitor termed PAI-2 which reacts well with two-chain forms of t-PA and u-PA but poorly with single-chain forms. PAI-2 may contribute to the reduced fibrinolysis found in pregnancy. The inhibitor can only be detected in placental extracts.

Plasma-mediated (intrinsic) plasminogen activation

The role of the contact factors and particularly factor XII in physiological fibrinolysis is debatable. *In vitro* it can be demonstrated that surface-enhanced fibrinolysis is diminished in the absence or reduction of factor XII, HMWK and prekallikrein. Kallikrein formed by the action of factor XIIa–HMWK on prekallikrein can be shown to result in plasminogen activation. It has been suggested that kallikrein-induced plasminogen activation is by the alternative route of the conversion of scu-PA to tcu-PA. Intrinsic plasminogen activation may be inhibited by C1 esterase inhibitor. The activation pathways are shown by *Figure 2.24*.

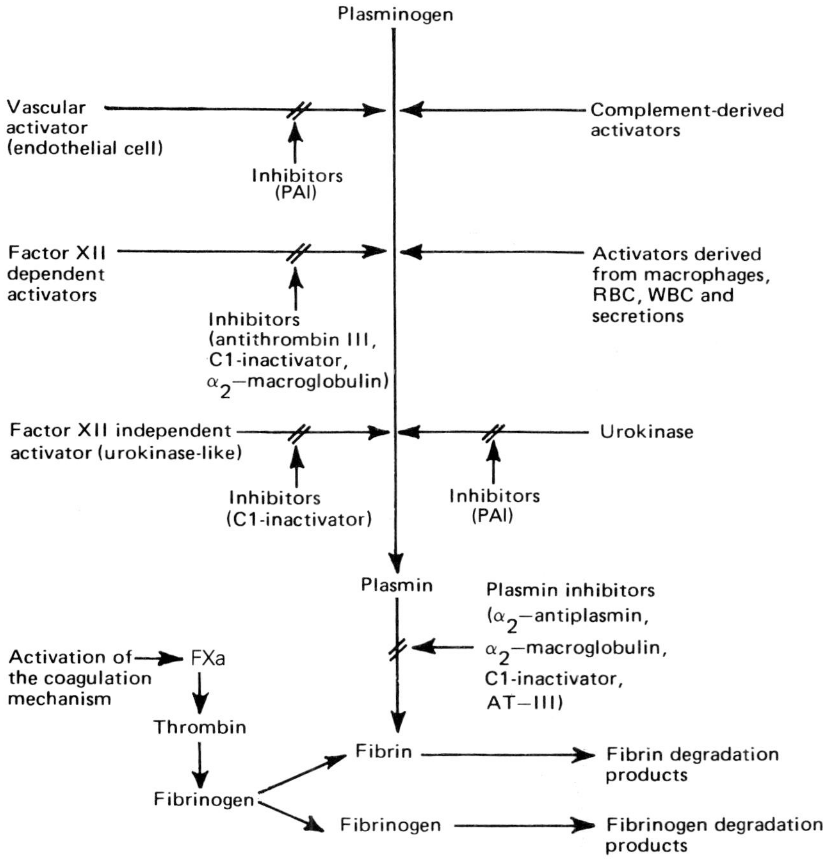

Figure 2.24 The fibrinolytic system

Plasmin inhibitors

Inhibition of plasmin or plasmin formation may be achieved by a variety of proteins with antiplasmin activity. The most important is by the action of the single-chain glycoprotein alpha-2 antiplasmin (α_2AP) which has a similar structure to ATIII. The inhibitor very rapidly forms a stable 1:1 complex with plasmin with resultant loss of protease activity. α_2AP has a role in preventing plasmin formation by blocking the lysine-binding sites of the plasminogen molecule, thus inhibiting the binding of plasminogen to fibrin. Covalent cross-linking of α_2AP to fibrin by factor XIIIa also inhibits plasmin activity in fibrin clot.

As the amount of plasminogen in plasma is greater than that of α_2AP, excess plasmin is inhibited by alpha-2 macroglobulin (α_2MG) which is a large tetrameric glycoprotein (725 000 d) capable of inactivating a wide variety of proteases including thrombin, kallikrein and plasmin. Plasmin and α_2MG rapidly form an equimolar complex probably initiated by plasmin-mediated modification of the α_2MG resulting in conformational change and plasmin binding.

Further inhibition of plasminogen binding to fibrin and potential plasmin formation is by the reversible binding of about 50% of plasma plasminogen to histidine-rich glycoprotein (HRG). Other described inhibitors of plasmin, including ATIII, are probably of minor significance *in vivo*.

Degradation of fibrin/fibrinogen by plasmin

Although the principal role of plasmin is the conversion of insoluble fibrin to soluble degradation products (FDPs) which are cleared from the plasma, there is evidence that in normal plasma there is limited plasmin cleavage of the Aα chains of fibrinogen resulting in a lower molecular weight form, and that further digestion contributes to plasma turnover of native fibrinogen. The progessive degradation of fibrinogen and non-crosslinked fibrin results in very similar degradation products.

The first stage of the proteolysis of fibrinogen results in the symmetrical removal of three small peptides, designated A, B and C, from the C-terminal of the Aα chains followed by the removal of the first 42 amino acids of the N-terminal end of the Bβ chains. In the case of fibrin, the first 14 amino acids (fibrinopeptide B) have already been cleaved by thrombin, resulting in a smaller 15–42 fragment. The remaining molecule is termed fragment X and has a molecular weight of 280 000. Fibrinogen will still have fibrinopeptide A and is therefore thrombin-clottable.

Asymmetric digestion follows with the splitting off from the C-terminal end of fragment Δ which consists of a portion of all three chains linked by disulphide bridges leaving the large fragment Y. This is followed by separation of a further fragment D from fragment Y leaving the N-terminal portion of all six, disulphide-linked, chains termed fragment E. Fragments D and E are resistant to further plasmin digestion. Thus one fibrinogen molecule is degraded to two fragment Ds and one fragment E plus the minor peptides. The sequence is shown diagrammatically by *Figure 2.25* [50].

The transglutaminase cross-linking of the γ or α chains of stable fibrin results in characteristic D-dimers and D-dimer:E fragments as well as X, Y, D and E fragments. Fragments X and Y may form large aggregates up to 2×10^6 molecular weight, termed X and Y oligomers.

Plasma proteins

Plasma proteins comprise a multiplicity of components and further advances in technology will no doubt reveal further complexity.

The early techniques of salt precipitation revealed the presence of 'globulin' and 'pseudo-globulin' fractions which were further separated by analytical ultracentrifugation, moving-boundary electrophoresis and later by solid-zone electrophoresis,

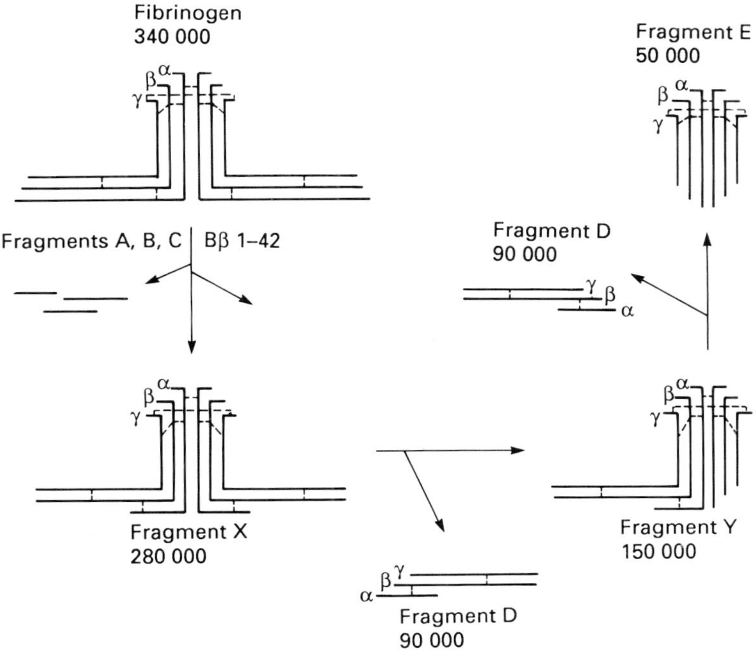

Figure 2.25 Schematic diagram of fibrinogen degradation [50]

which provides the relatively simple, but nevertheless valuable, separation into albumin and globulin and the further separation of the globulin fractions in order of their electrophoretic mobility into α_1, α_2, β or γ globulins. The introduction of immunological separation and identification, isolectric focusing, and determination of molecular weight by ultracentrifugation, polyacrylamide gel electrophoresis and gel filtration have permitted further characterization of the many protein fractions.

The separation of proteins by electrophoresis and molecular weight have shown that although some proteins of significance in practical haematology have similar characteristics, e.g. the immunoglobulins, in most instances proteins with functional relationships such as the components of the complement system or the haem-binding proteins have activities in more than one electrophoretic fraction, and have greatly differing molecular weights or differing isoelectric points. Consideration of the different plasma proteins in this section therefore follows a functional rather than an analytical approach, as has already been adopted in the section dealing with normal blood coagulation.

In addition to those involved in haemostasis, plasma proteins are divided into: (1) immunoglobulins, (2) the complement system and (3) transport proteins of haematological significance.

Immunoglobulins [51]

The antibodies in normal or pathological plasma are immunoglobulins (Ig), are mainly found in the γ-globulin electrophoretic fraction, and collectively constitute about 30% (by concentration) of the total serum proteins (i.e. excluding plasma fibrinogen).

The immunoglobulins consist of five major classes designated IgG, IgA, IgM, IgD, and IgE, each type being categorized by differences in structure.

Structure of immunoglobulins

Each class of immunoglobulin has a fundamentally similar structure consisting of four polypeptide chains held together by disulphide bonds. Two 'light (L) chains' (each having about 220 amino-acid residues) are linked to a pair of 'heavy (H) chains' (about 430 amino acids) by disulphide bonds. The basic structure is shown in *Figure 2.26*.

By determining the amino-acid sequences of the polypeptide chains it is recognized that the N-terminal half of the light chains and the N-terminal quarter of the heavy chains are extremely variable (V_L and V_H), while the remainder of the chains conform to a limited number of constant regions (C_L and C_H). The constant portion of the heavy chain is further divided into three parts C_H1, C_H2 and C_H3. The limited number of constant regions of the heavy chains determine the class of immunoglobulin and are designated γ, α, μ, δ, ε or G, A, M, D, and E. The variable portions of the molecule produce different secondary and tertiary structures which confer antibody specificity. The constant regions interact to hold the molecule together and determine the functions of complement binding, placental passage and binding to cell membranes.

The constant regions of the light chains are of two types, designated kappa (K or κ) and lambda (L or λ), and the normal immunoglobulin molecules of each heavy-chain class (G, A, M, D, E) have either kappa or lambda light chains (never both) with the ratio of immunoglobulin molecules having kappa or lambda subtypes being in the order of 3:2. Exposure of the immunoglobulin molecule to digestion by the proteolytic enzyme papain splits the molecule into three fragments: two fragments, each designated 'Fab' (ab = antibody), consisting of an entire light chain and part of the heavy chain, and one Fc fragment (c = crystallizable). The two Fab fragments are identical and retain antibody specificity. Treatment with pepsin cleaves the molecule at a different site on the heavy chain resulting in a large fragment known as Fab_2 which consists of the two Fab fragments with an additional section of the heavy chain still joined by a disulphide bond (*Figure 2.26*).

The immunoglobulins IgG, IgD and IgE are similar in that they exist as monomers. IgA in plasma is also a monomer but is present in body secretions as a dimer; the two monomers are linked at the Fc end by a J chain with an additional carbohydrate portion or secretory piece, which protects against digestion. IgM is a pentamer, i.e. consists of five monomers joined at the Fc sections by J chains; it is the pentamer structure that confers characteristic ability to bind complement.

The constant regions of the heavy chains of IgG, IgM and IgA have demonstrable variations which allow subclassification: IgG can be divided into four subclasses – IgG_1, IgG_2, IgG_3 and IgG_4 while IgM and IgA each have two subclasses. The biochemical, biological and physical properties of the plasma immunoglobulins are summarized in *Table 2.8*.

Complement system [52]

Complement is a complex system of proteins, many of which are proteinases, involved in host-defence against infection, initiation of inflammation and

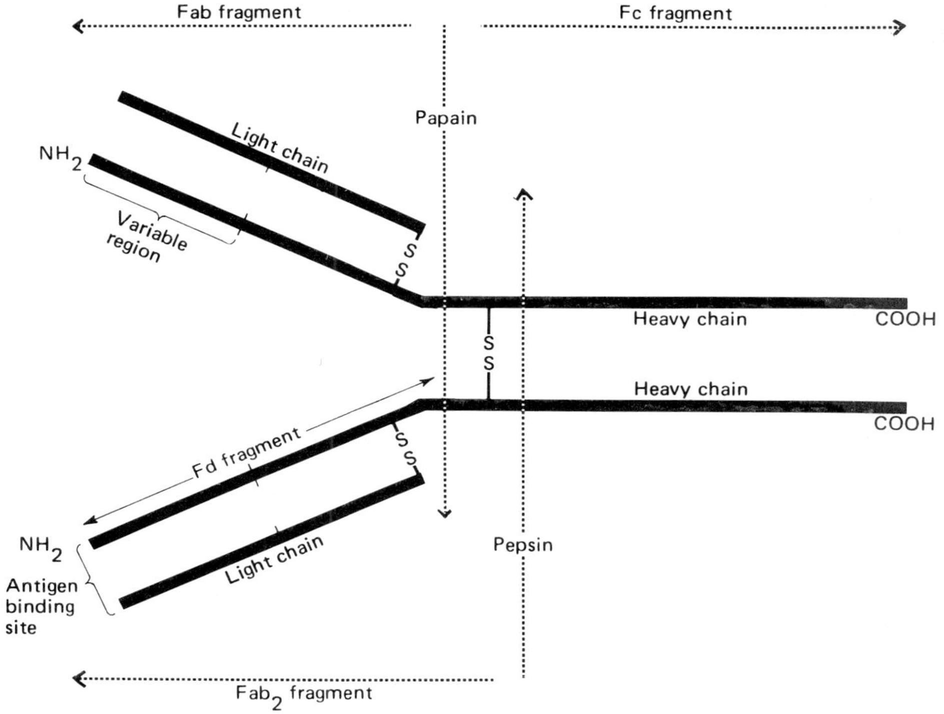

Figure 2.26 Diagrammatic representation of immunoglobulin monomer

Table 2.8 Properties of the plasma immunoglobulins

Property	*IgG*	*IgA*	*IgM*	*IgD*	*IgE*
Notation	$\gamma_2\kappa_2$ $\gamma_2\lambda_2$	$\alpha_2\kappa_2$ $\alpha_2\lambda_2$	$\mu_2\kappa_2$ $\mu_2\lambda_2$	$\delta_2\kappa_2$ $\delta_2\lambda_2$	$\varepsilon_2\kappa_2$ $\varepsilon_2\lambda_2$
Number of subclasses	4	2	2	–	–
Molecular mass	150 000	175 000	900 000	180 000	196 000
Sedimentation constant	7S	7S	19S	7S	8S
Concentration in serum (g/l)	8–17	1.4–4.2	0.5–1.8	0.03–0.4	0.01
Relative percentage	72	20	7	1	0.01
Half-life (days)	23	6	5	3	2
Antibody activity	Yes	Yes	Yes	No	Yes
Complement fixation	Yes	No	Yes	No	No
Placental transfer	Yes	No	No	No	No

destruction of certain bacteria and viruses. There is also involvement with the coagulation, kinin and fibrinolytic systems, and in platelet aggregation.

Complement activity depends on the sequential activation of a series of enzymes, each step resulting in a new enzyme activity. The system also incorporates a number of inhibitory factors to control unwanted activation. The proteins involved in the complement pathways represent about 10% of normal serum globulins and are mostly found in the β-globulin fraction.

Complement is classically activated by contact with altered Fc portions of immunoglobulin in an antigen–antibody complex (the classical pathway). Other activators of the classical pathway are enzymes such as trypsin, plasmin and the contents of lysosomes, polyanions (e.g. dextran sulphate, heparin and protamine sulphate), and a variety of substances which include endotoxins, cell membranes and viruses. The classical pathway consists of three functional units: recognition (C1), activation (C2, C3 and C4) and membrane attack (C5, C6, C7, C8 and C9). In additon to the nine complement components there are three main inhibitors or inactivators which are directed against C1 (C1 INH), C3b (C3b INA), C3a and C5a (anaphylatoxin inactivator). The classical pathway is illustrated in *Figure 2.27*.

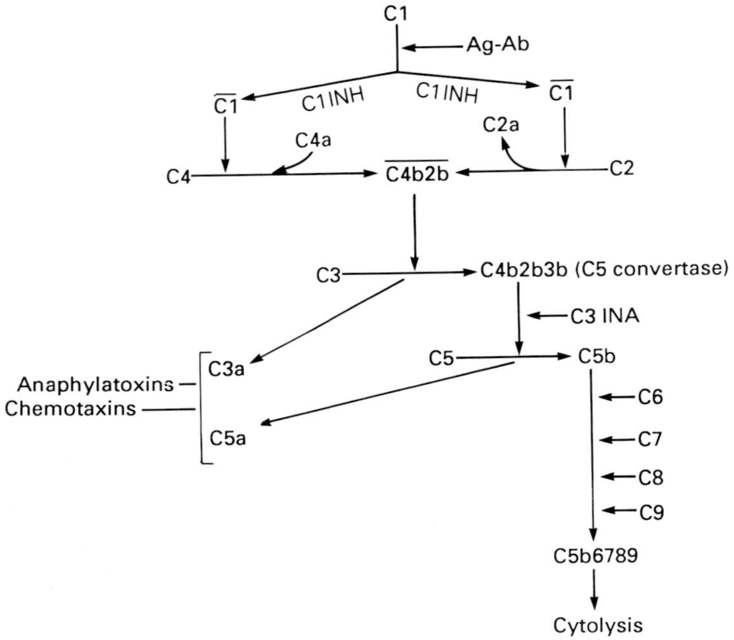

Figure 2.27 Simplified representation of the classical pathway of complement activation

The complement pathway may also be activated by an alternative route (alternative pathway) which does not depend on an antigen–antibody reaction, bypasses the C1, C4 and C2 components and converts C3 to C3b which in turn activates C5 and the remainder of the classical pathway. An important component of the alternative pathway is the feedback amplification loop of C3b acting with C3 proactivator (factor B). The alternative pathway is shown diagrammatically in *Figure 2.28*.

Biological activators of the alternative pathway are aggregated immunoglobulins, bacterial endotoxins, yeast cell walls, inulin and cobra venom. The only known association of the alternative pathway and a haematological disorder is the lysis of red cells in paroxysmal nocturnal haemoglobinuria (*see* page 322).

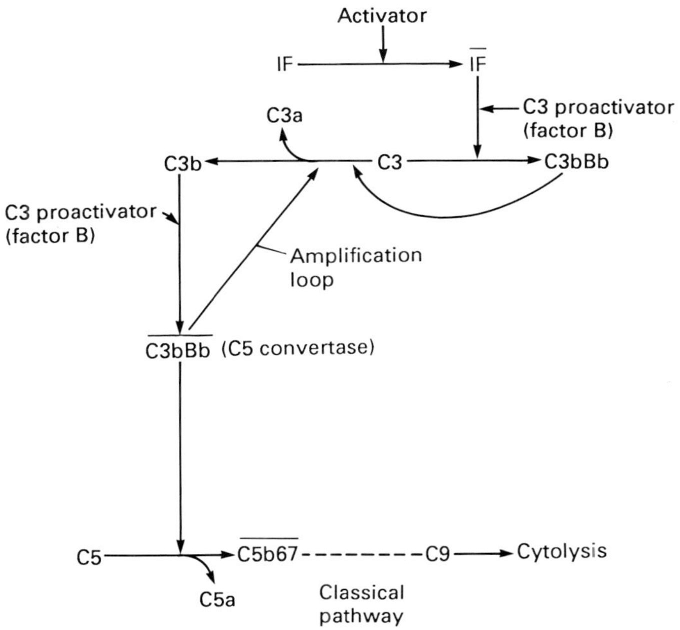

Figure 2.28 The alternative complement pathway. IF = initiation factor; $\overline{\text{IF}}$ = activated initiation factor

Transport proteins

Transferrin

Transferrin is a glycoprotein which migrates with the β_1-globulin fraction on electrophoresis. By starch gel electrophoresis considerable heterogeneity is apparent and at least 21 isotransferrins can be separated, which are assigned to groups C, B, and D, in order of decreasing mobility, with subscript numerals. All variants appear to function equally well in the binding, transport and release of ferric-iron molecules.

Transcobalamins [18]

The proteins transporting vitamin B_{12} are called transcobalamins. The two major classes are termed transcobalamins I and II (TCI, TCII).

TCI is an α-globulin of molecular weight 56–58 000 and is derived from the granulocytes and other tissues. It carries the major fraction of the B_{12} in plasma, being two-thirds saturated, but is apparently inactive in providing vitamin B_{12} to developing cells. It may serve by limiting availability of B_{12} to bacteria. Transcobalamin III (TCIII) is an iso-protein of TCI, differing in its carbohydrate content. Some workers refer to TCI and TCIII as R-proteins because of their similarity to the 'R' (rapid-electrophoretic-mobility) proteins in other body fluids.

TCII is the physiological carrier of B_{12}, is a β-globulin of molecular weight 38 000 and carries a minor fraction of the B_{12} in plasma but gives it up readily to the tissues. Heterogeneity of TCII has been described.

Albumin

Albumin is the most abundant (60%) of the plasma proteins. It is a small, globular protein of high mobility and its main function is to maintain homeostasis by its haemodynamic and transport functions, and to act as a protein reserve. Albumin can bind a host of molecules amongst which is the water-insoluble unconjugated bilirubin derived from the breakdown of haemoglobin. Excessive intravascular haemolysis can result in the liberation of haem which binds to albumin to form methaemalbumin which is transported to the liver for further degradation and iron salvage.

Haptoglobins

Haptoglobins (Hp) are glycoproteins which migrate with the α_2-globulins. They form stable complexes with haemoglobin (HpHb) but do not bind haem. Their biological function is in the metabolism of plasma haemoglobin by preventing its glomerular filtration and confining its uptake to the liver, thus acting as an iron-salvage mechanism. The HpHb complexes are rapidly removed by the liver with a half-life of between 9 and 30 minutes. Haptoglobin levels are usually expressed in relation to haemoglobin-binding capacity and normal plasma can bind 0.4–1.4 g Hb/l.

The haptoglobin molecule consists of two dissimilar chains and genetic variations of the smaller chains results in three allelic genes, Hp^{IF}, Hp^{IS}, and Hp^2, producing six commonly occurring haptoglobin genotypes, though the phenotypes are designated Hp 1–1, 1–2, and 2–2. The different phenotypes are associated with slightly different plasma haptoglobin levels. Complete, genetically determined, absence of haptoglobins (ahaptoglobinaemia) has been described and designated 0–0 and though rare in Caucasian populations is found in 4–20% of negroes. The molecular weight of the haptoglobins is about 85 000.

Haemopexin

Haemopexin (Hx) is a β_1-glycoprotein which binds haem (ferric-protoporphyrin) in an equimolar ratio. It is synthesized exclusively in the liver and consists of a single polypeptide chain with molecular weight of about 57 000. In normal plasma Hx concentration is 0.5–1.0 g/l and has a half-clearance time of about 1 day, but clearance is greatly accelerated when complexed with haem. Unlike serum haptoglobin, Hx is not an acute-phase reactant and therefore levels are not affected by inflammation or tissue destruction. The affinity of haem for Hx is greater than for albumin and there is active transfer of albumin-bound haem to Hx.

Table 2.9 summarizes the characteristics of the transport proteins.

Reference values

In order to interpret quantitative data it is necessary to relate observed values to defined reference values. It would be ideal if an observed value could be related to a value or range of values for that particular individual but this information is rarely available, and very few haematological parameters are constant, an exception being the mean red-cell volume (MCV) which remains remarkably stable in a 'healthy' individual even from year to year. Biological within-subject variation limits the value of population-based reference values[53].

Table 2.9 Physicochemical and biological properties of the transport proteins

	Transferrin	*Transcobalamins*		*Albumin*	*Haptoglobins*	*Haemopexin*
Notation	Tf	TCI, TCIII	TCII	–	Hp	Hx
Function	Iron transport	Plasma B_{12}	B_{12} transport	Homeostasis, bilirubin transport, haem binding, iron salvage	Hb binding, iron salvage	Haem binding, iron salvage
Electrophoretic mobility	β_1	α	β	Anodal fraction of plasma proteins	α_2	β_1
Molecular mass	77 000	56–58 000	38 000	66 300	85 000	57 000
Heterogeneity	Yes	No	Yes	Yes	Yes	No
Plasma concentration	1.9–2.7 g/l	800 ng/l	1000 ng/l	35–45 g/l	0.4–1.4 g/l (Hb binding capacity)	0.5–1.0 g/l

Using measurements from a reference population, a distribution of reference values may be obtained outside which it would be statistically improbable that a value will fall (reference limits). It is conventional to define the reference limits to include 95% (±2SD from the mean) of the reference values of the reference population. It follows that 5% of the reference values will fall outside the reference limits (false abnormal rate) and an indeterminate number of abnormal observed values will fall within the reference limits (false normal rate).

Establishment of reference values [54]

The establishment of reference values requires the selection of *reference individuals* who form the *reference population*; a statistically significant number of reference individuals is the *reference sample group* and represents the reference population. The selection of the reference individuals is of extreme importance. Haematological values show considerable variation in relation to age and sex and these factors must clearly be taken into account when defining the reference population. Less obvious influences are ethnic origin, socioeconomic class and environment. Physiological conditions also influence haematological values, and include exertion, stress, emotion, posture, food intake, smoking, pregnancy, stage of the menstrual cycle, etc. Additionally the intake of drugs such as oral contraceptives and alcohol influence certain measurements. The time of sampling and the methods of collection are also relevant and standardized procedures have been proposed [55].

If it is desired to study a specific population then the *reference values* must be obtained from a reference population of individuals within the specific population, e.g. values in pregnancy must be related to reference values of a pregnant reference population, or observed values in a population living at altitude must be related to reference values derived from a similar reference population.

In routine haematological investigation and diagnosis it would be impractical to demand reference values from matched reference populations. A convenient, frequently used and ostensibly 'healthy' population is that of hospital staff, but it is often difficult to obtain sufficient reference values to be statistically reliable, and age distribution is inevitably limited. Blood-donor panels have been used and although suitable for certain measurements, the age distribution is again limited, and donors are obviously not suitable for studies of red-cell parameters. Selected patient populations can be used if the parameters to be measured are not influenced by their clinical condition.

An alternative approach is to use measurements from a random patient population. Although these reference values will include many abnormal results, by suitable mathematical treatment reference limits can be derived. The advantage of this approach is the virtually unlimited number of measurements from a wide spectrum of age groups in both sexes. The reference values are divided into male and female sources, into decades in the adults and by years, months, weeks or even days in children, infants and neonates. The values are plotted as histograms and the *reference distribution* described mathematically. Biological variation is often Gaussian and *reference limits* containing 95% of the reference values within the distribution curve can be determined. Reference limits for haemoglobin concentration, red-cell numbers, MCV and other derived parameters can be readily determined in this manner. Even when the distribution is only approximately Gaussian the method is still useful.

Many reference values, however, do not have a Gaussian distribution and the application of conventional ±2SD limits will be misleading. In such instances plotting the reference values on a logarithmic scale will often convert the distribution to a 'near-Gaussian' form. An example is shown in *Figure 2.29* where a 'skewed' serum B_{12} distribution is transformed by plotting the reference values on a logarithmic scale. 'Log-normal' distributions are commonly found in the analysis of reference values of coagulation factors.

When the distribution is found to be heavily 'skewed', 'one-sided' limits are often appropriate. For example, the values for bleeding-time tests are only clinically significant when longer than normal. In such cases where all the 'false abnormal' values occur in one 'tail' of the distribution, the range can be expressed as $-\infty$ to mean +1.64SD ($-\infty$ stands for any low value)[56] .

When two values have some relationship, e.g. the MCV and Hb concentration, the reference values of each measurement may be studied by plotting one against the other to produce reference limits that are encompassed in a square or rectangle.

Reference limits should ideally be determined for each test in every laboratory. Only when a well-established method is used with reliable instrumentation and calibration is it justifiable to adopt reference limits determined elsewhere and only then if they conform to widely accepted values.

The relationship of the terms used in the above discussion is shown in *Figure 2.30*.

Reference limits for commonly determined blood values

The data presented are derived from several sources, including the authors' laboratories. It is again emphasized that reference limits are influenced by the reference population and the techniques and instrumentation used. Comprehensive data in infants and children are assembled in reference [57].

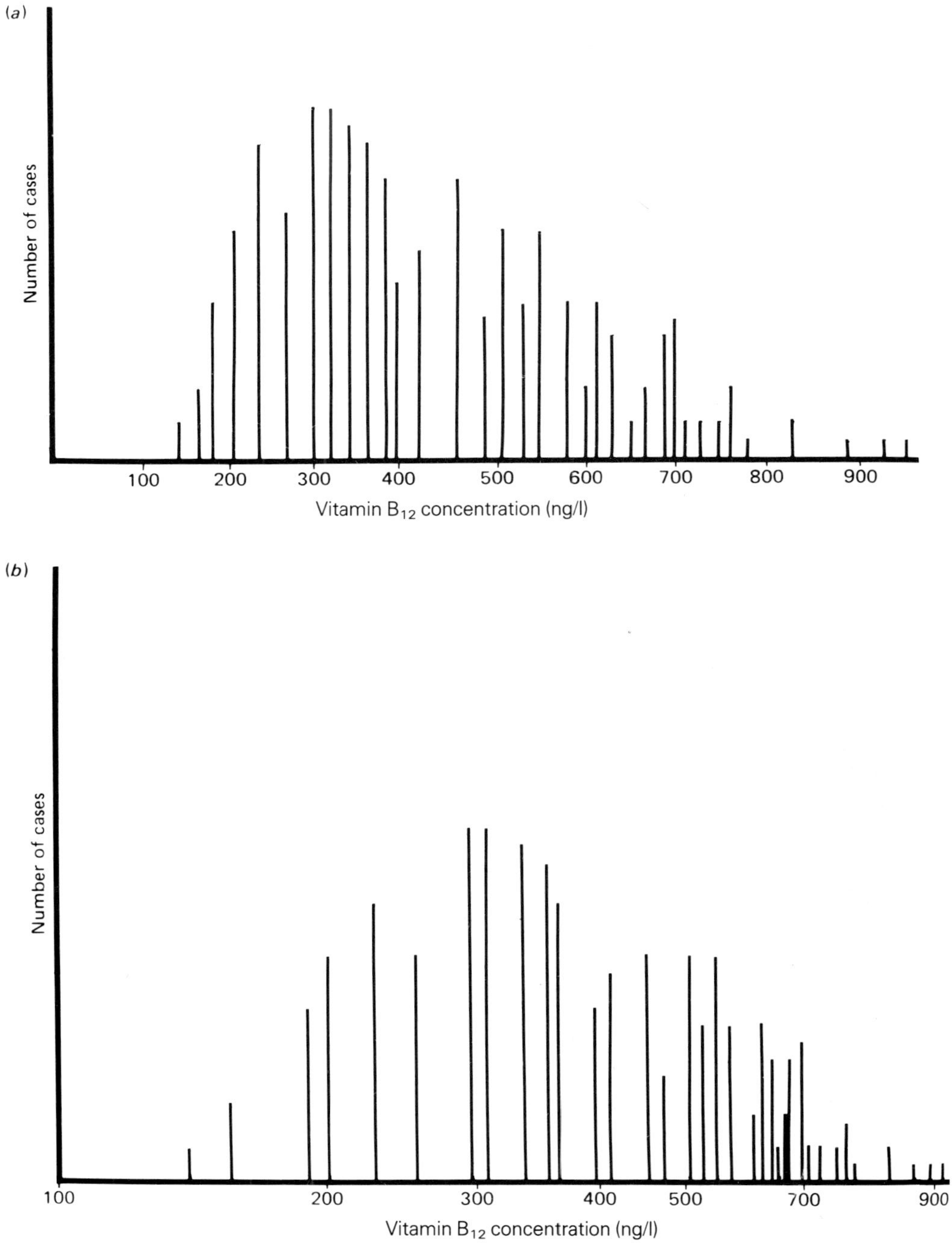

Figure 2.29 Frequency distribution of serum vitamin B_{12} levels of 300 subjects without anaemia. (*a*) Values plotted on an arithmetic scale; the distribution is clearly skewed. (*b*) The same data as in (*a*) plotted on a logarithmic scale; the distribution is near Gaussian

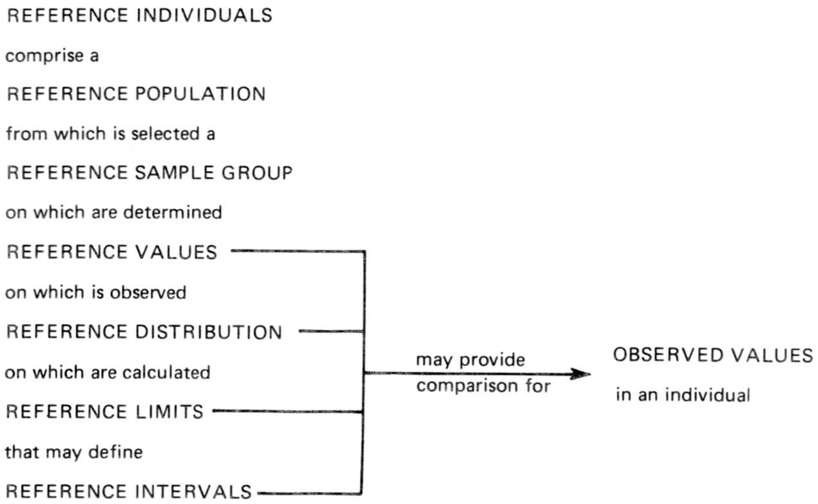

Figure 2.30 The relationship of recommended terms used with reference values [54]

Whole blood

Red-cell values

Group	*Hb* (g/dl)	*RBC* ($\times 10^{12}$/l)	*MCV* (fl)	*MCH* (pg)	*PCV* (l/l)
Infant:					
Full term	13.6–19.6	4.0–5.6	100–115	32–39	0.42–0.60
1 month	11.0–15.0	3.2–5.3	85–100	29–32	0.33–0.55
1 year	11.0–13.5	4.1–5.3	71–90	23–30	0.33–0.40
Children, 10 years	11.5–14.8	4.2–5.2	77–93	25–32	0.35–0.45
Adult:					
Male	13.5–17.5	4.6–6.5	83–95	27–32	0.41–0.50
Female	12.0–16.0	3.9–5.6	81–93	26–31	0.36–0.46
Female (post menopausal)	13.0–16.0	4.3–6.0	83–95	27–32	0.40–0.48

Leucocyte counts

Group	*Total* ($\times 10^9$/l)	*Differential* ($\times 10^9$/l)				
		Neutrophils	*Eosinophils*	*Basophils*	*Lymphocytes*	*Monocytes*
Infant:						
1 day	10.0–25.0	6.0–14.0	0.1–0.8	0.01–0.1	2.0–7.0	0.2–0.8
3 days	9.0–15.0	1.5–7.0	0.2–0.8	0.01–0.1	2.0–6.5	0.3–1.1
1 month	7.0–15.0	1.5–7.0	0.2–0.6	0.01–0.1	3.0–9.0	0.4–1.2
1 year	6.0–15.0	1.5–7.5	0.2–0.6	0.01–0.1	4.0–10.0	0.4–1.2
Children:						
5 years	6.0–14.0	2.0–8.0	0.2–0.5	0.01–0.1	1.5–7.5	0.7–1.5
10 years	4.5–12.0	2.5–8.0	0.1–0.5	0.01–0.1	1.5–6.5	0.5–1.0
Adult	4.0–10.0	2.0–7.5	0.04–0.4	0.015–0.1	1.5–3.5	0.2–0.8

Platelets
Cord blood and infants, 180–450 × 10^9/l. Adults, 140–340 × 10^9/l.

Reticulocytes
Cord blood, 2–6% of erythrocytes, 100–250 × 10^9/l. Adult, 0.4–1.6% of erythrocytes, 20–80 × 10^9/l.

Erythrocyte sedimentation rate (mm in 1 hour)
Westergren: males, 3–5 mm; females, 4–7 mm. Children have mean values approximately twice the adult ranges with a greater range of observed values.

Plasma

Plasma viscosity
Males and females, 1.5–1.72 cPa.
Physiological: birth–3 years, 1.25–1.47 cPa; pregnancy (3rd trimester), 1.5–1.8 cPa. Individual biological variation <0.05 cPa.

Ferritin (adult values)
Males, 28–220 μg/l, mean 103 μg/l. Females, 15–180 μg/l, mean 40 μg/l.

Iron (adult values)
Both sexes (higher in males), 9.0–27 μmol/l (50–150μg/dl).

Iron-binding capacity (adult values)
50–75 μmol/l (250–420 μg/dl).

Bilirubin (total)
All age groups other than neonates, 5–17 μmol/l (0.3–1.0 mg/dl).

Haemostasis screening tests
One-stage prothrombin time, 11–14.5 seconds; dependent on thromboplastin reagent.
Thrombin time, 12 ± 2 seconds; dependent on working concentration of thrombin.
Reptilase time, 15 ± 3 seconds; dependent on working concentration of reptilase.
Kaolin–cephalin clotting time (KCCT), 32–45 seconds; dependent on reagent and activation time.
Fibrin/ogen degradation products, less than 8 mg/l.

Reference values for factor assays in haemostasis are presented in Chapters 15–17.

References

1. Marchesi, V. T. (1983) The red cell membrane skeleton: recent progress. *Blood*, **61**, 1–11
2. Schrier, S. L. (1985) Red cell membrane biology – introduction. *Clin. Haematol.*, **14**, 1–12
3. Perutz, M. F. (1974) Mechanisms of denaturation of haemoglobin by alkali. *Nature*, **247**, 341
4. Bunn, H. F. (1987) Subunit assembly of haemoglobin: an important determinant of haematologic phenotype. *Blood*, **69**, 1–6
5. Beutler, E. (1985) How do red cell enzymes age? A new perspective. *Br. J. Haematol.*, **61**, 377–84

6. Zimran, A., Torem, S. and Beutler, E. (1988) The *in vivo* ageing of red cell enzymes: direct evidence of biphasic decay from polycythaemic rabbits with reticulocytosis. *Br. J. Haematol.*, **69**, 67–70
7. Snyder, L. M., Leb, L., Piotrowski, J., Saubeman, N., Liu, S. C. and Fortier, N. L. (1983) Irreversible spectrin-haemoglobin cross-linking *in vivo*: a marker for red-cell senescence. *Br. J. Haematol.*, **53**, 379–84
8. Snyder, L. M., Garver, F., Liu, S. C., Leb, L., Trainor, J. and Fortier, N. L. (1985) Demonstration of haemoglobin associated with isolated, purified spectrin from senescent human red cells. *Br. J. Haematol.*, **61**, 415–19
9. Fortier, N. L., Snyder, L. M., Garver, F., Kiefer, C., McKenney, J. and Mohandas, N. (1988) The relationship between *in vivo* generated haemoglobin skeletal protein complex and increased membrane rigidity. *Blood*, **71**, 1427–31
10. Alderman, E. M., Fudenberg, H. H. and Lovins, R. E. (1980) Binding of immunoglobulin classes to subpopulations of human red blood cells separated by density-gradient centrifugation. *Blood*, **56**, 817–22
11. Leb, L., Snyder, L. M., Fortier, N. L. and Andersen, M. (1987) Antiglobulin serum mediated phagocytosis of normal senescent and oxidised RBC: role of anti-IgM immunoglobulins in phagocytic recognition. *Br. J. Haematol.*, **66**, 565–70
12. Galili, U., Flechner, I., Knyszynski, A., Danon, D. and Rachmilewitz, E. A. (1986) The natural anti-alpha-galactosyl IgG on normal human senescent red blood cells. *Br. J. Haematol.*, **62**, 317–24
13. Clark, M. R. and Shohet, S. B. (1985) Red cell senescence. *Clin. Haematol.*, **14**, 223–57
14. Osterloh, K. R. S., Simpson, R. J. and Peters, T. J. (1987) The role of mucosal transferrin in intestinal iron absorption. *Br. J. Haematol.*, **65**, 1–3
15. Huebers, H. A. and Finch, C. A. (1984) Transferrin: physiological behaviour and clinical implications. *Blood*, **64**, 763–7
16. Worwood, M. (1982) Ferritin in human tissues and serum. *Clin. Haematol.*, **11**, 275–307
17. Bellotti, V., Arosio, P., Cazzola, M. *et al.* (1987) Characteristics of a ferritin-binding protein present in human serum. *Br. J. Haematol.*, **65**, 489–93
18. Begley, J. A. (1983) The materials and processes of plasma transport. In *The Cobalamins* (ed. C. A. Hall), pp. 109–33. New York: Churchill Livingstone
19. Lichtman, M. A. (ed.) (1975) Granulocyte and monocyte abnormalities. *Clin. Haematol.*, **4**, 483–722
20. Glasser, L. and Fiederlein, R. L. (1987) Functional differentiation of normal human neutrophils. *Blood*, **69**, 937–44
21. Rice, W. G., Ganz, T., Kinkade, J. M., Selsted, M. E., Lehrer, R. I. and Parmley, R. T. (1987) Defensin-rich dense granules of human neutrophils. *Blood*, **70**, 757–65
22. Butterworth, A. E. and David, J. R. (1981) Eosinophil function. *N. Engl. J. Med.*, **304**, 154–6
23. Church, M. K. and Holgate, S. T. (1988) The basophil leucocyte: morphological, immunological and biochemical considerations. In *Topical Reviews in Haematology*, Vol. 1 (ed. S. Roath), pp. 65–86. Bristol: Wright
24. Territo, M. C. and Cline, M. J. (1975) Mononuclear phagocyte proliferation, maturation and function. *Clin. Haematol.*, **4**, 685–703
25. Kimber, I. (1985) Natural killer cells. *Med. Lab. Sci.*, **42**, 60–77
26. Wright, J. H. (1906) The morphogenesis of blood platelets. *J. Morphol.*, **21**, 263–78
27. Hovig, T. (1989) Megakaryocytes and platelet morphology. *Clin. Haematol.*, **2**, 503–41
28. Eldor, A., Vlodavsky, I., Deutsch, V. and Levine, R. F. (1989) Megakaryocyte function and dysfunction. *Clin. Haematol.*, **2**, 543–68
29. Evatt, B. L., Kellar, K. L. and Ramsay, R. B. (1986) Thrombopoietin present and future. In *Megakaryocyte Development and Function* (eds R. F. Levine, N. Williams, G. Levine and B. L. Evatt), pp.143–155. New York: Alan R. Liss
30. Kroll, M. H. and Schafer, A. I. (1989) Biochemical mechanisms of platelet activation. *Blood*, **74**, 1181–92
31. Hutton, R. A. (1989) Normal haemostasis. In *Postgraduate Haematology*, 3rd edn (eds A. V. Hoffbrand and S. M. Lewis), pp. 560–97. Oxford: Heinemann
32. Gonias, S. L. and Pizzo, S. V. (1986) The biochemistry of haemostasis. *Clin. Lab. Haematol.*, **8**, 281–305

33. Walsh, P. N. (1987) Platelet-mediated trigger mechanisms in the contact phase of blood coagulation. *Sem. Thromb. Haemost.*, **13**, 86–94
34. Vroman, L. (1987) The importance of surfaces in contact phase reactions. *Sem. Thromb. Haemost.*, **13**, 79–85
35. Kluft, C., Dooijewaard, G. and Emeis, J. J. (1987) Role of the contact system in fibrinolysis. *Sem. Thromb. Haemost.*, **13**, 50–68
36. Gianelli, F. (1989) Factor IX. *Clin. Haematol.*, **2**, 821–48
37. Tuddenham, E. G. D. (1989) Factor VIII and haemophilia A. *Clin. Haematol.*, **2**, 879–96
38. MacGillivray, R. T. A. and Fung, M. R. (1989) Molecular biology of factor X. *Clin. Haematol.*, **2**, 879–918
39. Nemerson, Y. (1988) Tissue factor and haemostasis. *Blood*, **71**, 1–8
40. O'Brien, D. P. (1989) The molecular biology and biochemistry of tissue factor. *Clin. Haematol.*, **2**, 801–20
41. Marler, R. A., Kleiss, A. J. and Griffin, J. H. (1982) An alternative extrinsic pathway of human blood coagulation. *Blood*, **60**, 1353–8
42. Jenny, R. J. and Mann, K. G. (1989) Factor V: a prototype pro-cofactor for vitamin K-dependent enzyme complexes in blood clotting. *Clin. Haematol.*, **2**, 919–44
43. Furlan, M. (1988) Structure of fibrinogen and fibrin. In *Fibrinogen, Fibrin Stabilization and Fibrinolysis* (ed. J. L. Francis), pp.17–64. Chichester: Ellis Horwood
44. Miloscewski, K. J. A. and Losowsky, M. S. (1988) Fibrin stabilization and factor XIII deficiency. In *Fibrinogen, Fibrin Stabilization and Fibrinolysis* (ed. J. L. Francis), pp. 175–202. Chichester: Ellis Horwood
45. Lane, D. A. and Caso, R. (1989) Antithrombin: structure, genomic organization, function and inherited deficiency. *Clin. Haematol.*, **2**, 961–98
46. Dittman, W. A. and Majerus, P. W. (1990) Structure and function of thrombomodulin: a natural anticoagulant. *Blood*, **75**, 329–36
47. Dolan, G., Ball, J. and Preston, F. (1989) Protein C and protein S. *Clin. Haematol.*, **2**, 999–1042
48. Rao, L. V. and Rapaport, S. I. (1987) Studies of a mechanism inhibiting the initiation of the extrinsic pathway of coagulation. *Blood*, **69**, 645–51
49. Marsh, N. A. (1988) The fibrinolytic enzyme system. In *Fibrinogen, Fibrin Stabilization and Fibrinolysis* (ed. J. L. Francis), pp. 223–263. Chichester: Ellis Horwood
50. Hutton, R. A. (1989) Normal haemostasis. In *Postgraduate Haematology* (eds. A. V. Hoffbrand and S. M. Lewis), p.591. Oxford: Heinemann
51. Goodman, J. W. (1987) Immunoglobulin I: Structure and function. In *Basic and Clinical Immunology* (eds D. P. Stites, J. D. Stobo and J. V. Wells), pp. 27–36. Los Altos: Lange Medical Publishing
52. Roitt, I., Brostoff, J. and Male, D. (1985) Complement. In *Immunology*, Chapter 7. London: Gower Medical Publishing
53. Fraser, C. G., Wilkinson, S. P., Neville, R. G. *et al.* (1989) Biological variation of common haematologic laboratory quantities in the elderly. *Am. J. Clin. Pathol.*, **92**, 465–70
54. International Committee for Standardisation in Haematology (ICSH) (1981) The theory of reference values. *Clin. Lab. Haematol.*, **3**, 369–73
55. International Committee for Standardisation in Haematology (ICSH) (1982) Standardisation of blood specimen collection procedure for reference values. *Clin. Lab. Haematol.*, **4**, 83–6
56. Healy, M. J. R. and Ingram, G. I. C. (1978) The 'normal range' of tests of haemostasis. *Thromb. Haem. (Stutt.)*, **39**, 504–9
57. Hinchcliffe, R. F. (1987) Reference ranges and normal findings. In *Practical Paediatric Haematology* (eds R. F. Hinchcliffe and J. S. Lilleyman), pp. 359–97. Chichester: John Wiley and Sons

Chapter 3

Basic haematological practice

Advances in instrumentation and the development of computer-assisted technology have altered markedly the methodology of haematology laboratories. Whether the concept of 'totally automated routine haematology' can be achieved or is desirable is a matter for debate. Even in the most highly automated departments there are certain investigations which can only be performed manually and appearances which can only be determined visually, each of which depends upon individual skills and experience. Furthermore, the values of reference preparations for calibrating instruments or automated equipment are often dependent on reference techniques involving basic procedures performed manually. Some abnormal blood samples defy analysis or interpretation by instrumentation. To understand fully the principles behind automated techniques usually requires understanding and experience of the basic manual technique and therefore no apology is made for including in this section certain techniques that may be considered obsolete but which are a necessary aspect of laboratory haematology.

Collection and handling of blood samples

The objectives in blood sample collection are to obtain a representative sample of circulating blood in a form best suited to the invesigations required, with a minimum of artefact whether induced by the collection procedure, containers, anticoagulants or subsequent storage or handling, while showing proper concern for the well-being of the patient and the safety of the staff immediately or subsequently involved.

Collection of blood samples

Blood may be obtained from capillaries, veins or arteries by skin puncture, venepuncture or arterial sampling, respectively. The most satisfactory method is to obtain venous blood but in certain circumstances capillary puncture may be preferable. Blood from different sites may vary considerably, not only in respect of oxygen saturation but also in the relative proportions of plasma and cells, e.g. capillary blood has a lower ratio of cells to plasma than venous or arterial blood. Circulatory stasis at the extremities because of cold or circulatory failure may reverse the relationship, the ratio of cells to plasma being falsely increased. A similar situation may be produced by prolonged application of a tourniquet. Skin puncture is usually restricted to situations when venepuncture is difficult, e.g. in neonates, infants or young children, or in patients with extensive burns. In subjects where repeated sampling of larger volumes of blood is contraindicated, capillary puncture is also preferable, e.g. in premature infants. Venous blood is suitable for all purposes other than for blood-gas analysis, for which arterial blood is essential. The procedures are summarized in *Table 3.1*.

Table 3.1 Procedures for collecting blood samples

	Capillary	*Venous*
Site	Digit, ear-lobe, heel, toe	Arm, wrist, hand, groin
Volume	Up to 0.5ml	Up to 60 ml
Equipment	Minimal. Lancet, sample container, pipette or glass capillary	Syringe and needle or vacuum system. Sample containers
Disadvantages	Repeat testing restricted. Additional tests often not possible. Sample may only represent 0.002% of total blood volume. Local stasis may produce false results	Artefact may be introduced by the anticoagulant
Advantages	Cheap, quick, relatively easy. Direct measurement of sample	More representative sample. Suitable for majority of investigations. Repeat or additional tests possible

Technique of blood collection

Precise details of technique will not be given as operators have varied approaches. The general principles are outlined.

Skin cleansing

As this is usually performed with 70% isopropyl alcohol, cleansing is of doubtful value and is carried out mainly for aesthetic purposes. The brisk friction will, however, aid blood flow from capillary puncture and reduce the possible problem of contamination of the sample with fat globules or debris which can cause erroneous cell counts.

Capillary puncture

It is essential that a separate sterile lancet is used for each patient. The site should be warm and free from obvious circulatory stasis. The puncture should ideally produce a free flow of blood but often slight pressure is necessary and is acceptable practice. The first two or three drops may be discarded. Samples may be bled directly into a suitable container or collected by calibrated pipette with immediate measurement and dilution. Glass capillary tubes may be used which can be calibrated 'to contain' or have a 'break off' section of known volume. Plain glass capillaries may be used to collect small volumes of clotted blood, the tubes being centrifuged to separate the serum. Special precautions are necessary when collecting blood for platelet counting and are described on page 95. It is generally accepted that blood films made directly from fresh blood are superior to those made after contact with anticoagulants, though platelet clumping in fresh films may make assessment of platelet numbers difficult. The concept that satisfactory platelet counts can be perfomed only by using the first two or three drops of blood is fallacious.

Collection of blood samples in paediatric practice has been comprehensively described [1].

Venepuncture

An arm or hand vein is usually selected. Puncture is facilitated by application of a tourniquet to restrict the venous return. Prolonged application should be avoided as the haematocrit can increase by as much as 0.010 per minute. Furthermore, certain studies may be invalidated, e.g. for studies of fibrinolysis or for factor VIII assay. A 20-gauge, 25 mm needle appears to be the most suitable for collecting volumes of 10–20 ml, though 21-gauge, 37 mm needles are widely used. Flow-rate characteristics indicate that for volumes over 20 ml a thin-walled 19-gauge, 40 mm needle is to be preferred [2]. For volumes over 60 ml an even larger gauge should be used. Exceptionally, for fine veins, a 23-gauge needle is preferable. The object of selecting the most suitable needle is to obtain sufficient blood as quickly as possible while keeping artefacts in the specimen to a minimum.

The choice between a conventional syringe and needle procedure and a vacuum collection system is usually dictated by local practice though personal preference often supersedes the approved procedure! The problem of droplet formation by plug-type caps of certain vacuum systems has not been entirely overcome. The overall costs are similar though in experienced hands collection by vacuum systems is slightly quicker. Frothing should be avoided and in no circumstances should the blood be expelled from the syringe through the needle as distortion of the cells and haemolysis will result.

In addition to local circulatory stasis, posture and the time of sampling in relation to meals also influence the ratio of cells to plasma. Exertion and stress may produce transient changes in leucocyte number as well as subtle changes in the haemostatic mechanism. Ideally the patient should be fasting and at rest for 30 minutes, a situation that is usually impractical without prior preparation.

Collection of blood samples from patients in 'high risk of infection' category

Infection may be transmitted from patient to staff during the blood collection procedure. Viral agents are the greatest hazard and in some instances are potentially lethal. Certain categories of patients have a higher incidence of viral infection than the general population. 'High-risk' categories include liver disease and haemophiliacs, those receiving immunosupppressive therapy or multiple transfusions of blood products and 'long-stay' patients in institutions. Homosexuals and intravenous drug abusers are other risk groups. Patients with unexplained fever, particularly those who have travelled from or through areas associated with virulent viral agents, must also be considered to be in the 'high-risk' category. Previous negative results of tests for virus infection do not remove patients from the 'high-risk' category. Paradoxically, perhaps the highest risk samples are from symptomless carriers of viral agents.

The Advisory Committee on Dangerous Pathogens (ACDP) has categorized pathogens from 1 to 4 according to hazard [2] and has issued guidelines for the procedures for obtaining and the subsequent handling in specific circumstances [3,4]. Pathogens in group 4 incude the agents of viral haemorrhagic fevers, e.g. Lassa and Marburg viruses and the variola (smallpox) virus. Group 3 pathogens include the hepatitis B virus and the human immunodeficiency virus (HIV) formerly called LAV/HTLVIII and the cause of acquired immunodeficiency syndrome (AIDS). The incidence of symptomless hepatitis B carriers in the general population is in the order of 1 in 1000. The incidence of HIV infection varies; in certain categories it may be 1 in 10 or even more frequent. It can be argued therefore that sensible precautions should be adopted for the collection of all blood samples.

The most likely route of infection is skin puncture or 'needle-stick' injury, by a contaminated needle or 'sharp' or by blood contamination of a skin abrasion. All skin lesions must be covered by a waterproof adhesive dressing and, ideally, additionally protected by wearing surgical gloves. Surgical gloves do not afford protection against needle-stick injury and any procedure such as attempting to replace a needle guard must be avoided.

Certain infections may be transmitted via mucous membrane contamination. Face masks may be used to prevent droplet infection. The use of safety spectacles should be considered and a disposable apron may be used. Clearly a balance should be sought between reasonable precautions and creating unnecessary alarm in, or stigmatization of, an individual patient.

All swabs, used syringes and needles should be secured in suitable containers and disposed of by incineration. Working surfaces which may have been contaminated by droplets should be disinfected frequently. Specimens from possible hazard groups 3 and 4 must be individually and conspicuously identified as being a 'danger of infection' by using the standard black on yellow label, transported in similarly identified individual plastic envelopes and separated from the request form which must also clearly indicate the infection risk. If infection with a hazard group 4 pathogen is suspected the clinician should discuss the problem with the laboratory *before any specimens are despatched*. The further handling and transportation of blood samples are considered on page 90.

Anticoagulants

Many haematological tests demand blood that has not clotted and this is achieved by collection into tubes or bottles containing anticoagulant.

Ethylene-diamine-tetra-acetic acid (EDTA)

For cell counting the anticoagulant of choice is one of the salts of EDTA which in optimal concentration does not affect cell numbers or size and inhibits platelet clumping while changes in cell morphology are initially minimal.

EDTA acts as a chelating agent and reacts stoichiometrically with ionized calcium. EDTA is not readily soluble and therefore sodium, lithium or potassium salts are used. Di-potassium EDTA is the most commonly used because of its slightly greater solubility though there is evidence that the tri-potassium form is a better chelating agent. Although EDTA is the anticoagulant of choice for cell counting and morphology, occasionally problems arise due to EDTA-dependent agglutination of red cells, platelets and neutrophils which, although detectable by visual counting, can produce spurious low counts when using cell counting instruments (*see* Chapter 8).

Choosing the optimum amount of EDTA is difficult: 0.44 mg of EDTA is needed to chelate the calcium in 1 ml of normal whole blood, but allowance must be made for the larger amount of calcium in the increased plasma volume of anaemic blood samples. BS 4851 recommends 1.5 ± 0.25 mg of di-potassium EDTA per ml of blood, though the concentration of EDTA does not appear to affect the Hb, RBC, or total leucocyte count unless a concentration of 4 mg/ml is reached. The NCCLS recommends 1.5–2.2 mg/ml [5]. Such a concentration can be readily attained by adding insufficient blood. Sample containers *must* contain the appropriate volume of blood. Concentrations of EDTA in the order of 4 mg/ml will produce cell changes in 30 minutes which may otherwise take 24 hours in the presence of optimal concentrations of EDTA (*see* page 91). Inhibition of platelet function and the extreme lability of factor VIII make EDTA unsuitable for routine studies of haemostasis.

However, tri-potassium EDTA is the least suitable because it causes the largest red-cell shrinkage with increasing EDTA concentration, the largest change in red-cell volume on standing and results in lower MCV values [6]. Furthermore, transfer of red-cell water to the plasma compartment results in a measurable decrease in plasma viscosity (P. Basterfield, personal communication).

Tri-sodium citrate

Tri-sodium citrate is used mainly for studies of haemostatic function in the proportion of one volume of citrate to nine volumes of blood and for the standard Westergren erythrocyte sedimentation rate (ESR) test in the proportions of one volume of citrate to four volumes of blood. Citrate removes calcium by forming a loose ionic complex. The particular suitability of citrate for studies of haemostasis is that platelets retain their functional capability which is lost with EDTA and that coagulation factors are more stable, particularly factor V and factor VIII. The use of sodium oxalate has no apparent advantage and factor V is particularly unstable. There has been confusion over the optimum concentration of citrate. The original recommendation of 38 g/l (0.13 mol/l) used the dodecahydrate form which is no longer readily available. The dihydrate salt at a concentration of 32 g/l (0.109 mol/l) is a suitable alternative, though for ESR the ICSH reference method recommends 30.8 g/l (0.105 mol/l). Previous confusion between the concentration used in commercially available containers appears to have been resolved. Significant differences may undoubtedly be obtained in coagulation tests if excess citrate is present and this is particularly noticeable when the PCV is greater than 0.400 [7]. The addition of a buffer to tri-sodium citrate for coagulation studies has been recommended. The dipolar buffer N-2-hydroxyethyl-piperazine-N-2-ethane sulphonic acid (HEPES) at a concentration of 50 g/l in 32.0 g/l tri-sodium citrate dihydrate maintains the pH of the anticoagulated plasma at 7.4, stabilizes reference or control plasmas [8], and maintains the optimal pH for platelet aggregation studies.

Heparin

Heparin is a naturally occurring mucopolysaccharide obtained from tissues such as lung and placenta and has clinically useful anticoagulant properties. As a laboratory anticoagulant it has a limited value. Its action is by inhibiting the normal coagulation process by inactivation of factor Xa and IIa and is therefore useless for coagulation studies. Platelets and leucocytes show clumping and blood films stain with a bluish tinge. The use of heparin is confined mainly to collection of blood for assay of red-cell enzymes and for cell culture techniques. It has been recommended for studies where added salts could theoretically influence results, e.g. red-cell osmotic fragility tests. Lithium heparin is commonly used at a concentration of 1–5 mg (10-50 units) per 1 ml of blood.

Oxalates
The use of oxalates either singly or in combination is obsolete and will not be considered.

Defibrinated blood
If blood is briskly and continuously agitated during coagulation in the presence of material such as glass beads or paper clips, the fibrin collects around the bodies as it is formed and can be removed from the sample together with the platelets, leaving the red cells and leucocytes suspended in serum. The procedure is adopted when the use of anticoagulant is contraindicated and when it is desired to recover red cells and leucocytes in large numbers. It is also used when the removal of calcium is undesirable, e.g. when complement activity must be retained. An automated apparatus giving a maximal yield of cells with minimum haemolysis has been described[9]. The use of anticoagulants is summarized in *Table 3.2*.

Table 3.2 Anticoagulants

Property	*EDTA*	*Tri-sodium citrate*		*Heparin*
Colour Code (BSS)	Pink	Purple	Purple and white	Orange
Substance	Di- or tri-potassium EDTA	32.0 g/l Tri-sodium citrate solution	30.8 g/l Tri-sodium citrate solution	Lithium heparin Dried or fluid
Amount	1.5 mg/ml	1 volume to 9 volumes blood	1 volume to 4 volumes blood	10–50 units (1–5 mg/ml)
Mode of action	Stoichiometric chelation of Ca^{2+}	Binds Ca^{2+} in loose ionic complex		Anti-Xa and IIa
Uses	Routine 'cellular haematology'	Studies of haemostasis	Westergren ESR	Osmotic fragility. Cell culture
Advantages	Preserves morphology of RBC and WBC. No platelet clumping	Coagulation factors stable. Platelet function retained	Reference method recommendation	Ca^{2+} still present
Disadvantages	Not suitable for coagulation studies. Useless for platelet function	Not suitable for cell counting due to dilution		Unsuitable for blood films, WBC and platelet counting

Specimen containers

There are a wide variety of blood specimen containers commercially available. Materials used are glass, polypropylene or polystyrene. A container should be safe and reliable. BS 4851[10] and BS 6242 are specifications for such containers and detail the type of closure and the colour code for various anticoagulants and require an indication of the volume of blood to be added. The main aim of the specifications, however, is to reduce hazards due to leakage or breakage of the container. Ability to withstand centrifugation is important. For blood counting there is little to choose between glass and polystyrene though there is evidence that some platelet loss occurs with both materials compared with a siliconized glass container. For coagulation and platelet studies requirements can vary, ranging from siliconized glass to prevent contact activation, to plain glass when maximum thrombin production is required. The International Committee for Standardisation in Haematology recommends the use of plastic containers for blood samples for coagulation tests [11].

As most studies are carried out in a matter of hours, sterile containers are not necessary, but for cell culture or procedures requiring the incubation of the blood sample or its components, sterile containers are essential and aseptic technique imperative. When studies involve the incubation of samples or reagents for specified periods the heat conductivity of the container material can have considerable effect and may even be critical.

Handling of blood samples

All blood samples should be regarded as capable of transmitting infection and sensible precautions taken. This will include avoiding contact with broken skin, avoiding unnecessary droplet or aerosol formation and strictly observed prohibition of direct mouth pipetting. Discarded samples and containers should be incinerated. Contaminated glass-ware should be immersed in hypochlorite solution (1 in 1000) before cleaning. High-risk samples should be processed separately. Ideally a closed area should be set aside for centrifugation and serum or plasma separation and should be equipped with a protective cabinet and a centrifuge with buckets fitted with screw lids. Personnel should wear protective clothing, gloves, mask and protective spectacles. All glass-ware should be packaged and autoclaved before cleaning or disposal.

Any spills should be immediately dealt with by swabbing with hypochlorite solution as should all surfaces after completing operations. Equipment should be cleaned and disinfected (hypochlorite must never be in contact with metal). Subsequent handling of high-risk samples is inevitable. Sensible precautions should be adopted. These are based on operator protection, avoiding unnecessary droplet formation, use of disposable equipment when possible, disinfection of apparatus or equipment before cleaning and proper disposal of samples, containers and discarded apparatus. For infrequent examination of 'HIV specimens' a separate, defined work station is acceptable. When frequent or routine examination of HIV specimens is predicted, a separate room and equipment should be available [3]. The addition of β-propiolactone, a potent viricidal agent, is recommended to all specimens which may be infected with category 4 pathogens [4,12]. This procedure is also often adoped for category 3 hazards.

Transportation of blood samples [13]

Samples in transit within a hospital should ideally be in an upright position in racks to prevent leakage or damage, and to avoid unnecessary handling. Experience with pneumatic tube systems has shown that samples may be conveyed with little or no deterioration of sample quality. High-risk samples, suitably identified, should be in closed transparent envelopes separate from the request form though most hospitals transport all samples in individual transparent plastic bags. For specimens transported outside the hospital, other than by post, a transport box with fastenable lid must be used and must be leakproof if plastic bags are not used.

The principle of long-distance or postal transmission is protection of the specimen in a rigid secondary container with sufficient absorbent material to contain any leakage. The container must be labelled as 'danger of infection' and visible to anyone who unpacks the outer postal package, but should not be visible on the outer cover. The regulations for posting overseas are particularly detailed and stringent. Changes in sample quality during transit are described under appropriate sections.

Changes in blood during storage

Red-cell, leucocyte and platelet numbers are stable for a least 24 hours in EDTA, and haemoglobin is unchanged for many days if the blood does not become infected. Progressive morphological changes are, however, inevitable though they may be reduced or delayed by ensuring optimal EDTA concentration and by storage at 4°C. If delay in testing is unavoidable blood films should be made immediately and fixed in methanol.

Red cells swell gradually as judged by MCV measurement with automated counters, though storage a 4°C for 24 or even 72 hours does not produce significant change in volume [14,15]. Crenation and sphering is consistently produced after 24 hours at room temperature.

Neutrophils show vacuolation, swelling of the lobes of the nucleus and loss of granules, followed by loss of lobe bridges and ultimate disintegration.

Lymphocytes and monocytes develop a typical 'clover-leaf' appearance together with vacuolation.

Platelets tend to swell with loss of granules.

Changes in gross appearance and physical properties. Incubation at 37°C produces rapid degeneration and therefore blood should be kept at room temperature or 4°C. At low temperatures, autoagglutination is common and plasma viscosity is increased. All samples must be warmed and thoroughly mixed before testing. ESR is decreased after storage in sodium citrate even at 4°C. This is probably due to changes in cell shape reducing the facility to form rouleaux. Plasma viscosity is not affected by storage at room temperature for at least 48 hours and probably as long as 7 days. Changes in haemostatic function are dealt with in Chapter 15. Particular problems associated with delay in testing by automated instruments are dealt with in Chapter 8.

Visual blood-cell counting

Although in recent years visual cell counting has been largely replaced by instrumentation the technique is still important in the following circumstances:

1. When visual counts can still be regarded as the reference technique, e.g. platelet counting.

2. When very low leucocyte and platelet counts obtained by instruments may require confirmation.
3. When instruments fail to provide cell counts because of failure to satisfy mathematical or statistical criteria.
4. For absolute counts of certain cell types, e.g. eosinophils.
5. The counting of cells in body fluids other than blood, e.g. CSF.

Fundamental principles

Diluting fluids

Blood must be diluted to enable cells to be counted. The criteria of a suitable diluting fluid are that it should:

1. Prevent lysis or gross changes in the cells to be counted, i.e. be isotonic and possibly contain a fixative.
2. Ideally destroy unwanted cells.
3. Contain an anticoagulant.
4. Be free from debris.

Preparation of dilutions

The use of pipettes with a bulb containing a bead cannot be recommended because of problems of accurate calibration, inadequate mixing and the use of unnecessary small volumes of blood. Capillary pipettes or dispensing devices and stoppered tubes are recommended.

Counting chambers (haemocytometers)

Many patterns of ruling have been recommended but only two will be described, the Improved Neubauer and the Fuchs–Rosenthal. Rulings etched on metallized glass provide greater clarity. BS 748 covers all aspects of counting chambers and cover-slips. Chambers with double, or even four, compartments are useful.

Improved Neubauer This ruling is ideal for counting red cells and platelets and may be used for counting all but the very lowest number of leucocytes. The total ruled area is 9 mm^2 with the central 1 mm^2 divided into 400 squares each with a side of 0.05 mm and separated into 25 groups of 16 squares which are outlined by triple lines. This central area is used for red-cell and platelet counting, while the four corner 1 mm^2 areas, which are each divided into 16 smaller squares, are used for leucocyte counts. The depth of the chamber is 0.1 mm.

Fuchs–Rosenthal The ruled area is also 3×3 mm. Each 1 mm^2 is outlined by triple ruling and further divided into 16 squares. The chamber has a depth of 0.2 mm and therefore a greater volume can be examined. This is particularly suitable for counting small numbers of cells in order to reduce the inherent error (*see* page 93). The chamber is ideal for cell counts of CSF.

Technique of counting

The carefully cleaned chamber with the special, thick, flat and optically correct cover-slip firmly, centrally in place (as shown by refraction spectra), is filled with well-mixed diluted blood using a Pasteur pipette or disposable glass capillary. Care must be taken not to overfill the chamber which will result in overflow into the channels. Before attempting to count, the cells must be allowed to settle completely.

Although the counting of cells in a certain area will facilitate simple calculation, it is emphasized that the more cells counted the more accurate will be the count. Cells are counted in areas outlined by the triple rulings. It must be remembered that the centre of the triple lines delineates the limits of the squares. Inevitably some cells will touch or overlay the margin of the squares. To ensure that cells in adjacent squares are not counted twice, the cells touching the centre line on two sides are included in the count and cells touching the other two sides are excluded from the count. The number of cells in the area are then calculated, taking into account the area counted, the depth of the chamber and the dilution.

$$\text{Total cells per } \mu\text{l} = \text{cells counted} \times \frac{1}{\text{area counted (mm}^2\text{)}} \times \frac{1}{\text{depth (mm)}} \times \text{dilution}$$

Error in cell counting

Technical errors in cell counting may be introduced during sampling, dilution or mixing, by incorrect filling of the chamber and by inaccurate counting. They may be minimized by using accurately calibrated glass-ware and good technique. There is also, however, an *inherent error* in cell counting due to the random distribution of the cells in the chamber, resulting in variation in the numbers of cells in areas of equal size. The distribution, however, follows a mathematical pattern known as a Poisson series in which the SD $= \sqrt{n}$, where n equals the number of cells counted (in practice SD $= 0.92\sqrt{n}$). Thus if 500 cells are counted the SD $= \sqrt{500} = \pm 22$ and thus the 95% confidence limits of $\pm$2SD will be 456–544. The coefficient of variation (CV) will be $22/500 \times 100 = 4.4\%$.

It will be apparent that if a smaller number of cells is counted CV will be much greater, e.g. if 100 cells are counted it will be 10%. Conversely the only way to reduce the inherent error is to count more cells. Thus if 1000 cells are counted, CV will be reduced to approximately 3%. Larger numbers of cells may be counted by increasing the area, using additional chambers, preparing additional dilutions or using a chamber with a larger volume, e.g. a Fuchs–Rosenthal chamber.

Red-cell counting

Diluting fluid 32.0 g/l tri-sodium citrate dihydrate containing 10 ml 40% formaldehyde. This is a simple fluid to prepare, contains anticoagulant, is isotonic and contains a fixative. Leucocytes are not destroyed and although in most cases including them in the count will be insignificant, in some cases of leukaemia they will be a significant source of error. They can be recognized in the chamber and should be disregarded.

Dilution 20 µl of blood in 4 ml of diluting fluid in a stoppered 75 × 12 mm tube producing a 1 in 200 dilution (strictly 1 in 201). When the blood is known to be anaemic a 1 in 100 dilution should be prepared to enable more cells to be readily counted.

Counting Improved Neubauer chamber. An arithmetically convenient technique is to count the cells in five groups of 16 small squares in the central area, i.e. $0.2\,mm^2$ or $0.02\,mm^3$. At least 500 cells should be counted to reduce the inherent error. Then, if 500 cells are counted:

$$\begin{aligned} \text{total red cells} &= 500 \times \frac{1}{0.02} \times 200 \text{ (dilution)} \\ &= 500 \times 10\,000/\mu l \\ \text{or} &= 500 \times 10^4/\mu l \\ \text{or} &= 5.0 \times 10^6/\mu l \\ \text{or} &= 5.0 \times 10^{12}/l \end{aligned}$$

Leucocyte counting

Diluting fluid 2% acetic acid. A simple fluid which rapidly lyses the red cells. The fixative properties of the acetic acid denatures the nuclear proteins of the leucocytes and makes the differing nuclear characteristics readily identifiable. An approximate differential count may even be performed while counting the total leucocytes.

Dilution 0.1 ml of blood in 1.9 ml diluting fluid in a 75 × 100 mm stoppered tube. A 1 in 10 dilution should be made when the leucocyte count is less than $4.0 \times 10^9/l$.

Counting An improved Neubauer, or, when the count is low, a Fuchs–Rosenthal chamber.

Improved Neubauer chamber An arithmetically convenient system is to count the four corner $1\,mm^2$ areas ($0.4\,mm^3$). If 100 cells are counted:

$$\begin{aligned} \text{Total leucocyte count} &= 100 \times \frac{1}{0.4} \times 20 \text{ (dilution)} \\ &= 100 \times 50/\mu l \\ \text{or} &= 5000/\mu l \\ \text{or} &= 5.0 \times 10^3/\mu l \\ \text{or} &= 5.0 \times 10^9/l \end{aligned}$$

Fuchs–Rosenthal chamber A convenient technique is to count $5 \times 1\,mm^2$ areas ($\equiv 1\,mm^3$, as depth $= 0.2\,mm$). Then if 250 cells are counted:

$$\begin{aligned} \text{Total leucocyte count} &= 250 \times 10 \text{ (dilution)} \\ \text{or} &= 2.5 \times 10^3/\mu l \\ \text{or} &= 2.5 \times 10^9/l \end{aligned}$$

With the same diluted sample, the count using the improved Neubauer chamber would have a CV of 10%, whereas the Fuchs–Rosenthal chamber would produce a CV of approximately 6% which is entirely acceptable for clinical purposes.

Platelet counting

Many methods have been described for visual platelet counting and they undoubtedly reflect the difficulties in preventing platelet aggregation, as well as the problem of certain identification by conventional light microscopy. The introduction of EDTA as the routine anticoagulant with its ability to inhibit platelet aggregation has resolved much of the problem, though occasionally samples may show clumping with conventional EDTA concentrations of 1.5 mg/ml of blood. Problems may also be encountered with clumping due to platelet cold agglutinins[16] and falsely low counts due to the platelet–leucocyte rosetting phenomenon in EDTA blood[17]. Phase-contrast microscopy has been advocated and adopted to improve platelet recognition.

Blood samples

Blood obtained by clean venepuncture is the most satisfactory. Difficulty or delay in sampling can result in loss of platelets. Once mixed with EDTA, the blood may be handled and sampled without fear of significant platelet loss.

Capillary blood sampling for platelet counting presents problems which can, however, be overcome. The often quoted 'loss of platelets at the site of skin puncture' is not a serious difficulty. Free-flowing blood from skin puncture may be repeatedly sampled without significant loss, the count falling only immediately before the cessation of bleeding. The unmodified collection and measurement of capillary blood by capillary pipette will, however, result in serious less of platelets even when siliconized glass-ware is used. The loss is proportionally greater from higher platelet numbers and is due to the large surface area of the capillary relative to the volume of blood collected. The problem may be overcome by using capillary pipettes with graduations giving equal volumes. By drawing a solution of 0.1% EDTA to the first graduation followed by blood to the second graduation and then immediately expelling into an appropriate diluting fluid, loss of platelets can be minimal. Alternatively the less accurate bulb-dilution pipette may be used with a 'sandwich technique' of diluting fluid or EDTA solution to the 0.5 mark followed by blood to the 1.0 mark and diluting fluid to the 11 graduation to produce a 1 in 20 dilution which is immediately and thoroughly mixed.

Diluting fluids

Two approaches have been recommended, the difference being whether the red cells are lysed or not. Using the formal–citrate fluid described for red-cell counting the platelets are clearly identifiable and the absence of debris from lysed red cells is an advantage. However, it is necessary to dilute blood 1 in 100 to avoid overcrowding of the chamber with red cells, therefore when dealing with low platelet counts it is difficult to count sufficient platelets to reduce the inherent error. In practice the accurate determination of low platelet counts is important in the control of cytotoxic therapy and in other conditions, and therefore this method is not entirely suitable for routine use. The difficulty of excess red cells may be overcome by allowing blood to stand and using the supernatant platelet-rich plasma. The count is corrected for PCV. Blood samples that sediment slowly are a problem. Many fluids have been described that preserve the platelets while lysing the red cells. It does not appear necessary to go beyond a simple aqueous ammonium oxalate solution (10 g/l)[18]. Red cells are lysed, allowing counting over the whole range of possible platelet numbers; dilution may be reduced to allow increased accuracy with low platelet counts by counting larger numbers. Red-cell debris may cause difficulty in identification.

A diluting fluid that is suitable for both platelets and leucocytes is a definite advantage as both cells may be counted in one preparation. A suitable fluid is available commercially. Whichever fluid is used, it must be prepared using scrupulously clean glass-ware and freshly distilled water. Membrane filtration (pore size 0.22 μm) may be used.

Dilution

To 1.9 ml of diluting fluid is added 0.1 ml of blood (1 in 20 dilution) and mixed thoroughly.

Counting

An improved Neubauer chamber is used. Platelets settle slowly and to avoid drying the haemocytometer is placed in a moist chamber for 30 minutes. Premature counting before complete sedimentation will result in serious error[19].

An arithmetically convenient procedure is to count five groups of 16 small squares in the central area (0.02 μl). If 250 cells are counted then:

$$\text{Total platelet count} = 250 \times \frac{1}{0.02} \times 20 \text{ (dilution)}$$

$$= 250 \times 1000/\mu l$$

$$\text{or} = 250 \times 10^3/\mu l$$

$$\text{or} = 250 \times 10^9/l$$

To reduce the coefficient of variation at least 100 platelets should be counted.

Eosinophil counting

The absolute number of eosinophils may be determined indirectly from the differential leucocyte count of a stained film by reference to the total leucocyte count. A more accurate assessment can be made by direct counting in a haemocytometer after dilution in a suitable fluid. Although now seldom used, the eosinophil count before and after an ACTH injection can be an index of adrenal cortical function[20]. An accurate eosinophil count may be of value in predicting graft-versus-host disease after tissue transplantation.

Diluting fluid

A satisfactory fluid must lyse the red cells while enhancing eosinophil recognition by staining and perhaps lysis of the other types of leucocyte. A variety of fluids have been recommended. The acetone-containing solution suggested by Dunger is stable for up to 1 month if kept at 4°C. Mix 10 ml acetone, 10 ml aqueous eosin (200 g/l) and 80 ml water.

Dilution

0.1 ml of blood in EDTA is diluted in 0.9 ml of diluting fluid and mixed. The eosinophils slowly disintegrate; counts should be completed in 30 minutes.

Counting

A Fuchs–Rosenthal chamber should be used. Two or more chambers should be filled to enable sufficient cells to be counted to reduce the inherent error.

Reference range

This is 40–400 × 10^6/l. Eosinophil counts in normal subjects assume a log-normal distribution and there is considerable diurnal variation: counts are low in the morning and highest at night. Automated differential counting of large numbers of leucocytes indicates that the reference range is considerably narrower than that cited above. This illustrates the point that physiological ranges of normality, particularly those involving relatively small numbers of cells are, in part at least, a combination of normal variation and error due to random distribution.

Basophil counting

The absolute number of basophils may be obtained from the differential and total leucocyte counts. The infrequency of basophils makes this approach tedious and time consuming and requires the counting of at least 1000 leucocytes to obtain reasonable precision. Direct counting is more satisfactory and the method described is superior to those using toluidine blue and neutral red[21].

Principle

Blood is diluted in EDTA to prevent platelet clumping and further treated with cetyl pyridinium chloride to facilitate red-cell lysis, and Alcian Blue to stain the heparin-containing granules, with the addition of lanthanum chloride as a mordant. Hydrochloric acid is added to reduce the pH and increase staining contrast. This procedure is similar to that which was used by the Technicon Hemalog D and H6000.

Method

Reagents

1. Solution A: 0.1% EDTA in 0.9% NaCl.
2. Solution B: deionized water containing 0.076% cetyl pyridinium chloride, 0.7% lanthanum chloride $6H_2O$, 0.9% NaCl, 0.21% Tween 20 and 0.143% Alcian Blue 8 GN (colour index No. 74240) filtered through a 1 μm filter.
3. Solution C: 1 mol/l HCl.

Technique

0.1 ml of blood is diluted in 0.4 ml solution A and 0.45 ml solution B is added. After 1 minute of gentle agitation 0.05 ml of solution C is added and again mixed gently. The final dilution is 1 in 10. Cells are counted using a Fuchs–Rosenthal haemocytometer. To reduce the inherent error the total ruled areas of two chambers should be examined, i.e. 18 mm^2.

Significance

Elevated numbers of basophils are found in myeloproliferative disorders and untreated hypothyroidism. Reduced numbers are reported in thyrotoxicosis, infection and following steroid treatment.

Counting of cells in cerebrospinal fluid and body fluids other than blood

Although not strictly haematology, counting of cells in other body fluids is often performed by haematologists because of their expertise and availability of equipment. This aspect of cell counting is becoming increasingly important in monitoring the possible presence of leukaemic blast cells in the CSF of patients with acute leukaemia.

Samples of body fluids, particularly CSF, often contain blood, possibly as a contaminant introduced during collection. The technique described below enables leucocytes (and other nucleated cells) to be counted and related to the number of any red cells present.

Technique

Red-cell counting
An improved Neubauer chamber is filled with fluid. If the sample is grossly blood stained, dilution will be necessary, making it possible to obtain a more accurate count by instrument counting.

Nucleated cell counting
To four volumes of the CSF is added one volume of 10% acetic acid. This lyses any red cells that may be present and at the same time, by denaturing the cell nuclei, allows the ready identification of the neutrophil polymorphs and the lymphocytes. A Fuchs–Rosenthal chamber is used and $5 \times 1\,mm^2$ areas counted, a volume of 1 μl. The total count is multiplied by 5/4 to allow for the dilution by the acetic acid. Types of leucocyte may be expressed as percentages of the total count or as number per μl.

If the fluid is contaminated with blood during the collection procedure the number of leucocytes introduced from the blood will be in the order of 1 per 500–1000 red cells in a subject with a normal blood count. A more accurate assessment of blood-derived leucocyte contamination can be made by reference to the relative proportions of leucocytes and red cells in a blood sample collected at the time of sampling the body fluid. In certain cases where cells other than blood cells are present, a stained film prepared from a centrifuged deposit or by a Cytospin centrifuge may be necessary to allow cell identification. Considerable cell distortion may result from centrifugation techniques and a gravity sedimentation technique may be preferred[22].

Reticulocyte counting

A stage in the transformation of early erythroblast to mature erythrocyte is that, having lost its nucleus, the cell remains in the bone marrow for approximately 72 hours before release into the circulation where it takes a further 48 hours to transform into a mature red cell. During this non-nucleated, pre-red-cell stage, the immature red cell contains precipitable, ribosomal, RNA-containing material and the cell is termed a reticulocyte. The more immature the reticulocyte the greater the ribosome content, which is gradually lost as the reticulocyte matures. The number of reticulocytes is therefore an index of red-cell production by the bone marrow and as such is one of the most valuable observations in diagnostic haematology.

The recognition of the reticulocyte is based on the ability of certain non-toxic dyes to precipitate and stain the ribosomal material in unfixed reticulocytes. Though reticulocytes are larger than mature red cells and show polychromasia in Romanowsky-stained blood films, supravital staining techniques enable their number to be determined with sufficient accuracy. Staining with fluorochromes, e.g. acridine orange, can also be used [23].

Computerized image-analysis systems and flow cytometry allow automated reticulocyte counting.

Principle

Blood is mixed with an isotonic, anticoagulated solution of a suitable dye. After staining, a film is made of the cell suspension. The reticulocytes (containing a blue-staining filamentous network, strands or fragments) are counted and expressed as a percentage of the total number of red cells counted.

Alternatively they may be expressed as a corrected percentage by reference to the whole-blood haematocrit, and can be presented as an absolute number by reference to the number of red cells in the original sample. A reticulocyte production index may be derived by reference to the degree of anaemia shown by the whole-blood haematocrit.

Staining fluids

Cationic dyes such as Brilliant Cresyl Blue (BCB) and New Methylene Blue (NMB) are commonly used as vital stains. Unreliability of certain batches may be attributed to mis-identification by suppliers [24]. Certified batches of each dye are probably quite suitable for use although Azure B has been recommended as an alternative [25].

Stain

1.0 g of NMB is dissolved in 100 ml citrate-saline (20 ml 30 g/l trisodium citrate dihydrate, 80 ml 9 g/l sodium chloride). Filter before use.

Method

Blood should be less than 12 hours old as some degree of maturation takes place *in vitro*. Approximately equal volumes of blood and staining solution are mixed in a 75 × 12 mm tube and allowed to stand for 15 minutes. Warming at 37°C does not significantly improve the results. The cells are resuspended and films made in the usual way. Excessively thin films should be avoided as reticulocytes may be unevenly distributed. Excessive concentrations of EDTA inhibit staining. When perfectly dry the films are examined without fixation or further staining. Mature red cells stain greenish-blue without demonstrable inclusions. Reticulocytes are identified by precipitated material, staining deep blue, appearing as a filamentous network, strands or fragments. Other red-cell inclusions which must not be confused are Howell–Jolly bodies and Pappenheimer bodies which are, however, demonstrable after fixation and counter-staining. Of particular significance are the presence of Heinz bodies and precipitated Hb H which are only seen in supravital preparations which are not fixed or counter-stained. This is the main argument for not counter-staining reticulocyte preparations.

Counting

A 2 mm (× 100) oil-immersion objective is preferred. An area of the film where the cells do not overlap is selected. An eye-piece diaphragm may be used to reduce the field area. The *total* red cells in each field are noted, together with the number of reticulocytes. As in counting cells in chambers, the distribution of the reticulocytes is random, and again the more cells counted the more accurate witll be the result. A common practice is to count a total of 500 red cells noting the number of reticulocytes. The CV can be readily calculated, i.e. if 50 reticulocytes are seen in 500 red cells the SD = 7 and the CV will be 14%. For most purposes this would be acceptable but for lower reticulocyte counts, more cells should be counted. This is particularly important when investigating possible bone-marrow hypoplasia or mild haemolytic anaemias. Quality assurance studies suggest that the major discrepancy between the results of different observers is the problem of what is or is not a reticulocyte, particuarly when only a single dot or small fragment of material is present [26].

Expression of results

As a percentage of total red cells This is a common practice and is satisfactory if, when interpreting results, it is realized that the result is relative to the number of circulating red cells, for example:

1% of 5 $\times 10^{12}$ RBC/l = 5×10^{10} reticulocytes
2% of 2.5 $\times 10^{12}$ RBC/l = 5×10^{10} reticulocytes
5% of 1 $\times 10^{12}$ RBC/l = 5×10^{10} reticulocytes

Thus an apparent increased percentage of reticulocytes may reflect normal red-cell production associated with reduced numbers of red cells rather than increased bone-marrow release of reticulocytes.

As numbers/unit volume or as a corrected percentage These may be derived using the PCV.

$$\text{Corrected reticulocyte (\%)} = \frac{\text{Patient's PCV}}{\text{Normal PCV}} \times \text{Observed reticulocyte percentage}$$

This interpretation of the reticulocyte count assumes that the release of bone-marrow reticulocytes is occurring normally. Ferrokinetic data suggest that to obtain a truer index of bone-marrow red-cell production, account must be taken of a reduced reticulocyte transit time in the bone marrow, in that reticulocyte-stay in the marrow is reduced by the influence of anaemia. A maturation index is suggested by which the reticulocyte count should be divided to compensate for the presence of the so-called 'shift reticulocytes' [27].

Haematocrit	*Index*
45	1.0
35	1.5
25	2.0
15	2.5

Correction to the reticulocyte count is then made as follows:

$$\frac{\text{Observed reticulocyte count \%}}{\text{Maturation index}} \times \frac{\text{Observed haematocrit}}{45} = \text{Corrected reticulocyte \%}$$

Examples of applying this formula to observed reticulocyte counts is shown below:

Observed reticulocyte %	*Haematocrit*	*Corrected %*
1.0	45	1.0
6.5	35	3.0
14.0	25	4.0
24.0	15	3.2

The physiological limit for a corrected reticulocyte count is 6–8%, i.e. when the bone marrow produces approximately 6–8 times the normal numbers of red cells.

Measurement of haemoglobin

The haemoglobin content of blood may be determined by physical properties such as specific gravity, chemical compostion (i.e. iron content), by gas analysis or by spectral characteristics. For routine purposes photometric or spectrophotometric measurement is the most suitable and is widely used.

Since haemoglobin is a chromoprotein at high concentration the photometric or spectrophotometric measurement of haemoglobin in blood might have been expected to be established for many years as an accurate determination. The many techniques that have been recommended indicate that until recent years this has not been the case. Although the light absorption of a diluted blood sample could be accurately measured in the haemoglobin or oxyhaemoglobin (HbO_2) form there was no acceptable standard solution because of the tendency to fade. As alternatives, tinted glass, neutral density filters, or inorganic salt solutions of stable optical density were recommended and used, but considerable and unacceptable discrepancies between laboratories were not uncommon.

Conversion of haemoglobin to more stable derivatives such as carboxyhaemoglobin (COHb) and alkaline haematin have been used to overcome the instability of haemoglobin, but standard solutions of such derivatives are not wholly satisfactory. By exposure to potassium ferricyanide and potassium cyanide, haemoglobin is converted to the extremely stable cyanmethaemoglobin (haemiglobincyanide, HiCN, cyanferrihaemoglobin). The determination of the millimolar extinction coefficient of HiCN [28] provided the basis for international collaboration in establishing the International Haemiglobincyanide reference preparation in 1966 which was further modified in 1977 (ICSH standard EP 6/3: 1977), together with a recommended reference method for haemoglobinometry in human blood (ISCH Standard EP 6/2: 1977). More recently the Expert Panel on Haemoglobinometry of the ICSH has made further recommendations for a reference method for haemoglobinometry in human blood (ICSH standard 1986) and specifications for the international reference preparation (3rd edition) [29]. The HiCN method is now established as the reference method and other photometric techniques measuring Hb as HbO_2, methaemoglobin (Hi), or alkaline haematin should be calibrated and checked using blood samples in which the haemoglobin concentration has been determined accurately by the standard HiCN method. This also applies to haemoglobin estimations by iron determination or gas analysis. For routine purposes such methods are unsuitable and will not be considered further.

Haemiglobincyanide reference preparation [29]

The reference preparation is related to the molar absorption coefficient and relative molecular mass of one haem group and one quarter of the total globin moiety (the original standard related to the whole haemoglobin molecule). The preparation is manufactured at 3-year intervals on behalf of the ICSH. It is made from washed human red cells, haemolysed by toluene and centrifuged free from debris. The haemoglobin is converted to HiCN. The final product is equivalent to a haemoglobin content of approximately 600 mg/l. It is dispensed as a sterile solution by membrane filtration in sealed 10 ml ampoules of amber glass. Each batch is tested in laboratories nominated by the ICSH board in accordance with the principles described below.

Concentration

The HiCN (equivalent haemoglobin) concentration is calculated from the results of at least five laboratories using the equation:

$$c(\text{mg/l}) = \frac{A^{540}_{\text{HiCN}} \times 16\,114.5}{11.0 \times 1.000} = 1465 \times A^{540}_{\text{HiCN}}$$

where A^{540}_{HiCN} = absorbance of the solution at λ = 540 nm; 16 114.5 = relative molecular mass of haemoglobin derived from 64 458/4; 11.0 = e^{540}_{HiCN} (millimolar absorptivity); 1.000 = light path length in cm.

Using an appropriate blank, A^{540} is measured on a spectrophotometer, the wavelength scale of which has been calibrated with the aid of the Hg (or H, or D) emission spectrum, or holmium oxide in perchloric acid, and on which absorption checks have been performed using calibrated glass filters or other means which have been certified by a standardizing authority. The slit width is so chosen that the half-intensity band width is less than 2 nm. The cuvettes in which the solution is measured are plan-parallel with an inner wall-to-wall distance of 1.000 cm, tolerance 0.995–1.005 cm. The measurements are carried out at 20–25°C.

The arithmetic mean and standard error of the results of the laboratories are recorded after erratic results, if any, have been discarded in accordance with statistical practice. Experience with this procedure has shown that the confidence limits of the final results are within ±1%.

Purity

The purity is controlled by: (1) judging the shape of an absorption spectrum between 450 and 750 nm, light path 1.000 cm; (2) determining the quotient $A^{540}_{\text{HiCN}}/A^{504}_{\text{HiCN}}$; the value of this quotient should lie between 1.59 and 1.63; (3) measuring turbidity in the near infra-red (between 725 nm and 800 nm, e.g. at 750 nm). The absorbance should be less than 0.002 per cm light path length using an appropriate blank.

Stability

The standard is kept at 4°C and has a stability of at least 6 years.

Sterility

Sterility control is carried out aerobically and anaerobically at 22 and 37°C.

Labelling

The International Reference Preparation is labelled with batch number, the value of its haemoglobin concentration (mean and standard error) and an expiry date which is considered well within safe limits. The producer notifies all customers if continuing control of stability indicates that a particular batch is no longer acceptable.

Purpose and distribution

The Reference Preparation is used to assign values to secondary HiCN reference solutions or HiCN calibration solutions and as a reference against which to judge the purity of such HiCN solutions. It is made available for reference use only to national standards committees for haematological methods, to official government-nominated holders or to individuals approved by ICSH. The national holder must ensure that an opportunity is given to manufacturers and distributors to use the Reference Preparation as a reference material if so desired.

Reference method for haemoglobinometry (ICSH standard 1986)

It is recommended that at present the haemoglobin content of blood should be expressed as mass concentration in grams per litre though grams per decilitre (g/dl) is acceptable. If the substance concentration (mmol/l) is preferred, the elementary entity should be specified by the notation (Fe) or (4Fe).

Principle

The haemoglobin derivatives found in blood with the exception of sulphaemoglobin are converted to HiCN by dilution in an appropriate reagent, and the haemoglobin concentration measured photometrically by reference to the International Haemiglobincyanide Standard.

Reagent

A suitable reagent is prepared as follows. Dissolve 200 mg of potassium ferricyanide, 50 mg potassium cyanide and 140 mg potassium dihydrogen phosphate in water and dilute to 1 litre. Add 1 ml Nonidet P4O (or suitable alternative). The pH should be 7.0–7.4 checked by a pH meter and osmolality 6–7 mmol/kg. Store in a brown borosilicate glass bottle at room temperature, under which conditions the reagent is stable for 2 months. Plastic containers should not be used as there is evidence that the cyanide is absorbed from the solution. Freezing destroys the potassium ferricyanide but can be prevented by the addition of ethanol, methanol, ethylene glycol or glycerine[30]. The reagent has a conversion time of 3–5 minutes in contrast to the original or the modified Drabkin's reagents which have conversion times of 10 minutes or more. There must be no turbidity. The reagent has a low ionic strength and euglobulin fractions of plasma may precipitate, particularly if in increased concentration, causing turbidity and erroneously high Hb values. The addition of 5 g/l of NaCl has been recommended to prevent this problem. The turbidity due to grossly increased leucocyte numbers may also be reduced by this modification, though in extreme leucocytosis and in erythroblastosis, centrifugation is recommended[31, 32].

The conversion time of carboxyhaemoglobin to HiCN is up to 30 minutes[33].

Dilution

A suitable dilution is 1 in 251 for either a filter photometer or a spectrophotometer.

Photoelectric colorimeter

A narrow-band yellow-green filter with maximal transmission near 540 nm is used. The instrument must be calibrated and linearity verified (*see* below) using a HiCN calibration standard. The haemoglobin concentration is read from a previously constructed calibration graph, directly from the scale, or in some instruments from the digital display against a suitable blank.

Spectrophotometer

The extinction is measured at 540 nm against an appropriate blank. The instrument calibration and the cuvette specification should be as described for the preparation of the International Standard.

Haemoglobin concentration (c) is calculated from:

$$c(\text{g/l}) = \frac{A^{540}_{\text{HiCN}} \times 16\,114.5 \times F}{11.0 \times 1.000 \times 1000}$$

where A^{540}_{HiCN} = absorbance of the solution at 540 nm; 16 114.5 = relative molecular mass of haemoglobin; F = dilution factor used; 11.0 = millimolar absorption coefficient; 1.000 = light path in cm; 1000 = conversion factor for mg to g.

For a dilution (F) of 1:251, c (g/l) = 367.7 × A^{540}_{HiCN}.

Verification of linearity

Linearity should be verified through the clinical range of haemoglobin concentrations, i.e. 2–25 g/dl. The range above about 15 g/dl is not possible with the International Reference Preparation. A blood sample with a haemoglobin concentration of 10 g/dl (or similar known value) when diluted 1 in 100 will provide a HiCN solution equivalent to 25 g/dl of a 1 in 250 dilution. Appropriate dilutions of this solution may then be made to cover the whole clinically observable range of haemoglobin concentrations. It has been pointed out that simply plotting absorbance against concentration to demonstrate linearity and therefore conformance to Beer's law does not mean that accuracy is similar throughout the observed range. The plotting of absorbance (ordinate) against the log of the concentration (abscissa) over a wide range of values (a Ringbom plot) is recommended[34]. The accuracy is greatest at the point of inflection of the curve and where the curve has the steepest slope.

The performances of photocolorimeters differ considerably and the optimal range for accurate measurement may vary considerably, e.g. 5–15 g/dl for one instrument compared with 10–30 g/dl for another. 'Relative analysis error' will be greatest in those parts of the curve below or above the optimal reading range. Ideally blood samples should be appropriately diluted so that the absorbance falls within the optimum range. This is unlikely to be feasible in routine practice. However, when preparing secondary standards or when selecting an instrument, the Ringbom procedure should be considered.

Determination of packed red-cell volume

The packed cell volume (PCV) is the proportion of whole blood occupied by the red cells expressed as l/l. Determination of PCV by centrifugation is a reproducible procedure. The measurement assesses red-cell status in that the PCV depends essentially upon the number and volume of the red cells. It is the basis for the determination of the 'absolute values' of red-cell volume and haemoglobin content. The PCV became established as a reliable indication of anaemia when the accuracy of haemoglobinometry was questionable. Apart from measuring the PCV, the colour of the plasma can be observed and gross increases in leucocyte or platelet numbers are shown by increased thickness of the respective cell layers (the 'buffy coat'). The original Wintrobe tubes were spun for 30 minutes at 1500 *g* and under these conditions 0.030–0.040 of a PCV of 0.450 is occupied by plasma trapped in the red-cell column [35]. The volume of 'trapped plasma' can be reduced by extending the centrifugation time to 1 hour, or more effectively by increasing the centrifugal force.

The introduction of the 'micro-PCV' using suitable glass capillaries and high-speed centrifuges capable of applying 12 000 *g* enables the centrifugation time to be reduced to 5–10 minutes and reduces the trapped plasma of the red-cell column of normal blood with a PCV of 0.440, to 0.014. It is therefore possible to define the conditions for performing a micro-PCV which should produce reproducible and comparable results between different laboratories.

Although a relatively small volume is occupied by trapped plasma in the PCV of normal blood, there can be considerable plasma trapping in blood samples where there is abnormal red-cell shape and, perhaps more importantly, inflexibility of the red cells. This may amount to as much as 20% of the red-cell column in the extreme example of sickle-cell anaemia [36].

Although it has been suggested that the micro-PCV technique compresses the red cells [37], significant compression has been shown not to occur with the Wintrobe technique at 1400 *g* for 30 minutes [38]. The correlation between the results of 'macro' and 'micro' techniques suggests that compression is minimal. Nevertheless the term PCV should perhaps be applied only to values obtained by centrifugation.

Relationship of the 'spun' PCV to the PCV obtained by other techniques

PCV may be derived from PCV = MCV × RBC where MCV is mean red-cell volume determined by electrical impedance or light scatter technologies. Such methods eliminate the problem of trapped plasma but it is not yet possible to determine red-cell volume accurately from the physical performance characteristics of an instrument without recourse to a primary standard [39]. In practice therefore, instrument-derived red-cell volume measurements are obtained by calibration of an instrument using a blood sample, the MCV of which has been determined from a spun PCV! Furthermore, PCV calculated from MCV × RBC may be incorrect due to the problem of measuring the MCV of red cells of abnormal shape and deformability. This aspect is considered further in Chapter 8.

Although there are problems in obtaining the 'true' PCV, reproducible values can be obtained which can be used to calculate MCV and to measure red-cell mass and plasma volume. A reference range can be determined for MCV which, although possibly not based on 'true' values, is a valuable aid to haematological investigation. The discrepancy between the PCV of a sample of venous blood and the 'whole body' PCV is considered in the section on the measurement of blood volume (*see* page 482).

PCV by centrifugation

Collection of blood samples

Physiological variation in the proportions of red cells and plasma is summarized in *Table 3.3*.

Table 3.3 Physiological variation in the proportions of red cells and plasma

Activity	*Fall in PCV*	*Rise in PCV*
Ambulant	0.020–0.060	–
Recumbent	–	0.020–0.060
Exercise	–	0.020–0.050
Bed-rest	–	0.016 (mean)
Postprandial	0.015 (maximum at 2–4 h)	–
Local stasis	–	1 minute, 0.004 2 minutes, 0.010 3 minutes, 0.030

Anticoagulant

K_2EDTA, 1.5 mg/ml. The use of K_3EDTA in the same proportions causes red-cell shrinkage [40].

Reference method

Though the 'macro-haematocrit' or Wintrobe tube is rarely used for routine determination of PCV, the ICSH reference method for determination of PCV by centrifugation uses the Wintrobe tube because the dimensions and uniformity of the tube bore can be checked and the amount of trapped plasma may be measured using radioiodine-labelled human serum albumin [41].

Apparatus and materials

The Wintrobe tube should be made of glass and graduated with a uniform scale. The exact dimensions of the graduated part are not important, and tubes of length 100 mm and internal diameter of 2.5 or 3.0 mm may be used. The bore uniformity, to within 0.05 mm, should be checked with a suitable micrometer and the exact internal radius also determined. If tubes of the required bore uniformity are available but a micrometer is not, then the internal radius may be determined gravimetrically. The tube is filled to around the 0.1 mark with mercury and weighed, and the exact length of the mercury column is noted. Mercury is then added to around the 1.0 mark, the tube is re-weighed, and the new length is noted. If the difference in weight is w g and the difference between the lengths of the mercury columns is l mm, then the internal radius r (in millimetres) is $(23.41w/l)^{1/2}$.

The lower end of the tube must be sealed with a flat bottom, and the plane of the internal surface should be at right angles to the axis of the tube and aligned with the origin of the graduations.

Radioiodine-labelled human serum albumin solution, having a concentration of about 20 g/l and ideally >0.4 mCi/ml, should be used. Less than 2% of the label should be present as free iodide at the time of use. The ability of the preparation to bind to red cells should be assessed; if the material is to be satisfactory then the red-cell binding after four washes with isotonic saline should be less than 1% of the albumin that is in the trapped plasma when the method recommended below is used.

Method

A 5 ml blood sample (or red-cell preparation) is labelled by adding 10 μl of the albumin solution and is then used for the PCV determination.

The Wintrobe tube is filled from the bottom upwards with well-mixed blood, and the level of the meniscus is noted to the nearest one-third of a millimetre. It may be convenient to use a Pasteur pipette to fill the tube, which must then be sealed with paraffin wax paper to minimize evaporation.

The tube is centrifuged at room temperature so that the relative centrifugal force is 12 000–25 000 m s^{-2} (about 1200–2500 *g*) 50 mm from the base of the tube*. During the centrifugation period the temperature of the blood should not exceed 35°C. After 30 minutes the centrifuge is allowed to come to rest without braking, and the position of the upper end of the red-cell column is noted to the nearest one-third of a millimetre. The uncorrected PCV, expressed as a proportion, may then be calculated by dividing this value by the reading obtained for the blood meniscus before centrifugation.

To determine the plasma trapping correction, plasma is aspirated from the tube, and aliquots are retained for counting. The traces of plasma above the red cells and upon the wall of the tube are removed by gentle washing with isotonic saline and discarded. Next the red cells are aspirated, the tubes washed with saline and the washings added to the cells and counted.

Calculation

After the counts have been corrected for radioactive background, the plasma-trapping proportion is calculated as follows:

$$(\text{counts in red cells} \times 10^3)/(\text{counts/ml plasma} \times \pi r^2 h)$$

where r is the internal radius of the Wintrobe tube and h is the height of the red-cell column in millimetres. The PCV corrected for plasma trapping is then: uncorrected PCV × (1 − plasma trapping).

Micro-method

Glass capillary tubes conforming to BS 4316: 1968 are used. This should ensure uniformity of bore and the facility for flat, heat-sealing of the tubes. Well-mixed oxygenated blood is drawn into the tube by capillary flow leaving about 1 cm

* Acceleration in m s^{-2} is given by $1.1 \times 10^{-5} \times R \times N^2$ where R is the centrifugal radius 50 mm from the base of the tube expressed in millimetres and N is the number of revolutions/minute. The standard acceleration due to gravity is 9.807 m s^{-2}. This centrifugal force packs the red cells sufficiently and allows subsequent washing procedures to be completed without disturbing the top of the red-cell column.

unfilled. The unfilled end is carefully sealed in a fine flame or plugged with Plasticine or similar material. The tube is centrifuged for 5 minutes in a purpose-designed instrument producing 12 000 *g*. If the PCV is elevated a further 5 minutes' centrifugation to obtain maximum packing is recommended. The length of the red-cell column is expressed as a ratio of the total column. Specially designed 'PCV-readers' are available. Care must be taken not to include the leucocyte or platelets (the 'buffy layer') when measuring the red-cell column. Reproducibility should be within ±0.010. Correction may be made for trapped plasma (*Table 3.4*)[35] but in other than normal blood or that in which trapping has been characterized, correction may well be inaccurate. It is probably preferable to establish a method and recognize its limitations.

Table 3.4 Trapped plasma as a percentage of the red-cell column[36]

Group (no. of subjects)	*Range*	*Mean*
Controls (26)	0.8–4.2	3.2
Hypochromia (14)	3.6–6.2	4.4
Macrocytosis (14)	2.4–5.7	3.7
Sickle trait (1)	5.2	
Fully sickled	22.4	

Results are expressed as the ratio of red cells to whole blood in litres (l/l). By microcentrifugation it is only possible to measure results to two decimal places, e.g. 0.45. The addition of a third place, e.g. 0.450, is undesirable and unnecessary as it implies a degree of accuracy that is not possible due to the inherent error of reading the lengths of the red-cell column.

In addition to errors due to trapped plasma it has been demonstrated that the diameter and the type of glass of the capillary tube influences the micro-PCV[42]. The smaller the diameter the lower the PCV for a given blood sample and the decrease in PCV using soda-lime glass is twice that using borosilicate tubes. It is, however, suggested that the false low PCV due to diameter and type of glass fortuitously compensates for the overestimation due to plasma trapping!

Red-cell absolute values

The calculation of the size and haemoglobin content of red cells from the haemoglobin concentration of whole blood, PCV and red-cell count was introduced by Wintrobe as a basis for the classification of anaemias. Recognition of the inherent errors of red-cell counting together with the lack of standardization in haemoglobinometry, led to 'absolute values' falling into disrepute. With the introduction of electronic cell counting, the standardization of haemoglobinometry, and the use of the microhaematocrit technique, there has been a re-emergence in the use of red-cell absolute values in haematological diagnosis which has been reinforced by the use of fully automated blood analysers. The usual parameters measured are: mean red-cell volume (MCV), mean red-cell haemoglobin (MCH) and the mean red-cell haemoglobin concentration (MCHC).

The last phrase is a misnomer as it is not a 'mean' value but the concentration of Hb/dl of red cells as distinct from whole blood. The measurement of mean red-cell diameter (MCD) from dried blood films and the calculation of mean cell average thickness (MCAT) is artificial, has little to contribute to diagnostic haematology and will not be considered.

Calculation of absolute values

In each example the following parameters will be used:

Hb = 15 g/dl; PCV = 0.45; RCC = 5.0×10^{12}/l.

Mean cell volume

$$\text{MCV} = \frac{\text{PCV}}{\text{RCC}}$$

$$= \frac{0.45\,\text{l/l}}{5 \times 10^{12}/\text{l}} = \frac{0.09}{1 \times 10^{12}} = 0.09 \times 10^{-12}/\text{l}$$

$$= 90 \times 10^{-15} \text{ or } 90\,\text{fl}$$

Reference range = 82–95 fl; less than 82 fl = microcytic; greater than 95 fl = macrocytic.

Notes

1. It must be recognized that the MCV is a *mean* or average value and a normal value may be found when red cells are abnormal e.g. with anisocytosis or from a dimorphic population.
2. An abnormal MCV is usually reflected by change in red-cell diameter as seen in stained blood films. This is not always the case and obvious macrocytosis in the blood film may be associated with a normal MCV, i.e. the red cells must be thinner than normal. Conversely, red cells may have a smaller diameter but have a normal MCV in the presence of spherocytosis.
3. The MCV of an individual is remarkably constant in health and, indeed, may be used for reference purposes.
4. As the normal range for MCV is relatively wide, significant change may be seen in red-cell morphology while the MCV remains in the normal range. For example if MCV is usually 92 fl, the development of iron depletion with a falling MCV will be apparent by blood film changes, yet the MCV may be 84 fl, still in the reference range.
5. The MCV of reference materials used to calibrate electronic counters is often derived from a PCV corrected for trapped plasma. MCV calculations using an uncorrected PCV will give a higher value.

Mean cell haemoglobin

$$\text{MCH} = \frac{\text{Hb (g/dl)}}{\text{RCC/l}} = \frac{15 \times 10\ \text{g/l}}{5 \times 10^{12}/\text{l}} = \frac{30}{1 \times 10^{12}} \text{ or}$$

$$30 \times 10^{-12}\ \text{g/l or } 30\ \text{pg}$$

Reference range = 27–32 pg; less than 27 = microcytes; greater than 32 = macrocytes.

Note on MCH

The haemoglobin content of a red cell is determined by the volume of the cell and therefore there is a direct linear relationship between MCV and MCH. Slight loss of linearity found with some cell analysers is due to problems of MCV measurement of abnormal cells[43].

Mean cell haemoglobin concentration (MCHC)

$$\text{MCHC} = \frac{\text{Hb (g/dl)}}{\text{PCV (l/l)}} = \frac{15}{0.45} = 33\ \text{g/dl}$$

Reference range = 32–36 g/dl.

Notes on MCHC

Normal red cells have maximum haemoglobin content and results greater than 36 g/dl are unusual except in marked spherocytosis or loss of cell water. Low values for MCHC indicate hypochromia and an early fall in MCHC derived using a spun PCV is a valuable indicator of hypochromia when an MCV is not available. It is now clear, however, that a low MCHC is mainly an artefact due to a falsely high PCV caused by the trapped plasma associated with abnormal red-cell morphology. The early fall in MCHC is not seen in data obtained from instruments where MCV is measured and PCV calculated, thus eliminating the artefact of trapped plasma. Low values are seen, however, in moderate to severe hypochromia and may be due to the over-estimation of MCV as mentioned in the notes on MCH.

References

1. Hinchcliffe, R. F. (1987) Blood sample collection. In *Practical Paediatric Haematology* (eds R. F. Hinchcliffe and J. S. Lilleyman), pp. 1–15. Chichester: Wiley
2. Sacker, L. S. (1975) Specimen collection. In *Quality Control in Haematology* (eds S. M. Lewis and L. S. Sacker), pp. 211–19. London: Academic Press
3. Advisory Committee on Dangerous Pathogens (ACDP) (1983) *Categorisation of Pathogens According to Hazards and Categories of Containment.* London: HMSO
4. ACDP (1986) *LAV/HTVIII – The Causative Agent of AIDS and Related Conditions: Revised Guidelines.* London: HMSO
5. National Committee for Clinical Laboratory Standards (NCCLS) (1988) Additives to blood collection devices: EDTA. Proposed standard H-35-P. Villanova, PA
6. Koepke, J. A., van Assendelft, O. W., Bull, B. S. and Richardson-Jones, A. (1989) Standardisation of EDTA anticoagulation of blood counting procedures. *Labmedica*, Dec/Jan, 15–17
7. Koepke, J. A., Rodgers, J. L. and Ollivier, M. J. (1975) Pre-instrument variables in coagulation testing. *Am. J. Clin. Pathol*, **65**, 591–6
8. Zucker, S., Cathey, M. H. and West, B. (1970) Preparation of quality control specimens for coagulation. *Am. J. Clin. Pathol.*, **53**, 924–7
9. Bray, P. J., Ford, D., Glendhill, R. M. and Grimes, A. J. (1977) Defibrination of normal human blood *in vitro*: a method of giving a high recovery of untraumatised cells. *Br. J. Haematol.*, **35**, 551–9
10. British Standards Institution (1978) *Specification for Medical Specimen Containers for Haematology and Biochemistry.* BS 4851
11. Ingram, G. I. C. and Hills, M. (1976) Reference method for the one-stage prothrombin time test on human blood. *Thromb. Haemost*, **36**, 237–8
12. ACDP (1988) *Inactivation of Viral Haemorrhagic Fever Specimens with β-Propiolactone.* London: HMSO

13. Health and Safety Commission. Health Service Advisory Committee (1986) *Safety in Health Service Laboratories: The Labelling, Transport and Reception of Specimens*. London: HMSO
14. Lawrence, A. C. K., Bevington, J. M. and Young, M. (1975) Storage of blood and the mean corpuscular volume. *J. Clin. Pathol.*, **28**, 345–9
15. Cohle, S. D., Saleem, A. and Makkaoui, D. E. (1981) Effects of storage of blood on the stability of heamatologic parameters. *Am. J. Clin. Pathol.*, **76**, 67–9
16. Van Vliet, H. H. D. M., Kappers-Klunne, M. C. and Abels, J. (1986) Pseudo thrombocytopenia: a cold autoantibody against platelet glycoprotein $GPII^b$. *Br. J. Haematol.*, **62**, 501–11
17. Crome, P. E. and Barkhan, P. (1963) Platelet adherence to polymorphs. *Br. Med. J.* **ii**, 871
18. Lewis, S. M., Wardle, J., Cousins, S. and Skelly, J. V. (1979) Platelet counting – development of a reference method and a reference preparation. *Clin. Lab. Haematol.*, **1**, 227–37
19. Ashman, B. (1976) An assessment of platelet counting methods. *Med. Lab. Sci.*, **33**, 201–8
20. Hills, A. G., Forsham, P. H. and Finch, C. A. (1948) Changes in circulating leucocytes induced by the administration of pituitary adrenocorticotrophic hormone (ACTH) in man. *Blood*, **3**, 755–68
21. Gilbert, H. S. and Ornstein, L. (1975) Basophil counting with a new method using alcian blue. *Blood*, **46**, 279–86
22. Nishimura, K., Hosoya, R. and Nakajima, K. (1978) Sedimentation cytology in central nervous system leukaemia with a simple apparatus. *Br. J. Haematol.*, **40**, 583–6
23. Jahanmehr, S. A. H., Hyde, K., Geary, C. G. *et al.* (1988) Simple technique for fluorescence staining of blood cells with acridine orange. *J. Clin. Pathol.*, **41**, 926–9
24. Gadson, D., Hughes, M., Dean, A. and Wickramasinghe, S. M. (1986) Morphology of redox-dye treated Hb H containing red cells: confusion caused by wrongly identified dyes. *Clin. Lab. Haematol.*, **8**, 365–6
25. Wittekind, D. and Schulte, E. (1987) Standardised Azure B as a reticulocyte stain. *Clin. Lab. Haematol.*, **9**, 395–8
26. Gilmer, P. R. and Koepke, J. A. (1976) The reticulocyte: an approach to definition. *Am. J. Clin. Pathol.*, **66**, 262–7
27. Hillman, R. S. and Finch, C. A. (1969) The misused reticulocyte. *Br. J. Haematol.*, **17**, 313–15
28. Zijlstra, W. G. and van Kampen, E. J. (1960) Standardisation of haemoglobinometry. I. The extinction coefficient of hemiglobincyanide at $\lambda = 540$ nm: 540/HiCN. *Clin. Chim. Acta*, **5**, 719–26
29. ICSH Expert Panel in Haemoglobinometry (1987) Recommendations for reference method of haemoglobinometry in human blood (ICSH standard 1986) and specifications for international haemiglobincyanide reference preparation (3rd ed.). *Clin. Lab. Haematol.*, **9**, 73–9
30. Zweens, J., Frankena, H. and Zijlstra, W. G. (1974) Decomposition on freezing of reagents used in the ICSH-recommended method for the determination of total haemoglobin in blood, its nature, cause and prevention. *Clin. Chim. Acta*, **91**, 337–52
31. Vanzetti, G. and Franzini, O. (1972) Improved reagents and concentrated reference solutions in haemoglobinometry. In *Modern Concepts in Haematology* (eds A. Izak and S. M. Lewis), pp. 44–53. London: Academic Press
32. Matsubara, T., Okuzono, H. and Tamagawa, S. (1972) Proposal for an improved reagent in the hemiglobincyanide method. In *Modern Concepts in Haematology* (eds A. Izak and S. M. Lewis), pp. 29–43. London: Academic Press
33. Van Kampen, E. J. and Zijlstra, W. G. (1983) Spectrophotometry of hemoglobin and hemoglobin derivatives. *Adv. Clin. Chem.*, **23**, 199–257
34. Eilers, R.J. and Crocker, C. (1972) The value of Ringbom curves in haemoglobinometry. In *Modern Concepts in Haematology* (eds A. Izak and S. M. Lewis), pp. 58–65. London: Academic Press
35. Chaplin, H. Jr and Mollison, P. L. (1952) Correction for plasma trapped in the red-cell column of the haematocrit. *Blood*, **7**, 1227–38
36. England, J. M., Walford, D. M. and Walters, D. A. W. (1972) Re-assessment of the reliability of the haematocrit. *Br. J. Haematol.*, **23**, 247–56
37. Sirs, J. A. (1968) The measurement of the haematocrit and flexibility of erythrocytes with a centrifuge. *Biorheology*, **5**, 1–14
38. England, J. M. and Down, M. C. (1975) Determination of the packed-cell volume using ^{131}I-human albumin. *Br. J. Haematol.*, **30**, 365–70

39. Helleman, P. W. (1972) Chemical and physical aspects of electronic cell counting. In *Modern Concepts in Haematology* (eds A. Izak and S. M. Lewis), pp. 164–80. London: Academic Press
40. Crossland-Taylor, P. J. (1982) The micro-PCV. In *Advances in Haematological Methods. The Blood Count* (eds O. W. van Assendelft and J. M. England), p. 85. Boca Raton: CRC Press Inc.
41. ICSH Expert Panel on Blood Cell Sizing (1980) Recommendations for reference method for determination by centrifugation of packed cell volume of blood. *J. Clin. Pathol.*, **33**, 1–2
42. Karlow, M. A., Westengard, J. C. and Bull, B. S. (1989) Does tube diameter influence the packed cell volume? *Clin. Lab. Haematol.*, **11**, 375–83
43. England, J. M. and Down, M. C. (1976) Measurement of the mean cell volume using electronic particle counters. *Br. J. Haematol.*, **32**, 403–9

Chapter 4

Principles of quality assurance

Quality assurance is relevant to all aspects of patient care and is increasingly subject to scrutiny by the process of medical audit and accreditation.

Quality assurance in clinical laboratories is well established and can be defined as 'the activity of a laboratory to ensure reliability of test results, interpretation and relevance to clinical practice'. This demands the application of *internal quality control* (IQC) programmes and participation in *external quality assessment schemes* which can include aspects of education and training.

Internal quality control (IQC)

IQC is the set of procedures undertaken by the staff of a laboratory for continuous monitoring of operation and results, in order to decide whether the results are reliable enough to be released.

Since all measurements are subject to error, satisfactory IQC programmes should enable laboratories to measure, predict, calculate and control the variation in any measurement. A satisfactory programme involves the activities of setting standards, appraisal of performance, remedial action as necessary and retrospective analysis of errors to prevent recurrence. Indeed, IQC should be primarily designed to *prevent* errors as well as *detect* errors.

IQC does not start with the receipt of a specimen in a laboratory and finish with despatching a result. It includes positive identification of the patient, preparation of the patient, e.g. ensuring a fasting state for certain investigations, sample collection and quality, i.e. the *pre-analytical phase*, as well as analytical procedures, reagent quality, performance of equipment, standards and controls – the *analytical phase*, and reporting and ensuring the correct result is with the correct patient or the *post-analytical phase*. This concept has been termed *total quality control*.

The major day-to-day process of IQC is the monitoring of reproducibility and precision, to satisfy predetermined requirements by means of standards/reference preparations and controls and by the use of statistical procedures.

Definitions [1,2]

Accuracy: is the measure of agreement between the estimate of a value and the true value. It is measured as the amount, or degree, of inaccuracy.

Inaccuracy: numerical difference between the mean of a set of replicate measurements and the true value. This difference may be expressed in the units (positive or negative) in which the quantity is measured, or as a percentage of the true value.

Precision: agreement between replicate measurements. It has no numerical value but is recognized in terms of imprecision.

Imprecision: standard deviation (SD) or coefficient of variation (CV) of the results of a set of replicate measurements.

Examples of the concept of accuracy and precision are shown in *Figure 4.1*.

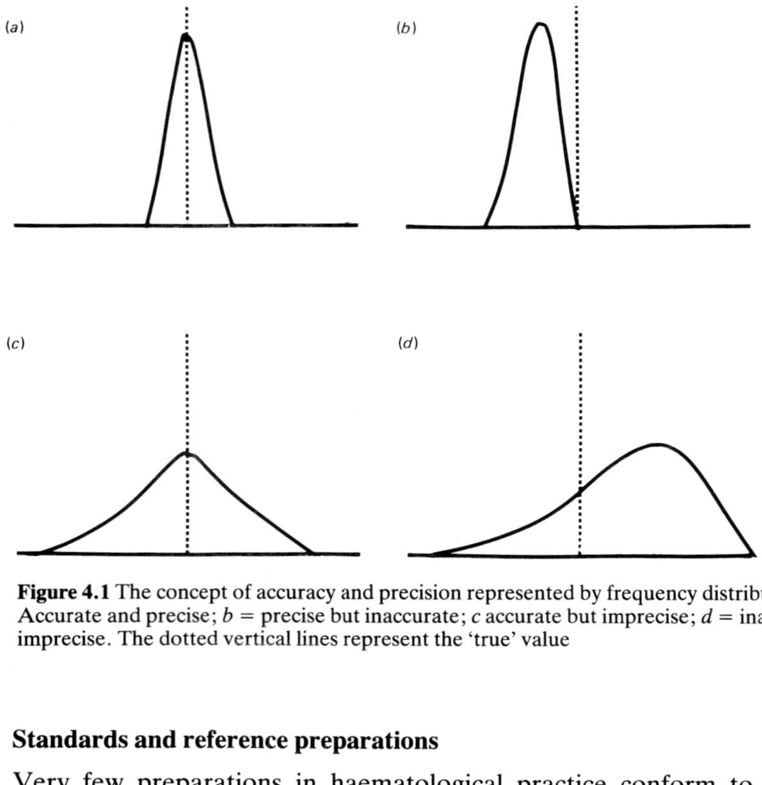

Figure 4.1 The concept of accuracy and precision represented by frequency distribution curves. *a* = Accurate and precise; *b* = precise but inaccurate; *c* accurate but imprecise; *d* = inaccurate and imprecise. The dotted vertical lines represent the 'true' value

Standards and reference preparations

Very few preparations in haematological practice conform to the criteria of a primary analytical standard. However, biological standards can have national or international status, a precisely defined content, long-term stability and be assigned an international unit of content or activity. When a preparation does not fulfil these criteria it may be accepted as a reference preparation. Reference preparations have values assigned by reference methods, usually by repeated testing by selected laboratories. They may be available as cell or particle suspensions, as lyophilized serum or plasma, haemolysates, etc., and are used for calibration or reference purposes.

Control preparations

These are ideally identical in nature to the samples being tested. There is no requirement for having preassigned values and they are used to monitor precision by assessing variance from the mean of a set of replicate measurements. Stability of the value(s) of a control preparation is a desirable objective.

Techniques of internal quality control

As previously stated the objective is to produce results of high validity to the clinician by *prevention* of poor quality rather the *correction* of poor quality. Investigations in haematology may provide *quantitative* or *qualitative* data.

Control of quantitative tests

Standardization or *calibration* is by the use of standard or reference preparations. It is desirable, and often essential, to employ standards at different levels throughout the measured range particularly when calibration is not linear. *Control* samples are used to determine the confidence limits (SD or CV) of a method and are included at intervals or from batch to batch to detect instrument, reagent or operator failure or to detect instrument or method 'drift'. With some techniques or instruments the control value may be affected by 'carry-over' from the previous specimen and therefore the control sample should be processed twice and the second value taken to be the more 'correct'.

Statistical and graphical representation of control data

Determination of confidence limits

At least 20 determinations are made on the control sample. The frequency distribution of the values should be plotted. If the distribution is 'normal' (Gaussian), standard deviation is calculated from the formula:

$$s = \sqrt{\frac{(\sum x - \bar{x})^2}{N - 1}}$$

where s = standard deviation, x = observed value, $\bar{x}$ = mean of observed values and N = number of determinations. With normal distributions 68% of values will fall within 1SD, 95% within 2SD and 99.7% within 3SD. Confidence limits of ±2SD are usual; only one in 20 determinations can be expected to fall outside this range. If there is a systematic tendency to lower or higher values the distribution will be 'skewed' and conventional calculation of SD will be misleading (*see* page 78).

Presentation and assessment of control data

The data from control samples can be plotted directly as a Levey–Jennings plot which shows the ±2SD confidence limits (*Figure 4.2*). When the control value lies within these limits the technique is considered to be 'under control'. On average one result in 20 can be expected to fall outside the 2SD limits and should be repeated. The chance against the repeat result falling outside the limits is 400 to 1 *if the estimation is still in control.*

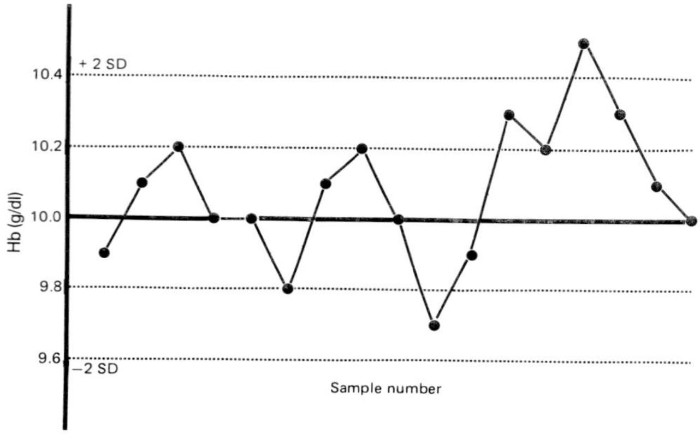

Figure 4.2 Levey–Jennings plot of control haemoglobin values. All values are within ±2SD except number 14 which might be expected once in every 20 values

The cumulative sum (Cusum) technique

This is the running total of a series of control values expressed as their difference from the arithmetic mean value of the control and taking into account their sign. The mean is subtracted from the control result and the value plotted. Subsequent differences of the control values from the mean are added to the preceding Cusum taking account of the sign and plotted. Thus, if the control values fluctuate about the mean, the Cusum will remain around zero with a horizontal plot. If the control values are consistently greater than the mean the graph will show a marked rise and conversely if consistently less will show a rapid fall. The data in *Table 4.1* are plotted by the Cusum technique in *Figure 4.3*. The results are plotted on 1 cm square arithmetic paper with each control sample at 1 cm intervals on the horizontal axis; 2 cm on the vertical axis is approximately 2SD. There is no significant trend in the cumulative values until sample 11, after which the plot rises. Precise evaluation of the Cusum is essential in determining whether the change of slope is significantly greater than 2SD which indicates a significant loss of accuracy. The use of a 'V mask' will provide a rapid and exact assessment of the Cusum [3]. With the graph scale described above and with a 'V' with an angle of 27 degrees and the line OP = 2.6 cm (*Figure 4.4*), if the control mean changes by 2SD the line joining the points of the Cusum will cut either arm of the 'V' (*Figure 4.5*).

Table 4.1 Repeated haemoglobin measurements on a control sample*

Measurement	*1*	*2*	*3*	*4*	*5*	*6*	*7*	*8*	*9*	*10*	*11*	*12*
Hb value	10.0	9.8	10.2	10.2	10.0	10.0	9.8	10.3	9.7	10.4	10.4	10.4
Difference from mean	0	−0.2	+0.2	+0.2	0	0	−0.2	+0.3	−0.3	+0.4	+0.4	+0.4

* Mean haemoglobin value = 10 g/dl

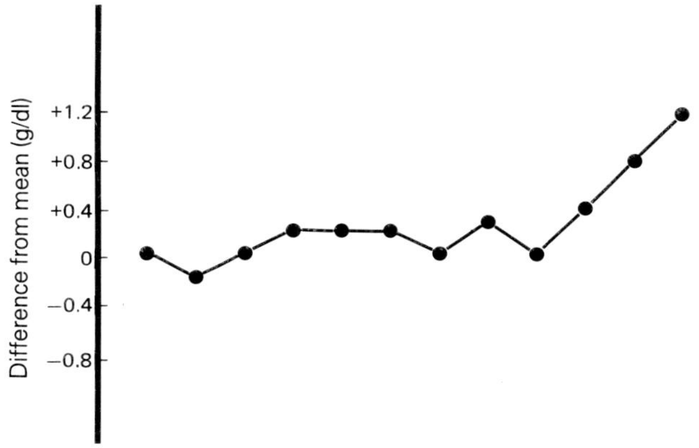

Figure 4.3 The data shown in *Table 4.1* plotted as a Cusum graph. There is no significant trend in the graph until samples 11 and 12. (Not drawn to scale)

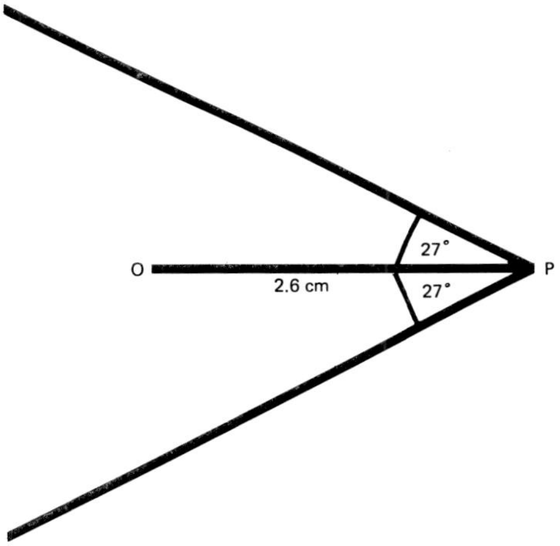

Figure 4.4 The construction of a 'V mask' for the assessment of significant trends in Cusum graphs constructed on the scale detailed in the text. (Not drawn to scale)

The 'two-sample' or Youden plot[4]

This method may be employed when two control samples of different content are assessed by the same method, or alternatively when one control sample is tested by two different methods. The standard deviation of each control or for each method is determined and the graph prepared by showing the mean and 2SD range of sample A on the abcissa and similarly for sample B on the ordinate (or methods A and B as appropriate) (*Figure 4.6*). Some adjustment of a scale may be necessary to obtain comparable presentation of the ±2SD ranges. The normal distribution of the values for A and B will fall on the diagonal dotted line. Points away from the diagonal, though within the square, indicate loss of precision and points outside the square indicate loss of accuracy (out of control). If the points are identified by their sequence of testing, any systematic tendency to 'drift' towards loss of control will be recognized.

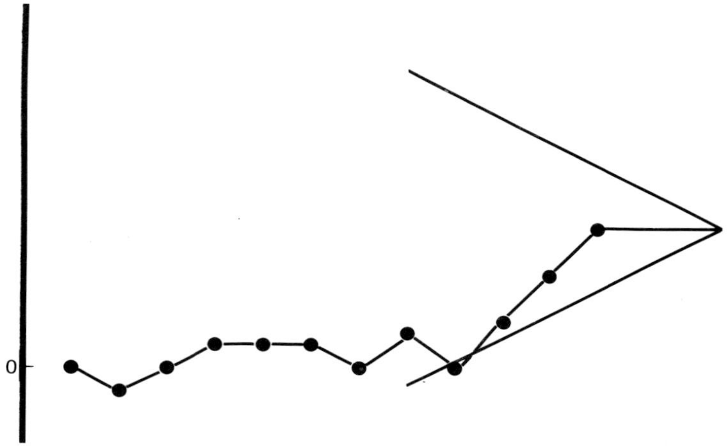

Figure 4.5 The 'V mask' applied to the Cusum graph shown in *Figure 4.3*. An arm of the 'V' cuts the graph, which indicates a significant loss of accuracy

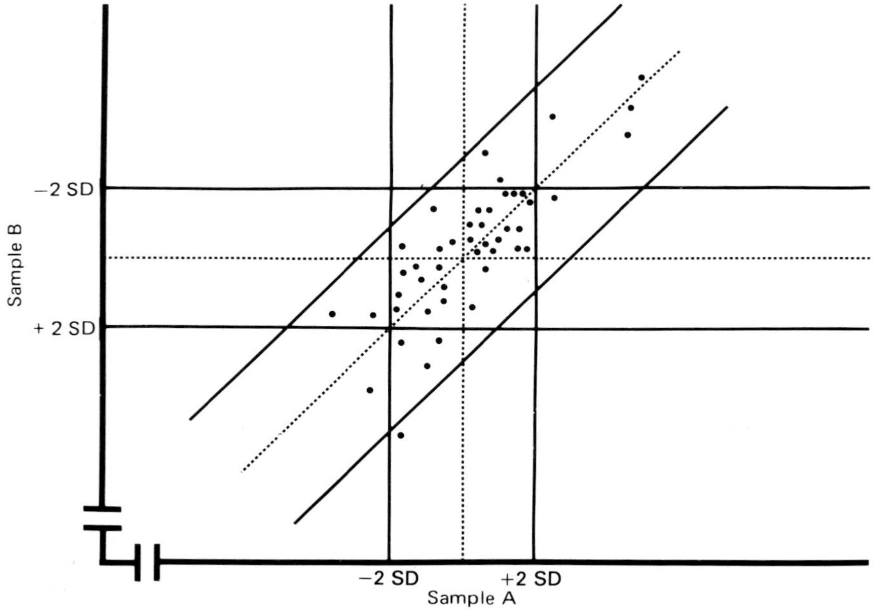

Figure 4.6 A 'two-sample' or Youden plot. For explanation, see text

Use of test results

Daily means

The arithmetic means of a series of large random samples will be similar. For example, the mean of all haemoglobin values determined in one day may be expected to be similar to the previous day's mean values, provided the method is under control. In practice, despite using very large numbers of samples, even up to several hundred each day, the variation in the source of the samples from day to day results in the standard deviation of the daily mean being too great. For example, samples from an antenatal, leukaemia, or thalassaemia clinic on any day would significantly lower the mean value for that day; conversely, to include the results from a polycythaemic group could sufficiently increase the mean value, making any consideration of whether the method was in control unreliable. To overcome such influences of the samples, only results falling within a restricted range (truncated range) are included in the analysis. For instance if haemoglobin values only between 12 and 17 g/dl are included, a series of daily mean values can be obtained from which the standard deviation can be calculated with narrow confidence limits. The 'daily mean' technique is too time consuming for manual processing but may be employed when data are computed 'on-line' with the instrumentation. It is inevitably a retrospective analysis and should be considered as additional to the use of control samples rather than being applied in isolation.

Batch means

When control preparations are not readily or cheaply available, the principle of 'batch mean' can be employed. Microbiological or radioisotopic assay of vitamins, one-stage prothrombin results for the control of anticoagulant therapy, plasma viscosity values or even ESR measurements are examples. Again a truncated range may be necessary to obtain meaningful results.

Bull [5,6] has suggested that the development of a 'robust estimator of the mean' can be used with as few as 20 samples per batch by incorporating information from the preceding batch of 20 samples. This has a 'smoothing effect' on the distribution of the data and is the principle underlying the calculations of a 'running mean' or 'moving average' which, together with the use of truncated values, is claimed to be able to detect loss of calibration of as little as 1%. The 'moving average' or Bull algorithm ($\bar{X}\beta$) was developed for the quality control of the red-cell parameters using the indices of MCV, MCH and MCHC produced by automated analysers and has been incorporated into the quality control software of such instruments. Not only will the $\bar{X}\beta$ value show loss of calibration ($>\pm3\%$ of mean indices) but the pattern of the displayed values for the indices can indicate the possible cause of the loss of control [5].

Advantages of the use of the $\bar{X}\beta$ include the use of fresh blood (patients' samples), the inherent stability of the mean indices, it is economical, involves frequent monitoring and preserved blood controls may be insensitive to instrument drift.

The use of the algorithm requires certain conditions to be met and has limitations:

1. The majority of samples must have normal indices. If not, randomization of samples is necessary, e.g. renal, neonatal, haematology and cytotoxic clinics or wards will, or may have, mean values which readily result in deviation $>3\%$ of the mean values.
2. The procedure controls instrument calibration drift and does not control or measure analytical precision.
3. The shifts detected by $>\pm3\%$ of the mean indices are greater than can be recognized by plotting results of a control sample as a Levey–Jennings plot and are certainly less sensitive than the Cusum technique.

4. 'Out of control' mean indices are more likely to be due to non-randomization of samples than loss of instrument calibration.
5. Blood counting is not confined to red-cell parameters.

Use of modal values

An alternative to determining the mean value of samples is the use of the modal value. The modal value of a sample population is stable and is not affected by the abnormal results which must be excluded when calculating the daily mean. The application of modal values to the quality control of automated blood counting has been described[7]. The claim that changes of as little as 0.1 g/dl in haemoglobin concentration or 0.02×10^{12}/l of red cells can be readily detected appears to be justified. It is emphasized that before using this approach it is necessary to establish the day-to-day stability of the modal values for a particular laboratory and during this period conventional quality control must be performed.

Use of samples from the previous day or previous batch

Retaining and re-testing samples from the previous day or previous batch is a procedure that has been advocated[8]. The technique can only be applied to parameters that are stable during storage. In the case of routine blood examination this will exclude the derived red-cell parameters dependent upon it. If results are examined critically the leucocyte and platelet counts are also not suitable, leaving only the haemoglobin and red-cell count. For other estimations any deterioration of samples due to exposure to light or by freezing and subsequent thawing would also be unsatisfactory. Slight progressive deterioration within the confidence limits of the method are not readily demonstrated and there appears to be no advantage in this approach, if adequate control preparations are available, other than economics.

Random errors

The techniques of quality control described above are designed to prevent errors of a *systematic* nature. More difficult to detect and potentially more serious are *random* errors. Indiscriminate erroneous reports can result from operator error, wrongly identified samples or by transcription errors. Undetected clots, sample carry-over, lipaemia, agglutination, haemolysis and spasmodic instrument fluctuation are other causes of random error and can be difficult to detect or prevent. An ideal way to detect random errors would be to re-test every sample after re-identification and changing the sequence of testing, followed by careful re-examination of the sample for clots, and for haemolysis and lipaemia after sedimentation. Such a procedure is clearly out of the question in most instances due to work load, time and cost. Four approaches are described to reduce the occurrence of random errors.

Further examination of samples

The poor quality of an individual sample is a frequent cause of isolated error. The commonest cause is probably the presence of undetected clots[9]. Straining of samples through a fine gauze after completing the investigations is a sensitive method of detection. Lipaemia, either endogenous or due to intravenous lipid infusion, may be observed after cell sedimentation as may the presence of haemolysis. When using automated analysers lipaemia and haemolysis may be suspected by aberrations in related parameters[10] as may the presence of agglutination due to cold agglutinins.

Duplicate testing of random samples

Carstairs[11] described the effect of instituting duplicate testing of random samples. The re-testing of about 5% of the daily work load reduced the incidence of random errors from 1.3% to 0.15% during a 4-year period. This was achieved by several measures including control samples at fixed intervals of less than 30 samples, introducing a formal operational log for instrumentation, revising transcription procedures, ensuring proper mixing of samples and revising the work allocation of personnel together with an awareness by staff that random checks were being made.

The difference between duplicates can be displayed in graphical form. The difference is calculated, given a positive value, and plotted on a chart showing 95% confidence limits, i.e. only 1 in 20 duplicate determinations should exceed the control limits.

Confirmation by related investigations

Microscopy of a stained blood film is routine practice. An experienced observer can estimate leucocyte and platelet count with reasonable assurance and any obvious discrepancy studied further. An absence of platelets in the film may be due to unsuspected clots in the sample as may a lymphopenia; the lymphocytes are unable to migrate from the clot. A low haemoglobin value without any abnormality in red-cell morphology suggests 'short-sampling'.

By comparison with previous results

The practice of relating data from previous samples to current results using computer storage, retrieval and display, by retrieval from a card index or by cumulative numerical or graphical display provides a further safeguard against random error. This procedure can be formalized using the concept of 'delta checks'[12]. Delta checking requires the establishment of limits beyond which the validity of a value is challenged. The limits must include analytical variance and physiological variation, to which can be added clinical significance. A laboratory can set its own limits for each parameter, e.g. for the blood count, WBC >25% of previous result, Hb >1 g/dl, MCV >2 fl. Limits can be set in coagulation testing, vitamin assays, plasma viscosity and so on. The procedure can be readily incorporated into the programmes of on-line data handling coupled with storage of patient records. Any unexpected or unexplained fluctuation should warrant a repeat determination and if confirmed a further sample should be obtained. This form of protection against random error may also be initiated at ward or clinic level.

External quality assessment (EQA)

Definition

This is a system of objectively checking laboratory results by an external agency. The checking is necessarily retrospective and comparison of performance with that of other laboratories is notified at a later date. The main objective of EQA is to establish between-laboratory comparability.

Format

EQA usually takes the form of distributing specimens, usually two or more, to participating laboratories who return the data to a central agency for assessment and subsequent return of the analysis to the participant with a consensus result, i.e. the survey or 'trial' approach.

Alternatively or additionally an 'inspectorate' approach can be adopted in which specimens are brought to the laboratory by an individual who observes the investigation of the samples and assesses the results by comparison with those obtained by a reference laboratory using a reference method.

A requirement for all EQA schemes is that the samples should be treated as if they were patient's samples, not necessarily handled by the most experienced members of staff, or assayed in replicate and a mean value submitted. An advantage of the 'inspectorate' method is that unlike the 'survey' schemes, the inspector can ensure that specimens are examined as part of the routine work pattern.

EQA may be international, national, regional or at a local level but the number of participants should not be less than 20 and may number several thousand. The inevitable delay in assessing the survey is minimized when the number of participants is relatively small but at the cost of less valid and limited conclusions.

Participation in EQA programmes may be voluntary or compulsory. In some countries, compulsory participation and satisfactory performance are the basis for accreditation or licence to practice. A lesser, though important sanction may be loss of approval for training.

Although the objective is essentially to achieve comparable performance between laboratories, additional valuable information regarding instrument performance or validity of methods can be obtained.

A requirement for EQA is that the material distributed must be stable during distribution to participants. Much of the organization of EQA surveys is in the development of suitable test materials.

Most, if not all, national EQA schemes (NEQAS) include assessment of performance which, as mentioned above, may be the basis for accreditation or licence to practice. It follows that there must be confidence not only in the scientific basis and operation of the scheme, but also in the assessment of performance.

Assessment

Assessment of performance may be based on comparison of participants' results with values or results obtained by a number of reference laboratories. Alternatively, comparison can be made with the mean or median of the values returned by the participants or, in the case of qualitative results, the consensus of the findings. The 'consensus mean' is the most widely used approach but is open to the criticism that the consensus value of *all* participants will be subject to bias depending on the number using a particular instrument, method or even reagent.

Current practice is to allocate participants to particular instrument, method and reagent groups and to determine a consensus for each group. This may result, however, in groups with insufficient data to be statistically valid, and furthermore may result in minority groups abandoning perfectly satisfactory procedures in order to be 'in consensus'. Differences between groups may be more apparent than real and reflect characteristics of the survery material rather than revealing unsatisfactory procedures.

Historically, assessment of 'satisfactory performance' and consequently the designation of 'poor or unsatisfactory performance' has been based on three approaches:

1. A statistical approach to *quantitative* data based on calculation of standard deviation or coefficient of variation from a consensus value.
2. *Qualitative* assessment by correct or incorrect results, for example, positive or negative results in screening for Hb S, identification of an abnormal Hb fraction or screening for enzyme deficiency *or* by assessment of clinical significance as low, borderline, normal or high.
3. A combination of the above, i.e. statistical analysis together with assessment of significance, e.g. assay of cobalamin and folate, G6PD or Hb A_2.

Statistical analysis of quantitative data [13]

Depending on the distribution of the data, the mean ($\bar{x}$) or population median (m) is determined. The median is particularly useful when the distribution is non-Gaussian and it is less affected by outlying results. For the blood count surveys of the NEQAS in haematology in the UK (UK NEQAS(H)), the median value is determined from which the percentiles which include 50% of data are used to derive the CV and a 'deviation index':

$$\text{Deviation index (DI)} = \frac{\text{Test result} - \text{median}}{\text{Standard deviation}}$$

The DI indicates how far a test result differs from the median as a multiple of the SD.

Variance index (VI) may be used instead of deviation and performance is compared with the best performance obtainable with a particular method:

$$\text{VI} = \frac{\text{V}}{\text{CCV}} \times 100$$

where CCV = chosen coefficient of variation calculated from the best performance by a routine laboratory under service conditions or by a referee under ideal conditions.

A value for the DI is used to determine poor performance. As the DI is based on the SD, one in 20 results can be expected to be >2DI and only when a participant exceeds this value for the same parameter on several occasions should the designation of 'persistent poor performance' be applied.

For some parameters a DI >3 is currently used to identify poor performance. This is unsatisfactory for two reasons. In a survey involving 1000 participants only three would fall outside >3DI which brings into question the validity of the exercise and, secondly, the range of values within 3DI can span the reference range of a parameter and the range of interpretation from 'low' to 'high'. Furthermore, it does nothing to encourage improvement in performance. On the other hand, the overall performance in a survey may be excellent with ±2DI well within the range of clinical relevance and 'poor performance' may be assigned when a laboratory is providing acceptable, clinically relevant results.

A further scenario is that a laboratory continues to provide reliable results and 'satisfactory performance' but due to an overall improvement in the performance of participants, perhaps due to the introduction of a new analyser, the laboratory may become 'poor performers' although their own performance has not deteriorated.

Alternative approaches to assessment

Peer comparison with statistical analysis is not the only way to evaluate quantitative data. Limits for acceptable performance or 'target values' may be based on physiological variation, a percentage of the reference range and clinically significant differences. Each of these approaches results in narrowing the acceptable limits of some parameters and widening others. Overall, however, they represent more meaningful assessment of performance. *Table 4.2* shows a comparison of alternative methods of determining acceptable limits of performance compared with the ±3DI limits of UK NEQAS(H)[14].

Table 4.2 Comparison of alternative methods of determining acceptable limits of performance with the >3DI limit of UK NEQAS(H)

	Hb	*RBC*	*MCV*	*WBC*	*Platelets*
Reference range					
10%	N	N	N	N	N
15%	W	N	N	W	N
Tonk's formula*	W	W	N	W	N
Physiological range	N	N	N	N	N
Clinical significance	W	S	N	W	N

* Tonk's formula: ± reference range × 0.25/mean reference value × 100
W = wider; N = narrower; S = same

Persistent poor performance

Statistical analysis based on SD, DI, VI or CV should result occasionally in results being outside defined limits. Criteria for categorization of 'persistent poor performance' (PPP) vary between different EQAS but in general depend on consecutive poor performance or poor performance in a defined number of surveys. Consideration should be given to the frequency of a survey. Poor performance in two out of three or three out of five surveys is acceptable if they are distributed at monthly intervals. When only four or even two surveys are performed each year, the criteria of PPP should be set accordingly. Non-participation in a survey for which a laboratory is registered should be considered as poor performance.

Hazardous performance

Qualitative tests often have a clear, correct or incorrect result of clinical importance; for example, blood group, testing for Hb S, detection of malaria parasites in a blood film. The results of certain quantitative tests may be of vital clinical significance, e.g. platelet count, factor VIII assay, tests for control of treatment such as the prothrombin time. In these circumstances incorrect results can have serious consequences and therefore even a single incorrect result in a survey should be designated as 'hazardous' and require contact between the scheme organizer and the participant.

The future of EQAS

There is no doubt that external assessment will continue and will expand. The present system in the UK of voluntary participation will probably be replaced by compulsory participation and satisfactory performance for the accreditation of a laboratory. The current code of confidentiality between the scheme organizer and a named contact in a participating laboratory must be relaxed to include senior managers and executives.

From a scientific viewpoint, the 'state of the art' is well within the limits of clinical relevance for certain parameters, and striving for further improvement in performance is unjustified and would not be cost-effective. Unfortunately there remain tests and parameters for which performance is alarmingly poor and not only those which are less commonly performed or for which surveys are infrequently carried out. There are also some tests which, overall, show poor performance and have not improved significantly over many years despite being identified by regular surveys.

A prerequisite for participation and satisfactory performance in external quality assessment is an adequate programme of internal quality control.

References

1. International Committee for Standardisation in Haematology (1984) *ICSH Handbook*
2. England, J. M. (1986) Internal quality control and calibration. In *Automation and Quality Assurance in Haematology* (eds R. M. Rowan and J. M. England), pp. 1–17. Oxford: Blackwell Scientific Publications
3. Cavill, I. and Ricketts, C. (1974) Automated quality control for the haematology laboratory. *J. Clin. Pathol.*, **27**, 757–9
4. Skendzel, I. P. and Youden, W. J. (1969) A graphic display of inter-laboratory test results. *Am. J. Clin. Pathol.*, **5**, 161–5
5. Bull, B. S. (1975) A statistical approach to quality control. In *Quality Control in Haematology* (eds S. M. Lewis and J. E. Coster), pp. 111–22. London: Academic Press
6. Bull, B. S. and Korpman, R. A. (1982) Intralaboratory quality control using patients' data. In *Quality Control* (ed. I. Cavill), pp. 121–50. Edinburgh: Churchill Livingstone
7. Prangnell, D. R. and Johnson, P. H. (1977) A new method of quality control for the Coulter Model S Counter. *J. Clin. Pathol.*, **30**, 487–91
8. Cembrowski, G. S., Lunetsky, E. S., Patrick, C. C. and Wilson, M. K. (1988) An optimised quality control procedure for hematology analysers with the use of retained patients' specimens. *Am. J. Clin. Pathol.*, **89**, 203–10
9. Lessels, S. E., Allardyce, M. and Davidson, R. J. D. (1977) Unwanted clots in the haematology department. *Med. Lab. Sci.*, **34**, 359–60

10. Lessels, S. E., How, J., Allardyce, M. and Davidson, R. J. D. (1978) Hyperlipaemia and distortion of the red cell profile. *Med. Lab. Sci.*, **35**, 389–92
11. Carstairs, K. C. (1977) Development and description of the 'random duplicates' method of quality control for a haematology laboratory. *Am. J. Clin. Pathol.*, **67**, 379–85
12. Nosanchuk, J. S. and Gottmann, A. W. (1974) CUMS and delta checks. *Am. J. Clin. Pathol.*, **62**, 707–12
13. Lewis, S. M. (1986) External quality control in Europe. In *Automation and Quality Assurance in Haematology* (eds R. M. Rowan and J. M. England), pp. 18–61. Oxford: Blackwell Scientific Publications
14. Hall, R. (1988) Current NEQAS surveys in haematology. In *Quality Control and Assurance in Clinical Laboratories. Three Years On* (ed. A. D. Farr), pp. 95–100. London: Institute of Medical Laboratory Sciences

Chapter 5

Preparation, staining and examination of blood films

Preparation of blood films

Routine morphological study of blood cells by light microscopy ideally requires the cells to be evenly distributed in a monolayer with a minimum of distortion. Until recently this has been difficult to achieve and blood films prepared by the 'wedge' technique have provided the basis for the accumulated knowledge of blood-cell appearances in health and disease. The introduction of automated instrumentation for blood-film examination by image analysis has been associated with preparation of 'spun' films. Earlier techniques using cover-slips are rarely employed.

Wedge films

Clean slides are essential. Suitable slides are available commercially, otherwise thorough cleaning followed by immersion in alcohol and polishing is necessary. The ideal film should occupy about half the length of the slide with margins within the width of the slide. The thickness of the film will decrease from 'head' to 'tail'. Excessively thin films will distort red-cell morphology, with a tendency to accumulate leucocytes at the margins and the tail. Thick films will have insufficient area where the red cells are spread without overlapping, and leucocyte morphology will be obscured.

A 'spreader' with a perfectly smooth edge and of a width rather less than the width of the slide is essential. Slides with polished margins are available, and a suitable width can be obtained by breaking 0.5 cm from the width. The thickness of the film is determined by the volume of blood, the angle of the spreader and the speed of spreading. A small drop of blood either directly from a skin puncture, from the tip of the venepuncture needle or by transfer from an anticoagulated sample is placed on the slide about 2 cm from one end. The spreader is placed on the slide in front of the drop of blood and drawn backwards to touch the drop to allow the blood to run along the width of the spreader by capillary attraction. The spreader is held between thumb and forefinger at an angle of about 30 degrees and with one smooth movement pushed along the slide to leave a film of blood. The film should be dried rapidly by waving the slide vigorously or by placing in a stream of cool air; heat is not normally used.

Thicker films can be produced by increasing the angle of the spreader and the speed of spreading, and vice versa to produce thin films (decreasing the angle and spreading slowly). The ability to produce satisfactory films from samples of varied cellularity is an essential skill. A number of gadgets, mechanical devices and automated instruments have been devised for preparing wedge films and have found variable acceptance. Usually films may be stained as soon as they are obviously dry, but thicker films may require a half-hour or more to dry thoroughly which is essential to avoid the cells being washed off during staining.

Spun films

Attempts to produce a monolayer blood film have gained impetus from the requirement of automated blood film analysers for sufficient numbers of leucocytes free from distortion and unnatural staining, and similarly for red cells without overlapping or loss of morphology due to excessive thinness of the film. These requirements can be achieved by equipment that rapidly rotates a slide on which a drop of blood has been placed; the thickness of the film is arbitrarily controlled by the time of spinning. Alternatively, a more sophisticated control of thickness can be achieved with a photoelectric device. Though cell morphology is generally good, certain blood-film changes that are of value in interpretation may be lost, e.g. rouleaux formation due to paraproteinaemia, autoagglutination and the characteristic rupturing of lymphocytes in chronic lymphocytic leukaemia. There is also a tendency to induce red-cell distortion. These possible disadvantages may be considered to be outweighed by the uniform quality of the spun films.

Thick films

This form of film preparation is used exclusively for the demonstration of malarial parasites which may be very scanty. The objective is to enable a larger volume of blood to be examined relatively quickly. A large drop of blood is spread into an area about 1 cm square, or a similar sized circle, and allowed to dry. A suitable thickness will just allow print to be seen through the film. It is *absolutely essential* that the film is completely dry before staining. This may take 2–3 hours at room temperature or about 30 minutes at 37°C. Temperatures up to 60°C may be used, shortening the drying time to 5 minutes. Films are stained unfixed and a partly dried film will be readily washed off the slide.

Concentration of nucleated cells (buffy-layer films)

Occasionally it is an advantage to prepare films of concentrated nucleated blood cells. Atypical and immature cells are found in small numbers in normal blood from adults and more frequently in neonatal blood samples. In certain disorders, however, characteristically abnormal cells may be demonstrated, for example, megaloblasts in pernicious anaemia and related disorders, erythrophagocytosis in certain autoimmune haemolytic anaemias and the presence of LE cells in systemic lupus erythematosus. Leucopenic blood samples can be processed to produce sufficient leucocytes for easier cytochemical assessment. The techniques of cell separation and concentration have also been used to demonstrate tumour cells in blood[1]. Centrifugation or sedimentation techniques may be used, but in the context of cell morphology the sedimentation techniques are less satisfactory. It must be remembered that any technique involving centrifugation will itself cause separation of the nucleated cells into layers because of their different densities. This could result in misrepresentation of the relative proportions of different cell types.

Centrifuge technique

Defibrinated or anticoagulated blood is suitable, though the agitation of the blood during defibrination causes cell distortion. On the other hand, platelets are removed during defibrination, which allows a 'purer' leucocyte preparation. Up to 10 ml of blood is centrifuged for 15 minutes at 1500 *g*. Most of the supernatant plasma or serum is removed using a Pasteur pipette and the topmost layer of cells together with some plasma is transferred to one or more Wintrobe haematocrit tubes and again centrifuged for 15 minutes at 1500 *g*. The 'buffy-layer' of leucocytes and other nucleated cells is carefully removed with a Pasteur pipette and transferred to a slide. After gentle but thorough mixing a series of films are made in the usual way and allowed to dry thoroughly before staining. This technique is rapid and simple requiring no special equipment or reagents.

Sedimentation techniques

The aim of these methods is to yield red-cell free leucocyte preparations. They usually use an additive, such as dextran, Ficol or methyl cellulose [2]. Density gradient solutions can be used to separate the different types of leucocytes.

'Wet films' or cells suspended in plasma

Techniques based upon the examination of blood cells suspended in plasma with or without the addition of supravital dyes had a considerable vogue in the early years of diagnostic haematology. Examination by direct, dark-ground and phase-contrast microscopy have been used and the motility of leucocytes and their precursors has been described in detail. With certain exceptions the 'wet preparation' adds little to modern diagnostic haematology, though valid applications are the demonstration of parasites (*see* pages 519, 521), the induction of red-cell sickling (*see* page 374) and the study of red cells by Nomarski interference microscopy after fixation in glutaraldehyde. Glutaraldehyde fixation is performed by adding 1 volume of blood to 10 volumes of 0.25% glutaraldehyde (10 ml/l of 25% glutaraldehyde) in isotonic phosphate buffer, pH 7.4.

Fixation of blood films

The purpose of fixation is to preserve cell structure and prevent disruption by subsequent procedures. Cell metabolism is halted by protein precipitation which also prevents lysosomal enzymes from inducing autocatalytic changes. Depending upon the procedures to be adopted, methanol, ethanol–formaldehyde and acetone are commonly used, sometimes at 4°C to ensure better preservation of cell enzymes. Unnecessarily prolonged fixation may eventually affect enzyme activity. The choice of fixative influences the optimum pH for subsequent staining; pH 6.8 is best for methanol-fixed films while formaldehyde fixation demands a lower pH. Unfixed films for malarial parasites stain better at pH 7.2.

Staining of blood films

The morphology of cells in blood and bone-marrow films is usually studied by light microscopy after staining with Romanowsky-type dyes. The most commonly used are those described by Leishman, Wright, May–Grunwald and Jenner, the last two being combined with Giemsa's stain.

Most workers profess a preference for a particular stain and technique, but there is little evidence that one stain is superior to another for routine purposes. Haematologists have long been aware, however, that stains from different manufacturers may show striking differences in quality of staining which may be apparent between different batches of the same stain from the same source!

The introduction of automated staining of blood films has highlighted stain variation and emphasized the need for standardization. This is particularly important for automated cell-recognition systems. Romanowsky-type stains are *compound dyes*, i.e. two or more dyes are mixed and interact to produce a new compound often with additional staining properties. Romanowsky dyes are also *neutral stains*, so-called because the compound dye is obtained by mixing an acid dye with a basic dye. Such stains are often insoluble in water when in equilibrium. Alcoholic solutions do not stain well and are used in 'on-slide' techniques which allow preliminary fixation by the alcoholic solvent. After dilution with water, dissociation of the acid and basic components occurs to produce the characteristic stained appearances which are very sensitive to pH.

Romanowsky mixed eosin and methylene blue solutions are stained at once. It was deduced that some compound dye was formed and it was noted that the quality of staining was variable and that methylene blue with a 'surface scum' gave good results. Nocht and Unna selected 'decomposed' or 'polychromed' methylene blue and obtained good results. Jenner mixed fresh methylene blue and eosin, collected the precipitate, the compound dye, which he dissolved in a solvent. Reuter and Leishman combined the techniques of Nocht and Jenner by mixing eosin and polychromed methylene blue and dissolved the precipitate in methanol. Wright's stain differs from Leishman's only in the technique of oxidizing the methylene blue.

The crux of producing a satisfactory stain is the oxidation of the methylene blue. Giemsa controlled the oxidation procedure to produce azure I (synonyms: azure B, methylene azure Bernthsen) to which he added methylene blue and eosin Y and dissolved the mixture in methanol with glycerol as a stabilizer. The controlled oxidation of the methylene blue and resulting uniformity of product gained Giemsa's stain its reputation as the stain of choice but there is little to choose between good examples of Leishman, Wright and Giemsa stains for routine blood films.

The International Committee for Standardization in Haematology (ICSH) have defined a Romanowsky stain as [3]: 'The stain consists of a mixture of the cationic dye azure B and the anionic dye eosin Y, in aqueous solution, in a ratio ranging from 6.5 to 7.3, with the two dyes acting separately or in conjunction on appropriately pre-treated biological substrates, to give a typical staining pattern which depends on the chemical and physical condition of the substrate'. The typical and unique staining pattern is the colour purple imparted to cell nuclei in contrast to the blue staining of the cytoplasm and the pink-orange colour of the erythrocytes.

Three mechanisms are involved in producing the characteristic staining of blood cells:

1. Coulombic attraction between dye and tissue substrate.
2. Metachromasia of azure B.
3. Dye–dye interactions between azure B and eosin Y.

Coulombic attractions are between molecules carrying opposite electrostatic charge. Thus a cationic dye is attracted to an acid substrate and an anionic dye to basic groups. Metachromasia depends on the property of certain dyes to form polymers which result in a colour change of the polymer. The colour purple seems to be the result of specific interactions between two molecules of azure B and one of eosin Y[4].

Thus the characteristic appearances of Romanowsky-stained structures in blood are: pink erythrocytes, purple chromatin, blue leucocyte cytoplasm, purple-black basophil granules, red-pink eosinophil granules, fawn to lilac neutrophil granules, purple platelet granules and blue nucleoli, with reticulocytes staining their characteristic polychromatic shades.

A commercial stain that has proved reliable over many years is powdered Leishman's stain from British Drug Houses which when dissolved in neutral methanol (solvent methanol BDH) has given consistently excellent results from batch to batch.

ICSH have published a reference method for staining blood and bone-marrow films by azure B and eosin Y[3] which is described below. It has been made possible by the relatively recent availability of purified dyes.

ICSH reference method

Preparation of staining solution

Azure B (comparable to C.I. 52010)

This dye must be the major fraction of any candidate material. It should comprise not less than 95% of the total dye content as demonstrated by chromatography and spectrophotometry. Purity is expressed by molar extinction coefficient, e = 85 000–94 000 (λ_{max} 641 nm)/M × cm; molecular mass of the dye cation, 270.24. This dye is available commercially as the thiocyanate and in other salt forms.

Eosin Y (C.I. 45380)

Purity of the dye is expressed by the molar extinction coefficient, e = 105 000 (λ_{max} 517 nm)/M × cm; molecular mass of the disodium salt, 691.9. Commercially available as the disodium salt or eosinic acid. In commercial samples of eosin Y, e should not be less than 85 000/M × cm^{-1}.

Azure B–eosin Y stock solution

3 g of azure B-thiocyanate and 1 g of eosin-disodium salt are dissolved in 1 litre of a methanol-dimethyl sulphoxide (DMSO) mixture. Dissolve the azure B by adding 400 ml of DMSO to the dye at 37 °C and ensure complete solution. Add 1 g of eosin Y to 600 ml of methanol, await complete solution of the dye then slowly mix the azure B-DMSO with the eosin-methanol. The stock solution is stable for about 3 months at room temperature if stored in a glass bottle in the dark and tightly stoppered when not in use. Increased stability can be achieved by lowering the pH to 3.5 by adding 80 µl of 1 mol H_2SO_4 to 100 ml of the stock solution.

Staining solution

The staining solution is prepared by mixing appropriate amounts of stock solution with buffer solution having a pH near neutrality; pH 6.8 is recommended for routine use but pH 7.2 is suggested for staining malarial parasites. A ratio of 1:15 stain to buffer is recommended.

Within certain limits the choice of buffer is discretional; HEPES buffer at a concentration of 10 mmol/l in distilled water is sufficient for maintaining pH with maximum stability [5]. The concentration may be increased to 100 mmol/l when the stock solution is pH 3.5 though stability may be decreased. Phosphate buffers may also be used but a low molarity should be specified as high concentrations of buffer ions can compete with the dyes for biological binding sites; 1.32 mmol/l is suitable.

Staining technique

1. Dry blood or bone-marrow films in air.
2. Fix by immersion in the stock solution for 5 minutes. Alternatively if staining is to be delayed, prefix in methanol for 5–10 minutes.
3. Rinse the fixed films briefly in distilled water.
4. Dilute the stock stain 1:15 in HEPES buffer pH 6.8, to which has been added 50 ml/l DMSO to delay precipitation of the stain.
5. Stain for 25 minutes or 35 minutes for bone-marrow films.
6. Rinse briefly in distilled water and dry in air.

Notes

1. The staining solution should be as fresh as practical.
2. Decay of staining capacity is indicated by blue nuclei rather than purple due to precipitation of eosin Y by azure B. The formation of precipitate makes the diluted solution unsuitable for further staining.
3. The addition of DMSO improves stability to over 4 hours.
4. When large batches of films are being stained, the staining solution should be changed at intervals.

Additional note

The methanol should be neutral, which implies freedom from acetic acid produced in the distillation process, and must also be water-free.

Preparation of Leishman's stain (commercial)

1.5 g of dried Leishman's stain (BDH) is dissolved in 1 litre solvent methanol (BDH) with the aid of agitation and if desired by warming to 50°C. Although Romanowsky dyes dissolved only in methanol are less stable than those dissolved in glycerol-methanol, the large volumes used and consequent rapid turnover makes deterioration an unlikely problem. The stain may be used at once.

Staining

'On-slide' technique

The slide is flooded with 1 ml of undiluted stain and left for 3 minutes. This is a combined fixation and partial staining period. 3 ml of phosphate buffer, pH 6.8 1.32 mmol/l is added, gently mixed, and left for 10 minutes. The stain is *washed off* (not tipped off) with buffer and allowed to differentiate for 1 minute. The slides are air dried and mounted if desired.

Sequential automatic staining

Multi-station machines are a great advantage in processing large numbers of slides in batches. A suitable timing cycle is 3 minutes in undiluted stain, 20 minutes in stain diluted 1 in 10 in phosphate buffer, pH 6.8, and 1 minute differentiation.

Notes

1. The combined fixation-staining stage is essential for good results. Pre-fixation in methanol followed by diluted stain does not produce similar appearances.
2. The 1 in 10 stain–buffer mixture is not only more economical, but when combined with a longer staining time produces better results than a lower dilution and shorter staining time.
3. Bone-marrow films are best stained by the 'on-slide' technique with extended fixation and staining to allow for the varied and usually increased cellularity.

Progressive automatic staining

Staining machines of this type follow the procedure of 'on-slide' staining, i.e. each slide is individually though automatically processed. Although not as economical as batch staining the process is not affected by the possibility of gradual 'exhaustion' of pre-mixed staining solution and eventual deterioration of staining quality.

Staining of thick films

The principle of staining thick films is that immersion of the unfixed, perfectly dry film in aqueous dyes will stain the parasites and liberate the haemoglobin from the red cells to allow the stained parasites to be seen readily. Field's method is a rapid technique using solutions of polychromed methylene blue and eosin either separately or in mixture, for a few seconds, with washing in water to elute excess dye and haemoglobin.

The use of diluted Giemsa's stain is also recommended, the unfixed film being immersed in diluted Giemsa followed by washing in buffer. Stain residue may be minimized by the use of 0.9% NaCl. Leishman's stain diluted 1 in 10 is also recommended.

Apart from being rapid there appears to be little advantage in Field's technique and for large numbers of films it is inconvenient. The diluted Giemsa or Leishman methods employ routine stains and can be used in association with sequential staining machines by placing the slides directly into the diluted stain.

Rapid staining of blood films

'On-slide' staining techniques take as little as 7 minutes to complete using standard stains. Whether the demand for more rapid staining is justifiable is debatable. Nevertheless the concept of a dip-technique completed in a few seconds has been supported and can be based on the Field's stain methodology. The results are usually inferior to standard methods and as such the advantage of saving a few minutes at the expense of quality does not appear justified.

Quality control of Romanowsky staining

Quality control of Romanowsky stains and staining in the haematology laboratory has been mainly empirical and based on the subjective assessment of the stained films. Progress in the purification of the essential components of a satisfactory stain as described earlier, and their assessment by thin-layer chromatography[6,7], allows preliminary selection of suitable dyes or final staining products.

Examination and interpretation of blood films

The morphology of blood cells in stained films is the basis of laboratory diagnosis of haematological disorders. A careful examination of a well-spread and stained film by an experienced observer can be more informative than a series of investigations.

A systematic approach to blood-film examination should be encouraged. Before embarking on microscopical examination the naked-eye appearance can be useful. Films showing a bluish tinge may reveal 'background' staining due to abnormal plasma proteins or gross leucocytosis, the latter being more noticeable at the edges and tail of the film. Examination with dry objectives is facilitated by cover-slip mounting or by spraying with vinyl. Alternatively, a thin film of immersion oil may be spread over the film. Preliminary examination at low magnification (about × 100) is useful. The number and distribution of leucocytes can be seen as can the presence of platelet clumps found normally in the tail of films prepared from fresh blood. Rouleaux formation or autoagglutination is readily seen at low magnification.

For routine assessment of red-cell morphology, leucocyte recognition and morphology and the numbers of platelets and their appearance, a magnification of approximately × 500 is best. This may be achieved with a 'dry' × 40 objective but a × 50 oil-immersion lens is preferred. A 2 mm (× 100) oil-immersion lens producing a final magnification of about × 1000 may be used for close study of structures in cells, the recognition of parasites and for counting reticulocytes.

A full report on blood-film appearances will include the size, shape and stained appearances of the red cells together with the possible presence of inclusions. Some important structures are not seen in Romanowsky-stained films and supravital staining is necessary for reticulocytes, Heinz bodies and precipitated Hb H. Leucocyte examination includes the differential leucocyte count, the presence of immature cells, changes associated with bacterial or virus infections and nuclear and cytoplasmic abnormalities whether inherited or acquired. Platelet numbers may be assessed in films of blood anticoagulated with EDTA. The presence of platelets of unusual size should be noted together with the number of granules and the presence of vacuoles.

Low-power appearance

In a well-spread film leucocytes are reasonably evenly distributed throughout the film though there is a tendency for cell types to predominate in particular areas. Neutrophils tend to be carried to the edges and tail leaving lymphocytes in higher numbers in the body of the film. If spreading is delayed or an uneven spreader is used this phenomenon is exaggerated to the point that an accurate differential count is impossible. Some degree of rouleaux formation is inevitable during drying of the film and if films are too thick or drying prolonged, rouleaux may extend almost to the tail of the film. Gross rouleaux may occur in the best-made films in the presence of paraproteins (*Figures 5.1* and *5.2*). Autoagglutination (*Figure 5.3*) is readily distinguished from rouleaux formation. Rarely, tumour-produced mucin may be seen in metastatic adenocarcinoma[8].

Routine examination

Using the × 50 oil-immersion objective an area of the film is selected where the red cells are just separated. In thick areas red-cell morphology cannot be seen and

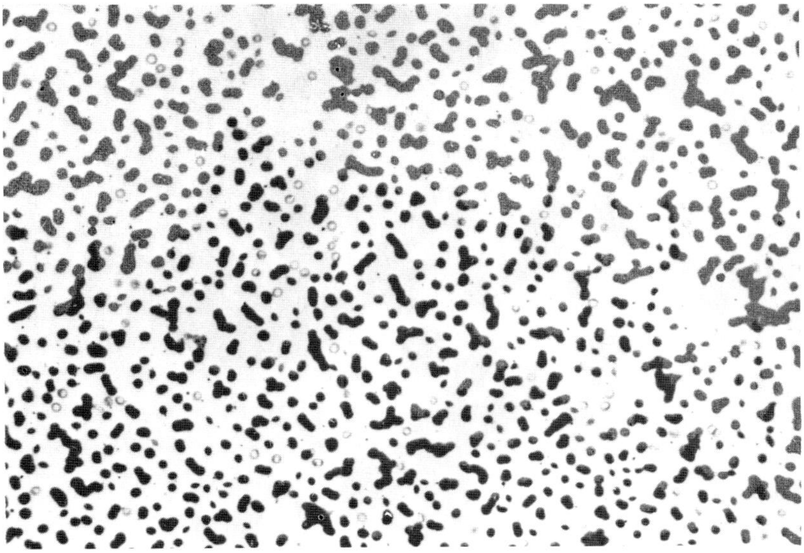

Figure 5.1 Blood film, with rouleaux formation due to paraproteinaemia. ×110

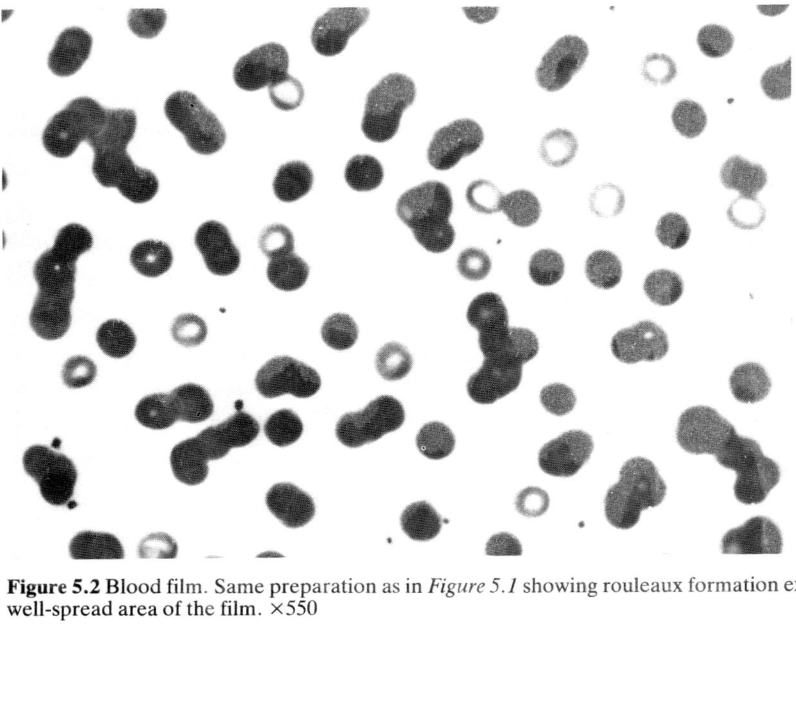

Figure 5.2 Blood film. Same preparation as in *Figure 5.1* showing rouleaux formation extending to a well-spread area of the film. ×550

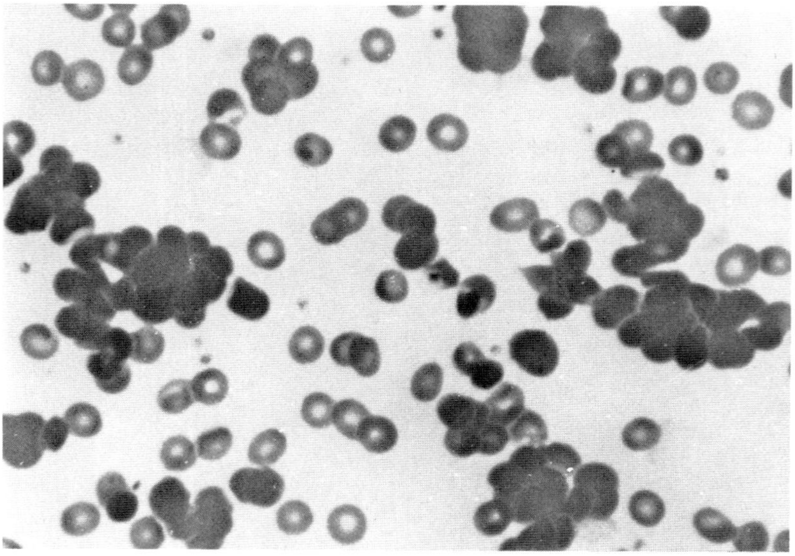

Figure 5.3 Blood film. Agglutination due to cold autoagglutinins. The appearances are clearly different from rouleaux formation. ×550

leucocytes are condensed and their morphology obscured. Towards the tail of the film red cells tend to assume false appearances; variations in shape are lost and cell thickness increases.

Red-cell morphology

The terminology used to describe red-cell appearances is derived largely from the Greek language as is the greater part of medical terminology. In some instances, however, descriptive terms in English are usual even though Greek derivations are available, e.g. 'sickle-cell' rather than 'drepanocyte' and 'target-cell' instead of 'leptocyte'. Usage of terminology may be cumbersome or convenient. For example, to write a report that 'red cells vary in size and shape' is simpler than 'red cells show anisocytosis and poikilocytosis' or even 'anisopoikilocytosis', but in the restricted space of a blood report form 'aniso-' is more convenient than 'variation in size'.

In health red cells are said to be *normocytic*. They are circular with only a very small proportion having an irregular outline and have a narrow range of size distribution around a mean diameter of about 7.2 μm. The haemoglobin stains with the eosin component and, owing to the biconcavity of the cell, stains more palely at the centre. This depth and distribution of staining is described as *normochromic*. Normal red cells are shown in *Figure 5.4*.

Abnormalities of red cells may be: (1) due to abnormal erythropoiesis; (2) acquired or induced in the circulation; (3) characterized by the presence of immature red cells in the blood. A convenient classification based on appearance are abnormalities of (a) size, (b) shape, (c) stain intensity or distribution, and (d) presence of inclusions.

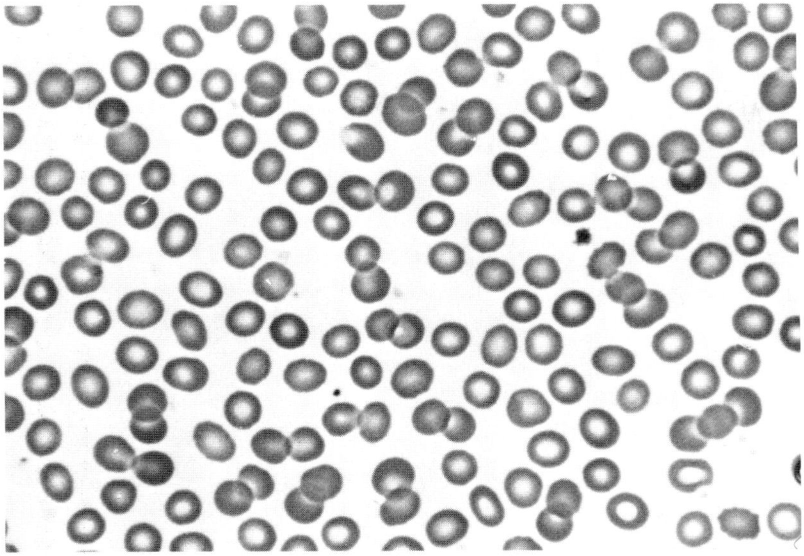

Figure 5.4 Blood film. Normal red cells. The cells are mainly circular with little variation in diameter. The area of 'central pallor' reflects the biconcave cross-section. ×550

Abnormalities in size

Macrocytes

These may be defined as cells with a diameter greater than 8 μm (*Figure 5.5*). It must be remembered that macrocytosis in the blood film does not necessarily mean that the cells have an increased volume. This is particularly important in the context of the measurement of MCV. Obvious macrocytosis in the film may be seen in blood with a normal MCV and is due to the cells being thinner than normal and is usually associated with a 'target-cell' appearance (*see* page 146). Macrocytes are usually the result of abnormal erythropoiesis but may also be due to modification of the cells in the circulation.

Microcytes

These are red cells with a diameter less than 6.4 μm and are usually associated with a reduced MCV (*Figure 5.6*). They are formed either as microcytes in the marrow or may be due to fragmentation of red cells in the circulation. Microcytes formed in the bone marrow contain less haemoglobin, are therefore thinner and stain palely. Those caused by fragmentation may stain palely, normally or often deeply. As in the case of macrocytes the altered diameter may still be associated with a normal MCV in which case the cells must be of a thickness greater than normal and will stain more deeply without 'central pallor'.

Anisocytosis

These are red cells of unequal size. This is the most common abnormality of red cells (*see Figure 5.5*). The variation in diameter is greater than between normal cells and may be marked. Anisocytosis is found in almost all red-cell disorders and is

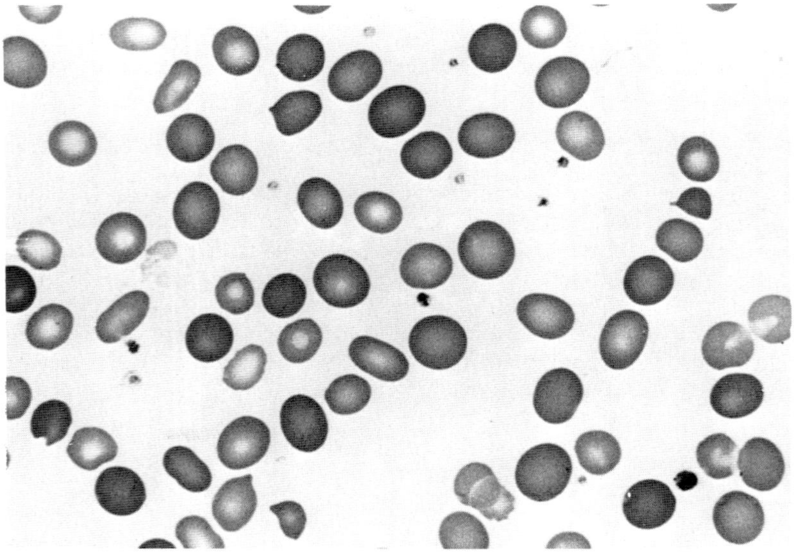

Figure 5.5 Blood film. The average cell diameter is greater than normal, or *macrocytic* (cf. *Figure 5.4*). *Anisocytosis*, increased variation in red-cell diameter, is also present and the picture may be described as showing *macroanisocytosis*. Also present is *anisochromasia* or variation in the intensity of staining. ×550

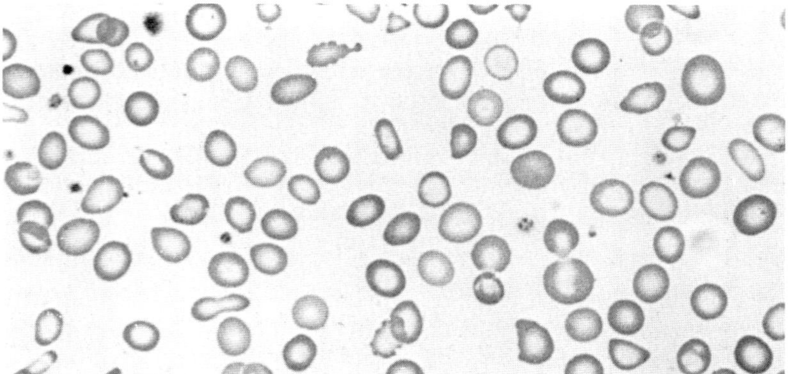

Figure 5.6 Blood film. The diameter of the red cells is decreased (cf. *Figure 5.4*) or *microcytic*. They are also *hypochromic* or pale-staining due to being thinner than normal. Some variation in shape, or *poikilocytosis*, is present. ×550

therefore non-specific. When the overall red-cell size is larger or smaller than normal the prefixes macro- or micro- may be used. Again it should be noted that marked anisocytosis may occur which, if distributed around the normal modal value, will give a normal MCV.

Abnormalities in shape

Poikilocytosis is the term used to denote abnormalities in shape. Its use is usually confined to changes in the outline of the red cell but can also be applied to red cells which, although circular in outline, do not have the normal biconcave cross-section, e.g. spherocytes, leptocytes and stomatocytes (*see* page 146). Although poikilocytosis describes any alteration in shape, in many instances the shape change is characteristic and descriptive terms are used. Poikilocytosis may be due to inherited structural or metabolic defects, abnormal erythropoiesis or by modification of cell shape in the circulation.

Poikilocytes with altered outline

Elliptocytes Oval and elliptical cells are found in a wide variety of red-cell disorders. The classic situation is in hereditary elliptocytosis when almost all the red cells are oval or elliptical to some degree (*Figure 5.7*). In megaloblastic anaemia oval macrocytes are characteristic. Large numbers may be seen in iron deficiency and are also a feature of myelofibrosis.

Tear-drop poikilocytes (dacryocytes) This characteristic appearance (*Figure 5.8*) is a feature of myelofibrosis or other conditions where the bone marrow is replaced by non-haemopoietic tissue and when associated with extramedullary erythropoiesis.

Sickle cells (drepanocytes) Sickle-shaped cells (*Figure 5.9*) coming to a point at each end are found only when the intracellular Hb S is in high concentration, i.e. in homozygous Hb S disease. Sickling is a reversible phenomenon associated with de-oxygenation of the haemoglobin, but in sickle-cell anaemia a variable population of red cells show irreversible sickling. Intermediate degrees of sickling are seen as rod-shaped elliptocytes, 'boat' shapes and 'oat' cells (*Figure 5.9*).

Red-cell fragmentation (schistocytes) Red-cell fragmentation may produce a variety of shapes. The fragments themselves are small and often appear spherical, triangular or irregular (*Figure 5.10*) and are usually the result of extreme physical or mechanical stress. The 'parent cells' from which fragments have been removed tend to become spherical, deeply staining and to have an irregular outline. The distorted spherocyte (*Figure 5.11*) gives the appearance of having had part of the cell 'torn out' or 'bitten' and is typical of drug or chemical damage or haemoglobin instability. The 'burr-cell' (*Figure 5.12*) as originally described[9] is probably the result of red-cell fragmentation, though a mechanism based on vacuole formation and rupture has been suggested[10]. The term has unfortunately been applied to other appearances, which has caused confusion.

Crenation Red cells showing numerous short, symmetrical projections are referred to as being crenated (*Figure 5.13*). This shape change has been extensively

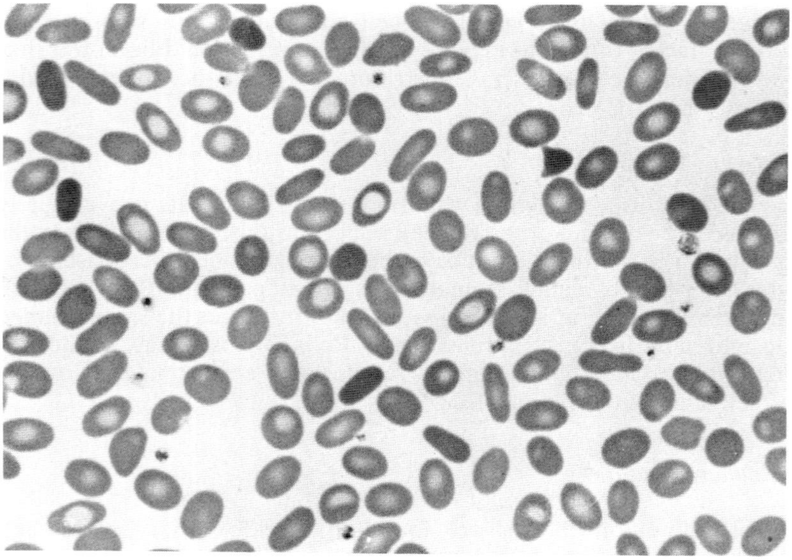

Figure 5.7 Blood film. Elliptocytosis. Virtually all the red cells are elliptical or oval. ×550

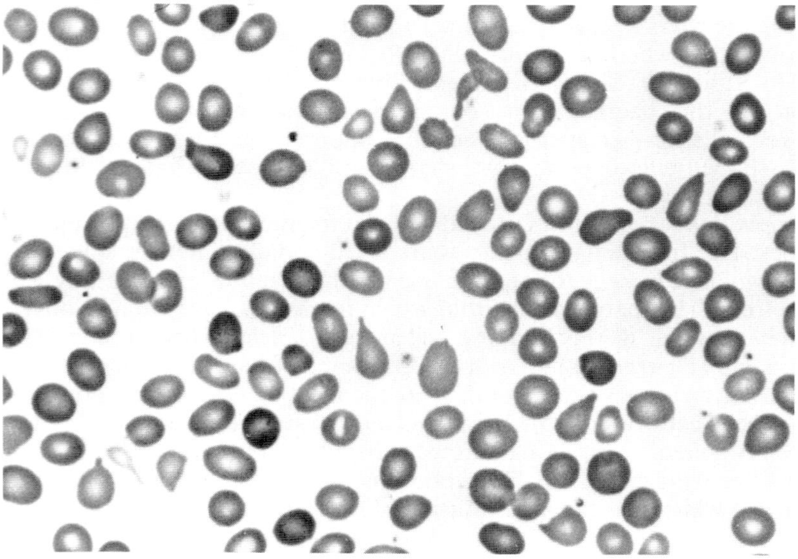

Figure 5.8 Blood film. Tear-drop poikilocytes in a case of myelofibrosis. ×550

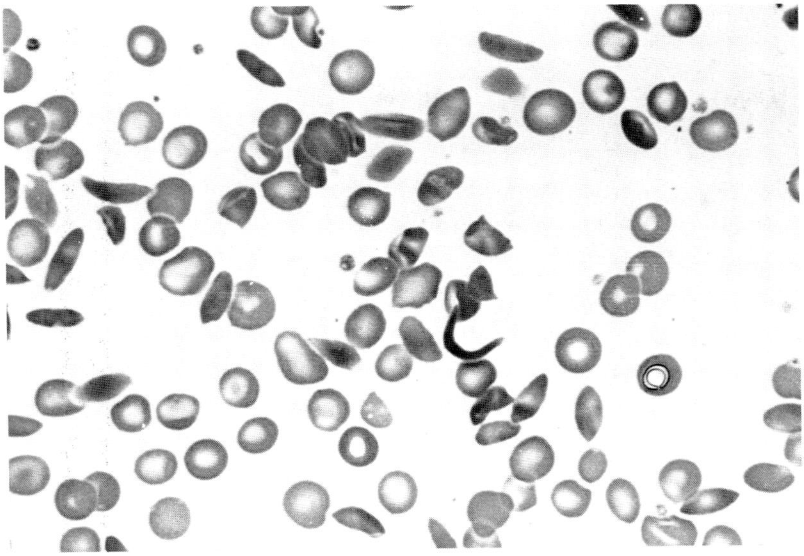

Figure 5.9 Blood film. Sickle cells (drepanocytes). Frequent 'boat' and 'oat-cell' shapes are present but only one true sickled cell. ×550

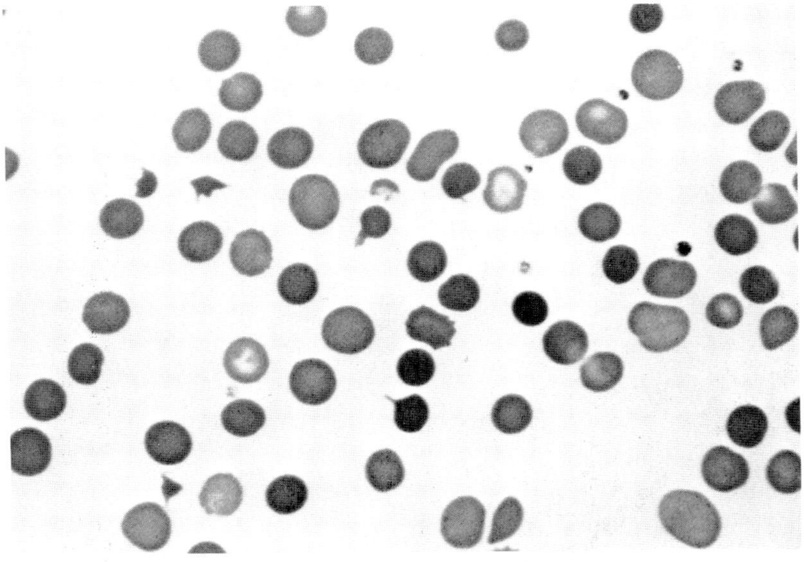

Figure 5.10 Blood film. Red-cell fragments (schistocytes). Several irregular red cells and fragments are shown. The deeply staining cells are spherocytic. Anisocytosis is obvious. ×550

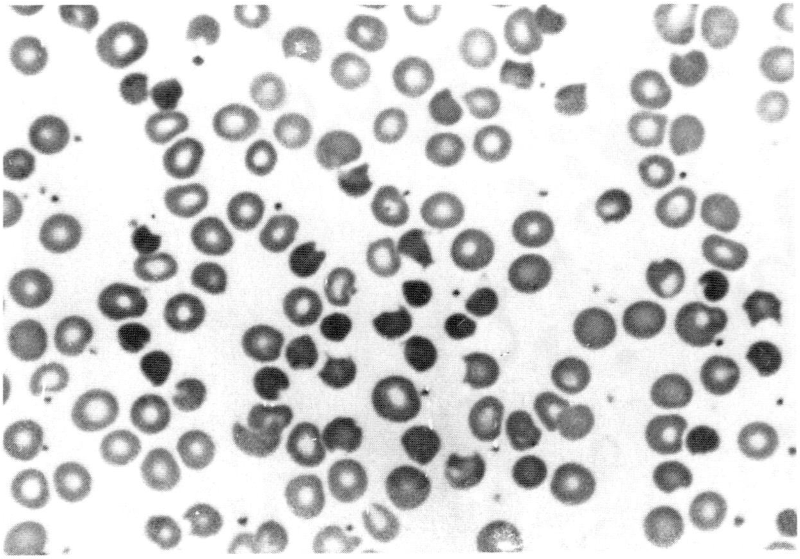

Figure 5.11 Blood film. Distorted red cells which are also spherocytic in a case treated with the oxidant drug 'dapsone'. The 'bitten' or 'torn-out' appearance is typically associated with haemoglobin denaturation and Heinz-body formation. ×550

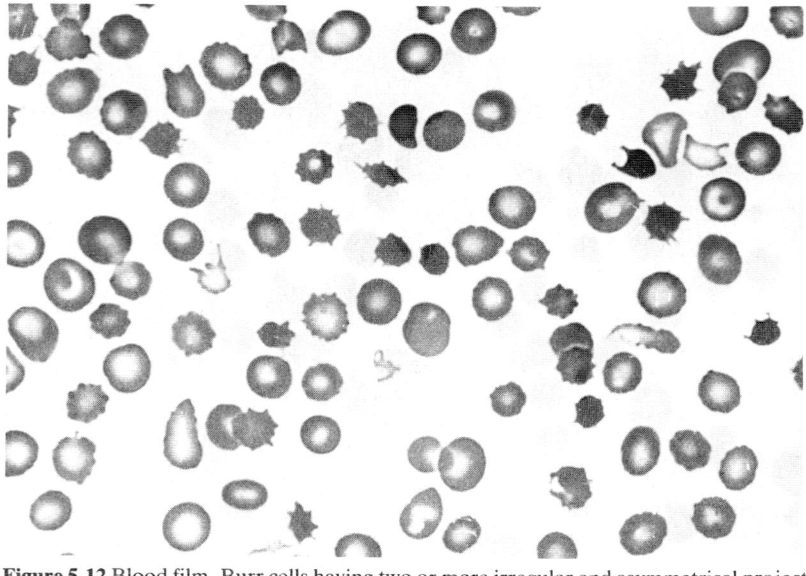

Figure 5.12 Blood film. Burr cells having two or more irregular and asymmetrical projections. The tendency of some of the cells to be spherocytic suggests loss of membrane. The cells with irregular but more symmetrical projections have specific designations (*see Figures 5.13* and *5.14*). ×550

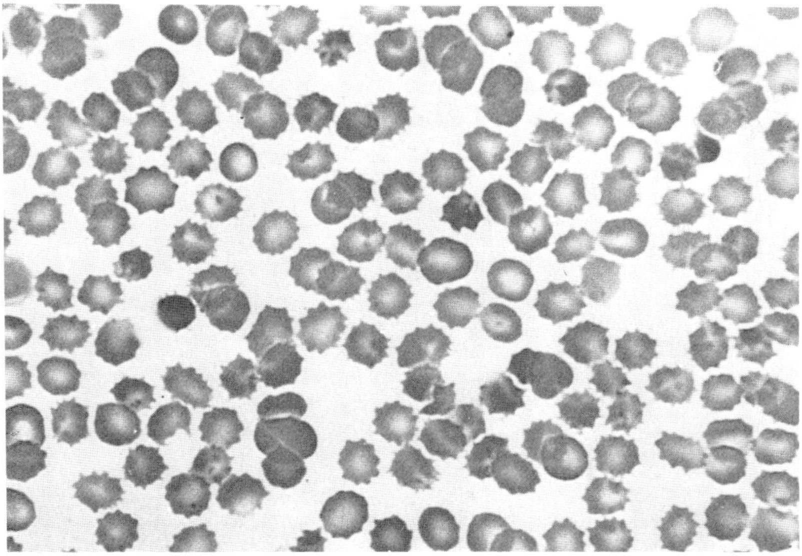

Figure 5.13 Blood film. Crenation. The majority of the red cells show multiple, short, symmetrical projections. ×550

studied and has many causes. It is probably the most common artefact in blood films and is consistently found in blood samples that have been stored for some hours at room temperature. Contact with glass surfaces induces crenation, particularly in cells washed free of plasma and is possibly due to a raised pH due to alkalinity of the glass. The addition of oleic acid and lysolecithin consistently produces crenation. The term echinocyte is suggested[11] and using the scanning electron microscope (SEM) the cell is seen as having 10–30 evenly distributed spicules of equal length. Though crenation is often an artefact it can occur *in vivo* in a variety of disorders[12], including gross electrolyte imbalance. Crenation is a stage in the transformation from disc to sphere and *in vitro* can be reversed as long as the cell has not lost surface area due to loss of membrane. The distinction between marked crenation and other cells with multiple projections has important diagnostic implications but can be difficult.

Acanthocytes (spiny cells) (*Figure 5.14*) Using SEM, these cells are defined as having 5–10 spicules of irregular distribution and unequal length[13]. In the blood film this definition is less easy to apply, and the term is often used loosely to include the cells distorted due to fragmentation, and irregular cells with rounded projections. The description of 'spur-cells' further complicates the terminology[14]. The classic association of acanthocytes is with abetalipoproteinaemia and is due to abnormal membrane lipids in which the lecithin content is markedly decreased[15]. The changes in red cells induced by splenectomy can certainly be described as acanthocytes and small numbers may be seen in a variety of disorders and may all be due to alteration of membrane lipids. An association with the McLeod phenotype of the Kell blood group system has been reported[16], and with the In (Lu) phenotype[17].

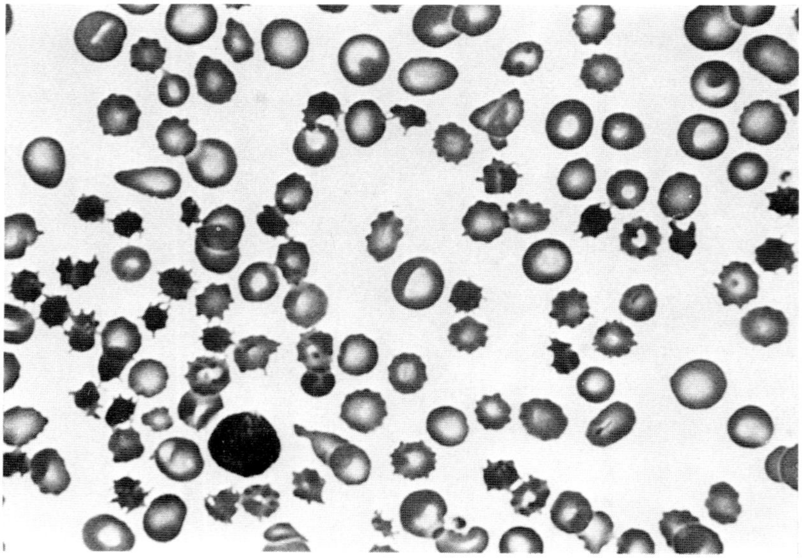

Figure 5.14 Blood film. Acanthocytes. Many red cells show 8–12 pointed projections. The tendency to spherocytosis suggests loss of membrane. Typical crenated cells are also present with some cells appearing to be intermediate between crenated and acanthocytic forms. ×550

Rhytiocytes (wrinkled cells) Irregular cells with undulating margin or long, rounded projections (*Figure 5.15*). In some films the changes appear to show progressive alteration eventually resulting in spherocytic acanthocytes. The lesser changes are found in untreated hypothyroidism [18], starvation [19], old age, heart disease and occasionally in pregnancy. The appearances may reflect subtle changes in membrane lipids.

Poikilocytes with circular outline
Deviation from the normal biconcave form can be recognized by altered staining appearances.

Spherocytes Loss of biconcavity and progression to a sphere is seen initially by loss of 'central pallor' and ultimately as a dense-staining (hyperchromatic) cell which has a smaller diameter than normal – the typical microspherocyte (*Figure 5.16*). The degree of spherocytosis may be slight or marked and often contrasts sharply with the non-spherocytic reticulocytes that are usually present. Spherocytosis may be hereditary or acquired but whatever the aetiology microspherocytosis is associated with loss of surface area (membrane) and usually results in shortened red-cell survival. In the hereditary form the spherocytosis develops after the reticulocyte stage and is due to abnormality of the cytoskeleton and is associated with lipid loss and excessive Na^+ flux across the membrane. A similar picture may be seen in antibody-mediated haemolytic anaemia. Chemicals or bacterial toxins may have a direct effect on the membrane causing gross spherocytosis. Smaller numbers of spherocytes are seen in a variety of haemolytic mechanisms due to mechanical or physical factors.

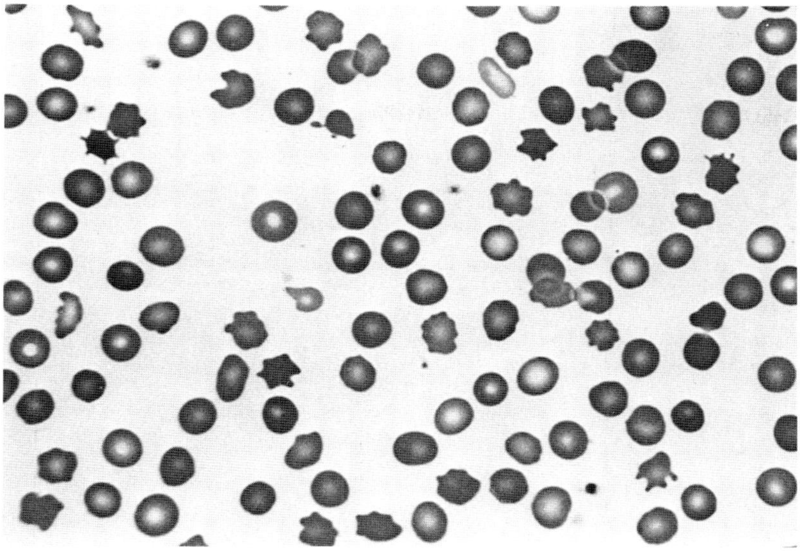

Figure 5.15 Blood film. Irregular cells with rounded projections are shown with stages suggesting progression to a typical acanthocyte. ×550

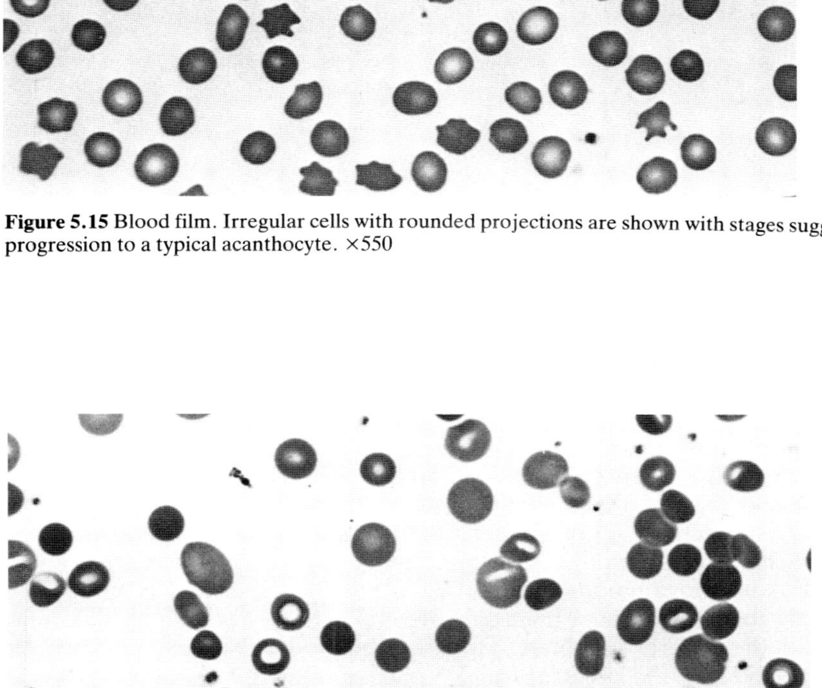

Figure 5.16 Blood film. Spherocytes. Frequent circular, deeply staining cells which tend to be microcytic. There is also marked anisocytosis and the staining of the larger cells, which are reticulocytes, contrasts sharply with the deep staining of the spherocytes. ×550

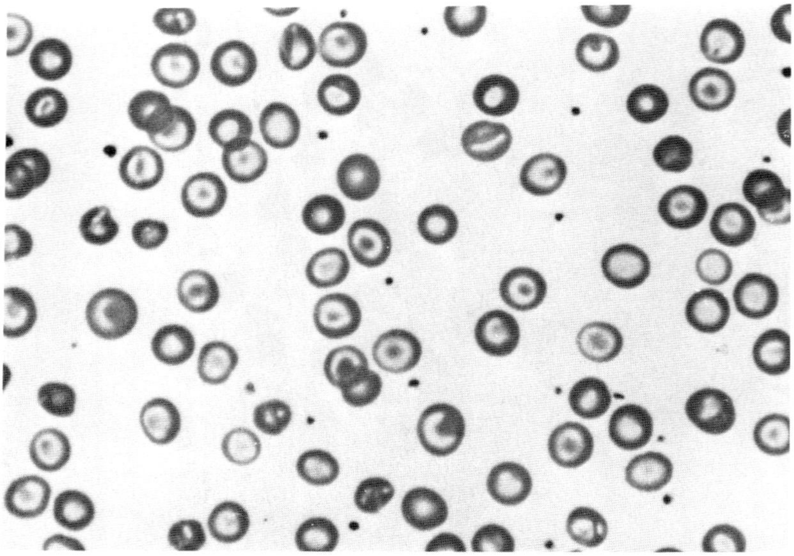

Figure 5.17 Blood film. Target cells (leptocytes). The area of central staining is clearly shown (from a case of obstructive liver disease). ×550

Target cells This descriptive term is applied to cells showing an area of central staining (*Figure 5.17*) which are abnormally thin cells or leptocytes. In wet preparations the cells can be seen to be cup shaped which is considered to de due to an increase in surface area while retaining the same volume. After drying, fixing and staining the cells assume the target appearance. They are a common finding in obstructive liver disease where the increased surface area is due to an accumulation of cholesterol and lecithin due to inhibition of plasma lecithin-cholesterol-acyl transferase (LCAT) activity by bile salts [20]. They are also a feature of the rare hereditary deficiency of plasma LCAT. Large numbers of target cells are seen in the homozygous haemoglobinopathies particularly in Hb C, D and E and in the double heterozygotes S/C, S/beta thalassaemia, etc. and may be due to abnormal Hb binding with the integral membrane protein, band 3. Variable numbers are seen in iron deficiency and thalassaemia. They appear after splenectomy and are probably associated with increased membrane surface-area [21]. Splenectomy in disorders such as thalassaemia produces gross target-cell formation.

Stomatocytes These cells have a narrow slit-like area of central pallor (*Figure 5.18*) and were originally described in a form of hereditary haemolytic anaemia [22]. Familial analphalipoproteinaemia (Tangier disease) with haemolytic anaemia is also associated with stomatocytes [23]. Like target cells, they are seen as cup shapes in wet preparations. They are also associated with liver disease particularly that associated with alcohol abuse. Even in the absence of demonstrable defects in hepatic function, stomatocytes may be found in association with alcohol intake over 50 g daily. The significance of stomatocytes in normal and pathological red cells is discussed by Weed and Bessis [24]. There is an association with the Rh^{null} genotype [25].

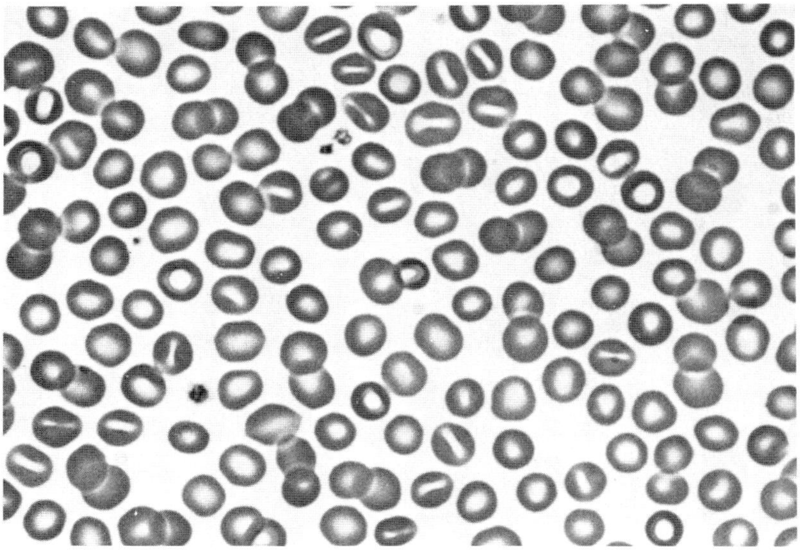

Figure 5.18 Blood film. Stomatocytes. Many cells show a 'stoma' or 'mouth' shown as a slit of central pallor (from a case of alcohol abuse). ×550

Xerocytes Cellular dehydration results in unusually high corpuscular haemoglobin concentration and typically gives the appearance of 'puddling' or pooling of haemoglobin to one side of the red cell. Cellular dehydration is a feature of the rare disorder of hereditary xerocytosis and more commonly in the Hb C syndromes (*see Figure 11.5*).

Combinations of poikilocytic change

It is not uncommon, particularly in haemolytic anaemias, to see combinations of poikilocytic change in the same cell. Spherocytic acanthocytes (*see Figure 5.14*) and fragmented spherocytes (*see Figure 5.11*) are examples. SEM has revealed the many permutations of red-cell shape which cannot be readily seen in the two-dimensional blood film [13].

Abnormalities in staining

The normochromic appearance of normal mature red cells has already been described as have the abnormal staining appearances of target cells, stomatocytes and spherocytes.

Hypochromasia

Pale staining of red cells is due to abnormally thin cells (*see Figure 5.6*). The concept that hypochromasia can simply be equated with a low cellular haemoglobin concentration is not valid. The hypochromic red cells seen in iron deficiency, thalassaemia or in sideroblastic anaemia are due to diminished haemoglobin formation resulting in microcytosis and leptocytosis and is often associated with target cells.

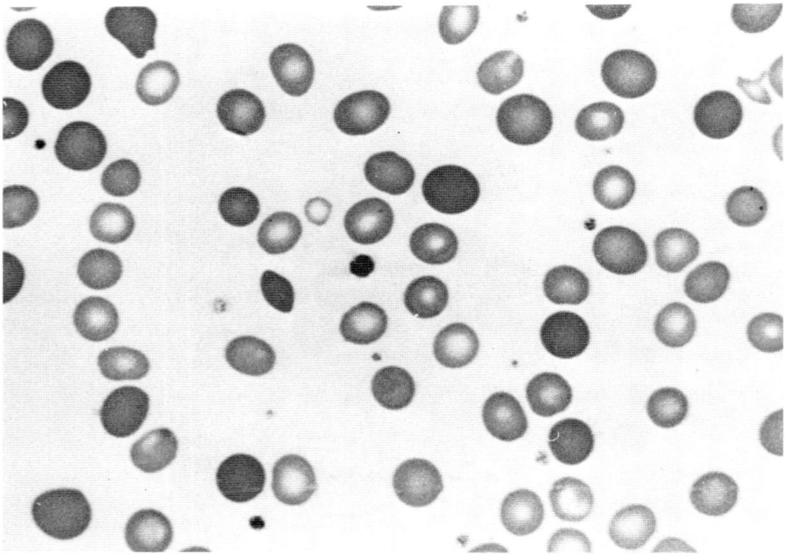

Figure 5.19 Blood film. Dimorphism. Hypochromic and normochromic red-cell populations. ×550

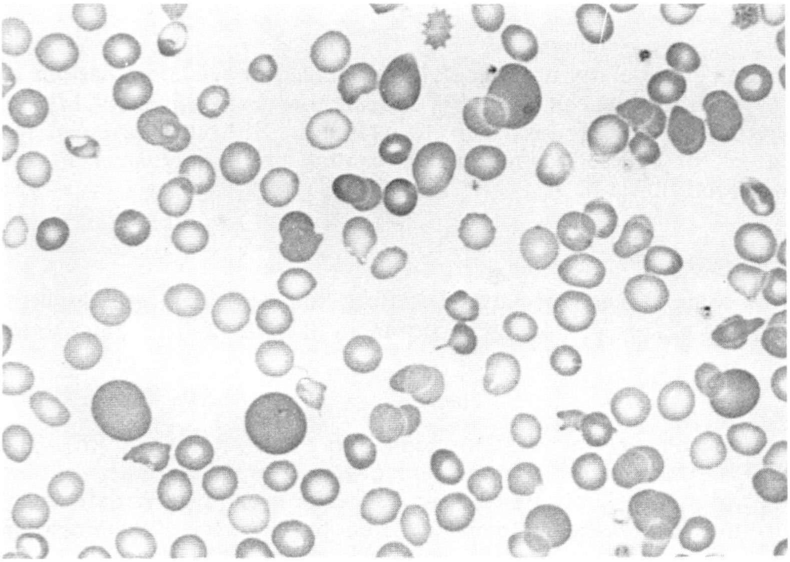

Figure 5.20 Blood film. Dimorphism in a case of treated iron-deficiency anaemia. ×550

Polychromasia
Mature red cells stain pink. As reticulocytes contain residual RNA they will have an affinity for the basic components of the stain and thus assume a degree of blue staining proportional to the amount of RNA. An increase in reticulocytes in the blood will be seen as a polychromatic red-cell population which is also often macrocytic. Although moderate to marked reticulocytosis is obvious, numbers up to 5% are often difficult to recognize and indeed may be missed.

Dimorphism
This means the presence of two populations of red cells in the same film. It is generally accepted that the term refers to staining appearance and is applied to hypochromic and normochromic populations (*Figure 5.19*). There are three well-recognized situations:

1. Iron deficiency after treatment. The 'new' population is normochromic and constrasts with the original hypochromic population. The normochromic cells usually show anisocytosis and tend to be slightly macrocytic (*Figure 5.20*).
2. After transfusion of blood to a patient with hypochromic anaemia. The normochromic population are of uniform size.
3. In sideroblastic anaemia. The picture is variable and depends on whether the disorder is hereditary or acquired.

A further example of dimorphism may be seen when a patient with normochromic anaemia becomes iron deficient during treatment, e.g. a patient with severe megaloblastic anaemia treated with vitamin B_{12} who is also iron deficient; the macrocytic, normochromic cells are the 'old' population and the hypochromic cells those appearing after treatment.

Red-cell inclusions

The varieties, nature and demonstration of red-cell inclusions are summarized in *Table 5.1*.

Table 5.1 Red-cell inclusions

Inclusion	*Nature*	*Demonstration*
Howell–Jolly bodies	DNA. Nuclear remnants	Romanowsky. Feulgen stain
Pappenheimer bodies	Fe^{3+} with protein	Romanowsky. Prussian-blue reaction
Basophilic stippling	Ribonucleoprotein. Precipitated residual RNA bases	Romanowsky
Protozoa	Malaria parasites. *Babesia* spp.	Romanowsky
Micro-organisms	*Bartonella bacilliformis*	Romanowsky
Reticulocytes	Ribonucleoprotein. Aggregated ribosomes	Supravital staining
Heinz bodies	Denatured haemoglobin	Supravital staining
Hb H inclusions	Precipitated Hb H	Extended supravital staining
Siderotic granules	Fe^{3+} in ferritin or mitochondria	Prussian-blue reaction

Romanowsky-stained preparations

Howell–Jolly bodies These are nuclear remnants and consist of DNA. They are usually single, deep purple and of varying size (*Figure 5.21*). They are consistently present after splenectomy and in splenic atrophy or whenever splenic function is greatly diminished. It is accepted that the nuclear remnants are normally removed by the 'culling' action of the spleen. When there is erythroid hyperplasia, Howell–Jolly bodies may be seen even in the presence of a normal spleen, particularly in the presence of dyserythropoiesis.

Pappenheimer bodies These consist of ferric iron complexed with protein, as evidenced by their demonstration by the Prussian-blue reaction and the basic dye components of Romanowsky stains. They occur when splenic function is absent and are seen as small dark-blue staining bodies of uniform size and usually occur singly, though splenectomy in disorders of haemoglobin synthesis such as the thalassaemias and sideroblastic anaemias may result in multiple inclusions of varying size which may stain less distinctly (*Figure 5.22*)

Basophilic stippling (punctate basophilia) This occurs as evenly distributed, multiple inclusions (*Figure 5.23*), stains blue-black and consists of aggregated ribosomes or pyrimidine nucleotides. Immature cells contain ribosomes that are evenly dispersed throughout the cell which, when stained with Romanowsky dyes in methanol, produce the homogeneous polychromasia of the reticulocyte. Under certain conditions such as incubation in dilute supravital dyes and by slow drying of blood films and subsequent staining with Romanowsky dyes, the ribosomes aggregate into coarse, irregular granules. In certain conditions such as thalassaemia and lead poisoning 'spontaneous' stippling is found in stained films and is of diagnostic significance. To some extent it may be considered as an *in vitro* artefact as the number and distribution in the film depends upon the speed of drying, though the possibility of disordered ribosomes in these disorders is likely. The use of EDTA-anticoagulated blood reduces the number of stippled cells in lead intoxication. Whether the stippled cells found in other conditions behave similarly is not clear. They are a notable feature in the hereditary haemolytic anaemia due to deficiency of pyrimidine-5-nucleotidase which is also depressed in lead poisoning[26]. Whether the stippled cells of thalassaemia and other dyserythropoietic states is also related to reduced enzyme activity is not known.

Protozoa These can parasitize circulating red cells, as is classically illustrated by malaria parasites (*Figure 5.24*), and their demonstration in blood films is necessary for diagnosis and differentiation. The subject is considered in detail in Chapter 14. Piroplasmosis or babesiosis in man is caused by organisms of the *Babesia* spp. which are normally confined to cattle. If splenic function is absent, the tick-borne infection may be acquired in humans.

Micro-organisms in red cells is a very rare occurrence, with the exception of bartonellosis (Oroya fever, Carrion's disease) which is confined to the South American Andes. The causative organism is *Bartonella bacilliformis* which belongs to the Rickettsiales. The protective influence of the spleen against *Bartonella* and *Babesia* can be shown in experimental animals. The organisms are seen as small rod-shaped or coccoid bodies which may be confused with malaria parasites (*see* Chapter 14).

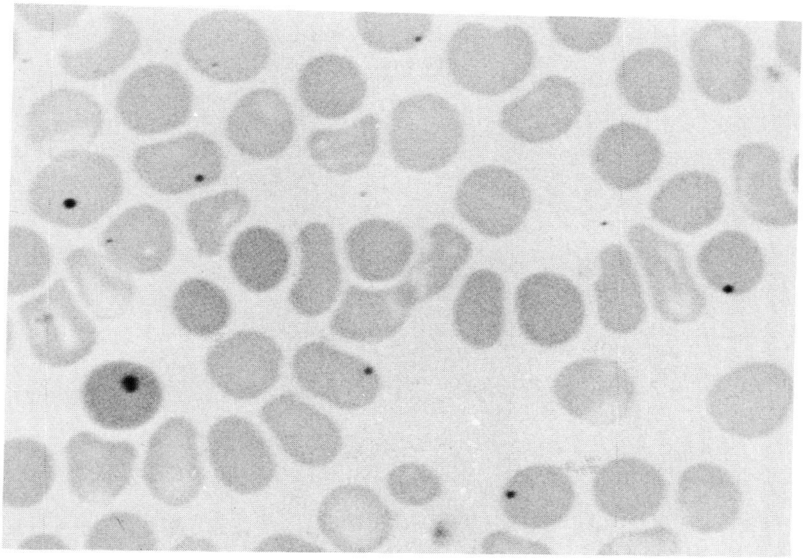

Figure 5.21 Blood film. Howell–Jolly bodies. The nuclear remnants are almost always found as single inclusions of regular shape. ×550

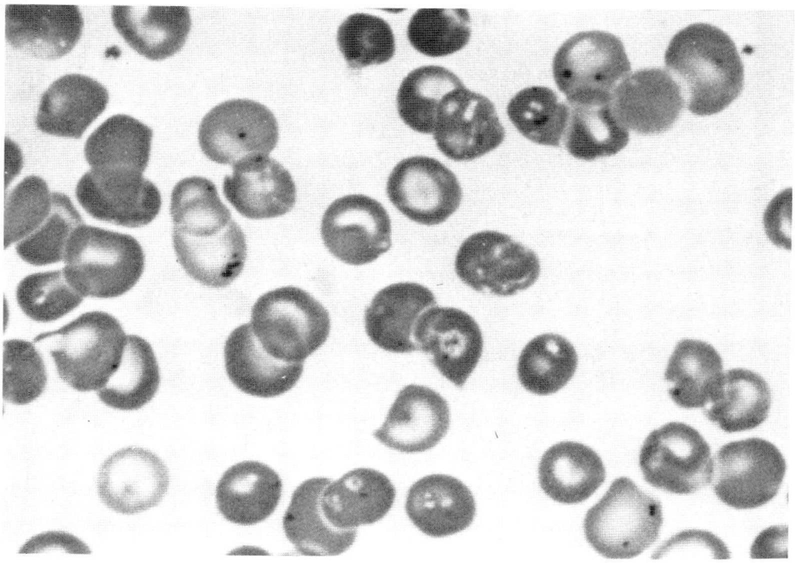

Figure 5.22 Blood film. Pappenheimer bodies. Single and multiple inclusions of variable size. From a case of iron overload and hyposplenism. ×825

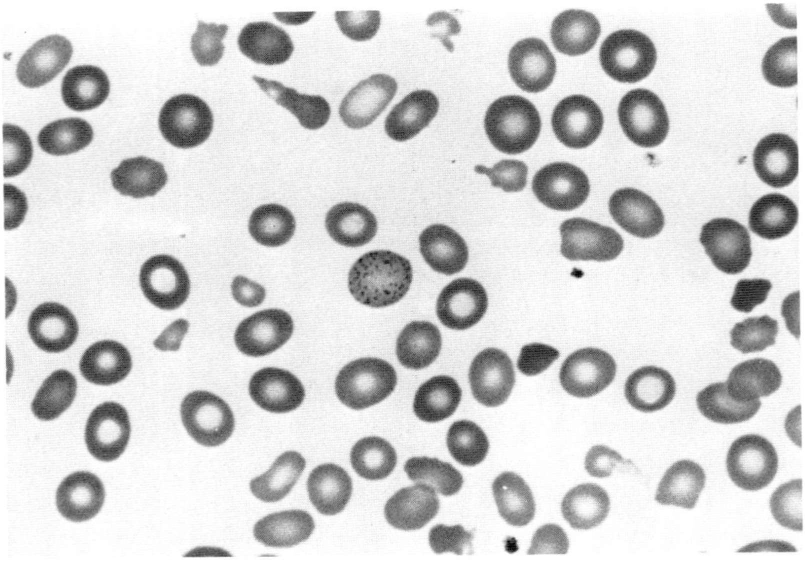

Figure 5.23 Blood film. Basophilic stippling. A single red cell showing multiple fine inclusions scattered throughout the cell. ×550

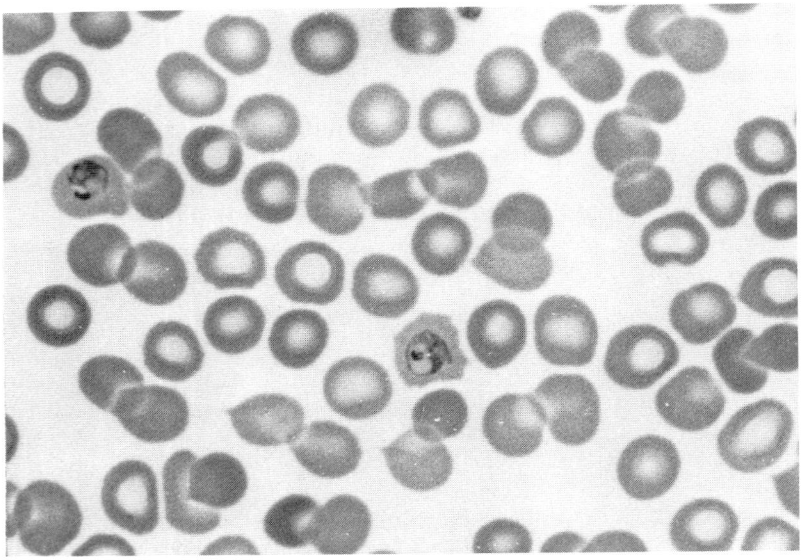

Figure 5.24 Blood film. Two mature trophozoites of *Plasmodium vivax*. ×825

Supravital staining

Reticulocytes are recognized by the aggregation of ribosomes into linear structures. The appearance and demonstration and significance is considered in detail in Chapter 3.

Heinz bodies are not seen in Romanowsky-stained films but require supravital staining. They can be demonstrated by the technique for reticulocytes but are more intensely stained by methyl violet. They are usually single, round structures, situated at the cell margin (*Figure 5.25*) and consist of denatured, precipitated haemoglobin bound to the cell membrane by disulphide linkages[27]. They are produced by the oxidant stress of drugs and chemicals, by an inherent instability of haemoglobin variants or by defects in the red-cell glycolytic pathways. Instability of haemoglobin resulting in loss of haem will result in 'white' Heinz bodies which can be seen as unstained areas in Romanowsky-stained films. The number of Heinz bodies will depend on the nature of the haemoglobin defect, the degree of oxidative challenge and on splenic function; they are particularly numerous after splenectomy or in hyposplenism. Confusion between Heinz bodies and other inclusions such as Howell–Jolly bodies and Pappenheimer bodies may occur. The substitution of brilliant green as the supravital dye has been recommended as specific to Heinz bodies[28]. The occurrence and significance of Heinz bodies is considered further in Chapter 11.

Hb H inclusions are precipitated tetramers of β-globin chains (β4) and are found when there is suppression of α-chain synthesis. They are demonstrated by incubating blood with brilliant cresyl blue to produce a 'golf-ball' appearance with multiple, evenly distributed, blue-staining bodies (*Figure 5.26*). Though they may be found in reticulocyte preparations, extending the staining time to 2 hours produces more consistent results. Numbers may be very small in the α-thalassaemia traits and require prolonged examination of the films (*see* Chapter 9).

Siderocytes are red cells containing aggregates of iron which can be demonstrated only by the Prussian-blue technique or by electron microscopy. Two types of siderocyte have been described. Siderotic granules associated with reticulocytes (the reticulated-siderocyte or R-S cell) are due to aggregates of ferritin which disappear as the cell matures. The non-reticulated siderocyte (S cell) represents non-ferritin iron located in the mitochondria and their removal is dependent upon splenic function. In normal blood the number of siderocytes (R-S + S) is less than 0.7%. Numbers of R-S cells greater than 1% have been recognized only in severe haemolytic anaemia and in sideroblastic anaemia with mild haemolysis. Increased S-cells are only seen when splenic function is reduced or absent[29].

Differential leucocyte count

The classified counting of leucocytes in the stained blood film and the expression of each cell type as a percentage and, by reference to the total leucocyte count, their 'absolute numbers' expressed as number × 10^9/l is an established procedure.

The limitation of the differential count is the inherent error of counting randomly distributed cells, together with the tendency of different cell types to predominate in particular areas of the film. Various counting patterns have been suggested to overcome the tendency, present even in the best-made wedge films, for the neutrophils to accumulate at the edges and in the tail of the film. In an attempt to represent fairly the neutrophils at the edge of the film the 'battlement' pattern includes the edges of the film which, if the film is poorly made, will result in

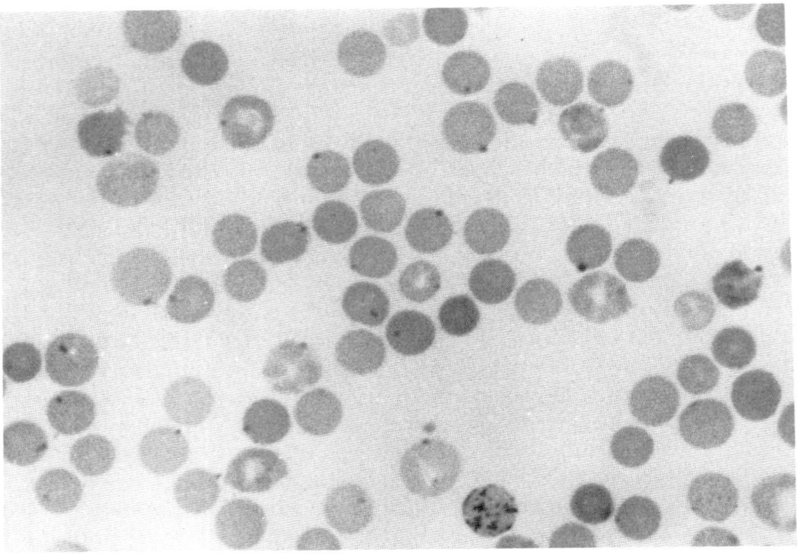

Figure 5.25 Blood film. Supravital staining with brilliant cresyl blue. Many red cells contain a single, membrane-associated inclusion. ×550

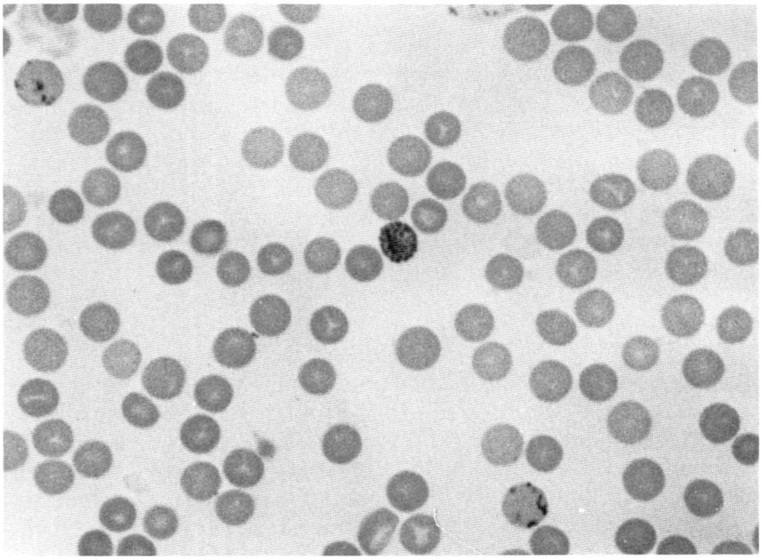

Figure 5.26 Blood film. Supravital brilliant cresyl blue preparation. A single red cell containing multiple, evenly distributed inclusions of precipitated Hb H. The appearance is clearly distinct from the two reticulocytes. From a case of α-thalassaemia trait. ×550

counting excess neutrophils. Counting all the leucocytes in a longitudinal strip from head to tail of the film has been recommended[30] on the premise that in a well-made film each strip will represent the blood drawn out from a small volume of blood when it has spread out between the slide and spreader. The disadvantage of this counting pattern is that in the thicker part of the film leucocytes appear smaller and condensed making identification more difficult. An alternative pattern is a series of lateral strips in the well-spread area of the film avoiding the edges.

The advantage of good morphology supersedes the objections of unequal leucocyte distribution which is minimal in a well-made film. It is emphasized that performing differential counts on badly spread films is a waste of time and could result in misleading conclusions. The use of 'spun-films' should eliminate the problem of leucocyte distribution but in comparison with well-spread wedge films may give at best only a 10% improvement in performance[31].

To reduce the inherent error of the differential count more cells would have to be counted. Routinely, at least 100 cells should be classified. There is no firm evidence that the improved confidence limits of counting 200 cells is clinically useful for the neutrophils and lymphocytes, but for normal numbers of minority populations – eosinophils, basophils and monocytes – the confidence limits are wide and exceed the accepted normal ranges. The confidence limits for 100 and 200 cell counts are shown in *Table 5.2*.

Table 5.2 95% Confidence limits for leucocyte differential counts*

Reported %	*Leucocytes counted*	
	100	*200*
0	0–4	0–2
1	0–6	0–4
2	0–8	0–6
3	0–9	1–7
4	1–10	1–8
5	1–12	2–10
6	2–13	3–11
7	2–14	3–12
8	3–16	4–13
9	4–17	5–14
10	4–18	6–16
15	8–24	10–21
20	12–30	14–27
25	16–35	19–32
30	21–40	23–37
35	25–46	28–43
40	30–51	33–48
45	35–56	38–53
50	39–61	42–58

* From reference[31]

Experienced observers are often capable of remembering the numbers of the five normal cell lines though many workers use a mechanical or electronic register for recording the count.

During counting any morphological abnormalities such as toxic or reactive changes are noted and of particular interest is the differentiation of neutrophils into segmented and non-segmented forms and the counting of the number of nuclear lobes. In the 'pre-antibiotic' era the classification of neutrophils by lobe counting and into 'band', 'stab' and metamyelocyte was considered a valuable diagnostic and prognostic procedure, and the terms 'shift to the left' and 'shift to the right' denote a tendency to immaturity or hypersegmentation, respectively. Though formal counts of the Arneth–Cooke or Schilling type are not commonly practised, the concepts are clinically useful. It has been shown that careful differentiation of segmented and non-segmented neutrophils is helpful in discovering early or mild inflammatory conditions in patients with normal total leucocyte counts and indeed normal numbers of neutrophils. The ESR, the nitroblue-tetrazolium dye (NBT) test and toxic granulation of the neutrophils are all less sensitive than the demonstration of non-segmented neutrophils[32]. Release of neutrophils from the marginating pool by the physiological mechanisms of stress, emotion, exercise etc. is not accompanied by a 'left shift'.

The value of neutrophil hypersegmentation as an early indicator of folate deficiency was recognized by Herbert[33] and a 'segmentation index'[34] obtained by the formula:

$$\text{Segmentation index} = \frac{\text{neutrophils with 5 lobes}}{\text{neutrophils with 4 lobes}} \times 100$$

appears to be a good discriminant[35], with an index of under 25 regarded as normal and an index of over 30 regarded as increased.

The problem of erythroblasts and the differential count

Erythroblasts are not uncommon in blood films in a variety of disorders. It is often recommended that the number of erythroblasts be related as NRC/100 WBC. However, all but the most mature erythroblasts are undoubtedly counted as leucocytes by automated electronic or optical systems. When erythroblast numbers are small their effect on the differential leucocyte count is insignificant and expression as number/100 WBC is adequate. When present in greater numbers they may seriously influence the interpretation of the total and differential leucocyte counts. Two options are available. The percentage of erythroblasts in the differential count can be used to correct the false 'WBC' to a more correct value and the differential count repeated expressing the normoblasts as number/100 WBC. Alternatively the erythroblasts are included in the differential count, reported as a percentage and the 'total WBC' expressed as the 'total nucleated cell count'. The absolute number of the leucocyte types can then be readily calculated. It is suggested that erythroblasts are included in the differential count and 'WBC' converted to 'nucleated cells' if the erythroblasts exceed 10% of the differential count.

Reference ranges for differential leucocyte counts

The normal adult range for differential counts is established by puberty. Thereafter, increasing age makes no significant difference to the values, nor are there significant sex differences. In childhood, infancy and in the neonate the normal ranges are influenced by age, and the data are summarized in Chapter 2.

With the introduction of automated leucocyte classification and the counting of larger numbers of cells it is becoming clear that though the values for neutrophils and lymphocytes are closely similar whether obtained by visual or instrument counting, at least a part of the normal ranges for the minority cell types are due to the inherent error of counting small numbers of cells. Whether the improved counting of basophils and eosinophils will be clinically useful is still unclear. It is again emphasized that much more information is obtained from the absolute number of a leucocyte type than the percentage value.

Abnormalities of leucocytes

Leucocyte abnormalities may be classified as cytoplasmic or nuclear. Combined nuclear/cytoplasmic changes are usually associated with malignant blood disorders and will not be considered in this section.

Abnormalities are usually acquired but, remarkably, several acquired changes have an inherited counterpart.

Cytoplasmic abnormalities of granulocytes (Table 5.3)

Hypergranularity

Toxic granulation This appears as coarse blue-black or purple stippling. The granules probably represent an abnormal staining reaction of the granules in toxic

Table 5.3 Abnormalities of neutrophils

Presentation	*Acquired state*	*Hereditary disorder*
Cytoplasmic:		
Hypergranularity	Toxic change	Alder–Reilly anomaly
RNA inclusions	Toxic change	May–Hegglin anomaly
Vacuolation	Toxic or degenerative artefact	Jordan's anomaly
Agranularity	Acute myeloblastic/myelomonocytic leukaemia. Pre-leukaemia	–
Giant granulation	Pseudo-Chediak–Higashi syndrome. Acute leukaemia. Myelodysplasia	Chediak–Higashi syndrome (CHS)
Nuclear:		
Hypersegmentation	Megaloblastosis. Uraemia. Heat stroke. Steroid therapy. Myelodysplasia	Hereditary hypersegmentation (Undritz anomaly)
Retarded segmentation	Acute myeloblastic/myelomonocytic leukaemia. Myelodysplasia. Drugs. Infection	Pelger–Huet anomaly
Nuclear appendages	Myelodysplasia	Klinefelter's syndrome. Multiple X chromosomes
Ring forms	Myelodysplasia. Chronic granulocytic leukaemia. Infections. Megaloblastosis	–

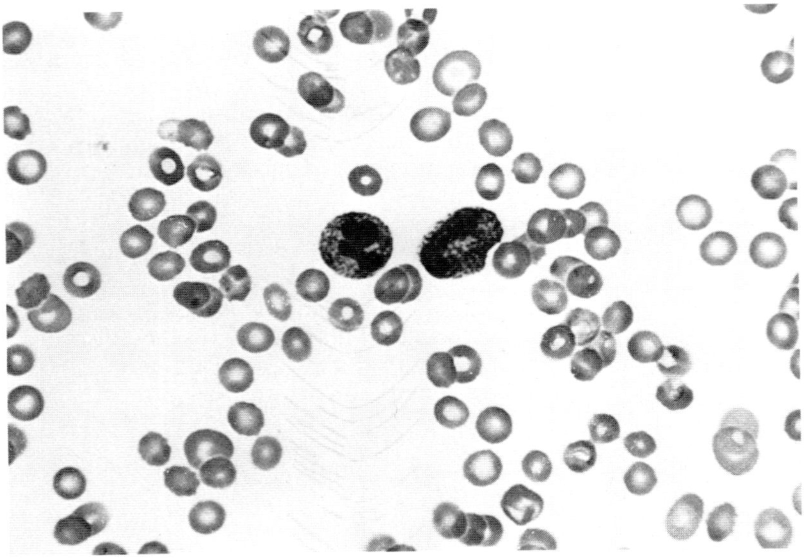

Figure 5.27 Blood film. A segmented and a band neutrophil showing coarse toxic granulation. From a case of septicaemia. ×550

cells and are not phagocytosed material, newly formed abnormal granules or autophagic bodies (*Figure 5.27*).

Alder–Reilly anomaly This is inherited as an autosomal recessive characteristic and is reflected in all leucocytes and in non-haemopoietic cells. Intense blue-violet granulation is seen in the 'complete' form and its presence in eosinophils is diagnostic. 'Incomplete' forms may involve neutrophils or lymphocytes or monocytes. Tissue basophils (mast cells) are involved in all types. The anomaly may be associated with the Pfaundler–Hurler syndrome (gargoylism). The granules are stored mucopolysaccharides and sphingomyelin due to a lysosomal deficiency of a hydroxylase [36].

RNA inclusions

Toxic states Döhle bodies are blue-staining, pyroninophilic, round or stranded structures with ill-defined margins and consist of rough endoplasmic reticulum containing RNA. Cawley and Hayhoe [37] believed that they represent focal failure of cytoplasmic maturation. The bodies are often associated with toxic granulation and bacterial infection.

May–Hegglin anomaly The inclusions are again blue staining and pyroninophilic of crescent or spindle shape in all types of granulocyte and also in monocytes. The inclusions tend to be at the periphery of the cell and more than one may be present. The structure is similar to the Döhle body of toxic states. The anomaly is inherited as an autosomal dominant trait and is associated with giant platelets, thrombocytopenia and a mild bleeding tendency. Electron microscopy shows that

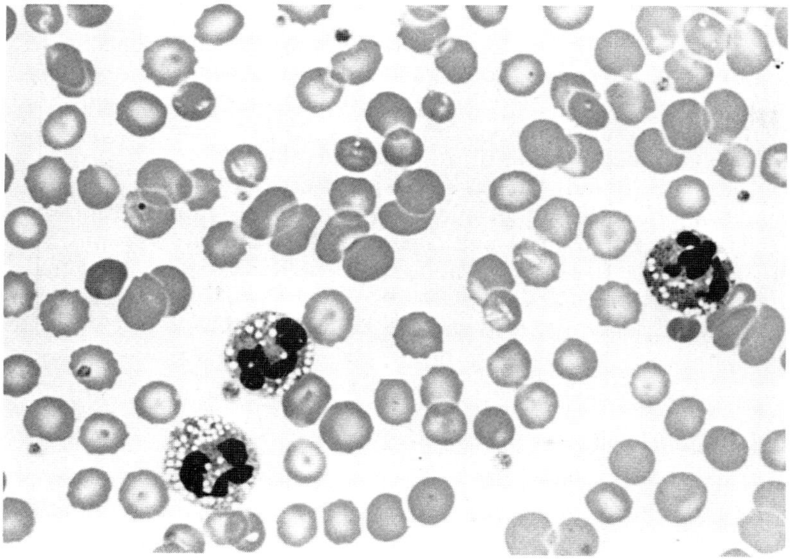

Figure 5.28 Blood film. Toxic vacuolation of neutrophils. ×550

they have a different structure to Döhle bodies and it is suggested that the term 'Döhle bodies' be confined to the inclusions associated with infection.

Vacuolation (Figure 5.28)

Toxic neutrophils may show clear vacuoles which increase in number if film preparation is delayed and probably reflect increased lysozyme activity. Normal neutrophils show increased vacuolation when film preparation is delayed[38] but at room temperature the numbers are small compared with those formed by toxic cells.

Jordan's anomaly is the presence of multiple large vacuoles in neutrophils, eosinophils, basophils and monocytes which stain positively for fat. The anomaly was first described in association with progressive muscular dystrophy and subsequently with ichthyosis. The vacuoles are not found in lymphocytes.

Agranularity

In *leukaemic, pre-leukaemic* or *myelodysplastic* disorders neutrophils devoid of granules and having a pale blue cytoplasm may be a feature. Enzyme activities are weak or absent and the PAS reaction reduced. The anomaly may be due to asynchronous nuclear/cytoplasmic maturation.

Giant granulation

The *Chediak–Higashi syndrome* (CHS) is probably inherited as an autosomal recessive characteristic. In the severe form neutrophils, eosinophils, basophils, lymphocytes and monocytes are involved and contain giant lysosomes of varying size up to 4 μm in diameter which stain variably as grey, blue, purple or orange and are strongly peroxidase positive. The bodies probably represent aggregations of normal azurophilic granules and in eosinophils may exhibit crystal formation.

Inclusions in the monocytes possibly represent phagocytosed material. Occasional large granules may be seen in lymphocytes. The anomaly is associated, in children, with severe chronic infections which are ultimately fatal. A frequent additional clinical finding is a form of albinism. In probable heterozygotes who are clinically normal, occasional large granules may be found in neutrophils and lymphocytes and may be similar to the 'incomplete' form of the Alder–Reilly anomaly.

'*Pseudo-CHS*' may be found occasionally in acute myeloid leukaemia, myelodysplasia and its variants. By light microscopy the giant granules represent those of typical CHS, but by electron microscopy, unlike the large granules of CHS, they can be shown to contain numerous microcrystalline structures resembling those of Auer bodies but with a different periodicity. Their occurrence may be associated with disseminated intravascular coagulation[39].

Nuclear abnormalities of granulocytes (Table 5.3)

Hypersegmentation (Figure 5.29)

Acquired The occurrence of neutrophils with six or more nuclear segments or lobes (as many as 10 or 12 may be found) is an important diagnostic observation and is an early, sensitive, though not specific, indication of megaloblastic erythropoiesis. Hypersegmentation is not an indication of maturity but is probably a reflection of increased nuclear mass even though the cells have a normal (2n) diploid content of DNA. Hypersegmentation is also found in uraemia but the neutrophils differ from the forms in megaloblastic anaemia in that they tend to be of normal size. It has been suggested that guanidosuccinic acid, a metabolite of urea, is the cause of uraemic hypersegmentation. In severe iron deficiency hypersegmentation may be observed in the apparent absence of vitamin B_{12} or folate deficiency or uraemia (*see* page 225). Occasional hypersegmented

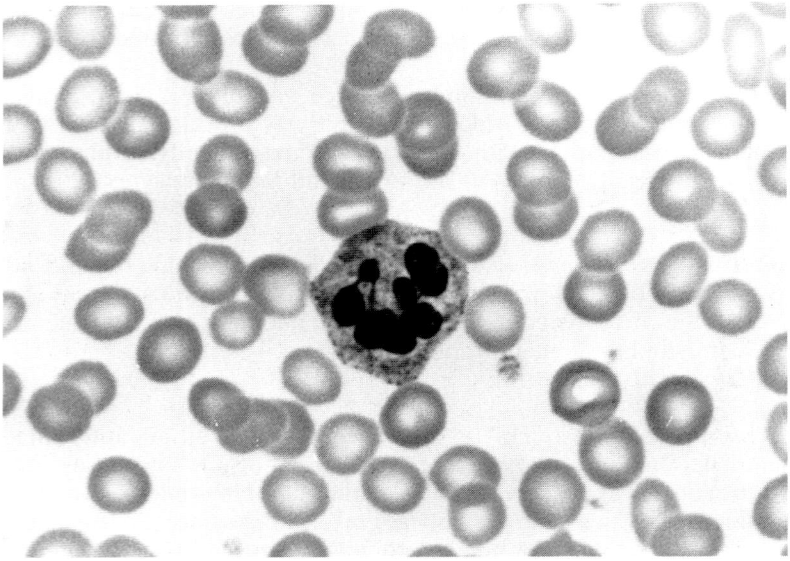

Figure 5.29 Blood film. Hypersegmented neutrophil showing at least seven nuclear lobes. ×825

neutrophils may be seen in toxic states. Hypersegmentation may be a feature in myelodysplasia, in heat stroke[40] and during treatment with glucocorticoids[41].

Hereditary hypersegmentation (Undritz anomaly) is a harmless condition inherited as an autosomal recessive in which the heterozygous state results in about 60% of neutrophils having four or more lobes. In the very rare homozygous state over 80% of neutrophils are hypersegmented (*Figure 5.30*). An inherited abnormality that may simulate hypersegmentation is Davidson's anomaly in which tetraploidy of the neutrophils is found, with cells having two segmented nuclei.

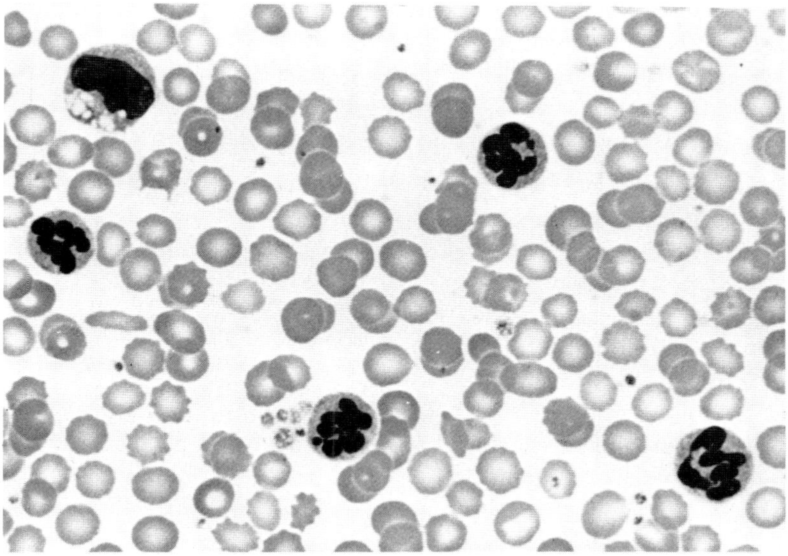

Figure 5.30 Blood film. Marked hypersegmentation. Virtually all neutrophils are hypersegmented. A probable example of hereditary hypersegmentation. ×550

Retarded segmentation

Acquired (Pseudo-Pelger) Neutrophils with round, unsegmented nuclei or segmentation limited to two lobes are not uncommon in acute or chronic leukaemia involving the granulocyte series. In myelodysplasia their numbers may be considerable. The bi-lobed cells often show the typical 'spectacle' appearance of the heterozygous form of Pelger–Huet anomaly (*see* below). There have been occasional reports of acquired Pelger anomaly in infections and drug reactions[42].

Pelger–Huet anomaly This benign abnormality is inherited as an autosomal dominant characteristic. The heterozygous form has a reported incidence ranging from 1 in 1000 to 1 in 10 000 and the neutrophils appear rod-like, dumb-bell or show the typical 'spectacle' or pince-nez form (*Figure 5.31*). In the rare homozygous form the nucleus is round and totally lacking any semblance of segmentation.

Nuclear appendages

The sex-specific, 'drumstick' appendages of the neutrophils in the female normally occur in 1–3% of cells (*Figure 5.32*). Absence of 'drumsticks' indicates the subject

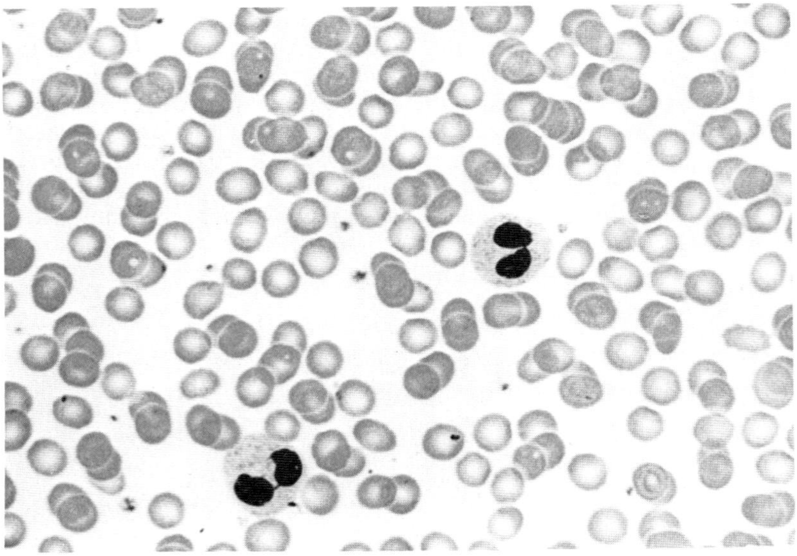

Figure 5.31 Blood film. Pelger–Huet anomaly (heterozygous form). The typical 'spectacle' appearance is shown. The microcytosis and hypochromia of the red cells is coincidental. ×550

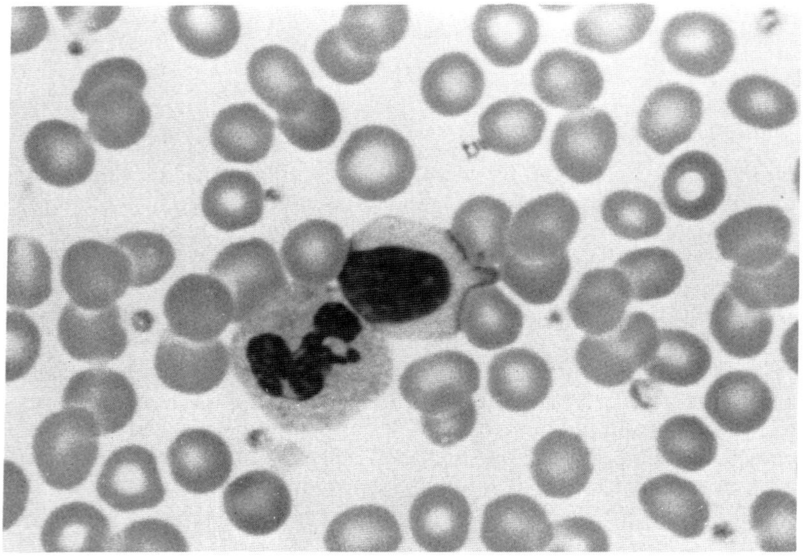

Figure 5.32 Blood film. Segmented neutrophil with a single 'drumstick' connected to nuclear lobe by a fine chromatin strand. ×825

is male (XY) or XO (Turner's syndrome) while the presence of drumsticks in Klinefelter's syndrome (XXY) reflects the additional X chromosome. A hereditary disorder has been described in females where as many as 35% of neutrophils show the characteristic appendages. More than one drumstick in a cell may represent additional X chromosomes, e.g. an XXX female.

The Seman anomaly shows cells with an increased number of non-specific appendages – small clubs, sessile nodules and rackets – which may be associated with D13–15 trisomy syndrome. Increased numbers of these appendages are probably induced by androgen and other hormones[43].

Ring forms

The nucleus in a ring, circle or 'dough-nut' form is normal in rodents but in humans has been described in association with megaloblastosis, myelodysplasia and other myeloproliferative disorders and in infections[44–46].

Abnormalities of eosinophils (Table 5.4)

Most of the hereditary abnormalities affecting the neutrophils are reflected in the eosinophils – a notable exception being the May–Hegglin anomaly. As nuclear segmentation in the majority of eosinophils is typically restricted to two lobes, heterozygous Pelger–Huet anomaly is more difficult to detect in eosinophils. The syndrome of hypersegmentation, hypogranularity and absent peroxidase activity described by Presentey[47] appears to be a distinct hereditary anomaly.

Table 5.4 Abnormalities of eosinophils

Presentation	*Acquired state*	*Hereditary disorder*
Cytoplasmic:		
Hypergranularity	–	Alder–Reilly anomaly
Giant granulation	–	Chediak–Higashi syndrome
Agranularity	Leukaemia	Inherited syndrome (*see* below)
Vacuolation	–	Jordan's anomaly
Nuclear:		
Hypersegmentation	–	Undritz anomaly (*see* below)
Retarded segmentation	Leukaemia	Homozygous Pelger–Huet
Combined nuclear/cytoplasmic abnormality:		
Hypersegmentation, Hypogranularity, Peroxidase negative		'Presentey' anomaly

Abnormalities of basophils

Alder's anomaly, Chediak–Higashi syndrome and Jordan's anomaly are seen in the blood basophils.

Abnormalities of monocytes

Alder's anomaly, Chediak–Higashi syndrome and Jordan's anomaly are also seen in monocytes. The inclusions of May–Hegglin anomaly are found in monocytes but are difficult to visualize by light microscopy.

As monocytes are phagocytic, stainable ingested material may be noted in various disorders. Of particular significance is the ingestion of other blood cells, notably erythrophagocytosis. Although the phenomenon is reported in various haemolytic anaemias it is particularly associated with complement-mediated haemolytic mechanisms.

Occasionally in lipid-storage disorders monocytes containing lipid may be seen in the blood. Unusual inclusions have been reported in the Hermansky–Pudlak syndrome[48].

Lymphocyte abnormalities

Nuclear changes

These have been described in various disorders but are not consistent or characteristic. Radial segmentation of lymphocyte (and monocyte) nuclei is an *in vitro* phenomenon associated with incubation at room temperature[49] or by heating at 41°C for 2 hours[50]. The nuclear clefting or notching of Rieder cells is considered to be a similar phenomenon.

Cytoplasmic abnormalities

The inclusions associated with the Alder–Reilly anomaly and the Chediak–Higashi syndrome are found in lymphocytes. A different type of inclusion has been described in a patient with rheumatoid arthritis[51].

Vacuolation

The vacuolation of Jordan's anomaly is *not* seen in lymphocytes. The cytoplasm of normal cells may contain a few small vacuoles. Marked, PAS-negative vacuolation is described in amaurotic idiocy. Vacuolated lymphocytes can be found in specific lipid storage diseases.

Table 5.5 Abnormalities of platelets

Appearance	*Acquired*	*Hereditary*
Aggregation of platelets in EDTA-anticoagulated blood	Faulty technique, autoagglutinins, platelet aggregation	–
Platelet satellitism	Presence of serum factor active in the presence of EDTA	–
Failure to clump in films of native blood	?	Thrombasthenia
Agranularity	Degranulation due to problems in collection. Platelet antibodies	Hemmeler anomaly May–Hegglin anomaly
Macrothrombocytes	Abnormal megakaryocytopoiesis. Extramedullary thrombopoiesis. Hyposplenism. Myeloid metaplasia	May–Hegglin anomaly or other ill-defined thrombopathies
Microthrombocytes	Acute leukaemias, aplastic anaemia	Wiskott–Aldrich syndrome

Abnormalities of platelets (*Table 5.5*)

The use of EDTA, with its property of preventing aggregation of platelets, as the anticoagulant of choice for routine blood samples permits better assessment of platelet appearances in blood films and an estimate of their numbers. Platelets appear as pale blue bodies with an irregular outline and contain numerous fine red granules which are centrally located. Their diameter measures 1.5–4 μm, most being about 2 μm and only about 10% being between 3 and 4 μm.

Platelet clumps in EDTA samples are usually due to faulty technique during collection but may be due to platelet agglutinins [52]. In some films the clumps may only be seen at the edges and tail of the film.

Platelet satellitism The encirclement of neutrophils with platelets may be seen in films of EDTA-blood. The number of platelets involved varies. Other granulocytes are not involved but occasionally a few lymphocytes may be affected. The phenomenon is only seen in blood anticoagulated with EDTA; samples in citrate, oxalate and heparin are normal. 'Native' blood also fails to show the effect. The pathogenesis of the satellitism is uncertain and its significance is unknown. It depends upon a plasma factor which only reacts in the presence of EDTA and when added to compatible EDTA-anticoagulated normal blood is incapable of inducing the phenomenon (*Figure 5.33*).

Failure to clump in films of native blood Though there may be a tendency to reduced platelet clumping in a variety of acquired platelet disorders the appearance is only typical in thrombasthenia (Glanzmann's disease). This is a rare disorder associated with a normal platelet count. The defect is due to an abnormality of the platelet membrane (*see* page 625).

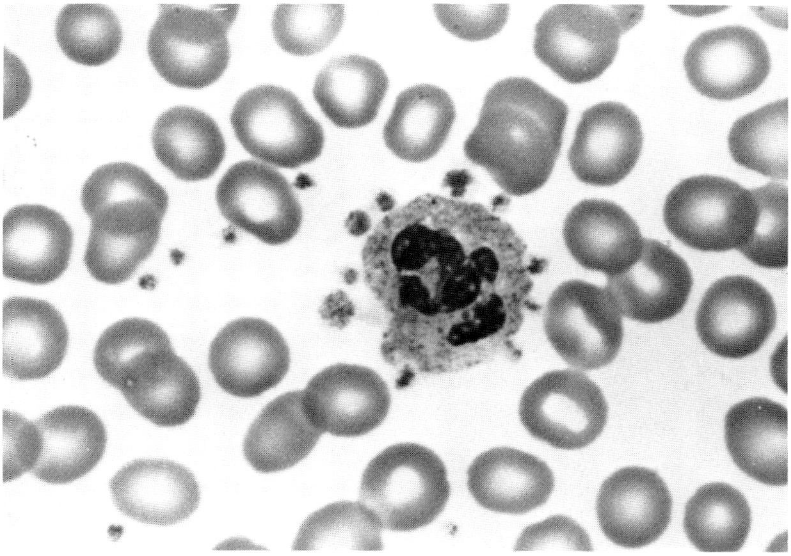

Figure 5.33 Blood film. Platelet satellitism around a neutrophil. ×825

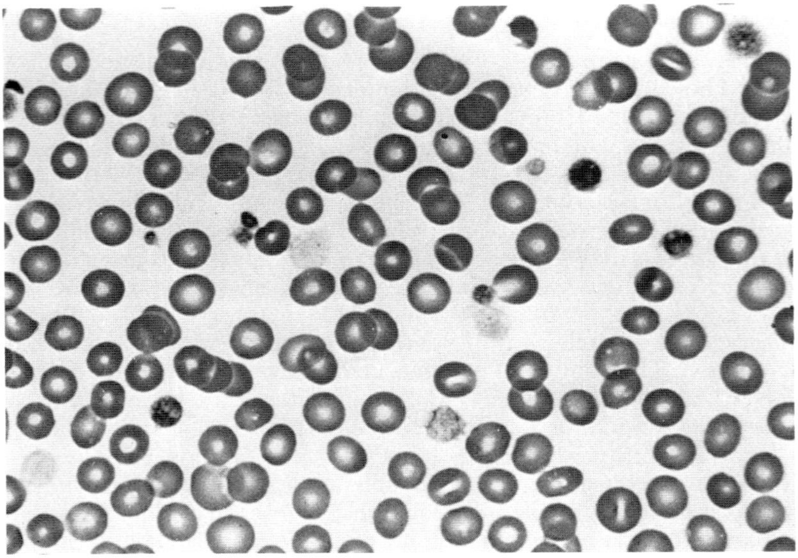

Figure 5.34 Blood film. Macrothrombocytes and agranular forms. From a case of Bernard–Soulier syndrome. ×550

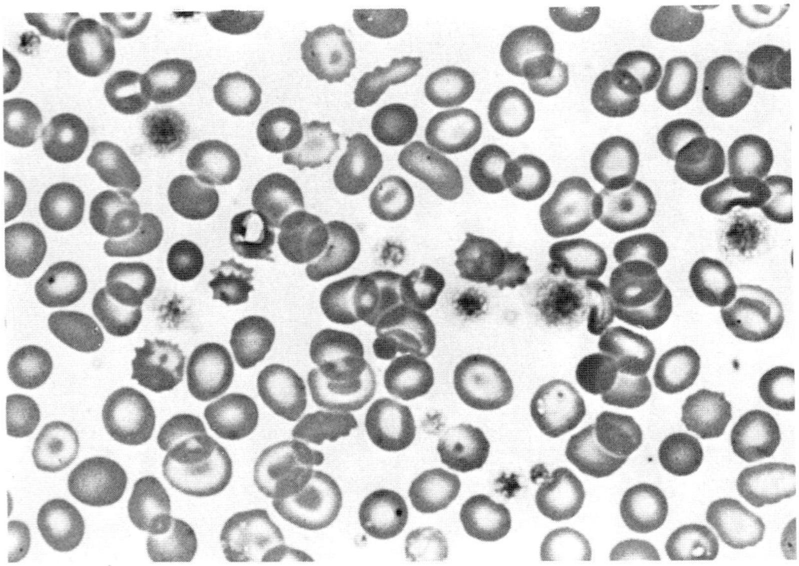

Figure 5.35 Blood film. Giant platelets, Howell–Jolly bodies, target cells and crenated or acanthocytic red cells. Post splenectomy. ×550

Agranularity (*Figure 5.34*) Problems in collection of the blood sample may initiate the release of granules from the platelets though clumping may be prevented by the action of the EDTA. Platelet antibodies are reputed to cause degranulation. Agranular platelets may also be seen in a variety of disorders affecting the maturation of the megakaryocytes in the bone marrow, particularly the myeloproliferative syndromes and in bone-marrow infiltration. The platelets in the May–Hegglin anomaly tend to have fewer granules than normal. In the Hemmeler anomaly there is no azurophilic granulation in the megakaryocytes or platelets. The platelet count is normal but there is a mild haemorrhagic diathesis.

Macrothrombocytes (giant platelets) Occasional giant platelets may be seen in normal blood but when more numerous than 5% they assume a definite significance. Giant platelets have been used as an index of thrombopoiesis in the marrow as it is claimed 'young' platelets are larger than normal and functionally more active[53], though this view is disputed[54]. When thrombopoiesis occurs outside the normal constraints of the marrow, large platelets are commonly found, e.g. in myeloproliferative syndromes[55]. The spleen acts as a reservoir for platelets and it is suggested that the young platelets are selectively sequestered until more mature. In patients who have had a splenectomy or in subjects with hyposplenism the absence of the spleen allows the larger, young platelets to circulate. In association with red-cell changes giant platelets are a valuable indication of reduced splenic function (*Figure 5.35*). Hereditary disorders with giant platelets include the May–Hegglin anomaly in which neutrophils with RNA inclusions are associated with a mild thrombocytopenia, bleeding diathesis and the giant platelets tend to be agranular. The Bernard–Soulier syndrome is a bleeding disorder characterized by a normal platelet count but the cells are markedly larger than normal (*see Figure 5.34*) and show defective adhesive and aggregating abilities (page 624). Other hereditary thrombopathies have been described which are less well characterized but in which giant platelets seem to be a recurring abnormality.

Microthrombocytes Normally about 10% of cells are small with diameters less than 1.5 μm. Increased proportions of small platelets are a feature of bone-marrow failure as is found in acute leukaemia and aplastic anaemia, though the associated severe thrombocytopenia is the more serious abnormality. Small platelets are also reported to be a feature of iron deficiency. Hereditary disorders associated with microthrombocytes include the Wiskott–Aldrich syndrome (thrombocytopenia with agammaglobulinaemia and infantile eczema). Some cases of platelet storage-pool disorders are also associated with small platelets.

References

1. Fleming, J. A. and Stewart, J. W. (1967) A critical and comparative study of methods of isolating tumour cells from blood. *J. Clin. Pathol.*, **20**, 145–51
2. Cufts, J. H. (1970) *Cell Separation: Methods in Haematology*. New York and London: Academic Press
3. International Committee for Standardisation in Haematology (1984) ICSH reference method of staining blood and bone-marrow films by azure B and eosin Y (Romanowsky stain). *Br. J. Haematol.*, **57**, 707–10
4. Allison, R. T. (1988) Romanowsky revisited. *Med. Lab. World*, June, 21–5

5. Bins, M., Huiges, W. and Halie, M. R. (1985) Stability of azure B–eosin Y staining solutions. *Br. J. Haematol.*, **59**, 73–8
6. Marshall, P. N. and Lewis, S. M. (1974) A rapid thin-layer chromatographic system for Romanowsky blood stains. *Stain Technol.*, **49**, 235–40
7. Marshall, P. N., Bentley, S. A. and Lewis, S. M. (1978) Staining properties and stability of a standardised Romanowsky stain. *J. Clin. Pathol.*, **31**, 280–2
8. Nosanchuk, J., Terzian, J. and Posso, M. (1987) Circulating mucopolysaccharide (mucin) in two adults with metastatic adenocarcinoma. *Arch. Pathol. Lab. Med.*, **111**, 545–8
9. Schwartz, S. O. and Motto, S. A. (1949) The diagnostic significance of 'burr' red blood cells. *Am. J. Med. Sci.*, **218**, 563–6
10. Bell, R. E. (1963) The origin of 'burr' erythrocytes. *Br. J. Haematol.*, **9**, 552–5
11. Bessis, M. and Lessin, L. S. (1970) The discocyte-echinocyte equilibrium of the normal and pathologic red cell. *Blood*, **36**, 399–403
12. Feo, C. J., Tcherna, G., Subtil, E. and Leblond, P. F. (1978) Observation of echinocytosis in eight patients: a phase contrast and SEM study. *Br. J. Haematol.*, **40**, 519–26
13. Brecher, G. and Bessis, M. (1972) Present status of spiculated red cells and their relationship to the discocyte–echinocyte transformation: a critical review. *Blood*, **40**, 333–44
14. Smith, J. A., Lonergan, E. T. and Sterling, K. (1964) Spur cell anaemia: haemolytic anaemia with red cells resembling acanthocytes in alcoholic cirrhosis. *N. Engl. J. Med.*, **271**, 396–8
15. Cooper, R. A. (1970) Lipids of human red cell membrane. Normal composition and variability in disease. *Semin. Haematol.*, **7**, 296–322
16. Symmans, W. A., Shepherd, C. S., Marsh, W. L., Oyen, R., Shohet, S. B. and Linehan, B. J. (1979) Hereditary acanthocytosis associated with the McLeod phenotype of the Kell blood group system. *Br. J. Haematol.*, **42**, 575–83
17. Udden, M. M., Umeda, M., Hirano, Y. and Marcus, D. M. (1987) New abnormalities in the morphology, cell surface receptors and electrolyte metabolism of In(Lu) erythrocytes. *Blood*, **69**, 52–7
18. Wardrop, C. and Hutchinson, H. E. (1969) Red cell shape in hypothyroidism. *Lancet*, **i**, 1243
19. Mant, M. J. and Fargher, B. S. (1972) The haematology of anorexia nervosa. *Br. J. Haematol.*, **23**, 737–49
20. Cooper, R. A. and Jandl, J. H. (1968) Bile salts and cholesterol in the pathogenesis of target cells in obstructive jaundice. *J. Clin. Invest.*, **47**, 809–22
21. De Hann, L. D., Werre, J. M., Ruben, A. M. Th. *et al* (1988) Alterations in size, shape and osmotic behaviour of red cells after splenectomy: a study of their age dependence. *Br. J. Haematol.*, **69**, 71–80
22. Lock, S. P., Sephton-Smith, R. and Hardisty, R. M. (1961) Stomatocytosis: a hereditary red-cell anomaly associated with haemolytic anaemia. *Br. J. Haematol.*, **7**, 303–14
23. Reinhart, W. H., Gossi, U., Butikofer, P. *et. al.* (1989) Haemolytic anaemia in analpha-lipoproteinaemia (Tangier disease): morphological, biochemical and biophysical properties of the red blood cell. *Br. J. Haematol*, **72**, 272–7
24. Weed, R. I. and Bessis, M. (1973) The discocyte–stomatocyte equilibrium of normal and pathologic red cells. *Blood*, **41**, 471–5
25. Sturgeon, P. (1970) Haematological observations on the anaemia associated with blood type Rh^{null}. *Blood*, **36**, 310–20
26. Valentine, W. N., Paglia, D. E., Fink, K. and Madokoro, G. (1976) Lead poisoning. *J. Clin. Invest.*, **58**, 926–32
27. Jacob, H. S. (1969) Mechanism of Heinz body formation and attachment to red cell membrane. *Semin. Haematol.*, **7**, 341–54
28. Schwab, M. L. L. and Lewis, A. E. (1969) An improved stain for Heinz bodies. *Am. J. Clin. Pathol.,* **51**, 673–5
29. Kurth, D., Deiss, A. and Cartwright, G. E. (1969) Circulating siderocytes in human subjects. *Blood*, **34**, 754–64
30. Dacie, J. V. and Lewis, S. M. (1975) *Practical Haematology*, p. 50. London: Churchill Livingstone
31. Koepke, J. A. (1977) A delineation of performance criteria for the differentiation of leucocytes. *Am. J. Clin. Pathol.*, **68**, 202–6

32. Mathy, K. A. and Koepke, J. A. (1974) The clinical usefulness of segmented vs. stab neutrophil criteria for differential counts. *Am. J. Clin. Pathol.*, **61**, 947–58
33. Herbert, V. (1964) Studies of folate deficiency in man. *Proc. R. Soc. Med.*, **37**, 377–84
34. Edwin, E. (1967) The segmentation of polymorphonuclear neutrophils. *Acta Med. Scand.*, **182**, 401–10
35. Bills, T. and Spatz, L. (1977) Neutrophilic hypersegmentation as an indication of incipient folate deficiency. *Am. J. Clin. Pathol.*, **68**, 263–7
36. Sandoz Ltd. (1973) *Atlas of Haematology*, 2nd edn. Basle: Sandoz
37. Cawley, J. C. and Hayhoe, F. G. J. (1972) The inclusions of the May–Hegglin anomaly and Döhle bodies of infections: an ultrastructural comparison. *Br. J. Haematol.*, **22**, 491–6
38. Lutas, E. M. and Zucker-Franklin, D. (1977) Formation of lipid inclusions in normal human leucocytes. *Blood*, **49**, 309–20
39. Gallardo, R. and Kranwinkel, R. N. (1985) Pseuso-Chediak–Higashi anomaly. *Am. J. Clin. Pathol.*, **83**, 127–9
40. Friedman, E. W., Williams, J. C. and Prendergast, E. (1982) Polymorphonuclear leucocyte hypersegmentation in heat stroke. *Br. J. Haematol.*, **50**, 169–70
41. Eichaker, P. and Lawrence, C. (1985) Steroid-induced hypersegmentation in neutrophils. *Am. J. Haematol.*, **18**, 41–5
42. Van Hook, L., Spivack, C. and Duncanson, F. P. (1985) Acquired Pelger–Huet anomaly associated with *Mycoplasma pneumoniae* pneumonia. *Am. J. Clin. Pathol.*, **84**, 248–51
43. Méhes, K. (1966) Nuclear projections in neutrophils. *Blood*, **28**, 598–601
44. Langenhuijsen, M. M. A. C. (1984) Neutrophils with ring-shaped nuclei in myeloproliferative disease. *Br. J. Haematol.*, **58**, 227–30
45. Peichen, M. (1986) Ring cells in infectious mononucleosis. *Br. J. Haematol.*, **62**, 397–8
46. Craig, A. (1987) Ring neutrophils in megaloblastic anaemia. *Br. J. Haematol.*, **67**, 247–8
47. Presentey, B. (1969) Morphological observations and genetic follow-up of a familial anomaly of eosinophils. *Am. J. Clin. Pathol.*, **51**, 458–62
48. White, J. G., Witkop, C. J. and Gerritsen, S. M. (1973) The Hermansky–Pudlack syndrome: inclusions in circulating leucocytes. *Br. J. Haematol.*, **24**, 761–5
49. Norberg, B. (1968) The influence of temperature on the formation of radial-segmented nuclei in human lymphocytes and monocytes. *Scand. J. Haematol.*, **5**, 255–63
50. Neftel, K. A. and Muller, C. M. (1981) Heat-induced radial segmentation of leucocyte nuclei: a non-specific phenomenon accompanying inflammatory and necrotising diseases. *Br. J. Haematol.*, **48**, 377–82
51. Hovig, T., Jeremic, M. and Stavem, P. (1968) A new type of inclusion bodies in lymphocytes. *Scand. J. Haematol.*, **5**, 81–96
52. Pegels, J. G., Bruynes, E. C. E., Engelfriet, C. P. and van dem Borne, A. E. G. Kr. (1982) Pseudothrombocytopenia: an immunologic study on platelet antibodies dependent on ethylene diamine tetra-acetate. *Blood*, **59**, 157–61
53. Karpatkin, S. and Garg, S. K. (1974) The megathrombocyte as an index of platelet production. *Br. J. Haematol.*, **26**, 307–11
54. Paulus, J. M. (1975) Platelet size in man. *Blood*, **46**, 321–36
55. Zeigler, Z., Murphy, S. and Gardener, F. H. (1978) Microscopic platelet size and morphology in various haematologic disorders. *Blood*, **51**, 479–86

Chapter 6

Bone-marrow biopsy

Bone-marrow biopsy is an important and indispensable aspect of haematological investigation and diagnosis. Cytological and histological examination are the basic aspects of bone-marrow investigation though in recent years the techniques of bone-marrow culture for cytogenetic and kinetic studies, isotopic labelling, processing for electron microscopy, clonal culture and other methods have become established. *Figure 6.1* summarizes the procedures that can be applied to bone-marrow samples.

Samples of bone marrow can be obtained by open surgical biopsy or open trephine, by percutaneous trephine using a needle of the Vim–Silverman, Gardner or Jamshidi pattern, or by aspiration using a special needle and syringe. Surgical biopsy is hardly ever carried out solely for haematological purposes and requires full operating-theatre practice. Bone trephines such as the Sacker–Nordin instrument requires skin incision and again full aseptic precautions are recommended. Most samples are therefore obtained by percutaneous biopsy, either by aspiration or needle trephine.

Aspiration biopsy

Precise details of technique[1,2] will not be given but an understanding of the principles involved is desirable.

Aspiration needles are stout with a well-fitting stillette and possibly an adjustable guard to control the depth of penetration. For many years the most favoured site for aspiration biopsy in the adult has been the sternum and needles of the Salah or Klima pattern which incorporate a depth guard are commonly used. Although the sternum is convenient when only aspiration is desired and the site is considered to yield the most cellular samples, there are disadvantages. The patient has a clear view of the procedure which may cause distress and the proximity of vital structures beneath the sternum has, very rarely, resulted in fatal complications. In infants and young children the sternum is naturally thin and an alternative site is preferable. The posterior iliac crest is most suitable though in the very young the presence of haemopoietic marrow in the long bones makes the tibia an alternative site.

There are few, if any, contraindications to aspiration biopsy and haemorrhagic complications are rare even in severe thrombocytopenia. Aspiration in subjects with severe coagulation disorders may be covered by the administration of coagulation factor concentrates.

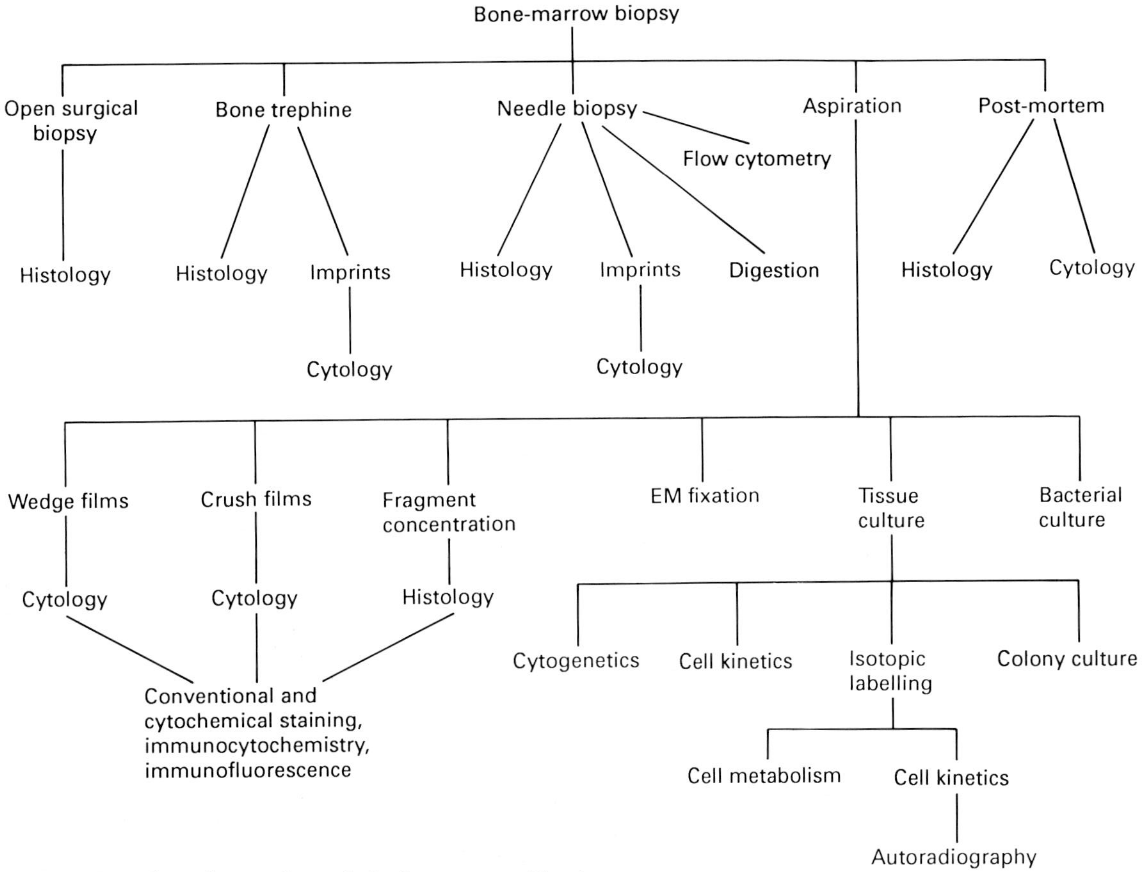

Figure 6.1 Procedures that may be applied to bone-marrow biopsies

A minimum volume of marrow should be aspirated. Volumes over 0.5–1.0 ml will almost certainly be diluted with blood, making interpretation and processing more difficult. In disorders associated with the replacement of haemopoietic marrow by other tissues or cells, marrow aspiration may be difficult or impossible – a 'dry-tap'. In such cases needle trephine biopsy is necessary. Furthermore, the recognition that infiltration of the marrow with malignant cells may be focal and that cellularity of the marrow may be 'patchy' has led to increased use of aspiration combined with needle trephine biopsy. The sternum is not a suitable site for trephine and therefore, increasingly, the posterior iliac crest is being used for aspiration biopsy. Aspiration needles of the Islam type [2] are particularly designed for the iliac crest in that there are a series of apertures extending almost 2 cm from the distal end of the biopsy needle. The advantage of this design is that marrow is aspirated from multiple sites and not simply from the tip of the needle. The needle is also well suited to harvesting large volumes of marrow for transplantation.

Preparation of marrow films

The aspirated marrow should be gently expelled on to a clean slide. The sample should contain small fragments of marrow from which films can be made. Excess blood is carefully drained to one side and the marrow particles picked off with the film-spreader and a series of films prepared as if using blood. In addition to spread films, some workers make crush preparations by gentle pressure of a second slide combined with the sliding apart of the two slides either in one movement or by a series of interrupted movements. Films should be fixed as soon as possible remembering that supplementary staining procedures may require special fixation. It is not recommended that the marrow sample be anticoagulated unless the amount of anticoagulant is appropriate to the volume of sample. Cellular artefacts and difficulties in staining will be experienced in the presence of excess anticoagulant.

In those cases where a 'dry-tap' is obtained any small amount of material in the needle may well be of diagnostic importance, particularly in the case of malignant disease.

Histological preparation of aspirated marrow

Histology of bone-marrow fragments provides a clearer picture of the architecture and cellularity and is superior to smears for demonstrating non-haemopoietic elements such as foci of malignant cells. The many techniques suggested for producing sections of aspirated marrow particles reflect the problem of obtaining maximum visualization of the fragments. The object is to concentrate the particles in one plane. An advantage of processing aspirated fragments is that the decalcification stage usually required for trephine samples is unnecessary.

Clot section technique

The aspirated marrow is expelled directly on to a siliconized watch-glass. The fatty marrow particles float to the surface and may be collected, together with a small amount of blood, using a pipette. Again the fragments tend to rise to the surface and blood clotting maintains their orientation in one plane, readily accessible to penetration by fixative, and facilitates orientation in embedding to allow the fragments to be presented for sectioning.

Sedimentation of bone-marrow particles [3]

Fixative

Absolute ethanol diluted with an equal volume of 15% formalin (150 ml/l 40% formaldehyde) is used. The specific gravity of the mixture is 0.93, almost exactly the same as human fat. When aspirated marrow is added the marrow particles rapidly settle leaving blood in suspension.

Method

0.25 ml of marrow is added to 20 ml of fixative and thoroughly mixed by inversion and allowed to fix overnight. The sediment is resuspended by inversion. After resettling for a few seconds the marrow particles are removed with a Pasteur pipette and transferred to 70% alcohol followed by two changes of absolute ethanol, each for 1 hour. The ethanol is replaced by toluene for 1 hour, replaced by toluene–paraffin wax and then by two changes of paraffin wax. After the wax has hardened the test tube is broken and the wax block recovered. The marrow particles will be concentrated into a small volume and can be readily sectioned.

Special handling of aspirated bone marrow

For electron microscopy

Aspirated bone marrow is fixed immediately in 4% glutaraldehyde in 0.1 mol/l Sörensen's buffer, pH 7.4, for 1 hour at 4°C. After washing in the same buffer the fragments are post-fixed for 1 hour in buffered 1% osmium tetroxide before dehydration and embedding in Araldite.

For cytogenetic studies

Aspirated marrow is transferred to one of a variety of suitable tissue-culture nutrient mixtures. Nutrient-mixture F10 is suitable and is available commercially (Gibco BioCult Ltd).

For isotopic labelling and metabolic studies

Aspirate is incubated in heparinized Hanks' (Hanks' Balanced Salt Solution, Gibco BioCult Ltd) solution to which penicillin and streptomycin may be added. The heparin must be preservative-free. If a cell suspension is required the marrow aspirate should be forced through a 21-gauge needle and then twice through a 25-gauge needle to break up cell clumps.

For colony culture techniques

Aspirate is transferred to a sterile container containing *preservative-free* heparin.

For immunofluorescent studies of malignant plasma cells

It is important to remove by washing any trace of plasma immunoglobulin which would inactivate the labelled anti-globulin sera. Collection into Hanks' Balanced Salt Solution and subsequent washing is a satisfactory approach. Clumps of cells may be broken up by force, using either a fine needle or a stainless steel screen.

Examination of post-mortem bone-marrow material

The rapid post-mortem autolysis of bone marrow is reflected in sectioned material and by disruption of cells in wedge-films. The protective effect of albumin was described by Berenbaum [4] who recommended that marrow be suspended in 5% bovine albumin, centrifuged, and the cells resuspended in an approximately equal volume of 5% albumin. Films are then made in the usual way. 'Spun-films' (*see* page 128) may produce satisfactory post-mortem preparations without the necessity for the albumin technique.

Trephine and needle biopsies

Although histology of aspirated bone-marrow particles can provide valuable information on the cellularity and architecture of the marrow, there is little doubt that a trephine or needle biopsy is superior (*Figure 6.2*). Not only may particle aspiration be difficult or impossible, in which case a trephine biopsy is essential, but in cases where both aspiration and trephine biopsies have been obtained, the sectioned sample shows a consistently higher rate of detection of malignant marrow infiltration [5,6]. The superiority of trephine biopsy over aspiration in the staging of patients with lymphomas has also been shown [7].

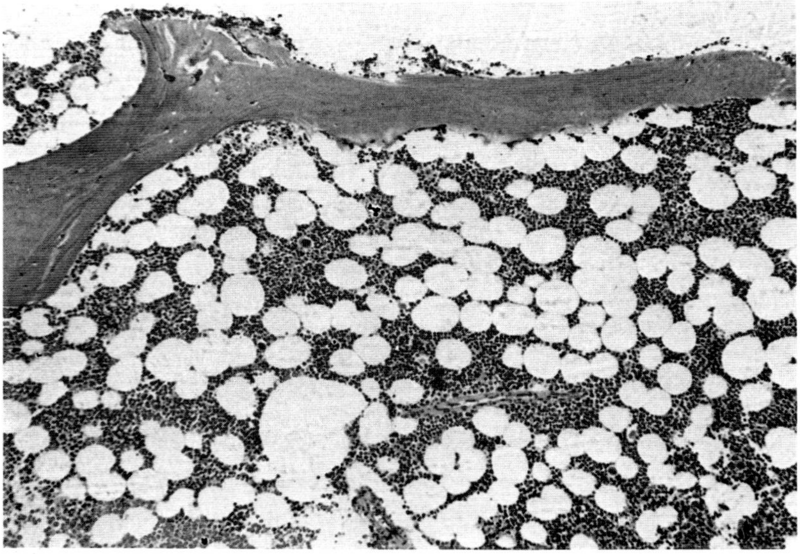

Figure 6.2 Trephine biopsy. Normal bone marrow showing areas of cellularity interspersed with fat spaces. ×110

When the marrow is replaced by fibrous tissue or bone, the trephine biopsy is the only means of obtaining a useful specimen. Assessment of iron stores is probably more reliable from a sectioned biopsy.

Although cytological preparations may be obtained by making an 'imprint' of the biopsy specimen on a slide by *gentle* pressure and the transfer of the surface cells, the preparation of sections for histological examination is the standard technique. An alternative and superior method to the 'imprint' technique is digestion of the trephine with collagenase, cytocentrifugation and subsequent staining[8]. Preparations can be completed 2 hours after biopsy. Paraffin sections are widely used but considerable shrinkage is inevitable. The choice of fixative and the method of decalcification affect the quality of the section and its subsequent staining. Mercuric chloride–potassium dichromate fixatives are widely used with the addition of acetic acid (Zenker's fluid) or formalin (Helly's fluid). Neutral buffered formalin has been recommended. The multiplicity of published techniques reflects the difficulties in obtaining first-class preparations. Plastic embedding, though time consuming and requiring utmost technical care, must be considered the method of choice due to better preservation, omission of decalcification and the ability to cut semi-thin sections. The technique of Burkhardt as modified and described by Te Velde *et al.* [9] is recommended. An evaluation of acrolein and neutral buffered formalin followed by methyl-methacrylate (MMA) embedding and its effect on subsequent staining has been reported together with recommended techniques[10]. For enzyme or immunohistology, methyl-methacrylate has shortcomings. Glycomethacrylate (GMA) is superior[11,12]. Immunocytochemical demonstration of cell-surface markers in sections of trephine biopsies prepared by cryotomy has been described[13].

Staining of bone-marrow preparations

The staining techniques that can be applied to bone-marrow preparations are summarized in *Table 6.1*.

Haematoxylin and eosin and reticulin staining is usually confined to histopathology departments. Cytochemical and immunological techniques are described in Chapter 13.

Table 6.1 Staining methods for bone-marrow preparations

Material	*Purpose*	*Staining*
Trephine biopsies, particle sections	Cellularity. Overall architecture. Non-haemopoietic elements.	Haematoxylin/eosin
	Assessment of iron stores.	Perls' Prussian blue reaction.
	Assessment of reticulin content.	Silver impregnation.
	Identification of haemopoietic cells	'Romanowsky'
Smears or imprints	Cytological identification.	'Romanowsky'
	Assessment of iron stores and distribution in erythroblasts.	Perls' Prussian blue reaction.
	Cytochemical identification	PAS, peroxidase, sudan black, esterases, acid phosphatase.

PAS = Periodic acid–Schiff.

Romanowsky staining

Bone-marrow sections

The many variations in technique make recommendations of any one method difficult as much depends on experience and personal preference. The choice between Giemsa, Leishman, May-Grunwald etc. is also very much one of personal choice and familiarity with the characteristics of the selected stain.

The general principle is to overstain the section in diluted stain and differentiate until the desired appearance is obtained. The dehydration stage preparatory to mounting must be as rapid as possible to avoid modification of the staining.

Bone-marrow films

Again the choice of Romanowsky stain is mainly dependent on personal preference and familiarity with the staining qualities of the dye selected. Because of the varied cellularity of bone-marrow films, automatic staining machines with staining cycles timed for blood films do not always give satisfactory results. It is recommended that either an 'on-slide' technique or staining jars be used to allow fixation, staining and differentiation to be varied according to the cellularity of the marrow film. The stained film should preferably be mounted under a cover-glass or alternatively may be sprayed with vinyl.

Perls' Prussian blue technique for ferric iron applied to blood or bone-marrow films

Ferric iron reacts with acidified potassium ferrocyanide to form the characteristic 'Prussian blue' of ferric ferrocyanide.

Method

Dry films are fixed for at least 30 minutes in absolute methanol and washed in running water for 15 minutes. A solution of 10 g potassium ferrocyanide in 1 litre of N/10 HCl is freshly prepared and warmed to 37°C in a staining jar. The fixed, washed films are immersed and stained for 20 minutes. The staining solution will develop a green coloration. The stained slides are again thoroughly washed for 15 minutes in running water, drained in the staining jar and counter-stained for 20–30 s with 0.1% aqueous safranin or eosin, again washed thoroughly and allowed to dry. Overstaining must be avoided. The films should not be blotted as marrow particles may adhere to the blotting paper. Ferric iron appears as dark blue particulate material.

Examination and assessment of stained bone-marrow preparations

Cellularity

The nucleated cell count of aspirated marrow is unreliable due to the variable dilution with blood even with samples of as little as 0.25–0.5 ml. Attempts to quantify cellularity by a volumetric approach are also unreliable. Qualitative assessment of cellularity from film preparations inevitably suffers from the problem of dilution with blood. Attention should therefore be concentrated on the examination of marrow fragments in the tail of the film and the 'trails' produced during spreading from the fragments. Crush preparations are also useful for assessing cellularity. Marrow of normal cellularity always contains fat and up to half the content of a marrow particle may be fat. Subjective assessment is not always reliable and reproducibility is poor [14]. Nevertheless the assessment of marrow cellularity is essential in marrow hypoplasia and aplasia and is of value in the differential diagnosis of erythrocytosis.

Histological preparations of aspirated bone-marrow fragments are preferred to film preparations and objective assessment by 'point-counting'[15,16] is probably superior to a subjective opinion. A variable is the non-random distribution of fragments because of their different rates of sedimentation during processing[15]. This problem is, of course, not found in trephine biopsies though 'patchy' marrow cellularity can be found.

Cytology

Cytological assessment other than overall cellularity should be performed systematically and include the pattern of maturation and morphology of the cells of each series, together with the numbers and appearances of the plasma cells and lymphocytes. Megakaryocytes will be found mainly at the edges of the films and in the vicinity of fragments and their number and maturation should be recorded. A careful search for non-haemopoietic elements such as neoplastic cells, tissue basophils (mast cells), lipid-loaded macrophages and other abnormal histiocytes should be made, particularly at the edges or tail of the film. The possible presence of parasites and micro-organisms should be considered and included in the report of the marrow appearances.

Myeloid–erythroid ratio (MER)

Opinion is divided on the value of routine differential counting of bone-marrow films but the MER is widely used as an expression of the myeloid and erythroid compartments relative to each other and is calculated after classifying at least 200 cells. In normal adult bone marrow the myeloid cells always outnumber the erythroid cells with a mean value of about 4:1. The ratio by itself does not, of course, indicate whether a series is hypo- or hyperactive. An increased MER may be due to increased numbers of 'myeloid' cells or depression of the erythroid series and similarly a reduced ratio may be due to erythroid hyperplasia or suppression of granulocyte activity. Confusion exists as to which cells to include in the 'myeloid' component. Most observers have apparently included granulocytes and lymphocytes, while others count granulocytes only. As a variable proportion of the lymphocytes and mature neutrophils are derived from the almost inevitable presence of blood, some workers exclude mature neutrophils and the lymphocytes from the count, in which case the normal MER is considerably lower.

Differential counting

Apart from the question as to whether a routine differential count is clinically helpful, the major objection is that the irregular distribution of the many types of cells in the marrow makes a count unreliable unless many cells are counted. If a differential count is to be attempted at least 200 cells should be studied and some authorities insist on a minimum of 500 cells.

Although differential counts are traditionally performed from the 'trails' of cells from marrow fragments in a wedge film, trephine biopsies can be used and have been considered to be more consistent[16].

The normal ranges for differential counts on aspirated bone marrow from adults are given in *Table 6.2*. The data illustrate the wide ranges found in health and indicate that minor changes associated with disease are difficult to identify. There

Table 6.2 Normal ranges for differential on aspirated bone marrow of adults

Myeloblasts	0.1–3.5%
Promyelocytes	0.5–5%
Myelocytes:	
Neutrophil	5–20%
Eosinophil	0.1–3%
Basophil	0–0.5%
Metamyelocytes	10–30%
Segmented:	
Neutrophils	7–25%
Eosinophils	0.2–3%
Basophils	0–0.5%
Lymphocytes	5–20%
Monocytes	0.1–1%
Macrophages	0.1–2%
Plasma cells	0.1–3.5%
Megakaryocytes	0.1–0.5%
Pronormoblasts	0.5–5%
Normoblasts:	
A, basophilic	2–5%
B, polychromatic	2–20%
C, pyknotic	2–10%

are certain exceptions, notably the number of myeloblasts in early or pre-leukaemic states and the number of plasma cells. Apart from the debatable value of expressing each cell type as a percentage, a differential count can illustrate the pattern of maturation of a cell series which might be overlooked in a qualitative assessment. In normal marrow the numbers of cells of each type in a series show a remarkably consistent pattern which can be readily seen when 'scoring' the differential count. Arrested maturation of granulocyte or erythroid series can be readily recognized. The break in maturation pattern in acute myeloblastic leukaemia, the 'hiatus leukaemicus', is typical. Hyperplasia of a cell series also alters the maturation pattern.

Iron content

Iron can be demonstrated in the bone marrow in both extra- and intracellular forms. Storage iron is reflected by both the amount of extracellular material and that found in macrophages. In normal marrow, storage iron will only be demonstrable in the marrow particles with occasional iron-containing macrophages. In iron depletion, particulate material is reduced or absent. Increased iron stores are reflected by increased iron in the fragments and increased numbers of macrophages with excess iron content. In haemosiderosis iron may be seen throughout the film and not confined to the fragments. Semi-quantitative scoring techniques have been suggested. That of Davidson and Jennison [17] relies on assessment of the number of iron-containing histiocytes while other workers have simply scored iron stores as: (+), (++) and (+++).

Erythroblast iron is assessed by the number of erythroblasts containing stainable iron and by the character, amount and distribution of the granules. The granules in the cytoplasm of normal erythroblasts are scattered, few, fine and difficult to see and are confined to the late or pyknotic cells. The original reports[18,19] that in normal marrow as many as 40% of late normoblasts contain stainable iron granules are difficult to support. Much depends on the resolution of the microscope. By definition iron-containing erythroblasts are 'sideroblasts'.

In iron depletion sideroblasts are absent. Iron-loaded states such as haemochromatosis and haemosiderosis are reflected in coarser more numerous granules. Increases in the number and size of the iron granules are of considerable importance and if distributed closely around the nucleus (peri-nuclear distribution), reflect iron-loading of the mitochondria. These 'ringed sideroblasts' are of special significance and their number and occurrence in each stage of erythroblast maturation should be noted. These aspects are considered in more detail in Chapters 9 and 12.

Reticulin

The connective-tissue framework of normal bone marrow consists of a network of fine reticulin fibres (*Figure 6.3*). The amount of reticulin may be variably increased in a wide variety of haematological disorders and when of normal pattern may simply reflect hypercellularity of the marrow. Of more importance is increased reticulin associated with an altered pattern. The fibres are thicker and the network coarser with the thick fibres aggregating into bundles with a wavy course and having the morphology of immature collagen. This pattern is essentially that described as 'fibroblastic' and is characteristically found in myelofibrosis though it may be observed to lesser degree in disorders such as chronic granulocytic leukaemia, polycythaemia vera and multiple myeloma[20]. Reticulin is usually decreased in aplastic anaemia.

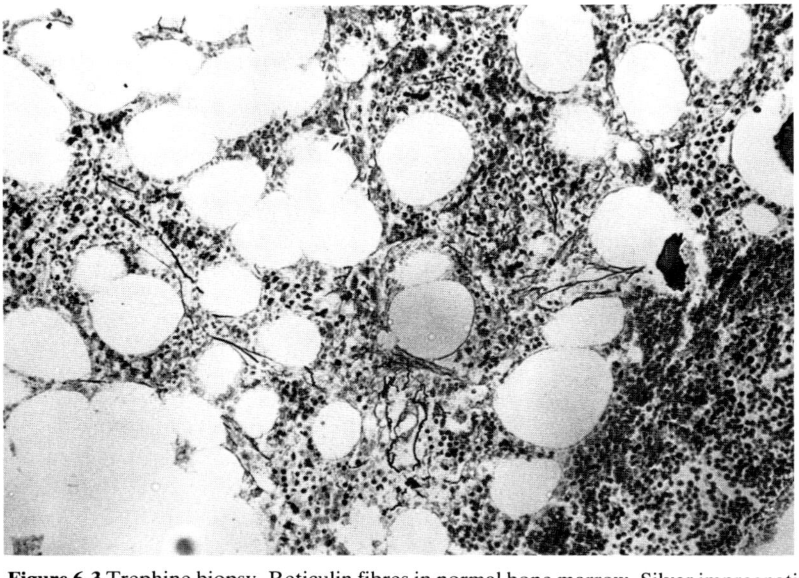

Figure 6.3 Trephine biopsy. Reticulin fibres in normal bone marrow. Silver impregnation technique. ×110

References

1. Knowles, S. and Hoffbrand, A. V. (1980) Bone-marrow aspiration and trephine biopsy. *Br. Med. J.*, **ii**, 280–1
2. Islam, A. (1983) A new bone marrow aspiration needle to overcome the sampling errors inherent in the technique of bone marrow aspiration. *J. Clin. Pathol.*, **36**, 954–8
3. Dacie, J. V. and Lewis, S. M. (1984) *Practical Haematology*, 6th edn, p. 123. London: Churchill Livingstone
4. Berenbaum, M. C. (1956) The use of bovine albumen in the preparation of marrow and blood films. *J. Clin. Pathol.*, **9**, 381–3
5. Contreras, E., Ellis, I. D. and Lee, R. E. (1972) Value of bone marrow in the diagnosis of metastatic cancer. *Cancer,* **29**, 778–83
6. Jacob, P. (1977) Discrepant bone marrow aspiration in leukaemia. *Lancet,* **i**, 356
7. Rosenberg, S. A. (1971) Hodgkin's disease of the bone marrow. *Cancer Res.*, **31**, 1733–6
8. Mononen, I. and Jansson, S. E. (1986) A rapid procedure, by collagenase treatment and cytocentrifugation, for the cytological evaluation of bone marrow biopsy specimens. *Clin. Lab. Haematol.*, **8**, 149–54
9. Te Velde, J., Burkhardt, R., Kleiverda, K. *et al.* (1977) Methyl-methacrylate as an embedding medium in histopathology. *Histopathology,* **1**, 319–30
10. Dancey, J. T., Denkelbeiss, K. A., Harker, I. A. and Greenaway, J. (1976) Section preparation of human marrow for light microscopy. *J. Clin. Pathol.*, **29**, 704–10
11. Beckstead, J. H. and Bainton, D. F. (1980) Enzyme histochemistry on bone marrow biopsies: reactions useful in the differential diagnosis of leukaemia and lymphoma applied to 2-micron plastic sections. *Blood,* **55**, 386–94
12. Islam, A. (1987) New instrument for longitudinal hemisectioning of undecalcified marrow cores for simultaneous processing and examination with useful and complementary techniques. *J. Clin. Pathol.*, **40**, 112–6
13. Phillpotts, C. J. and Smith, J. G. (1988) Treatment of bone marrow trephine biopsies prior to cryotomy for immunocytochemical demonstration of cell surface antigens. *Med. Lab. Sci.*, **45**, 52–6
14. Morley, A. and Blake, J. (1975) Observer errors in histological assessment of marrow hypocellularity. *J. Clin. Pathol.*, **28**, 104–8
15. Ho-Yen, D. O. and Slidders, W. (1978) Bone marrow cellularity assessed by point counting. *J. Clin. Pathol.*, **31**, 753–6
16. Wilkins, B. S. and O'Brien, C. J. (1988) Techniques for obtaining differential cell counts from bone marrow trephine biopsy specimens. *J. Clin. Pathol.*, **41**, 558–61
17. Davidson, W. M. and Jennison, R. F. (1952) The relationship between storage iron and anaemia. *J. Clin. Pathol.*, **5**, 281–5
18. Kaplan, E., Zuelzer, W. W. and Mouriquand, C. (1954) Sideroblasts. A study of stainable non-haemoglobin iron in blood. *Blood,* **9**, 203–13
19. Douglas, A. S. and Dacie, J. V. (1953) The incidence and significance of iron-containing granules in human erythrocytes and their precursors. *J. Clin. Pathol.*, **6**, 307–13
20. Burston, J. and Pinniger, J. L. (1963) The reticulin content of bone marrow in haematological disorders. *Br. J. Haematol.*, **9**, 172–84

Chapter 7

Erythrocyte sedimentation rate, plasma viscosity and blood rheology

Erythrocyte sedimentation rate (ESR)

When anticoagulated blood is allowed to stand undisturbed the red cells sediment. Discrete red cells sediment very slowly while aggregates of red cells settle more quickly. The rate of red-cell sedimentation is related to the size of the aggregates (Stoke's Law states that the rate of sedimentation is directly proportional to the square of the radius of the aggregate). Red-cell aggregation usually occurs as rouleaux formation in which the cells stack together in the manner of 'piles of coins' or 'chains', though aggregation may be in the form of agglutination due to antigen–antibody interaction. The chains of rouleaux form spherical aggregates of uniform size. The radius of the spheres is inversely proportional to the PCV[1].

The formation of rouleaux and spherical aggregates requires the presence of electrolyte, neutral or negatively charged macromolecules and metabolically active cells. Red cells possess a net negative charge due to sialic acid residues and therefore repel each other. The repulsive force, or zeta potential, increases with decreasing ionic strength of the suspending medium. To form rouleaux, macromolecules must be present to bridge the space between red cells. From experimental work, it has been suggested that the red cell binding site for negatively charged macromolecules is an active anion transport site or band 3 protein[1].

Alteration in the concentrations of hydrophilic protein fractions of the plasma, particularly asymmetric macromolecules, increases the rate of rouleaux formation, the formation of spherical aggregates and thus the rate of sedimentation. Changes in plasma proteins which affect the rate of rouleaux formation are associated with tissue damage and inflammation and are found in chronic disease processes. The rate of erythrocyte sedimentation (ESR) is therefore a non-specific index of the presence of organic disorder or disease activity.

The ESR is determined by filling a narrow tube of defined length and bore with well-mixed anticoagulated blood, placing it in a vertical position for a set time at the end of which the distance from the top of the column to the interface between the plasma and the sedimented red cells is recorded and expressed in mm/unit time.

Sedimentation follows an S-shaped curve with time, which can be considered as occurring in three phases. Phase 1 is a delay phase with no sedimentation, phase 2 is linear and sedimentation occurs at a constant rate, followed by phase 3 during which the rate slows as packing of the aggregates occurs and levels off to zero sedimentation.

Although the ESR is primarily a measure of plasma protein changes in disease, the sedimentation rate is also influenced by the viscosity of the plasma, red-cell factors, physical and technical variables and, in particular, the PCV of the blood sample.

Factors affecting the ESR

Effect of plasma proteins

Changes in plasma proteins occur rapidly following tissue injury or in response to inflammation, the 'acute-phase response' mediated by interleukin 1 [2]. Increased concentrations of fibrinogen, C-reactive protein (CRP), serum amyloid A-protein, α_1 proteins, haptoglobins and the third component of complement (C3) are followed by increases in α_2 macroglobulin and immunoglobulins. Albumin, which tends to counteract the rouleaux-forming properties of the macromolecular proteins, tends to diminish in concentration and further increases rouleaux formation. In the chronic pathological process changes in the 'acute-phase proteins' are generally less marked, fibrinogen being normal or slightly raised and the major influences probably being an increase in the IgG immunoglobulins. The anti-rouleaux influence of albumin must not be overlooked; normal or increased albumin concentrations will decrease the rate of rouleaux formation, while conversely hypoalbuminaemia will increase the sedimentation rate even when the macromolecular proteins are normal.

Influence of plasma viscosity

The rate of sedimentation of aggregated red cells is directly influenced by the viscosity of the plasma. Plasma viscosity is determined mainly by the concentration of the various plasma proteins; the higher the protein concentration the greater the viscosity. Although increased macromolecular proteins will increase rouleaux formation and hence the rate of sedimentation, gross immunoglobulin increases such as can occur in the paraproteinaemias may increase plasma viscosity to the extent of masking the full rouleaux-forming effect of the paraprotein.

Effect of red-cell factors

Efficient rouleaux formation depends upon the red cells having a normal shape and metabolic activity. Anisocytosis or poikilocytosis will reduce the ability to form rouleaux thus reducing the sedimentation rate. Storage of blood samples results in changes in shape and metabolism and reduces the ESR, although to an unpredictable degree.

The influence of the PCV in determining the size of the spherical aggregates has been referred to earlier, the lower the PCV the greater the size of the spherical aggregates which therefore results in an increased *rate* of sedimentation. The lower PCV must also affect the total *distance* of sedimentation. Conversely an elevated PCV, even with quite modest increases, results in a decrease in ESR.

Effect of physical variables

The conditions under which the ESR is performed may influence the results. The most consistent influence is the perpendicularity of the sedimentation tube. Slight deviations from the vertical will increase the rate of sedimentation; a 3-degree 'list' can increase the ESR by 30%. Racks for sedimentation tubes should be fitted with levelling devices to ensure the tubes are vertical. The use of an angle of 60 degrees has been suggested as a modification of the standard test to achieve greater sensitivity.

Temperature influences the ESR although variation in the ambient temperature of a laboratory is unlikely to be a significant problem unless the tubes are placed in direct sunlight. Higher temperatures cause falsely elevated results due to a reduction in plasma viscosity.

It has been claimed that vibration can reduce the ESR by retarding the rate of rouleaux formation. However, the vibration that might be encountered in practice, for example by a centrifuge on the same bench, has been shown to have a very limited influence on results[3].

Choice of technique

Two basic methods have been recommended and have gained wide acceptance, the Wintrobe and Lansberg and the Westergren techniques. The Wintrobe technique uses a tube closed at one end, 110 mm long with a bore of 2.5 mm and having a graduated scale from 0 to 100 mm, the Wintrobe haematocrit tube. Dry anticoagulant is used, originally an ammonium–potassium oxalate mixture, later replaced by dipotassium EDTA. The tube is filled using a capillary pipette and sedimentation read after 1 hour. An advantage claimed for the Wintrobe method is that the tube can be subsequently centrifuged to determine the PCV and the ESR corrected for anaemia by reference to a graph or nomogram.

The Westergren method employs an open glass tube similar to a graduated pipette with an overall length of 300 mm with a bore of 2.5 mm. The graduated portion measures 200 mm. Blood anticoagulated by the addition of one volume of sodium citrate to four volumes of blood is drawn up to form a column 200 mm in length and sedimentation is noted after 1 hour. Some workers have recommended taking an additional reading after 2 hours.

Comparisons have been made between the two techniques and it has been concluded that the Wintrobe method is more sensitive when the ESR is low and when the disease is in the acute stage, while the Westergren method more reliably reflects the clinical state[4]. The Wintrobe method loses sensitivity at high ESR values simply because of the shorter tube length while the Westergren is non-linear at lower values but is clearly superior for monitoring changes in subjects with active disease. It has been suggested that the Wintrobe method or the ZSR (*see* p. 186) is best for screening and the Westergren for monitoring the disease process[5]. The International Committee for Standardization in Haematology recommends the Westergren method[6,7].

ICSH reference method for the ESR on human blood

Materials

Anticoagulant–diluent solution Tri-sodium citrate dihydrate ($Na_3C_6H_5O_72H_2O$) 30.88 g; distilled water to 1 litre. The solution is filtered through a sterile membrane, maximum pore diameter 0.22 mm, into a sterile container and kept *without preservatives*. It must be discarded if turbid.

Westergren–Katz tube (1) The tube must be made of thick-walled glass tubing, which is straight, colourless, free from visible defects and internal strain. The upper end must be ground smooth, square with the longitudinal axis and have a suitable bevelled edge; the lower end must be tapered, finely ground and similarly square to the axis. (2) The tube must conform to the following dimensions: overall length, 300 ± 1.5 mm; tube bore, 2.55 ± 0.15 mm; uniformity of tube bore, ±0.05 mm. (3) The tube must possess the following markings: the inscription 'Westergren'; the scale, graduated in mm, extending over the lower 200 ± 0.35 mm. Maximal tolerated error between two subsequent mm markings is 0.2 mm. Graduations should be fine, clearly marked lines of uniform thickness (0.2 mm) and numbered from 200 at the bottom up to 0 in steps of 10 or less.

Method

Blood is obtained by clean venepuncture over a maximum period of 30 s, and thoroughly mixed in a proportion of four volumes of blood to one volume of filtered solution of sodium citrate. At room temperature the test must be set up within 2 hours, or at 4°C within 6 hours. Any sample showing evidence of agglutination when checked with a magnifying glass should be discarded. The blood-citrate is thoroughly mixed by gentle repeated inversion and a clean, dry, standard Westergren–Katz tube is filled and adjusted to the '0' mark. The tube is then placed in a strictly vertical position under room temperature conditions (18–25°C), not exposed to direct sunlight and free from vibrations and draughts. After this time period the distance from the bottom of the surface meniscus to the top of the column of sedimenting red cells (where the full density is apparent) is read in mm and recorded as the ESR value. The result is expressed as follows: 'ESR (WESTERGREN 1 h) = x mm'.

Appendix

1. Contamination with skin-cleaning materials during the venepuncture should be avoided.
2. If the laboratory ambient temperature is other than 18–25°C, it should be noted with the ESR value.
3. Blood samples for ESR test can be obtained without regard to the patient's circadian rhythm or meals.
4. For reutilization, the glass tubes must be cleaned in an acetone–water system. Use of dichromate and detergent mixtures is not recommended.
5. When evaluating an ESR test, additional factors should be considered such as haemoglobin level, age, sex, menstrual cycle, pregnancy, drugs taken (corticoids, contraceptive pills, etc.).
6. Values for 'normal' ESR are not given in the international recommendation.

Additional technical notes

1. *Anticoagulant* Blood collected into K_2EDTA may be used for ESR provided that one-fourth volume of sodium citrate is added. The substitution of 0.9% NaCl for the citrate is a satisfactory alternative.
2. *Delay in testing* The reference technique specifies that the test should be performed within 2 hours or 6 hours if the sample is kept at 4°C. Tests may be carried out on samples *in EDTA* kept for 24 hours at 4°C provided that citrate or NaCl is added immediately before testing.

3. *Sedimentation tubes other than glass* The trend towards disposable equipment, reinforced by the requirement to avoid unnecessary contact with potentially infective samples, has promoted the use of disposable plastic tubes often to be used with special sample container systems and devices for filling the tubes. Evaluations of these systems have mostly demonstrated results comparable with the reference method, provided that the technical criteria are met. Static electrical charge on plastic tubes does not affect the results[8].
4. *Micro-methods* Modifications to the standard technique have been suggested in order to reduce the volume of blood required, an approach of particular importance in paediatric work. The usual method has been either to shorten the tube, reduce the bore, or both. Shortening the tube must reduce the range over which readings can be obtained. Several studies have shown that slightly elevated values are obtained in the higher range by using narrow bore polystyrene 'Westergren' tubes. The differences are unlikely to be of clinical importance[9]. Any modification of the tube dimensions must be accompanied by a revised reference range and an appreciation that the results may not be comparable with the reference technique.
5. Occasionally the top of the column of sedimented cells is not clear-cut, possibly due to the presence of increased numbers of reticulocytes or the formation of amorphous aggregates by positively charged macromolecules. Readings are inevitably arbitrary and subjective.

Despite the recognized flaws in the technique the ESR continues to be widely used because of its simplicity and because it responds to the changes in asymmetrical macromolecules associated with inflammatory disease, and its value in diagnosis and as a means of monitoring the progress of disease. Automated ESR systems are available.

Interpretation of results [10]

Normal ranges Men, 3–5 mm in 1 hour; 7–15 mm in 2 hours. Women, 4–7 mm in 1 hour; 12–17 mm in 2 hours. In the elderly, many normal subjects have increased ESR readings due to reduced plasma albumin concentrations.

Physiological variations

(i) Normal infants: low readings are found due to low globulin levels and elevated PCV.

(ii) Normal pregnancy: increases into the pathological range are found in the last trimester due to the reduced PCV associated with hypovolaemia, an increase in α globulin and an increase in fibrinogen concentration.

Pathological variations

(i) Normal readings in the presence of active disease:
   (a) Erythrocytosis associated with an elevated PCV.
   (b) Cryoglobulinaemia. Cryoproteins precipitating at room temperature produce a low ESR. A marked increase in the value is found after warming and carrying out the test at 37°C.
   (c) Gross poikilocytosis such as that associated with sickling phenomena or marked spherocytosis may produce a falsely normal value.

(ii) Increased readings:
   (a) Anaemia, due to the low PCV.
   (b) Acute and chronic inflammation due to (i) changes in plasma macromolecules, (ii) hypoalbuminaemia, (iii) certain hyperlipidaemic states.
   (c) Cold agglutination, producing high ESRs at room temperature and normal values at 37°C.

'Corrected' ESR values
The influence of the PCV on the ESR which results in sex differences in the reference range and, more importantly, the difficulty in interpreting ESR results when the PCV is abnormal, has resulted in attempts to correct ESR values to a 'standard' PCV value.

As stated earlier, an advantage of the Wintrobe method is that the same tube for measuring ESR can be centrifuged to determine PCV and a 'corrected' ESR value obtained. A revised method of reading the ESR with correction to a PCV of 0.400 has been recommended[1]. Adjustment of the PCV to 0.350 before measuring ESR has been suggested[11] which can be incorporated into a quality control scheme. These approaches would be time-consuming and are unlikely to be adopted as routine procedures.

Zeta sedimentation ratio

The disadvantages of the ESR are the effect of the PCV, the time taken to obtain the result, the health hazard of filling and cleaning the tubes (or alternatively the cost of disposable systems), the volume of blood required and differing normal ranges between the sexes. Bull and Brailsford[12] described the measurement of the zeta sedimentation ratio (ZSR) as an indication of the effect of plasma macromolecules in decreasing the zeta potential of adjacent red cells. The technique measures the closeness with which red cells approach one another under a standard stress which is applied by a special centrifuge to blood contained in a vertical capillary tube. The standard stress is applied by four alternate cycles of compaction and dispersion to produce a degree of compaction known as the zetacrit (Zct) which is divided into the true haematocrit (PCV) obtained by further conventional centrifugation or from Coulter Counter Model S data.

Normal individuals have a ZSR of 40–51%. The ZSR technique eliminates the disadvantages of the ESR but 'consumer' resistance to an alternative unit, %, rather than mm/h and the reluctance to depart from established technique has resulted in only limited use of the method. A further disadvantage is the need to purchase new equipment and special capillary tubes. Correlation between the ZSR, ESR and clinical assessment of disease activity has been reported but the technique has not found general clinical acceptance. The clinical and laboratory aspects of the ESR with reference to the ZSR have been comprehensively reviewed[12].

Plasma viscosity (PV)

Viscosity is the resistance offered by a liquid to attempt to change its shape and may be defined as the ratio of shear stress to shear rate. The rate of shear is the tangential force exerted across a unit area between two parallel planes of the fluid under consideration, unit distance apart, one plane being fixed whilst the other moves at unit velocity. If the planes are x apart and move at relative velocity v then the velocity gradient is v/x. This velocity gradient is called the shear rate. If v is measured in cm s^{-1} and x in cm then v/x is expressed in reciprocal seconds, s^{-1}. The force per unit area that produces this rate of shear is the shear stress. If the ratio of shear stress to shear rate is constant the liquid is said to be 'Newtonian' in character, i.e. if the flow rate is to be doubled, twice the force will be required to bring this about[13]. The original unit of viscosity is the 'poise' – named after Poiseuille who formulated the relationship between the variables determining the flow of fluids through narrow tubes. The SI units of shear stress are pascals and the units of viscosity are millipascal seconds (mPa s): 1 millipascal-second is equivalent to 1 centipoise.

Plasma is considered to be Newtonian in behaviour and though doubts have been expressed they may have arisen through inadequate techniques. Viscosity depends upon the concentrations of plasma proteins, particularly the macromolecules. In solution, weight-for-weight, fibrinogen has a greater viscosity than IgG immunoglobulin which in turn has a greater viscosity than albumin. Thus the increases in plasma macromolecules in response to inflammation or tissue damage will result in an increase in plasma viscosity.

Measurement of plasma viscosity

Capillary viscometers are suitable for measuring the viscosity of Newtonian fluids and therefore for the study of plasma viscosity. The principle is to determine the time taken for a measured volume of plasma to flow through a capillary tube of standard bore and length, under a standard force at a controlled temperature.

The ICSH have published recommendations[14] for the measurement of plasma viscosity and a selected method using the Harkness Viscometer (Coulter Electronics Ltd) which is a convenient, rapid, precise and accurate instrument. The standard force is provided by a mercury manometer, electronic timing by the mercury moving between two electrical contacts and the temperature controlled by immersing the glassware in a thermostat-controlled water-bath maintained at 25 ± 0.1°C. Coefficient of variation (CV) is in the order of ±1% and measurements are made within 1 minute using 0.5 ml of plasma.

An alternative approach is used by the Luckham Clinical Viscometer (Luckham Ltd) by which 0.5 ml of plasma is drawn through a metal capillary thermostatically maintained at 25°C in an oil-bath. The time is measured by the interval between the leading and trailing edges of the plasma column passing a transducer. The CV is also in the order of ±1% and 120 samples can be tested in 1 hour.

A different approach is adopted by the Coulter Viscometer II (Coulter Electronics Ltd). Viscosity is determined by measuring the pressure required to force the plasma through the capillary, with correction of ambient temperature to 25°C or 37°C. A carousel is available which permits automatic sampling and a printer records the results; throughput is in the order of 50–60 per hour. Each of the above instruments produces comparable results.

Although plasma viscosity is routinely measured at, or corrected to, 25°C, the ICSH recommend that results should be expressed at 37°C. This recommendation has not yet been widely adopted in routine practice.

EDTA plasma is preferred and should be stored in capped tubes to prevent evaporation. Slight haemolysis has no effect. Plasma samples in capped tubes may be stored for at least 48 hours and probably up to 7 days at room temperature. On no account should samples be refrigerated since this can lead to irreversible denaturation of macromolecules. Ideally, centrifuged plasma should be used though plasma containing leucocytes and platelets obtained by gravity sedimentation of blood may be used; results in this case, however, are slightly higher than in cell-free plasma.

Interpretation of results

Adult reference ranges:

1.5–1.72 mPa s at 25°C
1.16–1.35 mPa s at 37°C.

Physiological variation

Age: birth–3 years = 1.25–1.47 mPa s at 25°C due to low immunoglobulins.
Pregnancy (3rd trimester): 1.5–1.8 mPa s at 25°C.
Individual variation: varies little over many years in healthy subjects; a change of >0.05 mPa s at 25°C can be clinically significant.

Diet, time of day, menstruation, posture and exercise can result in small changes of <0.03 mPa s at 25°C.

Plasma viscosity in disease

Acute infection or tissue damage are reflected by a prompt increase in PV. In chronic disease PV will be raised often within the range 1.75–2.00 mPa s. Invasive malignancy is associated with moderate or very high values. Terminal illness may be accompanied by a fall in PV to the normal range. Highest viscosities are found in the paraproteinaemias, those associated with myeloma to around 3.0 mPa s, while macroglobulinaemia may show extreme hyperviscosity, even as high as 20 mPa s. The disorders may be differentiated by adding mercaptoethanol to the plasma which causes disruption of the macroglobulin molecule with a consequent fall in viscosity.

PV is claimed to provide a better indication of the progress of a disease, particularly in response to drug therapy. PVs below the lower reference value can be found in the elderly due to reduced immunoglobulin levels[15], in hepatic disease due to reduced protein synthesis and in lymphoproliferative disorders with reduced immunoglobulins which show a correlation with the incidence of infections (P. Basterfield, personal communication). Measurement of plasma viscosity also allows rapid monitoring of plasmaphoresis in the treatment of hyperviscosity syndromes.

Comparison between the measurement of plasma viscosity and erythrocyte sedimentation rate

Changes in plasma proteins directly influence PV and indirectly the ESR by influencing the rate of rouleaux formation. The merits of the two methods can be considered from the laboratory aspect and by their predictive value in clinical practice. As might be expected there is a direct correlation between ESR and

PV[17]. When correlation of the two techniques with individual protein fractions are considered the ESR gives a much lower correlation than PV even when anaemic patients are excluded. The number of false results of both PV and ESR may be attributed to the contrary influence of albumin concentration on the two measurements or modest elevations of the PCV.

Further clinical comparisons are shown in *Table 7.1* and technical comparisons in *Table 7.2*. *Figure 7.1* shows the relationship between ESR and PV[16].

Table 7.1 Further clinical comparison

Plasma viscosity	*ESR*
Normal range narrow: 1/50th of total range	Normal range much wider
Normal range same for both sexes	Sex differences
Increase in pregnancy regular and predictable	Increase irregular and erratic
Results become abnormal earlier in the disease	Results abnormal later
Incidence of false normal values is low	Incidence of false normal values is high
Steroids alone will not return PV to normal	Steroids alone may return result to normality
Salicylates do not return PV to normal	Salicylates in sufficient concentration can produce a false normal value
Polycythaemia does not interfere	PCV >0.500 reduces the ESR and may mask disease
Myeloma and macroglobulinanaemia can be distinguished	ESR results similar
Low values can be clinically informative	'One-sided' measurement

Table 7.2 Technical comparisons

Plasma viscosity	*ESR*
Samples may be examined up to 7 days. Postal samples possible	4-hour storage in citrate, 24-hour storage in EDTA
Anaemia has not to be considered	No agreement as to whether correction for anaemia is possible or desirable
Red-cell factors have no effect	Red-cell surface differences affect rouleaux formation
Results from different laboratories are comparable	Not widely comparable despite ICSH recommended method
Standard conditions can be assured before each batch is tested	Technical errors which cannot be checked readily
Takes under 1 minute to complete	At least 1 hour to complete
Urgent results readily available	At least 1 hour to complete

Comment

Despite the overall superiority of the measurement of PV over the ESR there is resistance to abandoning an established technique with familiar expression of results. The initial cost of the equipment would be more than offset by the savings made by not purchasing the widely used disposable ESR equipment. Guidelines on the selection of laboratory tests for monitoring the acute-phase response have been drawn up[17].

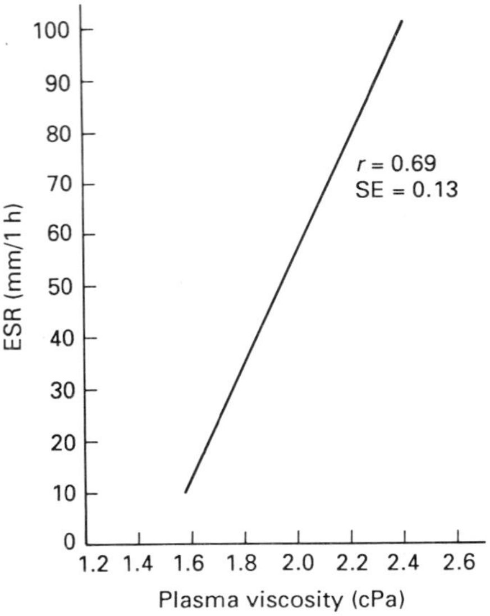

Figure 7.1 Relationship between ESR and PV in non-anaemic subjects [17]

Blood rheology

The flow of blood through the vascular system depends, not only on cardiac output, the structure of the vasculature and local conditions of stasis, but also on the flow resistance or viscosity of the blood.

Blood viscosity is determined by several factors: plasma viscosity, red-cell aggregation, PCV, red-cell and white-cell deformability. The combined effects of these determinants can be measured by whole-blood viscosity. The relative contribution of each of the above factors to whole-blood viscosity is different and in recent years there has been movement towards studying individual components rather than viscosity of whole blood although there is better correlation between clinical status and whole-blood rheology.

The measurement of red-cell aggregation (ESR, ZSR) and plasma viscosity, in the context of the diagnosis and monitoring of organic disease, has been described. This section considers the measurement of whole-blood viscosity and the contribution of the various components.

Whole-blood viscosity

The viscosity of whole blood is complex, the suspension of red cells in plasma behaving in a non-Newtonian manner which is shear-dependent.

At high shear rates ($>200\,s^{-1}$) blood viscosity is determined mainly by the plasma viscosity, temperature, induced deformability of the red cells and by the PCV. High shear-rate viscosity can be measured by either capillary or rotational viscometers. The PCV makes the greatest contribution to high shear blood viscosity and results should be corrected to a standard PCV of 0.450 or compared with a reference curve from PCVs in the range 0.200–0.700. It should be noted that the important determinant of blood rheology, red-cell aggregation, does not contribute to viscosity at high shear rates.

At low shear-rate viscosity ($1\,s^{-1}$), red-cell aggregation is a major determinant. Measurement of low shear-rate viscosity requires meticulous technique and reliable and sensitive instrumentation. A major problem is rapid sedimentation of red-cell aggregates immediately before or during the procedure.

Red-cell deformability [18]

Deformability is determined by shape, the ratio of surface-area to volume, membrane flexibility and internal viscosity. In addition to viscometry, deformability can be studied by laser diffractometry using the Ektacytometer (Technicon International) in which red cells are suspended in a high-viscosity medium and exposed to rotational shearing where they diffract a laser beam. The alternative approach is by filtration through polycarbonate or metal filters with pore sizes similar to the diameter of red cells. A pore size of 5 μm is probably preferable; results with smaller pore diameters are influenced by the MCV of the red cells. Filtration is influenced not only by the deformability of the red cells but also by the force applied, temperature, PCV, plasma viscosity, red-cell aggregation, leucocytes and by platelet clumps. Suspension of washed red cells in buffer is recommended to eliminate most of the interference.

The contribution of normal numbers of leucocytes to blood viscosity is very small. Their resistance to filtration compared with red cells is considerable, however, and can be projected to the *in vivo* situation of having to negotiate small vessels.

The ICSH has produced guidelines for the measurement of blood viscosity, and red-cell deformability [19] and blood rheology *in vitro* and *in vivo* has been reviewed [20].

The clinical applications of the measurement of whole-blood viscosity potentially encompass a wide variety of disorders. Apart from conditions such as peripheral vascular disease, diabetic microangiopathy, pre-eclampsia etc., of particular interest to haematologists are changes in blood rheology associated with polycythaemia, sickle-cell disease and other haemolytic anaemias, the hyperviscosity syndrome associated with paraproteins and the effect of gross leucocytosis. Viscosity measurements are also helpful in assessing the effect of drugs on blood flow.

References

1. Fabry, T. L. (1987) M ... n of erythrocyte aggregation and sedimentation. *Blood*, **70**, 1572–6
2. Dinarello, C. A. (1984 ... eukin-1 and the pathogenesis of the acute phase response. *N. Engl. J. Med.*, **311**, 1413–18
3. Hazleton, J. J. (1968) ... ocyte sedimentation rate: some observations under adverse conditions. *Med. Lab. Technol.* ... 0–3
4. Bull, B. S. and Bre ... (1974) An evaluation of the relative merits of Wintrobe and Westergren sedimentation met ... cluding haematocrit correction. *Am. J. Clin. Pathol.*, **62**, 502–10
5. Mosely, D. L. and ... B. S. (1982) A comparison of the Wintrobe tube, the Westergren and the ZSR erythrocyte ... ntation rate (ESR) methods to a candidate reference method. *Clin. Lab. Haematol.*, **4**, 16 ...
6. International C ... e for Standardisation in Haematology (1975) Reference method for the erythrocyte sed ... ion rate (ESR) test on human blood. *Br. J. Haematol.*, **24**, 671–3

7. International Committee for Standardisation in Haematology (1977) Recommendation for measurement of erythrocyte sedimentation rate of human blood. *Am. J. Clin. Pathol.*, **68**, 505–7
8. Roddie, A. M. S. and Pollock, A. (1987) Plastic ESR tubes: does static electricity affect the results? *Clin. Lab. Haematol.*, **9**, 175–80
9. Hackett, M. C., Hinchcliffe, R. F., Laycock, B. J. and Lilleyman, J. S. (1983) Erythrocyte sedimentation rate: evaluation of a commercial capillary-ESR tube in a paediatric haematology laboratory. *Med. Lab. Sci.*, **40**, 183–5
10. Eastham, R. D. (1977) *Clinical Haematology*, 5th edn. Bristol: Wright
11. Bull, B. S. (1981) Clinical and laboratory implications of present ESR methodology. *Clin. Lab. Haematol.*, **3**, 283–98
12. Bull, B. S. and Brailsford, J. D. (1972) The zeta sedimentation ratio. *Blood,* **40**, 550–9
13. Phillips, M. J. and Harkness, J. (1976) Plasma and whole blood viscosity. *Br. J. Haematol.*, **34**, 347–52
14. International Committee for Standardisation in Haematology (1984) Recommendation for a selected method for the measurement of plasma viscosity. *J. Clin. Pathol.*, **37**, 1147–52
15. Basterfield, P. (1975) Plasma viscosity as a routine replacement for the ESR. Presented at the Tenth Coulter Electronics Symposium
16. Hutchinson, R. M. and Eastham, R. D. (1975) A comparison of the erythrocyte sedimentation rate and plasma viscosity in detecting changes in plasma proteins. *J. Clin. Pathol.*, **30**, 345–9
17. Stuart, J. (1985) Erythrocyte rheology. *J. Clin. Pathol.*, **38**, 965–77
18. International Committee for Standardisation in Haematology (1986) Guidelines for measurement of blood viscosity and erythrocyte deformability. *Clin. Hemorheol.*, **6**, 439–53
19. Lowe, G. D. O. (1987) Blood rheology *in vitro* and *in vivo*. *Clin. Haematol.*, **1**, 597–636
20. ICSH Expert Panel on Blood Rheology (1988) Guidelines on selection of laboratory tests for monitoring the acute phase response. *J. Clin. Pathol.*, **41**, 1203–12

Chapter 8

Automated blood-cell analysis

In the great majority of haematology laboratories blood-cell counting and analysis are performed by semi and fully automated analysers. Early instruments were designed to count only one cell type at a time from pre-diluted blood samples. These have developed over 30 years into multi-parameter instruments with more than one analytical channel and accepting whole blood samples with automatic sampling and, theoretically, walk-away capability.

It is natural that advances in technology are often based on established principles. One of the earliest instruments for counting red cells simulated visual counting and used a counting chamber and diluted blood but replaced the visual counting with automated scanning and projection of the cell images onto a photomultiplier tube with digital display of the number of cells counted. Up to 10 000 cells could be counted, thus reducing the inherent error of random cell distribution, but a count took 2 minutes for a single cell type which, by modern standards, is desperately slow and cumbersome. Later instruments adopted the principle of drawing or propelling the cell suspension through a detection system, the concept of flow cytometry. Although the term 'flow cytometry' has been particularly associated with those instruments which count or identify particular characteristics of cells by the use of fluorescence excitation, it is arguable that all the present generation of analysers counting, sizing or identifying cells in 'moving' suspension are 'flow cytometers'.

The concept of 'continuous flow' analysis by which multiple samples, separated by air bubbles and at different stages of analysis, characterized by the Technicon systems of the 1960s and 1970s, has not survived. The current generation of instruments are discrete analysers though there may be some overlap of sample processing. Nevertheless they are capable of handling large numbers of samples at rates between 60 and 130 per hour, thus coping with the 4–5-fold increase in samples for blood counts in the last 20 years. It is debatable whether the increased workload is a consequence of rapid automated analysis rather than the analysers being developed to handle the increase in requests.

Initially the criteria for introducing or extending automation were based mainly on workload. It is now clear that there are other considerations:

1. Improved precision leading to:
2. Improved accuracy.
3. Production of data not otherwise routinely available.
4. Data not otherwise available.

The purpose of this chapter is to state the principles used in automated blood-counting instruments, to describe the interrelationships and significance of the various parameters and the erroneous results which may be produced. Calibration procedures and quality control preparations will also be considered.

A recent survey indicated at least 25 manufacturers of blood-cell analysers, though many use the same principle and produce similar information. Clearly, consideration of all types of analyser is neither useful nor desirable in a general haematology textbook and in the context of continuing technological development. In general, analysers count total leucocytes, red cells and platelets and measure haemoglobin concentration. In addition to the number of cells, the volume of the cells is determined and a variety of parameters describing the distribution of the measured volumes can be derived. Because there are several different technologies used to count and size the blood cells, the derived parameters are not necessarily comparable.

Electrical impedance technology

Particles (cells) suspended in electrolyte can be sized and counted by passing them through an orifice through which flows a low frequency current. As a cell passes through the orifice and displaces a volume of electrolyte, the lower conductivity of the cell causes a voltage change or pulse of a magnitude directly proportional to the volume of the cell. The number of cells is counted by the number of pulses per unit time. As more than one cell may be present in the sensing zone of the orifice, measurements must be corrected for 'coincidence', the correction formula being unique to the characteristics of the orifice and the volume counted. The volume of the cell cannot be accurately calculated from the physical constants of the system and recourse must be made to reference particles of known volume for calibration of the instrument.

Although the number of cells can be counted accurately, the measured volume may not reflect the true volume of the cell due to the shape of the cell. This is particularly relevant in the case of red cells which normally adopt a 'cigar shape' under the flow conditions of the orifice. Alteration of red-cell flexibility will therefore influence the apparent volume. This aspect is considered further in the section on measurement of the MCV.

The principle of measuring and counting by electrical impedance was pioneered by Coulter[1], is referred to as the 'Coulter principle', is used by Coulter Electronics and has been adopted by many other manufacturers (*Figure 8.1*).

Light-scatter technology

An optical detection system to count cells in diluted blood drawn through a fine capillary and detected by a photocell was an early development. The optical principle was extended by the Technicon Corporation by introducing dark-field optics and detection of scattered light[2]. The present generation of instruments use tungsten (non-coherent) light, a laser source (coherent or monochromatic light) or both. Tungsten light and dark-field optics are suitable for counting and sizing leucocytes but for determining red-cell and platelet volumes a laser source is preferable[3].

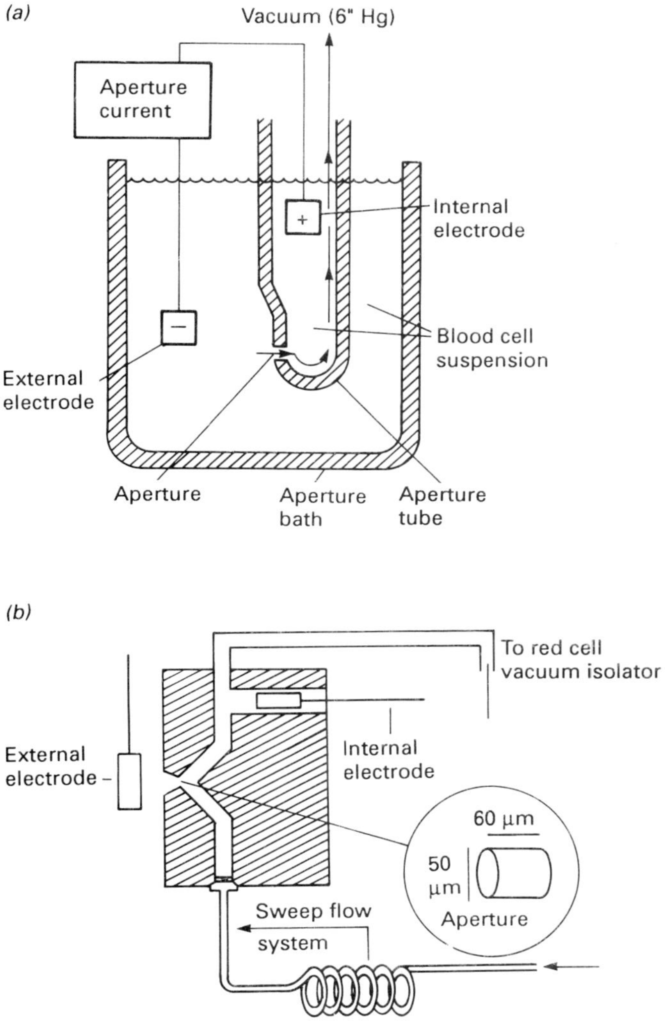

Figure 8.1 (*a*) Aperture impedance. The 'Coulter principle' of counting and sizing. The passage of a cell drawn through the aperture momentarily increases the resistance of the electrical path between electrodes located on each side of the aperture. (*b*) The aperture impedance orifice of the Coulter S Plus IV. The sweep flow system removes cells from the rear of the aperture and prevents recirculation. By permission of Coulter Electronics

Light-scatter detection requires that cells pass the detection point singly. The cell suspension is introduced into a stream of fluid which draws the cells into single file. This is known as 'sheath-flow' or 'hydrodynamic focusing' (*Figure 8.2*) and is also used in impedance technology to overcome the problem of 'coincidence' when measuring cell volume.

Laser light scattering is used not only for counting and sizing cells. The angle of scatter depends on the optical density of the cell and the detection of 'wide angle'

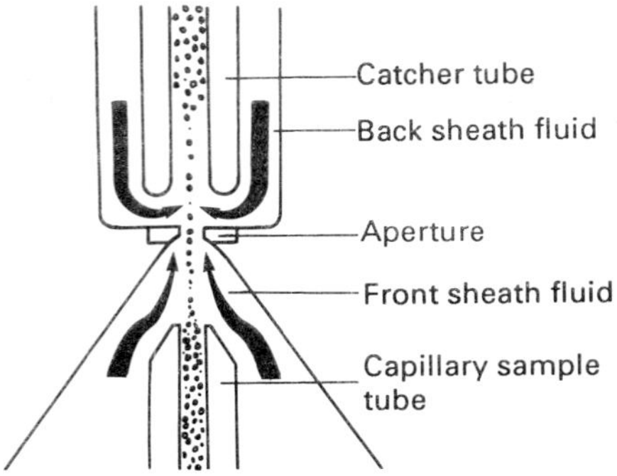

Figure 8.2 Hydrodynamic focusing. As cells are ejected from the sample tube, the flow of front sheath fluid surrounds the particle column, restricts the width and aligns the cells in single file. As the cells pass beyond the aperture they are surrounded by the flow of back sheath fluid which prevents recirculation. Sysmex/Toa NE8000. By permission of Toa Electronics

scatter is used in the Technicon H1 analyser to determine the haemoglobin concentration of each cell detected (*Figure 8.3*). Similarly, laser scatter is used to provide data of leucocyte structure in the Coulter VCS flow cytometer and in the STKS analyser.

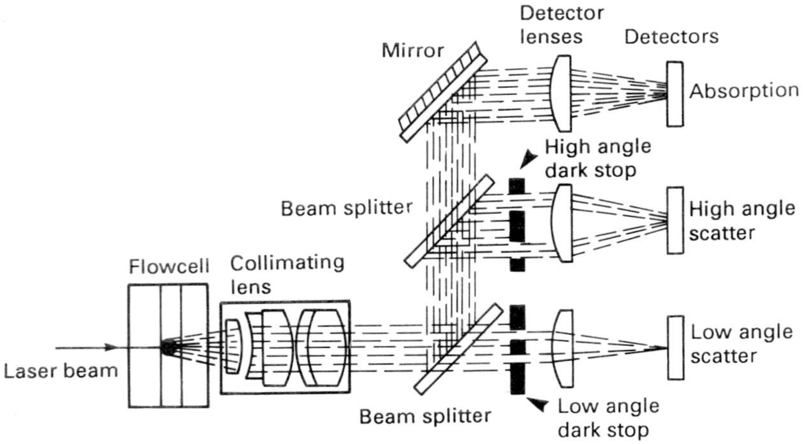

Figure 8.3 Laser light scatter. Cells passing through the flow cell under sheath flow conditions interrupt and scatter the laser beam. The angle of scatter is determined by the volume (low angle) and density (high angle) of the cell. Technicon H1. By permission of Technicon Corporation

Fluorescence-activated flow cytometry

Cells stained or labelled with fluorochrome enter a flow chamber in single file using 'sheath-flow', are struck by a focused laser beam and emit scattered and fluorescent light which is separated according to wavelength by mirrors and filters. An advanced instrument may have three fluorescence detectors and make two scatter

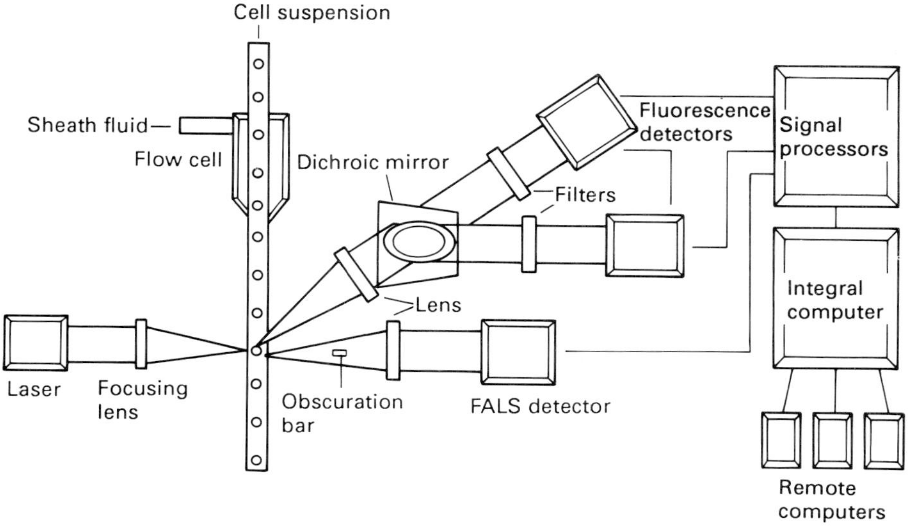

Figure 8.4 Fluorescence-activated flow cytometer. Stained cells enter the flow chamber in single file under sheath flow conditions. They are struck by the laser beam and emit scattered and fluorescent light which is separated, according to wavelength, by filters and mirrors to fluorescence detectors. The forward angle light scatter (FALS) counts the number of cells

measurements[4] (*Figure 8.4*). The FACScan (Becton Dickinson) and EPICS (Coulter) are examples of dedicated instruments.

Fluorochromes used for staining or 'marking' the cells include fluorescein isothiocyanate (FITC), phycoerythrin and thiazole orange. Antibodies conjugated with fluorochromes can be used to identify cells with specific antigens. The wide range of monoclonal antibodies now available allows recognition not only of specific cell lines but also cell subsets and stages of differentiation. FITC is the most widely used for antibody labelling though the use of different fluorochromes allows multiple antibody labelling of a cell suspension.

Fluorescence flow cytometry for lymphocyte subtyping has been combined with conventional cell counting and sizing in a single instrument, the Technicon H1. Fluorochromes which are specific for RNA, acridine orange, thiazole orange and auramine O, are used to identify reticulocytes and the cells are not only counted accurately but their relative maturity determined by quantitation of the amount of RNA[5–7]. An instrument designed solely for reticulocyte counting is available (R1000, Sysmex-Toa)[8].

Fluorescence flow cytometry has expanded from the research to the clinical laboratory and has a wide range of applications in diagnostic haematology and in the other disciplines of pathology[9].

Parameters of automated blood counting

Haemoglobin concentration

The ICSH reference method for haemoglobin measurement is based on conversion to cyanmethaemoglobin (HiCN). Automated instrument manufacturers often claim to measure haemoglobin in the HiCN form. However, the short time of exposure, even to concentrated reagents, and the admixture with reagents to facilitate leucocyte counting, does not allow for full conversion to HiCN. The reaction product is probably denatured globin haemichrome [10]. This does not invalidate measurement if the conversion time is constant and the effect of incomplete conversion is minimized by the use of a wide absorption band width of up to 60 nm. In the presence of the Hb derivatives relatively resistant to conversion to HiCN, carboxyhaemoglobin and sulphaemoglobin, discrepancies may occur with certain reagent systems. Variably extended time of exposure to the haemoglobin converting reagents during additional platelet counting cycles can result in errors of up to 0.4 g/dl (R. Hall, unpublished data) which, although probably not of clinical significance, can cause problems if control preparations do not have stable platelet numbers.

Red-cell count

All current systems are capable of accurate red-cell counting with CV $<1\%$. This pertains with both impedance and light-scatter technologies with or without correction for coincidence. The electronic editing of small 'pulses' due to debris, electronic 'noise' or large platelets must not exclude microcytic red cells or cell fragments which can be as small as 30 fl or even less.

Mean red-cell volume (MCV)

The differing technologies used to determine red-cell volume demand separate consideration.

Electrical impedance with pulse editing

A cell traversing the electrical field of the aperture creates an electrical 'shadow' and pulse, relative to its volume and deformability. Normal red cells will behave in a uniform manner but the histogram of the volume distribution is positively skewed. The MCV is the arithmetic mean of the measured cell volumes. Cells of abnormal shape create pulses disproportionate to their volume, e.g. a sphere produces a pulse 1.5 times its 'true' value and a fixed biconcave disc a value 1.2 times greater [11]. In addition, the internal viscosity of the cell due to the concentration of Hb will also influence the ability to deform. Increased Hb concentration will therefore decrease deformability thus overestimating the volume, and cells with low Hb concentration will deform more readily, underestimate the MCV and PCV and falsely increase the MCHC. Additional aspects influencing apparent cell volume are whether the cell is passing through the axis or margin of the aperture, or is sensed while in the electrical field surrounding the aperture; the position of the cell determines the pulse height. The coincidence of two or more cells measured simultaneously is corrected arithmetically in the cell count. In volume measurement doublet or triplet pulses are excluded by electronic editing.

Electrical impedance with hydrodynamic focusing

Because cells pass the transducer aperture in single file the chances of coincidence are greatly reduced. As the cells are aligned at the central axis of the aperture the variance in pulse heights due to variant position of the cell within the aperture is eliminated. The problem of accurate sizing of cells of different shapes and deformability remains.

The volume histogram of normal blood is more truly Gaussian with this measurement system. In the Sysmex/Toa systems the MCV is derived from the 'haematocrit' (Hct) and red-cell count (*see* below).

Light scatter

Cell volume measurement by light scatter is determined by cell shape and orientation as well as volume. These variables are eliminated by inducing isovolumetric sphering and fixation so that scatter is largely a function of volume. However the refractive index of the cell also influences the degree of scatter. This problem is overcome in the Technicon H1 system by measuring forward low-angle (2–3°) scatter. Variation in deformability is eliminated by the fixation of the cells. The MCV is the mean of the measured volumes and a volume histogram of normal blood is near-Gaussian.

Packed cell volume (PCV, Hct)

Most systems derive the PCV from MCV × RBC ($\times 10^{12}$/l)/1000.

In the Sysmex/Toa the Hct is computed by integration of pulses between upper and lower discriminators of the red-cell distribution curve, multiplied by a constant factor involving the dilution ratio and expressed as a percentage. The MCV = Hct%/RBC ($\times 10^{12}$/l) × 10.

In all systems the PCV is dependent on the measurement of MCV. The falsely low PCV obtained by impedance technology in the presence of hypochromic cells [12], is probably eliminated by light-scatter measurement of the MCV.

Haemoglobin distribution width (HDW)

This parameter is unique to the Technicon H1 system. In addition to measuring red-cell volume by low-angle forward light scatter, the density, i.e. haemoglobin concentration, of the cells is determined by detecting wide-angle (5–15°) scatter [13]. The haemoglobin concentration of each cell is measured directly and 'cellular haemoglobin concentration mean' (CHCM) is the mean of these measurements. The haemoglobin distribution width (HDW) is the standard deviation of the haemoglobin concentration histogram which shows a Gaussian distribution.

The volume and haemoglobin concentration values are also shown as an erythrogram or 'Mie map', with low-angle scatter (volume) on the y axis and wide-angle scatter (Hb concentration) on the x axis. Characteristic patterns are seen in several haematological disorders. The haemoglobin distribution histogram can illustrate hypochromic or less dense cell populations, dimorphic populations and, of particular importance, dense cells due to cell dehydration [14], spherocytosis or fragmentation. The percentages of cells with normal, low and high Hb concentration are calculated, the latter correlating well with blood film observations.

Red-cell distribution width (RDW)

The histogram of red-cell volumes indicates the degree of anisocytosis and a variety of quantitative parameters of anisocytosis have been derived from the volume distribution. The parameter of RDW is common to all systems but is derived in different ways making comparison difficult between different types of instrument.

Technicon and Coulter systems simply express the RDW as the CV of the distribution, i.e. SD/mean × 100. Sysmex/Toa use two derived measurements, RDW–CV and RDW–SD. RDW–CV is computed by determining the median value around which 50% of the area of the histogram lies on each side and 68.26% of the area around the median represents ±1SD; RDW–CV is SD/mean × 100. RDW–SD is the arithmetic distribution width at 20% relative height level of the histogram and is expressed in femtolitres (fl).

The RDW is a precise measurement and is more reliable than microscopic assessment in demonstrating anisocytosis[15]. It must be appreciated, however, that the RDW represents cell volumes and microscopy looks at cell diameters and there is no doubt that cells of similar volume can show obvious anisocytosis in the blood film. RDW has been recommended as a discriminator between iron deficiency (RDW increased) and thalassaemia trait (RDW normal)[16]. The combination of MCV and RDW has been advocated as a means of improving the diagnostic classification of anaemias[16]. Although this might be helpful as a preliminary indication of the type of anaemia, their use as diagnostic parameters appears simplistic and the general value has been questioned[17,18].

Mean corpuscular haemoglobin (MCH)

An unequivocal parameter obtained by Hb/RCC ($\times 10^{12}$/l) × 10. There is a clear correlation between MCH and MCV and as the measurement of Hb and red-cell count can be extremely precise, the use of MCH as an alternative to the problematical determination of MCV has many advocates. The close correlation between MCH and MCV is lost in certain recognized circumstances (other than instrument malfunction or inaccurate calibration) which include marked spherocytosis, dimorphism, hyperosmolar states and erroneous measurements due to characteristics of the blood sample such as lipaemia, haemolysis and paraproteinaemia.

Mean corpuscular haemoglobin concentration (MCHC)

Derived from Hb/PCV (l/l). Clearly the major possible variable is the PCV measurement which in all automated instruments is directly dependent upon measurement of red-cell volumes. There now seems little doubt that the normal or near-normal values for MCHC obtained by electrical impedance counters in iron deficiency anaemias is due to falsely low-volume measurements of cells with increased deformability due to reduced haemoglobin concentration and lowered internal viscosity. This results in underestimation of MCV, leading to a lower PCV and consequently a higher MCHC. Even if a 'true MCV', PCV and MCHC could be obtained, the MCHC has been effectively consigned to use as a quality control parameter and has little interpretive value in comparison with other red-cell parameters.

Total leucocyte count

All technologies depend on dilution of whole blood and lysis of red cells. The leucocytes may be counted as intact cells or have the cytoplasm 'stripped' from or 'collapsed' upon, the nucleus of the cells. Displayed counts are usually linear within the range 0.5–50 or even 99×10^9/l. Below 0.5×10^9/l, different systems show different degrees of accuracy, much depending on the 'background' count though accurate counts as low as 0.1×10^9/l can be achieved. Nucleated red cells will usually be counted as leucocytes.

Platelet count

Normal platelets show a log-normal volume distribution. This characteristic distribution is used by several systems as the basis for determining the platelet count. All systems use the distribution curve as a basis for determining the validity of the platelet count. Sysmex/Toa use three discriminators – a fixed point at 12 fl, a floating lower discriminator (LD) between 2 and 6 fl and an upper discriminator (UD) between 12 and 30 fl. The histogram of platelet volume distribution is monitored by the relative height of the upper and lower discriminators, the arithmetic distribution width and the existence of two or more peaks. The platelet count in 1 μl of whole blood is the number of cells >LD and <UD corrected for coincidence. Various 'flags' are generated by deviation from a log-normal distribution.

Coulter systems classify cells between 2 and 20 fl as platelets. Using a least-squares fit for a log-normal curve, a curve is fitted to the histogram over the range 0–70 fl. A variety of computer checks are made on the criteria of the fitted, smoothed curves from each of the three counting apertures. If any of the criteria is not met a 'no-fit' condition is generated. This may be due to a count <20 000, total 'vote out' of the fitted curve or unacceptable volume distribution. Up to four additional counting periods are instituted when the number of platelet pulses is below a predetermined value. The Technicon H1 system spheres and fixes the platelets. The platelets are detected in the laser channel and the platelet histogram derived from measurements made with the high-angle scatter detector. The platelet count is the actual number of pulses corrected for coincidence. Deviation from log-normal distribution and the presence of large platelets are 'flagged'.

All fully automated systems display platelet distribution histograms in the log-normal form which are difficult to assess visually. Distributions transformed by plotting on a logarithmic *x* axis could be easier to interpret.

Derived platelet parameters

These parameters depend greatly on the technology and their methods of derivation. Furthermore, the anticoagulant and the time elapsed before testing influences the significance of the measurements[19–22]. Consequently, derived platelet parameters must be interpreted with care.

Mean platelet volume (MPV)

On the Coulter system this represents the arithmetic mean volume of the platelets within the fitted curve. The product of each channel within the range 0–70 fl is summarized, divided by the total of platelets within the fitted curve, multiplied by a constant and the MPV expressed in femtolitres (fl). The reference range for MPV varies, dependent on the observed platelet count[23]. A nomogram has been described which shows the relationship between platelet numbers and MPV[24].

Sysmex/Toa compute MPV as:

$$\text{MPV} - \frac{\text{'Platelet crit'\%} \times 1000}{\text{Platelet count} \times 10^9/\text{l}}$$

where 'platelet crit' is computed by 'adding a factor to the height of the platelet pulses'.

The Technicon H1 system apparently uses the mode of the platelet distribution as the 'mean' platelet volume.

Platelet distribution width (PDW)

This use of this parameter is limited as the Federal Drug Administration of the USA have not approved the parameter for clinical use.

The Coulter systems express PDW as the CV of platelet distribution. The PDW as used by Sysmex/Toa is the arithmetic distribution width measured at 20% relative height level taking the histogram peak as 100%. The histogram of normal blood crosses the 20% level twice. PDW is reported in femtolitres (fl). The Technicon H1 literature does not provide the derivation of the parameter.

Automation of blood film examination and the differential leucocyte count

Blood film examination

Visual microscopy of blood films is a labour-intensive procedure which made it an obvious objective for automation.

Examination includes assessment of overall appearances, red-cell morphology, platelet number and morphology, leucocyte morphology and the differential leucocyte count. An approach to automation which addresses most of these aspects uses the principle of digital image processing or image-recognition (Hematrak). Several systems have been developed for conventionally prepared and stained films and there are differences in the manner by which the cell images are analysed. Essentially, the microscopical images of size, shape, nuclear and cytoplasmic features, and staining characteristics are converted into a larger number of recognition parameters which are processed by computer-based algorithms. Normal, immature or abnormal leucotyes and nucleated red cells can be positively classified. Red-cell features including size, shape and staining appearances can be identified and platelet numbers assessed. Up to 90 slides an hour can be processed by the Hematrak 590 system (Geometric Data) with automatic loading, oiling, focusing and examination. The films can be returned for manual review and identification of specific 'flagged' cells. Image analysis remains the only system of automation which conveys most of the information obtainable by visual microscopy. For a differential leucocyte count, up to 400 cells can be classified, the number specified by the reference method, though at the expense of speed of throughput.

The relatively high cost of image recognition systems, together with the incorporation of differential leucocyte counts into whole blood analysers, has resulted in the virtual withdrawal of manufacturers from this approach to automated haematology.

Differential leucocyte counting

Several approaches to the automation of this aspect of blood cell analysis have been made or have become established. Image analysis has been considered above. Pattern recognition of geometric parameters has not been accepted[25]. Volume measurement combined with cytochemistry has been the approach of the Technicon Corporation since 1974 and is now supplemented by laser light scatter in the Technicon H1 system. Differentiation of leucocyte volume measured by the aperture impedance principle is used by Coulter Electronics in the S Plus II–VI and STKR series, by Sysmex/Toa in the E5000 multiparameter analyser and by numerous other manufacturers.

Volume measurement together with analysis by 'radio-frequency' alternating current is used by Sysmex/Toa to improve classification in the NE8000 instrument. Volume measurement, 'high-frequency' alternating current and laser light scattering are combined in the dedicated VCS analyser of Coulter and is incorporated in the STKS multiparameter analyser.

Differentiation by volume and cytochemistry

This was developed by the Technicon Corporation using continuous-flow technology, was available in the dedicated Hemalog D analyser[26], and incorporated into the multi-parameter H6000 system[27]. A feature of the Hemalog D, which is now common to all flow cytometers, was the analysis of up to 10 000 leucocytes in each counting channel resulting in a very high degree of precision, though the hourly, daily and weekly physiological variation in the differential count[28,29] questions the need for such precision in routine counts.

The Hemalog D had three counting channels, peroxidase to identify neutrophils and eosinophils, esterase for monocytes and Alcian Blue for basophils; the lymphocytes were characterized as relatively small unstained cells. The cell distribution was presented as a scattergram or cytogram, volume by forward light scatter on the y axis and light absorption on the x axis. Boundaries or 'thresholds', fixed or moving, enclosed the cell clusters. Characteristic cytograms are produced by proliferative disorders and the instrument found particular application in the diagnosis and monitoring of acute leukaemias. As with the dedicated image analysis systems, the high cost plus the high revenue consequences of the Hemalog D confined the instrument to large haematology laboratories, and the combination of routine blood analysis and differential counting in the H6000 resulted in the withdrawal of the 'stand-alone' differential counter.

The H6000 abandoned the esterase channel and modified the pH of the peroxidase reaction to allow detection of monocytes by their weaker peroxidase reaction compared with neutrophils and eosinophils. A variety of 'flags' are generated by either abnormal cells or characteristics of the blood sample other than the leucocytes. Of particular relevance is the LUC flag (large unstained cells). This indicates large lymphocytes or other peroxidase-negative cells including cells in various lymphoproliferative disorders, acute monocytic or myelomonocytic leukaemia and infectious mononucleosis. Peroxidase-deficient neutrophils and monocytes are also classified as LUCs. Unlysed red cells due to haemoglobinopathies, the presence of uraemia and from neonatal samples, particularly from premature infants, are also recognized as LUCs.

The introduction of laser light scatter in the Technicon H1 has allowed replacement of the expensive Alcian or Astra Blue channel by basophil counting based on the resistance of these cells to disruption by a surfactant at low pH. The basophil/lobularity (nuclear) channel measures the conformation of the nuclei of leucocytes and nucleated red cells. The membrane and cytoplasm of leucocytes other than basophils are removed leaving the bare nuclei. The intact basophils are counted by low-angle light scatter. The volume of the intact basophil is greater than the bare nuclei of other leucocytes and is delineated by a fixed horizontal threshold. High-angle light scatter is responsive to the lobularity of the nucleus; the more lobulated the nucleus the larger the signal. Polymorphonuclear nuclei (PMN) are separated from mononuclear nuclei (MN) by a valley and a vertical threshold separates the two clusters (*Figure 8.5a*). The ratio of PMN:MN is the 'lobularity index' (LI). A low value suggests a 'left shift'. Blast cells appear to the left of the normal MN cluster. Nucleated red cells appear within the PMN cluster.

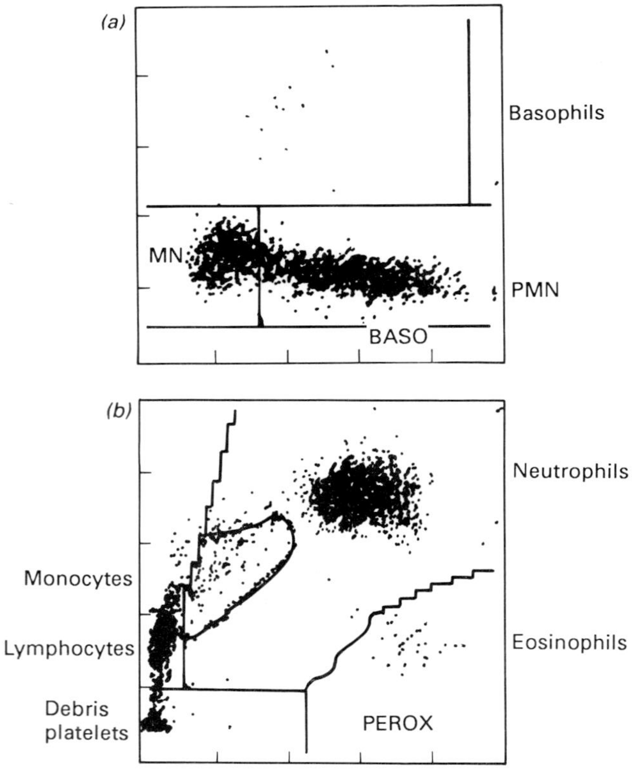

Figure 8.5 (*a*) Basophil/lobularity (nuclear) channel of the Technicon H1. See test for explanation. (*b*) Peroxidase channel of the Technicon H1. See text for explanation

As in the H6000, the peroxidase channel lyses the red cells and the volume and peroxidase activity of the fixed leucocytes are measured by dark-field light scatter and absorbance respectively. The fixed and moving linear thresholds for neutrophils, monocytes and eosinophils in the H6000 are replaced by 'cluster analysis' and delineation by curvolinear boundaries and displayed as an *x–y* scattergram (*Figure 8.5b*). The mean peroxidase activity of the neutrophils is assessed as the 'mean peroxidase index' (MPXI).

The performance and results of the leucocyte differentiation and counting is monitored and 'flags' are generated if distribution, peroxidase activity or nuclear lobularity are abnormal.

Differentiation by volume alone

Leucocyte volumes can be determined by analysis of the pulse heights generated by aperture impedance technology. The differentiation into lymphocytes and 'non-lymphocytes'[30] following partial lysis of the cytoplasm became available on the Coulter S Plus II with display of volume distributions and computed percentages. It was recognized that changes in shape of the distribution curves might be related to abnormal leucocytes[31]. The 'two-population' or 'abridged' differential had the greatest value in monitoring immunosuppressive and cytotoxic therapy.

By modifying the lytic system and computer analysis, the cells can be separated into three categories – lymphocytes, 'mononuclears' and granulocytes. This 'three-population' or 'histogram' differential has been adopted by several instrument manufacturers, notably Coulter Electronics in the S Plus IV (*Figure 8.6*), the Sysmex/Toa E5000 and other related instruments.

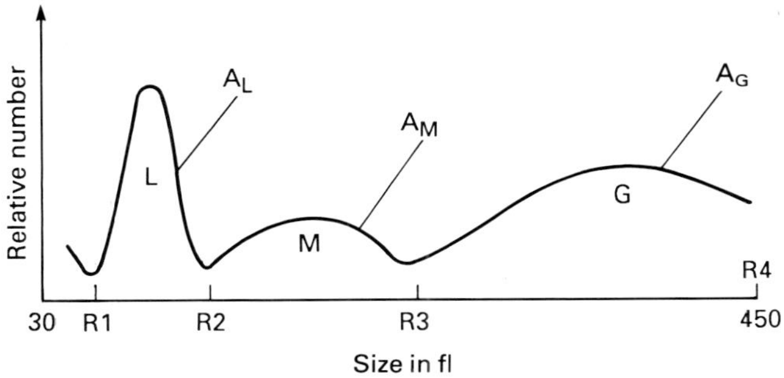

Figure 8.6 Diagrammatic representation of the WBC histogram of the Coulter STKR. The three cell populations of granulocytes (G), mononuclear (M) and lymphocytes (L) are defined by the 'valleys' R1–R4 which generate the corresponding flags in the event of abnormal distribution

This approach to differential counting has been widely evaluated and compared with alternative technologies[32–36]. These evaluations may be summarized as follows. In normal blood, lymphocyte counts correlate well with manual counts though a small proportion are classified as mononuclears and vice versa; most of the eosinophils are included in the granulocytes, the mononuclears include most of the monocytes, the basophils and a significant proportion of eosinophils. However, as a method for screening for abnormalities, the flagging systems monitoring the distribution peaks and 'valleys' between the cell populations appear capable of detecting abnormal cell distribution and cell types if present in sufficient quantity, though the incidence of false negative results is significant[35]. Testing of samples from an acute care environment may result in up to 75% flagged reports requiring further evaluation[37]. The effects of the type of anticoagulant and the time between collection and testing influence the histogram and the rate of flagging.

Differentiation by volume and light scatter

The combination of volume measurement and assessment of cell content by laser light scatter was used by Ortho Instruments in the ELT15 and 1500 analysers as a means of producing a 'three-population' differential separated by moving thresholds.

The granulocyte cluster was claimed to contain the eosinophils and basophils in addition to the neutrophils. The monocyte percentage appeared to be superior to the 'mononuclear' count determined by volume alone. Lymphocyte numbers correlated well with visual counts. This series of instruments is no longer in production.

Differentiation by volume, conductivity and light scatter

An innovative approach to differential counting has been developed by Coulter Electronics. Low-frequency impedance measurement of volume (V) has been combined with high-frequency measurement of conductivity (C) and laser light scatter (S) in a dedicated differential counter, the VCS. Measurement of V, C and S determine the cell volume, content and structural characteristics.

This combination of technologies provides a three-dimensional analysis of cell populations and subpopulations. A two-dimension scattergram of volume (V) and, primarily, light scatter (discriminant function 1 or DF1) is presented as a colour monitor display and colour or monochrome printout (*Figure 8.7a*). Scatterplots of volume and conductivity (DF2) and a three-dimension, rotatable display are obtainable. Single parameter histograms are also available. The DF1 scatterplot display of cell populations is divided by self-adjusting linear thresholds. Each cell type is counted in its own compartment. Basophils are located behind the upper right quadrant of the lymphocyte area. The percentages of the five normal cell types are presented and absolute counts are displayed if the total leucocyte count is entered via the keyboard of the computer.

The cell distributions are analysed by the computer program to provide a primary assessment: 'negative' shows a normal distribution; 'positive' indicates an irregular, atypical or abnormal population(s); and 'incomplete' that there were insufficient cells to perform an analysis. In addition, there are seven 'X' flags labelled X1–X7 (*Figure 8.7b*) which accompany the 'positive' flag; these flags are triggered by qualitative irregularities.

The initial software version resulted in excessive flagging (34%) of normal samples (R. Hall, unpublished data) though later versions show reduced false-positive flagging[37]. There is no requirement to allow samples to stabilize before testing though delay in testing (>6 hours) results in significant alterations in both percentages and the frequency of flags. Samples with total leucocyte counts $<1.0 \times 10^9/l$ will not provide a result and are flagged as 'incomplete'.

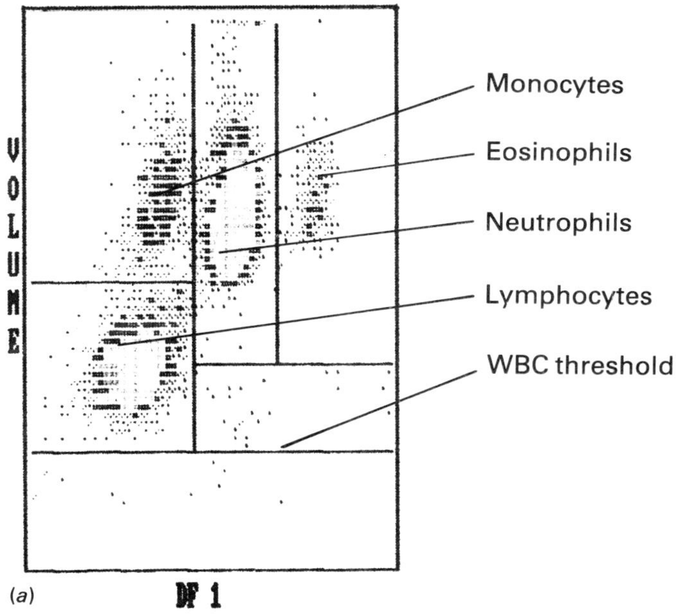

(*a*)

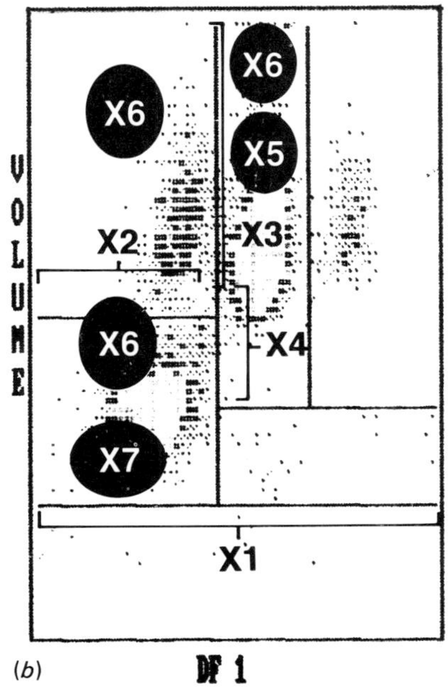

(*b*)

Figure 8.7 (*a*) Coulter VCS. The volume/DF1 scatterplot of normal blood showing the various cell populations separated by moving and fixed linear discriminators. The basophils are in the 'third dimension' behind the upper right quadrant of the lymphocytes. (*b*) The same scatterplot showing the monitoring of cell distributions by the flags X1–7. X1, WBC analysis threshold; X2, Floating discriminator between lymphocyte/monocyte region; X3, Floating discriminator between monocyte/ neutrophil region; X4, Floating discriminator between lymphocyte/neutrophil region; X5, Upper area in neutrophil region; X6, Tri-regional flag; X7, Lower area of lymphocyte region. By permission of Coulter Electronics

The operational requirement that VCS technology would be most advantageous if incorporated into a single multiparameter analyser has been met by the production of the Coulter STKS system capable of processing 100 samples/hour and providing all routine blood-count parameters.

Differentiation by volume and radio-frequency impedance

The use of high-frequency electromagnetic energy to examine cell content is also used in the Sysmex/Toa NE8000 multiparameter analyser. The lymphocyte, monocyte and granulocytes are counted and sized after 'gentle' lysis which does not greatly distort the cells. Resistance to direct current (DC) measures the volume of the entire cell while, simultaneously, radio-frequency alternating current (RF) impedance provides information on nuclear size and density. The DC size distribution corresponds to the three-population or 'trimodal' histogram with overlapping population distributions (*Figure 8.8a*). A two-dimensional scattergram of RF sizing and DC sizing is also generated (*Figure 8.8b*) which separates the overlapping distributions. A complex computer program, using eight floating discriminators, separates the lymphocyte, monocyte and granulocyte clusters.

The eosinophils are sized and counted by direct current (DC) resistance after time and temperature-dependent lysis, which shrinks all cell types except the eosinophils. The basophils are also sized and counted by DC resistance in an individual detector block after shrinkage of all cells except the basophils. The % neutrophils is determined by subtracting the % eosinophils + % basophils from the % granulocytes, i.e. %N = %G – (%E + %B).

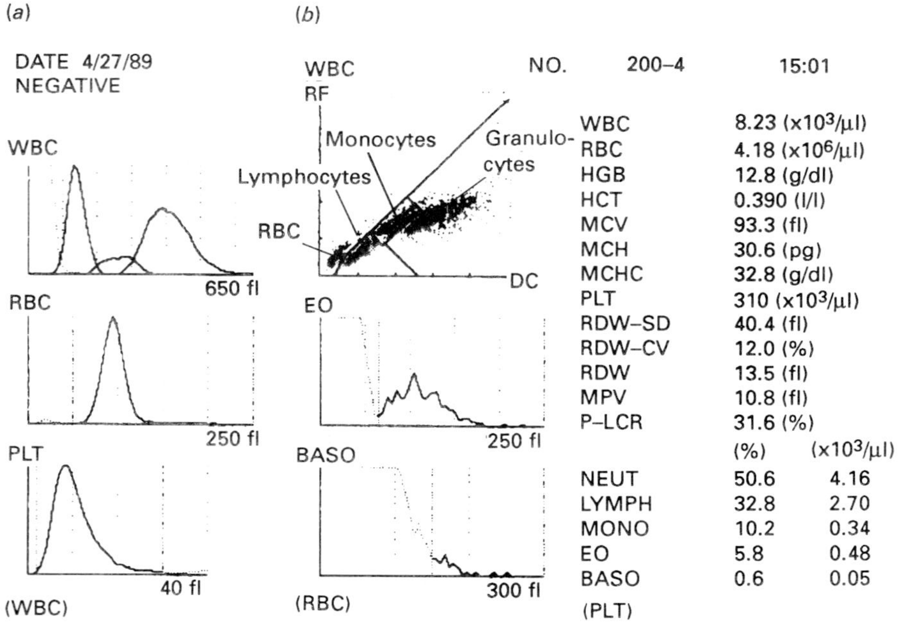

Figure 8.8 (*a*) Sysmex/Toa NE8000. The 'trimodal' histogram of leucocyte volume analysis obtained by direct (DC) analysis. (*b*) Sysmex/Toa NE8000. The radiofrequency (RF)/DC scattergram showing the distribution of the five normal leucocyte populations. By permission of Toa Electronics

The moving discriminators eliminate red-cell ghosts and are specified to exclude platelet clumps and to categorize atypical lymphocytes, left shift, immature granulocytes and blast cells.

Summary

There is little doubt that the present generation of analysers with full differential counting technologies is capable of differentiating the leucocytes of normal blood. It is in the handling of samples with abnormal morphological characteristics as distinct from quantitative abnormalities that differences in performance can be identified.

Semi-automated platelet counting

Platelet counts are largely obtained from multiparameter automated systems. In small laboratories and for use as 'back-up' to multiparameter instruments, dedicated, single parameter counters using the technologies of the larger analysers are widely used.

Such instruments can be separated into two types: those accepting prediluted whole-blood suspensions and those requiring preliminary separation of red cells from platelets. The diluted whole-blood analysers can provide accurate results with similar or better precision than their larger and more versatile counterparts. External quality assessment surveys (EQAS) have repeatedly shown that the instruments and methods involving separation and predilution of platelet-rich plasma perform poorly overall and may be regarded as providing hazardous results.

The problem appears to be a combination of incorrectly set-up or calibrated instruments and the techniques of separating red cells from platelets. This appears to be the case whether differential centrifugation or sedimentation is used. There is little doubt that instruments dependent upon separation procedures should be regarded as obsolete.

Erroneous results using automated analysers

Despite accurate calibration and a reliable quality control program producing satisfactory data, random errors will occur. Apart from incorrect handling of the sampling and 'short sampling', most of the incorrect results are related to characteristics of the blood samples and are therefore repeatable. Some errors can be recognized by deviation of the pattern of related parameters; others can be detected only in relation to other investigations; blood film examination is particularly important in this context.

Incorrect results may only be apparent with particular instrument systems and can be due to constituents of instrument-specific reagents, time of exposure to the action of reagents, temperature of the reaction, etc. Other false results are common to most analyser systems and the causes identified here are mainly confined to errors of this type.

Leucocyte count

Falsely high values can be due to:

1. Platelet clumping. Samples collected by poor technique may show platelet clumping or aggregates, the clumps being counted as leucocytes. Aggregation due to platelet agglutinins can result in higher leucocyte counts but the agglutinates are likely to break up during dilution and mixing. EDTA-dependent platelet clumping can also produce higher counts[38].
2. The introduction of epidermal cells and skin contaminants during capillary blood collection; this is particularly evident in leucopenic samples.
3. Cryoproteins with precipitation at room temperature can cause spuriously high leucocyte counts which may be recognized by the discrepancy in the number of leucocytes in the blood film[39]. The phenomenon is overcome by warming the blood to 37°C before processing.
4. Non-lysis of red cells can occur in samples from neonates and particularly from premature infants, in the presence of target cells and in association with red-cell clumping due to powerful red-cell agglutinins.
5. Mucin agglomerates from adenocarcinomas and certain other tumours[40] can mimic leucocytes.
6. Nucleated red cells will usually be included in the total leucocyte count. Current instruments will 'flag' the consequent abnormal volume distribution if present in sufficient numbers.

Falsely low values may be due to:

1. Aged samples in which leucocytes have disintegrated.
2. Clumping due to agglutinins or non-specific aggregation[41].

Haemoglobin concentration

Apart from samples containing clot or due to 'short sampling', falsely low haemoglobin values do not occur. Falsely high results can be due to:

1. Hyperlipidaemia, whether metabolic[42] or due to intravenous (parenteral) lipid infusion. This causes turbidity which is reflected by the haemoglobin value. The high reading results in an MCH value above that expected for the MCV and a high MCHC would also be expected. The Technicon H1 can be expected to show a 'comparison error' flag between the CHCM and MCHC. A corrected haemoglobin value can be obtained by gentle centrifugation or sedimentation of the sample, aspiration of the plasma and replacement with an equal volume of particle-free diluent.
2. Elevated leucocyte counts in the order of 100×10^9/l. The true Hb value is most easily obtained by manual determination after dilution in cyanmethaemoglobin reagent and centrifugation to remove the leucocytes from suspension. Alternatively the leucocytes may be removed by passing the whole blood through wool filters[43].
3. Unlysed red cells in the presence of marked target cell formation in liver disease and certain haemoglobinopathies.
4. Gross bilirubinaemia may slightly increase the Hb value.
5. The presence of marked *in vivo* haemolysis can produce a significantly higher Hb value due to the contribution of the free Hb in the plasma and would result in elevated MCH and MCHC.

6. Cryoglobulins and paraproteins may precipitate due to the relatively low ionic strength of reagents, pH and presence of quaternary ammonium salts[44,45].

Red-cell count

Falsely high values may be due to:

1. Red-cell counts include the contribution due to leucocytes. This always occurs but has a negligible effect in the presence of normal or modestly elevated leucocyte counts. Gross leucocytosis will obviously have a significant effect and the true red-cell count can be obtained by subtraction. However, the other red-cell parameters can also be obtained by filtration as mentioned above[43].
2. Giant platelets could be counted as red cells but are unlikely to be of sufficient volume or numbers to be significant.

Falsely low values may be due to:

1. Gross microcytosis or fragmentation, the very small cells being excluded from the count of instruments with fixed lower-volume threshold. Visual counting or an instrument with an adjustable lower threshold is indicated.
2. Agglutinins active at ambient temperature can result in cell aggregates being counted as single cells accompanied by a falsely high MCV. As the agglutinins are almost always more active at lower temperature, warming to 37°C before sampling will resolve the problem unless the thermal amplitude of the agglutinin is unusually high. EDTA-dependent agglutination which is not dispersed by warming has been described[46]; collection into heparin or ACD is indicated.
3. *In vitro* lysis due to incorrerct handling, storage or delay in testing. The Hb value will be correct but the remaining red-cell parameters will not be valid.

Mean corpuscular volume

Falsely high values may be due to:

1. Apart from increases due to prolonged storage and imperfect operating conditions[47,48], the most common cause is agglutination as discussed above.
2. In hyperosmolar states such as hyperglycaemia the red cells will rapidly take in water and increase the MCV when suspended in non-isotonic medium and tested immediately[49–51]. Predilution in reagent followed by standing for 30 minutes will allow equilibration and correct measurement of the MCV. The phenomenon is particularly a feature of Coulter systems. It has been suggested that uncorrected serial determinations may be of clinical value[49]. Unexplained high MCV which are not in accord with the MCH or reflected in the blood film appearances should be prediluted, allowed to stand and repeated. Alternatively, if there is no predilute facility on the instrument, the MCH can be used as the index of cell volume.

Falsely low values may be due to:

1. Hypo-osmolar states can be expected to have the opposite effect from the hyperosmolar conditions described above and results can be obtained by the same procedure.
2. Other causes of falsely low values are the inherent characteristics of certain instruments considered previously in this chapter and an increase in ambient temperature after calibration, thus reducing the conductivity of electrolyte in impedance counters[48]

Packed cell volume

As the PCV is derived from red-cell count and volumes in all instruments, incorrect results will be inevitable in the situations influencing those parameters.

Platelet count

Falsely high values may be due to:

1. Contamination of capillary samples with skin debris, food remnants with fat globules or subcutaneous fat droplets. Thorough cleaning of the site of capillary puncture is essential.
2. Microcytic or fragmented red cells can have volumes which extend into the distribution of platelet volumes. The problem can be suspected from the red-cell volume and/or platelet histograms, together with instrument flagging and, of course, the blood film. Manual counts are indicated. A correct platelet count can be obtained from the Technicon H1 showing the SR (small red cell) flag by reference to the P COUNT parameter [52].
3. Cytoplasmic fragments of leucocytes and particularly of leukaemic cells can simulate platelets. This is particularly difficult to resolve as the fragments are hard to differentiate from platelets in visual counting and even by blood film examination. After all, platelets are cytoplasmic fragments!
4. Cryoglobulinaemia with precipitation can result in pseudothrombocytosis [53].
5. Bacteraemia. It would be expected that bacteria in blood would be sized and counted as platelets and that if in sufficient number could result in spurious high counts [54]. *In vitro* contamination of samples by bacteria and their subsequent replication has been demonstrated.
6. *In vitro* haemolysis can result in red-cell ghosts being counted as platelets.

Falsely low counts may be due to:

1. The commonest causes are undoubtedly aggregation due to imperfect sample collection or undetected small clots.
2. Aggregation due to either IgG or IgM agglutinins which are EDTA-dependent or independent, temperature-dependent or independent, or interact with a further immunoglobulin, is well described [55] and not uncommon. Collection into ACD instead of EDTA may resolve the problem.
3. Platelet satellitism around neutrophils and, sometimes, lymphocytes is also EDTA-dependent.
4. Macrothrombocytes may be excluded from the count by certain instruments if they constitute a distinct population.

Instruments may fail to flag platelet clumping and cannot be considered reliable. All unexpected low platelet counts should be validated by a check of the sample for small clots and fibrin strands, and by blood film examination for clumps in the body and tail of the film, and for the presence of satellitism.

Calibration and quality control preparations for automated blood-cell counters

Automated instruments for measuring the various components of the blood count are not capable of direct measurement without reference to an external procedure or measurement. They are therefore 'comparators' which require calibration and ongoing quality control.

Calibrators and calibration

Calibration has been defined[56] as: 'the determination of a bias conversion factor of an analytical process under specified conditions in order to obtain accurate measurement of results. The accuracy over the operating range must be established by appropriate use of reference methods, reference materials and/or calibrators'.

Calibrators are materials with assigned values of defined accuracy which are traceable to determination by reference methods. They can be produced from fresh human and animal blood, artificial materials or mixtures of some or all of these. Values can be directly assigned to fresh blood by haematological reference techniques but its use as a calibrator is confined to a few hours. The values of the fresh blood are therefore usually used to assign values, via automated blood counters, to preserved blood or artificial materials to be used as calibrators or controls[57].

The assignment of values to fresh blood calibrators has been defined by the ICSH. The detailed description of the procedures[58] includes:

1. Haemoglobin measurement by the ICSH (1987) reference method;
2. PCV measured by ICSH (1988) selected method by microhaematocrit without correction for trapped plasma;
3. Red-cell count using a single-channel semi-automated electronic counter;
4. Red-cell indices by calculation;
5. White-cell count using a single-channel semi-automated electronic counter;
6. Platelet count derived from the results on an instrument capable of analysing whole blood.

Calibration of automated counters is therefore performed with fresh blood to which values have been assigned by reference techniques, or, by using preserved material the values of which have been determined with an automated counter that has been calibrated to the values of fresh blood.

No proposals have been made for calibration for the derived platelet parameter, the MPV, or for the parameters of the automated differential leucocyte count.

Control materials

Control preparations to which values may or may not have been assigned are used to ensure continued satisfactory performance after calibration. Ideally they should be of identical nature to the samples being tested, not only in its cellular constituents but also in its physical properties such as viscosity, mixing characteristics and tendency of the cells to stick together.

To achieve these requirements, while conferring stability, is difficult if not impossible. The cellular constituents are labile both in quantitative and qualitative terms. In order to maintain cell numbers and cell volume and retain as far as possible the characteristics of fresh blood during analysis, various stabilizing procedures have been recommended. In formulating the preparation of control material the stability of the individual parameters of untreated blood should be first considered.

Haemoglobin concentration is stable for many weeks if bacterial contamination is avoided.

Red cells collected into ACD, CPD or Alsever's solution remain intact for 5–6 weeks though changes in shape and volume occur. Red-cell volume increases during the first few days and then becomes reasonably constant though changes in temperature and oxygenation cause fluctuations in the MCV. Stabilization by mild fixation, but still allowing lysis during analysis, is a definite requirement.

Leucocytes are not stable in stored blood, the number being unpredictable during the first 7 days and then falling to low levels; a stable alternative is therefore necessary. As residual leucocytes will continue to decline, leucocyte-free blood is desirable as a starting material. Passage through a cotton wool filter can remove over 90% of white cells (and over 50% of the platelets). Inert synthetic particles, yeasts, fixed leucocytes or human red cells, or avian red cells have been used to simulate leucocytes.

Platelets are unstable in whole blood collected into ACD, CPD or Alsever's solution. Platelet-free blood should be used as a starting material and centrifugation of filtered blood and removal of the buffy layer is satisfactory. The 'platelets' to be added to the preparation must be stable and have a size distribution similar to that of human platelets; this is particularly important when using instruments which depend on a log-normal volume distribution for counting. This effectively excludes the use of latex and plastic particles. Fixed human, equine and porcine platelets appear suitable.

In summary, a satisfactory starting material is human blood collected into CPD-A, passed through a cotton wool filter and centrifuged to allow removal of the buffy layer. Red cells are stabilized by mild fixation and surrogate leucocytes are added together with fixed platelets. A bacteriostatic is added to prevent bacterial contamination. The method described below is based on that described by Morgan and Hunt [59].

Preparation of control material

Human blood collected into a standard CPD-A donor pack and unsuitable for transfusion or from a therapeutic venesection and tested negative for hepatitis B, C and HIV, is a suitable starting material. Concentrated cells or whole blood can be used. The blood is filtered through an Imugard IG 500 filter (Terumo Corporation) after priming with physiological saline; a new filter is used for each unit of blood.

Reagents

1. Phosphate buffered saline (PBS) pH 7.3 containing 30 g/l mannitol, 20 g/l D-glucose, 0.25 g/l sodium azide, sterilized by autoclaving at 10 lb/sq in for 10 minutes.
2. 50% glutaraldehyde.

Red cell preparation

To the filtered blood add a half volume of the PBS solution with 0.3% glutaraldehyde added. Mix, stand for 5 minutes and centrifuge at 3000 *g* for 10 minutes. Remove the supernatant and any residual buffy layer. Repeat the washing and centrifugation three times. Add sufficient PBS to give a final haemoglobin concentration of 12–14 g/dl and add 10 mg/ml di-sodium EDTA. The product is a suspension of gently fixed red cells which still allows lysis during haemoglobinometry and leucocyte counting.

N.B. The original method resuspended the cells in plasma protein fraction with added mannitol, D-glucose and azide.

Pseudo-leucocyte cell preparation

Approximately 20 ml of the untreated filtered blood is washed three times in PBS. To 10 volumes of PBS containing 0.5% glutaraldehyde, slowly add 1 volume of washed cells. After 18 hours at room temperature with occasional mixing, wash three times in PBS and resuspend in PBS to give a PCV of 0.50 l/l. Add di-sodium EDTA 10 mg/ml and sodium azide 0.25 mg/ml. At 4°C the fixed cells have a shelf life of over 6 months. Resuspend by thorough vortex mixing.
N.B. After fixation the cells tend to be 'sticky'. Excessive centrifugation will cause difficulty in resuspension; 200–300 *g* is adequate.

Preparation of fixed platelets

Units of time-expired human platelet concentrates are suspended overnight; those with excessive sedimented red cells are discarded. Pool the accepted units after filtration through a standard platelet administration set. Add an equal volume of PBS containing 0.2% glutaraldehyde and allow to fix for 20 minutes. Centrifuge at 700 *g* for 15 minutes, remove the supernatant, resuspend in PBS and repeat the centrifugation and resuspend in twice their volume with PBS. After dilution as required, the platelet suspension is processed on the analyser to check that the volume distribution and the numbers of residual leucocytes and red cells are not excessive. Excess leucocytes and red cells can be removed by sedimentation after standing overnight at 4°C and collection of the supernatant. This step may be repeated as necessary.
N.B. The method for preparing fixed, washed platelets for the assay of vWf:RiCoF (page 643) is also suitable for control platelets.

Preparation of composite control material

The red cells, pseudo-leucocytes and platelets are usually combined to give approximately normal values but can be adjusted to also provide values in the low and high ranges. The combined material is thoroughly and continuously mixed during dispensing into sterile vials. The volume dispensed should be sufficient to provide control sampling for 24 hours. Each batch is stored at 4°C for 4–6 weeks to allow stabilization of the MCV. The stabilized material has a shelf life of at least 6 weeks, the limiting parameters being the MCV and RDW. The haemoglobin concentration, cell counts and derived parameters of MPV and PDW are stable for longer periods provided that bacterial contamination does not occur.

Suitability

Although originally formulated for the Coulter series of analysers, the preparation has been used successfully with the Technicon H1 and Sysmex E5000.

References

1. Coulter, W. H. (1956) High-speed automatic blood cell counter and cell size analyser. *Proc. Natl. Electron Conf.*, **12**, 1034–40
2. Sturgeon, P. and McQuiston, D. T. (1965) A fully automated system for the simultaneous

determination of whole blood red cell count and hemoglobin content. *Am. J. Clin. Pathol.*, **43**, 517–22
3. Groner, W. and Epstein, E. (1982) Counting and sizing of blood cells using light scattering. In *Advances in Haematological Methods: The Blood Count* (eds. O. W. van Assendelft and J. M. England), pp. 73–84. Boca Raton: CRC Press
4. Shapiro, H. M. (1984) *Practical Flow Cytometry*. New York: Alan R. Liss
5. Tanke, H. J., Rothbarth, P. H., Vossen, J. M. J. J. *et al.* (1983) Flow cytometry of reticulocytes applied to clinical haematology. *Blood,* **61**, 1091–7
6. Carter, J. M., McSweeney, P. A., Wakem, P. J. and Nemet, A. M. (1989) Counting reticulocytes by flow cytometry: use of thiazole orange. *Clin. Lab. Haematol.*, **11**, 267–71
7. Koepke, J. F. (1989) Flow cytometric reticulocyte counting. *Labmedica*, June/July, 27–32
8. Kojima, K., Niri, M., Setoguchi, K., Tsuda, I. and Tatsumi, N. (1989) An automated opto-electronic reticulocyte counter. *Am. J. Clin. Pathol.*, **92**, 57–61
9. Quirke, P. and Dyson, J. E. (1986) Flow cytometry: methodology and applications in pathology. *J. Pathol.,* **149**, 79–89
10. Theodorsen, L. (1987) Haemoglobinometry and automated haematology analysers. *Clin. Lab. Haematol.,* **9**, 377–85
11. Rowan, R. M. (1983) *Blood Cell Volume Analysis*. London: Albert Clark
12. Guthrie, D. L. and Pearson, T. C. (1982) PCV measurement in the management of polycythaemic patients. *Clin. Lab. Haematol.,* **4**, 257–65
13. Tycko, D. H., Metz, M. H., Epstein, E. A. and Grinbaum, A. (1985) Flow-cytometric light scattering measurement of red blood cell volume and haemoglobin concentration. *Appl. Optics,* **24**, 1355–65
14. Mohandas, N., Johnson, A., Wyatt, J. *et al.* (1989) Automated quantitation of red cell density distribution and hyperdense cell fraction in RBC disorders. *Blood,* **74**, 442–7
15. Simel, D. L., De Long, E. R., Feussner, J. R., Crawford, J. and Weinberg, J. B. (1987) Peripheral blood film interpretation of anisocytosis versus quantitative assessment by RDW. *Clin. Res.*, **35**, 92A
16. Bessman, J. D., Gilmer, P. R. and Gardner, F. H. (1983) Improved classification of anemias by MCV and RDW. *Am. J. Clin. Pathol.,* **80**, 322–6
17. Simel, D. L. (1987) Is the RDW–MCV classification of anaemia useful? *Clin. Lab. Haematol.*, **9**, 349–59
18. Brittenham, G. M. and Koepke, J. A. (1987) Red blood cell volume distribution and the diagnosis of anemia. *Arch. Pathol. Lab. Med.*, **111**, 1146–8
19. Reardon, D., Hutchinson, D. and Trowbridge, E. A. (1987) Automatic measurement of platelet volume. *Med. Lab. Sci.,* **44**, 190–1
20. Reardon, D., Hutchinson, D., Preston, F. E. and Trowbridge, E. A. (1985) The routine measurement of platelet volume: a comparison of aperture-impedance and flow cytometric systems. *Clin. Lab. Haematol.,* **7**, 251–7
21. Lippi, U., Cappalletti, P., Schinella, M. and Signori, D. (1985) Mean platelet volume: fact or artefacts. *Am. J. Clin. Pathol.,* **84**, 111–3
22. Lippi, U., Schinella, M., Modena, N. and Nicoli, M. (1987) Unpredictable effects of K_3EDTA on mean platelet volume. *Am. J. Clin. Pathol.,* **87**, 391–3
23. Giles, C. (1981) The platelet count and mean platelet volume. *Br. J. Haematol.,* **48**, 31–7
24. Bessman, J. D., Williams, L. J. and Gillmer, P. R. (1982) Platelet size in health and disease. *Am. J. Clin. Pathol.,* **78**, 150–3
25. Smit, J. W., Gelsema, E. S., Huiges, W., Nawrath, R. F. and Halie, M. R. (1979) A commercially available interactive pattern recognition system for the characterization of blood cells: description of the system, extraction and evaluation of simple geometric parameters of normal white blood cells. *Clin. Lab. Haematol.,* **1**, 109–19
26. Pierre, R. V. and O'Sullivan, M. B. (1974) Evaluation of the Hemalog D automated differential leucocyte counter. *Mayo Clin. Proc.,* **49**, 870–4
27. Hasty, T., Harris, L. G., Stonacek, S. M. and Frazier, B. (1982) Evaluation of an automated continuous-flow haematology instrument. The Technicon H6000. *J. Clin. Lab. Automat.,* **2**, 408–15

28. Statland, B. E., Winkel, P., Harris, S. C., Birdsall, M. J. and Saunders, A. M. (1978) Evaluation of biologic sources of variation of leukocyte counts and other hematologic quantities using very precise automated analysers. *Am. J. Clin. Pathol.*, **69**, 48–54
29. Winkel, P., Statland, B. E., Saunders, A. M., Osborn, H. and Kupperman, H. (1981) Within-day variation of leukocyte types in healthy subjects as assayed by two automated leukocyte differential counters. *Am. J. Clin. Pathol.*, **75**, 693–700
30. Hughes-Jones, N. C., Morley, N., Young, J. M. S. and England, J. M. (1974) Differential white cell counts by frequency distribution analysis of cell volumes. *J. Clin. Pathol.*, **27**, 623–5
31. Wycherley, P. A. and O'Shea, M. J. (1978) Abridged differential counts provided by a Coulter Channelyser in a routine haematology department. *J. Clin. Pathol.*, **31**, 271–4
32. Clarke, P. T., Henthorn, J. S. and England, J. M. (1985) Differential white cell counting on the Coulter Model S Plus IV (three population) and the Technicon H6000; a comparison by simple and multiple regression. *Clin. Lab. Haematol.*, **7**, 335–51
33. Griswold, D. J. and Champagne, V. D. (1985) Evaluation of the Coulter S Plus IV three-part differential in an acute care hospital. *Am. J. Clin. Pathol.*, **84**, 49–57
34. Lai, A. P., Martin, P. J., Richards, J. D. M., Goldstone, A. H. and Crawley, J. C. (1986) Automated leucocyte differential count in acute leukaemia: a comparison of the Hemalog D, H6000 and Coulter S-plus IV. *Clin. Lab. Haematol.*, **8**, 33–41
35. Bain, B. J. (1986) An assessment of the three-population differential count on the Coulter Counter Model S Plus IV. *Clin. Lab. Haematol.*, **8**, 347–59
36. Pierre, R. V., Payne, B. A., Lee, W. K. *et al.* (1987) Comparison of four leucocyte differential methods with the National Committee for Clinical Laboratory Standards (NCCL) reference method. *Am. J. Clin. Pathol.*, **87**, 201–9
37. Barnard, D. F., Barnard, S. A., Carter, A. B. *et al.* (1989) An evaluation of the Coulter VCS differential counter. *Clin. Lab. Haematol.*, **11**, 255–66
38. Savage, R. A. (1984) Pseudoleukocytosis due to EDTA-induced platelet clumping. *Am. J. Clin. Pathol.*, **81**, 317–22
39. Abela, M., McArdle, B. and Qureshi, M. (1980) Pseudoleucocytosis due to cryoglobulinaemia. *J. Clin. Pathol.*, **33**, 796
40. Schaub, C. R. and Fahri, D. C. (1987) Circulating mucin in Wilms' tumor; a cause of artificial elevation of leucocyte counts. *Am. J. Clin. Pathol.*, **87**, 413A
41. Epstein, H. D. and Kruskall, M. S. (1988) Spurious leukopenia due to *in vitro* granulocyte aggregation. *Am. J. Clin. Pathol.*, **89**, 652–5
42. Nonsanchuk, J. S., Roark, M. F. and Wanser, C. (1974) Anemia masked by triglyceridemia. *Am. J. Clin. Pathol.*, **62**, 838–9
43. Francis, D. A., Francis, J. L. and Roath, O. S. (1985) Improved assessment of haemoglobin and red cell indices in blood samples with high white cell counts. *Med. Lab. Sci.*, **42**, 285–6
44. Nicholls, P. D. (1985) Haemoglobin measurement and blood protein precipitation with automated cell counters. *Med. Lab. Sci.*, **42**, 196–8
45. Wallis, J. P. and Ford, J. M. (1987) Incorrect haemoglobin estimation on the Coulter S+ IV in some patients with IgM paraprotein. *Clin. Lab. Haematol.*, **9**, 95–9
46. Reid, M. E., Bottenfield, L. K., Toy, P. T., Ellisor, S. S. and Hart, C. A. (1985) Agglutination of an EDTA blood sample caused by an EDTA-dependent panagglutinin. *Am. J. Clin. Pathol.*, **83**, 534–5
47. Lawrence, A. C. K., Bevington, J. M. and Young, M. (1975) Storage of blood and the mean corpuscular volume. *J. Clin. Pathol.*, **28**, 345–9
48. Young, M. and Lawrence, A. C. K. (1975) The influence of extraneous factors on Coulter S measurement of the mean corpuscular volume. *J. Clin. Pathol.*, **28**, 12–15
49. Allen, S. C., Balfour, I. C. and Wise, C. C. (1980) The red cell osmometer. *J. Clin. Pathol.*, **33**, 430–3
50. Davidson, R. J. L., Evan-Wong, L. A. and Lean, M. E. J. (1981) The Coulter MCV in diabetic ketoacidosis. *Clin. Lab. Haematol.*, **3**, 90–1
51. Savage, R. A. and Hoffman, G. C. (1983) Clinical significance of osmotic matrix errors producing spurious macrocytosis. *Am. J. Clin. Pathol.*, **80**, 861–5

52. McVeigh, D. J. and Van der Weyden, M. B. (1989) Correction of spurious haematological results using Technicon H1-derived data. *Clin. Lab. Haematol.,* **11**, 369–73
53. Patel, K. J., Hughes, C. G. and Parapia, L. A. (1987) Pseudoleucocytosis and pseudothrombocytosis due to cryoglobulinaemia. *J. Clin. Pathol.,* **40,** 120–1
54. Gloster, E. S., Strauss, R. A., Jiminez, J. F., Neuberg, R. W., Berry, D. H. and Turner, E. J. (1985) Spurious elevated platelet counts associated with bacteremia. *Am. J. Haematol.,* **18**, 329–32
55. Lombarts, A. J. P. F. and De Lieviet, W. (1988) Recognition and prevention of pseudothrombocytopenia and concomitant pseudoleucocytosis. *Am. J. Clin. Pathol.,* **89**, 634–9
56. Van Assendelft, O. W. and England, J. M. (1982) Terms, quantities and units. In *Advances in Haematological Methods: The Blood Count* (eds. O. W. van Assendelft and J. M. England), pp. 1–9. Boca Raton, Florida: CRC Press
57. England, J. M., Chetty, M. C., Garvey, B. *et al.* (1983) Testing of calibration and quality control material used with automated blood counting apparatus: application of the protocol devised by the British Committee for Standardization in Haematology. *Clin. Lab. Haematol.,* **5**, 83–92
58. International Committee for Standardisation in Haematology. Expert Panel on Cytometry (1988) The assignment of values to fresh blood used for calibrating automated blood cell counters. *Clin. Lab. Haematol.,* **10**, 203–12
59. Morgan, L. O. and Hunt, A. (1984) A whole blood control for Coulter electronic particle counters. *Med. Lab. Sci.,* **41**, 209–18

Chapter 9

Anaemias. I. Microcytic anaemias

Definition and concept of anaemia

It is difficult to formulate a definition of anaemia that is all embracing but for practical purposes anaemia may be stated as being 'a reduction in oxygen-carrying capacity due to a lower haemoglobin concentration than is usual for that individual'. However, a reduction in oxygen availability depends not only on haemoglobin concentration but also on the oxygen dissociation curve and the speed of dissociation, the amount of inactive haemoglobin, rate of blood flow and capillary function. Thus the presence of structural haemoglobin variants with altered oxygen affinities, a reduced 2,3-DPG level or the presence of inactive forms of haemoglobin will influence oxygen availability even though the haemoglobin mass may not be reduced.

An additional aspect is the wide range of haemoglobin values found in healthy populations; a significant reduction in haemoglobin concentration may occur in an individual and yet show a level within the reference range. Alteration of plasma volume may also result in misleading values as will haemoglobin estimation determined during the 48 hours following acute blood loss before the blood volume returns to normal. A compensated haemolytic anaemia may also result in a haemoglobin concentration within the normal range.

With the exception of those anaemias due solely to diminished haemoglobin synthesis, haemoglobin concentration is dependent on red-cell mass. Red-cell production and destruction (or loss) is normally finely balanced, i.e. production equals destruction. Anaemia will occur when production is less than destruction irrespective of whether production is increased, perhaps even many fold. The rate of progression of the anaemia and its ultimate severity will depend on the rate of destruction or loss of red cells and on the ability of the bone marrow to compensate by increased red-cell production. In a compensated anaemia when increased production is equal to increased destruction the haemoglobin concentration will reach a steady state but at lower than 'normal' level.

Classification of anaemias

Various systems of classification can be adopted:

1. By clinical associations.
2. By aetiology.
3. On the basis of red-cell parameters.

4. On the basis of bone-marrow erythropoietic activity.
5. A combination of two or more of the above.

Clinical association

An approach based on clinical observation, symptoms or associations such as acute or chronic, congenital or acquired, or primary and secondary are not suitable in the context of laboratory investigation, though they are useful in secondary classification.

Aetiology

A classification of anaemia on the basis of cause is commonly used in textbooks of medicine and is useful in the clearly defined situations of anaemia due to haemorrhage, due to shortened red-cell survival, in bone-marrow failure and in deficiency states. In those anaemias where there is more than one component or mechanism or when the cause is unknown, classification becomes imprecise, e.g. the thalassaemias, megaloblastosis and severe iron deficiency. Recourse is made to groupings such as 'dyshaemopoietic' or 'miscellaneous'.

Red-cell parameters

The introduction of red-cell 'absolute values' led to a system of classification based on the MCV and the apparent haemoglobin concentration or content as reflected by the MCHC and MCH, respectively. Three classes were recognized:

1. Macrocytic anaemia – having a raised MCV.
2. Normocytic–normochromic anaemias – with normal MCV and MCHC.
3. Microcytic anaemias – those with a low MCV.

This approach results in the grouping of anaemias of varied aetiology and mechanism. For example the 'normocytic–normochromic' anaemias will include acute blood loss, many haemolytic anaemias with widely differing mechanisms, the anaemias associated with acute or chronic proliferative disorders and often those associated with bone-marrow failure. Nevertheless the introduction of automated blood counting with the production of routine, potentially accurate and readily available measurement of MCV has made this approach to classification useful, particularly for the 'microcytic' and 'macrocytic' disorders.

Bone-marrow erythropoietic activity

The determination of erythropoietic activity by bone-marrow cellularity and corrected reticulocyte counts, supplemented perhaps by study of iron kinetics, allows division into two classes of anaemia:

1. Associated with erythroid *hyper*plasia.
2. Associated with erythroid *hypo*plasia.

These can be further subdivided by incorporating aetiological aspects:

1. With erythroid hyperplasia:
   (a) effective erythropoietic response – (i) haemorrhage, (ii) haemolysis;
   (b) ineffective erythropoietic response – (i) nuclear maturation and defects, e.g. megaloblastosis, and/or (ii) cytoplasmic maturation defects, e.g. defective haem or globin synthesis.

2. With erythroid hypoplasia:
   (a) decreased marrow stimulation – (i) reduced erythropoietin levels, e.g. renal disease, infection, neoplasia, endocrine disorders;
   (b) decreased bone-marrow response – (i) marrow failure, e.g. replacement or damage, (ii) severe iron depletion.

This classification allows for three basic erythropoietic states: effective hyperplasia, ineffective hyperplasia and hypoplasia and represents a pathophysiological classification of the mechanisms producing anaemia which is based on measurable or observable blood and bone-marrow parameters and is recommended as the most suitable for the laboratory haematologist to understand the *mechanisms* of anaemia.

Mechanisms of anaemia

Anaemia with erythroid hyperplasia

Anaemia with effective erythroid hyperplasia

Haemorrhage

Acute blood loss After acute blood loss the haemoglobin concentration will initially be normal because the red-cell mass and plasma volume are reduced in proportion. The immediate symptoms are therefore related to the reduced blood volume. Anaemia does not develop until fluid enters the circulation to restore the plasma volume. A minor fall in the haemoglobin concentration may occur in the first few hours due to water and salt adjustments but the major volume replacement is not achieved for up to 3–4 days. This is effected by an influx of pre-formed albumin and water. Final restoration of blood volume and its constituents is by replacement of other plasma proteins and regeneration of erythrocytes as shown by bone-marrow hyperplasia and a reticulocytosis.

Subacute blood loss When blood loss is in the order of perhaps 50 ml daily, clinical signs may be minimal and the patient presents with a mild to moderate anaemia with a compensated plasma volume and an established erythropoietic response. If a balance between blood loss and regeneration is achieved then a compensated state will be present until iron stores become depleted and a microcytic, hypochromic anaemia develops.

Chronic blood loss In the early stages of the anaemia of chronic haemorrhage there is erythroid hyperplasia which with increasing iron depletion develops into ineffective erythropoiesis and eventually results in a lack of bone-marrow response and a hypoplastic erythroid series.

Haemolysis
Haemolytic anaemias are caused by a shortened red-cell life span which is reflected by increased erythropoietic activity and reticulocytosis. Most haemolytic anaemias are associated with efficient conservation of iron and the anaemia is therefore usually normochromic and normocytic (there are exceptions), though the reticulocytosis may result in slight macrocytosis. The mechanisms leading to, or causing, a shortened red-cell survival may be classified in several ways but the fundamental reason is damage or 'loss of integrity' of the red-cell membrane.

Anaemia with ineffective erythroid hyperplasia

Radioisotope studies show that approximately 80–90% of normal erythropoiesis results in the delivery to the circulation of competent red cells. The remaining 10–20% of erythropoiesis is ineffective, i.e. the erythroblasts do not mature and are retained in the bone marrow with eventual cell death and destruction with liberation of enzymes and catabolic haem pigments. In certain anaemias the proportion of ineffective erythropoiesis is greatly increased. Various mechanisms have been implicated. Autoradiographic and microspectrophotometric studies of cells in interphase indicate that erythroblasts may be arrested in G_2 phase and show excessive DNA content. Additionally, cells may not enter the S phase. The formation of inclusion bodies with marrow trapping, mitochondrial damage and cell-membrane abnormalities are also possible mechanisms. Those cells that do reach the circulation usually have a shortened life span.

Ineffective erythropoiesis may be congenital or acquired, caused by defective protein or enzyme pathways, deficiency of essential metabolites, toxic chemicals or other uncertain mechanisms. The disorder may involve defects in nuclear or cytoplasmic maturation or a combination of both.

Nuclear maturation defects
Disordered synthesis of nucleic acids Deficiency of folate or of vitamin B_{12} which are essential for the synthesis of pyrimidines and purines results in megaloblastic erythropoiesis (*see* Chapter 10) which has long been used as a model for studying ineffective erythropoiesis. The features of ineffective erythropoiesis are erythroid hyperplasia, low reticulocyte count and macrocytosis.

Abnormalities of the nuclear membrane The recognition and classification of hereditary dyserythropoietic states associated with abnormalities of the erythroblasts such as multinuclearity, nuclear bridging, giant-megaloblast development with marked ineffective erythropoiesis is relatively recent. EM studies have indicated that abnormalities of the cytoplasmic or nuclear membranes may be the primary defects in such cases. Again, erythroid hyperplasia, a low reticulocyte count and macrocytosis are characteristic.

Defective cytoplasmic maturation
Maturation of erythroblast cytoplasm is associated with haemoglobin synthesis. Abnormal or reduced haemoglobin synthesis may be due to disordered haem or globin synthesis.

Disordered haem synthesis This may be due either to defective protoporphyrin production caused by enzyme defects, or to failure of iron incorporation into protoporphyrin. Such a failure may be caused either by iron deficiency or by interference with the enzymatic control of the insertion of iron into protoporphyrin. Drugs or chemicals can interfere at many of the intermediate stages of haem synthesis. Lead, anti-tuberculous therapy, alcohol and chloramphenicol all cause defective haem synthesis. Mitochondrial iron overload paradoxically also results in failure of haem synthesis.

Disordered globin synthesis A reduced though balanced production of the polypeptide chains forming the globin molecule would probably have a similar effect to that of iron deficiency. Imbalanced chain synthesis results not only in reduced haemoglobin synthesis but, more importantly, in the presence of unstable free polypeptide chains which precipitate and aggregate and cause intramedullary destruction of erythroblasts and membrane defects in those cells that do reach the circulation. Red-cell life span is consequently reduced. This sequence of events is characteristic of the thalassaemia syndromes.

Anaemia with erythroid hypoplasia

Due to decreased marrow stimulation

Direct hormonal control of erythropoiesis can only be attributed to erythropoietin. The erythropoietic changes associated with pituitary, thyroid, adrenal and gonadal function are probably exerted through effects on metabolism and oxygen requirements and not by direct effect on the bone marrow. Reduced erythropoietin stimulation of the bone marrow is due to low levels of plasma erythropoietin caused by either a failure of synthesis or by an inhibition by autoimmune mechanisms, as can occur in pure red-cell aplasia.

Due to decreased bone-marrow response

Marrow failure
Quantitative failure of erythropoiesis despite adequate erythropoietin stimulus is a fundamental defect typified by aplastic anaemia, whether 'idiopathic' or due to chemical or radiation damage. Replacement of the bone marrow by neoplastic cell proliferation – either haemopoietic as in leukaemia or non-haemopoietic such as in carcinoma, fibrous replacement or bone overgrowth – are other causes of failure to respond to erythropoietin.

Severe iron depletion
As stated previously the spectrum of iron depletion ranges from latent to severe with erythropoietic changes progressing from minimal to proliferative, to ineffective and eventually to hypoplasia.

Microcytic anaemias

If the MCV is used to define microcytosis the assigned value will depend on whether automated equipment is calibrated to a PCV corresponding to a spun haematocrit with or without adjustment for plasma trapping. Interlaboratory quality assessment surveys clearly show that the great majority of laboratories adjust the PCV to a lower value to allow for trapped plasma thus reducing the calibration of the MCV by about 5 fl and in this situation microcytosis is defined as a MCV less than 83 fl or a MCH less than 27 pg.

Microcytic hypochromic anaemia is by far the commonest type of anaemia and is due to defective synthesis of haemoglobin, the usual reason being depletion of iron stores. In certain ethnic groups, however, there is a high incidence of inherited disorders of globin-chain synthesis, the thalassaemia syndromes, and accurate laboratory differentiation is important not only for the purposes of treatment but also to allow effective genetic counselling to reduce the medical and socioeconomic effects of the severe forms of thalassaemia. Microcytosis is also associated with

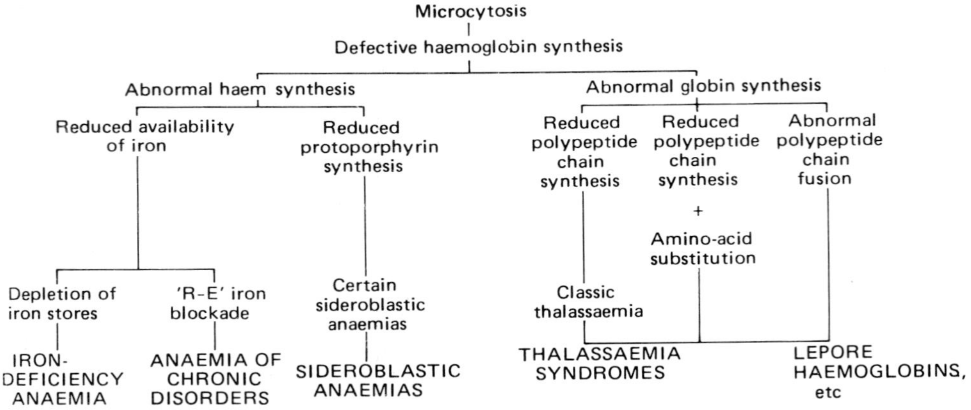

Figure 9.1 Causes of microcytosis

'chronic disorders' and with the anaemias characterized by the presence of 'ringed sideroblasts'. A diagrammatic representation of the causes of microcytosis is shown in *Figure 9.1*.

Iron-deficiency anaemia

The iron content of the body is normally maintained by efficient conservation mechanisms. The small uncontrolled losses via urine, sweat, bile and cell desquamation are replaced by controlled iron absorption which is normally sufficient to balance the loss. If iron loss or demand is excessive or absorption insufficient, iron stores will be depleted and result in a microcytic hypochromic anaemia.

The commonest cause of iron deficiency in the adult is blood loss which is physiological, as in the menstruating female, or pathological due to haemorrhage from the gastrointestinal tract, menorrhagia or, less commonly, from other sites. Poor diet or malabsorption of dietary iron due to gastric surgery or intestinal malabsorption are also common causes of iron depletion. Iron deficiency in pregnancy is common unless iron supplements are taken. The demand of an extra 1–2 mg of iron per day during the pregnancy, plus the loss by lactation, will result in a 'negative iron balance' of between 400 and 900 mg of iron though there is a 'saving' of 250–300 mg due to the amenorrhoea during pregnancy. The growth of children creates an extra demand for iron which is perhaps reflected by the lower 'normal ranges' for haemoglobin concentration and MCV during childhood.

In summary, depletion of iron stores is brought about by the *increased demand* of growth, pregnancy and lactation, by *blood loss* whether physiological or pathological, or by *reduced absorption* due to dietary deficiency or intestinal malabsorption. An unusual mechanism of iron depletion is loss of particulate iron in the urine (haemosiderinuria) due to chronic intravascular haemolysis.

The stages of iron deficiency may be defined as follows:

1. Pre-latent deficiency – reduced availability of storage iron (lowered plasma ferritin).

2. Latent deficiency – reduced serum iron, increased iron-binding capacity, low plasma ferritin.
3. Changes in red-cell morphology with a fall in haemoglobin concentration.

Blood changes

Changes in red-cell morphology are preceded by demonstrable reduction of storage iron. A falling MCV is an early indication of iron deficiency even though the value may still be within the normal range. A reduction in red-cell haemoglobin concentration (CHC) as determined by the Technicon H1 system may be the first cellular indication of iron depletion. Microcytosis and hypochromia develop with progressively more obvious poikilocytosis, small numbers of target cells and some cells showing basophilic stippling particularly when the anaemia is severe [1]. The MCV may fall as low as 50 fl or exceptionally even lower. The parameter 'red-cell distribution width' (RDW) is usually increased reflecting the presence of anisocytosis (cf. RDW in the microcytosis of thalassaemia trait). The abnormal blood picture due to poor diet, malabsorption or very slow blood loss develops insidiously and there is little evidence of an attempt by the bone marrow to compensate by increased output as evidenced by a significant reticulocytosis. When blood loss is greater or in its earlier (subacute) stages with mild to moderate anaemia, there is often a reticulocytosis in the order of 5% and the blood-film appearances may be interpreted correctly. The platelet count is often increased above $400 \times 10^9/l$ in moderate to severe iron deficiency irrespective of the aetiology.

Leucocytes are usually unremarkable but an eosinophilia may indicate the presence of intestinal parasites causing blood loss or malabsorption of iron. Neutrophil hypersegmentation is well documented in iron-deficiency anaemia and may be due to covert deficiency of folate even though the vitamin assays are in the normal range. The deoxyuridine suppression test on lymphocytes from patients with iron deficiency and neutrophil hypersegmentation has shown a high proportion of such patients to be folate deficient [2].

Biochemical abnormalities of iron-deficient red cells include elevated levels of δ-aminolaevulinic acid dehydratase [3] and erythrocyte protoporphyrin [4]. It has been suggested that erythrocyte protoporphyrin may be of value in retrospective diagnosis after iron therapy as the levels remain increased some months after restoration of haemoglobin concentration to the normal range. Iron deficiency results in the reduction of certain normal and abnormal haemoglobin fractions, notably Hb A_2, Hb F, Hb H and more positively charged β-globin chain variants. There is conflicting evidence whether the free α-chain pool is decreased or increased in iron deficiency [5–7].

Red-cell deformability is reduced in iron deficiency possibly due to increased lipid peroxidation.

Bone-marrow changes

Erythroid hyperplasia is common in the early stages but with progression of the anaemia there is considerable ineffective erythropoiesis followed by hypoplasia. Erythroblasts at all stages of maturation are smaller than normal with delayed haemoglobinization and ragged cytoplasm. Additional morphological and biochemical abnormalities probably reflect dyserythropoiesis. There is considerable reduction or complete absence of stainable iron which reflects the depleted iron stores. Sideroblasts are also greatly reduced or absent.

Plasma iron status

In iron depletion there is a fall in plasma iron associated with a rise in the transferrin level which is reflected by an increased total iron binding capacity (TIBC) and decreased percentage saturation. When the percentage saturation falls below 16% there is failure of adequate iron supply to the erythroblasts. The fall in plasma iron and decreased saturation precedes the appearances of anaemia. A disadvantage of plasma iron estimation as an index of iron status is the considerable diurnal and day-to-day fluctuation.

Plasma ferritin

In adults with normal iron balance, plasma ferritin levels for men are in the range 28–220 μg/l with a mean of 103 μg/l and for women 30–185 μg/l (mean 70 μg/l). In pre-latent deficiency, as assessed by ^{59}Fe absorption, values in men decrease on average to 24 μg/l and in women to 27 μg/l (range 8–65 μg/l). The mean values are clearly different though there is overlap at the extremities.

In latent iron deficiency where plasma iron is low and TIBC increased but haemoglobin levels are normal, plasma ferritin levels of 9 μg/l for males and 15 μg/l for females (range 5.3–32 μg/l) are found. In overt deficiency ferritin levels range from 2.7–12 μg/l with little difference between sexes. It may be concluded that depleted iron stores are reflected by a plasma ferritin value of less than 30 μg/l in the absence of inflammation, malignancy, liver disease etc., and that a level less than 15 μg/l is associated with iron-deficiency anaemia (*Table 9.1*). Plasma ferritin levels do not show diurnal, day-to-day or week-to-week changes in the normal subject [8] although there is a wide normal range. As plasma ferritin concentration is usually a reliable index of iron stores it should supersede the invasive bone-marrow biopsy as a means of assessing the amount of storage iron.

Table 9.1 Relationship between parameters of iron status and the development of iron-deficiency anaemia

Stage of development	*Marrow iron*	*Plasma iron*	*Mean plasma ferritin* (μg/l)	*Hb*
Normal	N	N	85 (N)	N
Pre-latent iron deficiency	↓	N	25 ↓	N
Latent iron deficiency	↓ ↓	↓	12 ↓ ↓	N
Overt iron deficiency	↓ ↓ ↓	↓ ↓	6 ↓ ↓ ↓	↓

N = Normal value; arrows indicate degree of decrease.

Red-cell ferritin

Although plasma ferritin is a reliable indicator of iron depletion, elevated ferritin levels are commonly due to inflammation, neoplastic disease and tissue necrosis. Measurement of red-cell ferritin is reported to be a more accurate reflection of iron supply. In the 'anaemia of chronic disorders' (*see* below) concomitant iron deficiency may be demonstrated by red-cell ferritin assay even when the plasma ferritin is normal or increased due to tissue damage [9].

Anaemia of chronic disorders (ACD)

Anaemia associated with chronic disease or inflammation is common and is found in disorders such as chronic infections, rheumatoid arthritis and malignancy. Although blood loss or a haemolytic mechanism may contribute to anaemia in these disorders there remains an anaemia which has been defined as 'that anaemia usually mild and not progressive which is characterized by decreased plasma iron, decreased TIBC, decreased transferrin saturation, decreased stainable iron in the erythroblasts and normal or increased reticuloendothelial iron'. 'Anaemia of chronic disorders' gives no indication of the haematological features of the anaemia and the more descriptive 'sideropenic anaemia with reticuloendothelial siderosis' has been suggested. Immunoreactive plasma erythropoietin levels are raised in inverse relationship to the degree of anaemia.

Pathogenesis

Three mechanisms have been implicated: (i) shortened red-cell survival, (ii) poor marrow response to anaemia, (iii) impaired flow of iron from R-E cells to bone-marrow erythroblasts – the so-called 'R-E block'. There is *in vitro* evidence that cell–cell interactions may play a part in ACD.

Normal cells transfused to patients have a shortened survival but patients' red cells survive normally in normal subjects, indicating an extracorpuscular mechanism. Increased phagocytic activity of the R-E system has been suggested as the possible cause. The bone-marrow response to the stimulus of the anaemia is impaired, as indicated by ferrokinetic studies. This is apparently due to the failure of the anaemia to stimulate the production of erythropoietin, as in rats the administration of exogenous erythropoietin elicits a marrow response, as does an additional hypoxic stimulus. In 'chronic disorders' a normal haemoglobin level may not be desirable and the mild anaemia may be part of a beneficial homeostatic compensation. Ferrokinetic techniques show little evidence of increased ineffective erythropoiesis.

The concept of the 'R-E block' was formulated from studies of patients with malignant neoplasms. Non-viable red cells labelled with radio-iron were transfused and the amount of injected radioactivity reincorporated into the circulating red cells measured. In normal subjects, 55–70% of radio-iron was reutilized whereas in the patients less than 40% appeared in the circulating red cells [11]. Confirmation of these findings has been obtained by using radioactive iron dextran as an index of reticuloendothelial-cell release of iron in patients with a variety of chronic diseases [12]. The R-E block theory can explain the low plasma iron value, the reduction in erythroblast iron and the increase in erythrocyte protoporphyrin in the presence of adequate iron stores. Although transferrin levels fall in acute infection the mechanism for the low transferrin levels in chronic disease is not clear. It must be emphasized that the 'chronic disorders' are a heterogeneous group of diseases and the pattern of iron redistribution may vary. For example, in rheumatoid arthritis bone-marrow iron is reduced but there is marked accumulation in synovial membranes, and in lymphoma, lymph nodes may show increased iron content. In rats, inflammation results in increased ferritin synthesis which may divert iron into ferritin stores with resulting reduced availability for erythropoiesis [13]. Whether this mechanism applies to the chronic disorders of humans is uncertain.

The anaemia of chronic disorders is often normocytic and normochromic but when the percentage saturation of transferrin falls below 15%, delivery of iron to erythroblasts is impaired and a microcytic hypochromic anaemia will develop. It is for this reason, together with the changes in iron status, that it is appropriate to consider the 'anaemia of chronic disorders' along with other microcytic anaemias particularly as oral iron therapy is of no benefit and differential diagnosis therefore of importance.

Changes in red cells

The anaemia is usually normocytic and normochromic and when microcytosis develops the MCV is usually between 70 and 80 fl unless overt iron deficiency supervenes. Morphology is unremarkable and the reticulocyte count is not significantly raised. Erythrocyte protoporphyrin levels and ALA-D activity are increased.

Bone-marrow changes

Cellularity is usually normal and slight increase in activity is not readily recognizable. Erythropoiesis is normoblastic and sideroblasts are absent or greatly reduced in number. In contrast, extracellular iron is present and is often increased.

Plasma iron status

Plasma iron is low, transferrin concentration is in the low normal range or reduced (cf. increased transferrin in iron depletion). Transferrin saturation is normal or low. Plasma ferritin levels are usually normal or increased.

Sideroblastic anaemias

This group of anaemias is characterized by iron loading of the erythroblast mitochondria resulting in the characteristic perinuclear distribution of iron staining, the 'ringed sideroblast'. In contrast to the iron granules in the cytoplasm of the normal sideroblast, mitochondrial iron is not ferritin.

Sideroblastic anaemias can be classified according to their aetiology (*Figure 9.2*).

In this section only the hereditary and the secondary types induced by drugs, chemicals, etc. will be considered for the reasons set out in *Table 9.2*. Primary acquired sideroblastic anaemia is dealt with in Chapter 12.

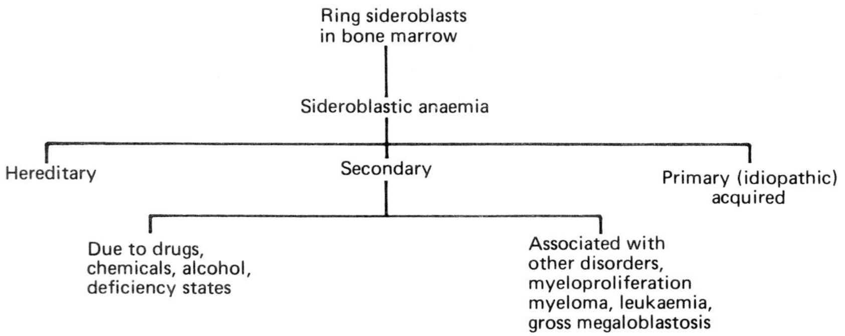

Figure 9.2 Classification of sideroblastic anaemias

Table 9.2 Differing characteristics of the various sideroblastic anaemias

Variable	*Hereditary sideroblastic anaemia*	*Secondary sideroblastic anaemia due to drugs, etc.*	*Primary acquired sideroblastic anaemia*
MCV	Reduced	Reduced	Normal or increased
RBC	Increased, normal or slightly decreased	Usually slightly decreased	Low
Erythropoiesis	Normal or slightly increased	Normal or slightly increased	Hyperplastic
Dysplasia	No or ±	No or ±	++
Distribution of sideroblasts	Predominantly in late normoblasts	Predominantly in late normoblasts	Typically occur at all stages of erythroblast maturation
Number of ring sideroblasts	10–40%	Occasional – 40%	Typically 20–80%
Ineffective erythropoiesis	Minimal	Minimal	Marked
Mechanism of anaemia	Defect in haem synthesis	Defect in haem synthesis	Defect in synthesis of DNA, RNA and haem

Sideroblastic anaemia. 1. Hereditary

The first authenticated example of hereditary sideroblastic anaemia (HSA) was described in 1958[14]. The disorder is rare and inherited as an X-linked abnormality with variable penetrance best shown by the large family reported by Losowsky and Hall[15]. Affected males have remarkably constant and similar blood and bone-marrow pictures. The female carriers show morphology ranging from that indistinguishable from the affected male to no morphological abnormality in blood or bone marrow. Typically the anaemia is mild and is usually discovered by routine screening.

Pathogenesis

The disorder is clearly one affecting the haem synthesis pathway as evidenced by reduced activity of ALA-synthetase and partial response to treatment with pyridoxal-phosphate, the prosthetic group of ALA-synthetase. It is likely, however, that HSA is a heterogeneous group in that in some examples ALA-synthetase activity is normal but shows reduced haem synthetase activity[16]. Biochemical heterogeneity is also suggested by the differing influence of added haem or δ-ALA on *in vitro* globin synthesis in reticulocytes from subjects with congenital sideroblastic anaemia[17]. Clearly, dyserythropoiesis and ineffective erythropoiesis is not a significant mechanism in HSA as shown by the normal red-cell count, normal reticulocyte count and by ultrastructural and kinetic studies[18].

Blood changes

In the male the blood film is characteristically dimorphic and the normochromic population is normocytic (*Figure 9.3*). The microcytic hypochromic population is unremarkable and shows no tendency to target-cell formation or basophilic

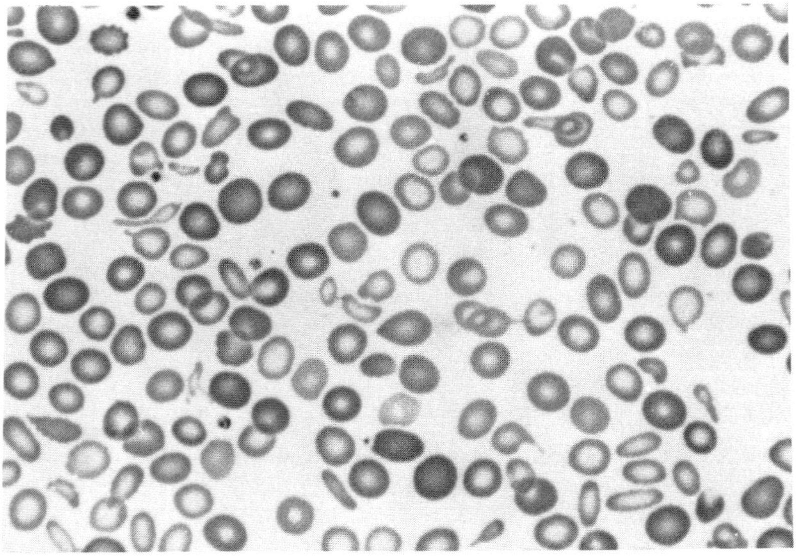

Figure 9.3 Blood film. Hereditary sideroblastic anaemia, showing the clearly dimorphic appearance of the affected male. ×550

stippling. The average volume of the two cell populations produces an MCV of 70–80 fl. The basic red-cell parameters simulate thalassaemia trait using most discriminant functions (page 247). However, the dimorphic population results in a raised RDW and the bimodal red-cell volume histogram could be confused with iron-deficiency anaemia after treatment or transfusion. The female heterozygote may exhibit a similar picture or be completely normal. Reticulocytes are not significantly increased. No abnormal haemoglobin components have been demonstrated though Hb A_2 levels may be reduced due to asynchronous globin-chain synthesis and excess $\alpha\beta$ dimers [19].

Bone-marrow appearances

Erythropoiesis is normoblastic with normal or slightly increased cellularity. Micronormoblasts are present and show delayed haemoglobinization. Dysplasia is not a feature. Iron staining shows normal or increased stores and characteristically 10–40% of normoblasts are ringed sideroblasts. In the female heterozygote the appearances may be identical with the affected male, show a smaller proportion of ring sideroblasts or be quite normal. The ring sideroblasts are confined mainly to late normoblasts [20].

Plasma iron status

The defect in haem synthesis results in progressive iron accumulation and therefore plasma iron is elevated and transferrin levels are normal with a high percentage saturation. Plasma ferritin levels are normal or increased.

Sideroblastic anaemia. 2. Secondary

Induced by drugs

The occurrence of ringed sideroblasts secondary to other disorders is not rare. They may be found in pernicious anaemia, myeloproliferative disorders, myeloma, leukaemia, carcinoma, renal disease, etc.[21], but the association is inconsistent, numbers are usually small and probably make a minor contribution to the mechanisms of the anaemia.

Of greater importance is the association of ringed sideroblasts with the administration of drugs such as the anti-tubercle agents isoniazid, cycloserine and pyrazinamide, the antibiotic chloramphenicol and as a result of alcohol abuse. All these agents reduce ALA-synthetase activity either by influencing pyridoxal-5-phosphate availability, or by inhibiting pyridoxal-5-phosphate catalysed reactions. Chloramphenicol inhibits the synthesis of mitochondrial enzymes such as cytochrome oxidase, ALA-synthetase and haem synthetase[22]. The association between secondary sideroblastic anaemia and alcohol abuse has been mentioned in this section for convenience. The red-cell change due to alcohol is typically macrocytosis and is considered further in Chapter 10.

Withdrawal of drug treatment or stopping alcohol intake results in reversal of the abnormal blood picture and disappearance of the ringed sideroblasts. A rare cause of secondary sideroblastic anaemia due to auto-antibody mediation has been described[23]. Sideroblastic anaemia due to nutritional deficiency or malabsorption of pyridoxine is extremely uncommon.

Blood and bone-marrow changes

The blood picture of drug-induced sideroblastic anaemia is characteristically dimorphic and microcytic. The bone-marrow changes are similar to that of hereditary sideroblastic anaemia. The ringed sideroblasts are confined mainly to the late normoblasts and less frequently to the dividing intermediate normoblasts and rarely involve the early (basophilic) cells.

Lead poisoning

Lead has no known physiological role and therefore its presence in blood and tissues may be regarded as potentially harmful. Lead enters the body by ingestion or inhalation and most passes to the bones though some remains in soft tissues, including the blood and bone marrow, where it is particularly associated with red cells and their precursors. Inorganic lead is associated with haematological effects while organic lead, notably tri-ethyl lead, affects the central nervous system.

Severe anaemia due to lead poisoning is uncommon but may occur, particularly in children, and may prove fatal. Pica in children is a well-documented route of lead poisoning.

Mild anaemia with clinical symptoms in adults is usually associated with industrial or accidental exposure or due to water supply via lead pipes in a soft-water area.

Haem synthesis in lead poisoning

Lead accumulates in the mitochondria of the erythroblasts and results in non-specific disturbances of mitochondrial enzymes with consequent disordered haem synthesis due to enzyme inhibition at several points in the synthesis pathway.

Urinary excretion of the metabolic intermediates ALA and coproporphyrin show that ALA dehydratase and coproporphyrinogen oxidase are probably the enzymes mainly inhibited, though the rate-limiting enzyme ALA synthetase and haem synthetase are also affected together with the intermediary enzymes porphobilinogen deaminase and uroporphyrinogen decarboxylase. Reduced ALA dehydratase activity in red cells is probably the most sensitive index of the presence of lead poisoning and indeed may be too sensitive for the investigation of occupational exposure or in the differentiation of the microcytic anaemia.

Most of the protoporphyrin in red cells is bound to zinc and measurement of zinc protoporphyrin in relation to MCV and Hb level has been recommended for distinguishing between iron deficiency anaemia, β thalassaemia trait and lead poisoning [24].

Globin synthesis in lead poisoning

In normal erythropoiesis the synthesis of haem and globin is balanced and under the control of one or more sensitive feedback mechanisms. Studies of globin-chain synthesis in reticulocyte-rich preparations from a case of lead poisoning [25] indicate that there is unbalanced chain synthesis leading to a pool of free β chains. It is uncertain whether abnormal globin synthesis is a direct effect of lead or is due to defective haem synthesis as has been described in other sideroblastic anaemia [19].

The role of pyrimidine-5-nucleotidase activity

The observation that red-cell pyrimidine-5-nucleotidase activity is inhibited in subjects with lead poisoning can explain the presence of basophilic stippling of the red cells as being due to accumulation of pyrimidine nucleotides as is seen in hereditary deficiency of the enzyme [26]. The haemolytic component of the anaemia of lead poisoning may be explained on the basis that the excess nucleotides divert ATP activity from other metabolic functions with resulting red-cell membrane damage (*see* page 313).

Blood findings

The blood picture is typically microcytic but is not dimorphic. There is an increased reticulocyte count which reflects the shortened red-cell survival. Classically there is basophilic stippling and though this is not a reliable or sensitive index of sub-clinical lead poisoning, in patients with anaemia and clinical symptoms 1% or more of red cells may show stippling.

Bone-marrow appearances

Erythropoiesis is hyperplastic and normoblastic. The ringed sideroblasts are confined mainly to the late normoblasts which may also show diffuse PAS positivity.

Biochemical findings

Red-cell protoporphyrin is consistently and markedly increased; a finding that has been used as a screening test, though smaller increases are also found in microcytic anaemias not due to lead, notably those caused by iron deficiency.

Red-cell enzymes associated with the haem synthesis pathway – particularly ALA-D, ALA-S, haem synthetase and coproporphyrinogen oxidase – show reduced activity. Pyrimidine-5-nucleotidase shows low activity resulting in the accumulation of pyrimidine nucleotides (CMP and UMP) which may be demonstrated spectrophotometrically using deproteinized red-cell extracts[27]. *In vitro* experiments[28] demonstrate that lead inhibits the hexose-monophosphate shunt and may contribute to the shortened red-cell survival in lead poisoning.

Urine δ-ALA is excreted in increased amounts and has been used in screening for occupational exposure to lead. Coproporphyrin is also elevated and in severe cases porphobilinogen may be present. The excretion of lead in urine is often normal even in established lead overload but is grossly elevated after treatment with chelating agents and has diagnostic significance.

Blood lead levels Subjects with red-cell abnormalities will usually have blood levels over 5 μmol/l (100 μg/dl). Though the normal range for blood lead is 0.7–1.9 μmol/l (15–40 μg/dl), workers with industrial exposure will have higher levels and 3.8 μmol/l (80 μg/dl) has been suggested as the upper acceptable level. Although increased amounts of haem precursors in urine, bone marrow and circulating red cells or deficient activity of enzymes involved in the haem pathway may strongly suggest lead-poisoning, the definitive diagnosis of lead intoxication requires the demonstration of an increased level of blood lead or a concentration of urinary lead higher than would be invoked in normal subjects after the administration of EDTA.

Haemoglobin components The abnormal rates of synthesis of β and α chains and apparent reduction of available α chains results in a lowered level of Hb A_2. This is also the case, however, in other microcytic anaemias due to defective haem synthesis and low levels are also found in iron depletion and secondary sideroblastic anaemias other than that due to lead poisoning.

An anodal or 'fast' minor haemoglobin component has been described in the anaemia of lead poisoning. Its occurrence is apparently not a consistent finding and is more common in severe anaemia. The relation of this 'Hb Pb' to the other normal minor haemoglobin components such as Hb Al_c is not clear.

The thalassaemia syndromes

The thalassaemia syndromes are a heterogeneous group of inherited anaemias. They are characterized by a reduction or total absence of synthesis of one or more of the globin chains of haemoglobin. The haematological consequences depend mainly on whether the disorder is inherited in the homozygous or heterozygous form. In the heterozygous form or trait the presentation is typically microcytic and hypochromic due to diminished haemoglobin synthesis. In the homozygous or major form, in addition to the diminished haemoglobin synthesis, there is ineffective erythropoiesis and a shortened red-cell survival. The severe forms could therefore have been considered in the sections on the haemolytic anaemias or the dyserythropoietic disorders. Furthermore, the geographical and racial distribution of the thalassaemia syndromes correlates strikingly with the distribution of abnormal haemoglobins due to amino-acid substitutions and frequently results in the interaction of the two types of haemoglobin disorder.

The thalassaemia syndromes are included in this section on the microcytic anaemias for the following reasons:

1. Thalassaemia traits are characteristically microcytic and hypochromic.
2. The blood-film appearances are similar to the changes in iron-deficiency anaemia.
3. The high incidence of thalassaemia in certain populations makes positive diagnosis important.
4. The more severe forms of thalassaemia are typically microcytic despite ineffective erythropoiesis and the haemolytic component.

The thalassaemia syndromes can be classified broadly by the globin chain or chains affected: α, β, δβ, δ or γ. Interaction with haemoglobin variants due to amino-acid substitutes increases the complexity. A classification of the thalassaemia syndromes is as follows:

1. α-thalassaemia syndromes:
   - (i) Heterozygous α-thalassaemia-1.
   - (ii) Heterozygous α-thalassaemia-2.
   - (iii) Hb Constant Spring trait.
   - (iv) Hb H disease (i + ii or iii).
   - (v) Hb Barts hydrops or α-thalassaemia major (homozygous α-thalassaemia-1).
2. β-thalassaemia syndromes:
   - (i) Heterozygous β thalassaemia.
     - (a) Reduced or absent β-chain synthesis.
     - (b) δβ thalassaemia, absent β-chain synthesis.
     - (c) Silent type.
     - (d) Hb Lepore trait.
   - (ii) Homozygous β thalassaemia.
     - (a) Homozygosity of a β-thalassaemia defect.
     - (b) Double heterozygosity of any two different β-thalassaemia defects.
     - (c) Certain double heterozygotes – thalassaemia intermediate.
3. α + β thalassaemia.
4. Rare forms of thalassaemia:
   - (i) γ thalassaemia.
   - (ii) δ thalassaemia.
5. Interacting thalassaemia:
   - (i) α thalassaemia + α-chain variant.
   - (ii) β thalassaemia + β-chain variant.

The molecular basis of the thalassaemia disorders

The molecular biology of protein synthesis is a complex process which theoretically at least provides several possible stages at which a defect could give rise to the absent or diminished synthesis of a polypeptide chain. Briefly, it could be due to gene deletion, defective transcription of mRNA, reduced or abnormal mRNA, abnormality of the ribosomes, defective tRNA, or failure of initiation, elongation or termination of the polypeptide chain.

All the evidence, however, indicates a defect or deficiency of the mRNA for the affected polypeptide chain as the cause of the imbalanced chain synthesis.

The defect of mRNA is heterogeneous. Failure to synthesize polypeptide chains can occur when mRNA production is absent, when mRNA is non-functional, or when mRNA is produced but cannot be utilized due to defective translation.

Furthermore, absent mRNA may be due to gene deletion as in α-thalassaemia-1 or a failure of production in the presence of intact genes as occurs in most examples of β^0 thalassaemia. Partial expression of β-chain genes as evidenced by reduced β-chain synthesis (β^+ thalassaemia) further illustrates the heterogeneity of the molecular defect in thalassaemia.

Another defect in the rate of chain synthesis is due to the formation of elongated chains as typified by Hb Constant Spring (Hb CS). This abnormal α-chain variant has an additional 31 amino acids due to a single base change in the terminator codon of the α_2-globin gene, thus allowing further chain assembly until another stop codon is reached. The elongated chain has a reduced rate of synthesis and thus behaves as a thalassaemia gene.

The Lepore haemoglobins consist of normal α chains combined with an abnormal chain consisting of the N-terminal ends of the δ chain fused to C-terminal ends of β chains which arise from unequal crossing-over between δ- and β-chain genes and the formation of δ-β fusion genes. The synthesis of the δ-β chain declines steadily during erythroblast maturation and is not found in reticulocytes, thus following the pattern of normal δ-chain synthesis. The alternative 'cross-over' of N-terminal β chains with C-terminal δ chain (the anti-Lepore haemoglobin) also shows no synthesis in reticulocytes. The diminished synthesis of the Lepore haemoglobin therefore simulates the effect of a β-thalassaemia gene. Single amino-acid substitutions resulting in haemoglobin variants with diminished chain synthesis have been reported [29].

It is emphasized that haematological consequences of the thalassaemia syndromes are not due to diminished haemoglobin synthesis *per se* but to the imbalance between α- and β-chain production which results in the formation of unstable dimers or tetramers of the excess chains with consequent ineffective erythropoiesis, haemolytic anaemia and, in the case of the β thalassaemias, iron loading of the tissues.

α thalassaemia

Absent or reduced α-chain synthesis produces the widest spectrum of clinical effects, ranging from normality in one of the heterozygous forms, to the homozygous state which is invariably fatal *in utero* or soon after birth and accompanied by gross abnormalities of haemoglobin composition (*Table 9.3*).

The wide variation in severity is because the two α-globin genes (α_2, α_1) on each of the pair of chromosome 16 (*see* page 26) allow one, two, three or all four genes to be affected. The commonest forms of α thalassaemia are due to deletion of one of a pair of α genes (α–/ or α^+) resulting in diminished α-chain synthesis, or both genes (––/ or α^0) resulting in absent α-chain synthesis. The deletion forms of α thalassaemia are heterogeneous and can be characterized by the extent of the deletion, e.g. $-\alpha^{3.5}$, $-\alpha^{3.7}$, $-\alpha^{4.2}$, the number indicating the number of deleted bases $\times 10^3$ or kilobases (kb). Less common forms of α thalassaemia exist in which the structural genes are grossly intact but contain mutations resulting in defective initiation, RNA processing or stability, polyadenylation or termination (Hb CS). Non-deletional forms have been expressed as α^{Th}. Triplication ($\alpha\alpha\alpha$) or quadruplication ($\alpha\alpha\alpha\alpha$) of α genes on a single chromosome result in excess α-chain production which is harmless in otherwise normal globin synthesis but in heterozygotes for β thalassaemia results in further excess of α chains and a more severe haematological and clinical presentation.

Table 9.3 The commoner α-thalassaemia syndromes, described by genotype, haemoglobin composition and general blood picture

Type of thalassaemia	*Genotype*	*Haemoglobin composition*	*Blood picture*
Normal	αα/αα	A, F, A_2	Normal
α thalassaemia-2 trait	αα/α–	A, F, A_2, 1–2% Barts in cord blood	Slight microcytosis
α thalassaemia-1 trait	αα/– – α–/α–	A, F, A_2, 5–10% Barts in cord blood, occasional Hb H inclusions	Microcytic, hypochromic, slight anaemia
Hb H disease	α–/– –	A, 5–30% H, small amount Barts	Moderate anaemia, anisocytosis, hypochromic, target cells, Hb H inclusions
Hb Barts hydrops (α-thalassaemia major)	– –/– –	Barts, H, Portland. No A, F, A_2	Erythroblastosis, moderate to severe anaemia
Hb H with Hb Constant Spring	– –/csα	A, H, 2–3% CS	As for Hb H disease
Hb Constant Spring trait	α cs/αα	A, trace CS, trace Barts in cord blood	
α thalassaemia-1/Hb Q	– –/Q–	H + Q	As for Hb H disease

The various molecular defects of α thalassaemia have differing frequencies in different ethnic groups or geographical areas. For example, the α^0 (– –/) defect is rare in negroes while the α^+ (α–/) abnormality is relatively common and results in a frequency of α_1 thalassaemia trait (α–/α–) in the order of 5–7% but only rare examples of Hb H disease (α–/– –) and the virtual absence of Hb Barts hydrops (– –/– –). In contrast both α^0 and α^+ have a significant frequency in Mediterranean populations and Hb H disease is more common. In south-east Asia the α^0 and α^+ defects occur in high frequency and as Hb CS, α chain Hb variants and β thalassaemia are also found, over 50 genotypic variants of the thalassaemia syndromes are found[30, 31]. *Table 9.3* shows the commoner thalassaemia syndromes with particular reference to south-east Asia.

Suppression of α-chain synthesis, the chain common to all the normal haemoglobin components, results in excess γ and β chains which form the tetramers γ4 (Hb Barts) and β4 (Hb H). Hb Barts has a high oxygen affinity and lacks Bohr effect and therefore cannot supply oxygen to the tissues. Hb H also has a high oxygen affinity and is useless in supplying oxygen. It is also unstable which results in reduced red-cell survival. It has no affinity for haptoglobin which results in increased urinary iron loss.

Laboratory findings

α thalassaemia-2 trait

The MCV is slightly, though significantly, reduced though red-cell changes are not characteristic and discriminant functions (*see* page 247) do not differentiate from mild depletion[32,33]. Hb H inclusions are rarely seen and their absence does not exclude the trait. Detection is easier at birth when about 1–3% Hb Barts is present in the cord blood[34] and may be detected by electrophoresis though quantitation at this level is unreliable. In adults diagnosis may be possible by measuring the relative rates of α- and β-chain synthesis though overlap of results with α thalassaemia-1 and normal subjects may be found. The definitive method is by DNA mapping. Hb Constant Spring trait presents as α thalassaemia-2.

α thalassaemia-1 trait

The blood picture is typically microcytic and hypochromic with a normal or slightly increased red-cell count, mild anaemia and moderate reduction in MCV. The discriminant function usually gives a negative value[32]. Occasional cells containing Hb H inclusions may be found after incubation with brilliant cresyl blue though an exhaustive search may be necessary. The inclusions are more numerous in the 'reticulocyte-rich' top layer of centrifuged red cells. Coexistent iron deficiency may result in the disappearance of Hb H. Hb A_2 and Hb F show slight but significantly lower levels than normal. The blood of neonates with α thalassaemia-1 contains 3.5–8.5% Hb Barts. Osmotic fragility is decreased. Serum iron levels are usually normal. Again the definitive studies are α/β-chain synthesis ratio, which is less than unity and DNA mapping.

Hb H disease (α thalassaemia-1/α thalassaemia-2)

Hb H disease shows considerable variation in severity. At birth, despite a near normal Hb concentration, the red-cell morphology suggests a thalassaemia disorder. There is microcytosis with anisopoikilocytosis and target cells. About 20–40% Hb Barts is detected, the remainder being Hb A and Hb F with a small amount of Hb H. As γ-chain production switches to β-chain synthesis, Hb H gradually replaces Hb Barts together with the disappearance of Hb F and by the end of the first year the typical picture of Hb H disease is established.

There is moderate anaemia with marked microcytosis and hypochromia, anisocytosis with target cells and distorted microcytes. Basophilic stippling is always seen. Reticulocytosis is usually slight except during acute haemolytic episodes. Fluctuations in Hb concentration may be marked, with severe anaemia associated with infection and acute haemolysis.

The haemoglobin pattern is Hb A + Hb H, the Hb H being the minor component (usually ranging from 5 to 25%). Hb Barts may persist into adult life. Hb A_2 levels are slightly reduced. Hb F level is normal or slightly increased though it must be remembered that Hb Barts is alkali resistant. Incubation of blood with brilliant cresyl blue produces multiple inclusions of precipitated Hb H but not necessarily in all cells (*Figure 9.4*). Splenectomized patients show preformed large single Heinz bodies quite distinct from the Hb H inclusions.

Bone marrow shows erythroid hyperplasia though ineffective erythropoiesis is less marked than in the severe forms of β thalassaemia. Iron loading, so typical of the β thalassaemias, is not a feature of Hb H disease. This is probably due to the lack of affinity of Hb H for haptoglobin, which causes iron loss. Again an important diagnostic point is that the presence of iron depletion in the α-thalassaemia syndromes is associated with a significant reduction in or even an absence of Hb H[35].

The pathophysiology of Hb H disease is therefore multifactorial; a degree of ineffective erythropoiesis, defective haemoglobin synthesis, a haemolytic component, the ineffective oxygen transport of Hb H and, not uncommonly, iron depletion. Nevertheless, most patients reach adulthood and may not present for diagnosis until they are elderly.

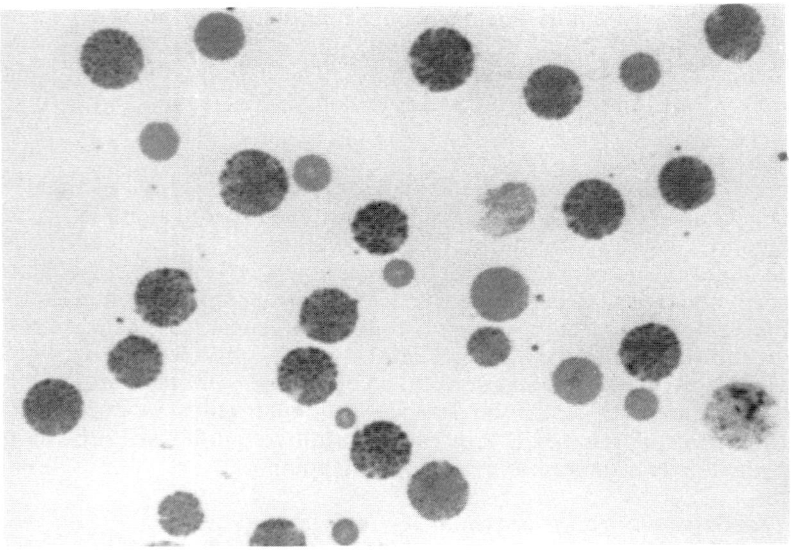

Figure 9.4 Brilliant cresyl blue preparation. Multiple inclusions of intracellular precipitated Hb H are seen in the majority of red cells. A single reticulocyte is also shown. A case of Hb H disease. ×825

The high incidence of Hb Constant Spring in south-east Asia means that approximately 40% of patients with Hb H disease have the double heterozygosity of the α-thal-1 and Hb CS genes; haemoglobin constitution is Hb A + Hb H + 2–3% Hb CS.

The interaction of α thalassaemia-1 with the α-chain variant Hb Q produces a clinical picture and blood film identical with those of Hb H disease with 75–85% Hb Q and 15–20% Hb H. No Hb A or Hb A_2 is formed; small amounts of Hb Barts and Hb Q_2 are present.

The interaction of α thalassaemia genes with β-chain substitutions such as Hb E produces a wide variety of clinical and haematological expression [30].

Hb Barts hydrops fetalis disease (*α-thalassaemia major*)
As previously stated, this disorder is uniformly fatal *in utero* or shortly after birth. Cord-blood studies show moderate to severe anaemia, with marked erythroblastaemia producing an MCV as high as 180 fl which masks the marked anisopoikilocytosis, hypochromic macrocytes and microcytes. Reticulocytosis is variable.

Haemoglobin constitution consists of 70–80% Hb Barts with a trace of Hb H. No Hb A, A_2 or F is present. The remaining haemoglobin is Hb Portland ($\zeta_2\gamma_2$). How the affected fetus manages to survive *in utero* to term with the presence of 80% inactive Hb Barts is not clear. Hb Portland may contribute to oxygen transport.

β thalassaemias

As in α thalassaemia the β thalassaemias show marked clinical and haematological variability due to the heterogeneity of the molecular defects affecting β-chain synthesis, together with the associated defect of δβ thalassaemia and the chain suppression associated with chain fusion abnormalities characterized by Hb Lepore. Unlike the α thalassaemias, most forms of β thalassaemia are not due to gene deletion.

Although subjects with homozygous β thalassaemia can survive infancy and childhood, the effect of the imbalanced peptide-chain synthesis and consequent excess of unstable chains which do not form tetramers, results in a complex pathophysiology shown in *Figure 9.5*.

It should be remembered that although the haematological manifestations may be severe, the major pathologies are (i) tissue siderosis leading to cardiac failure, endocrine failure and liver damage; (ii) skeletal deformity, hypermetabolic state, gout and folate deficiency; (iii) splenomegaly and hypersplenism.

Clinically, β thalassaemia may be classified into the severe form or β-thalassaemia major (Cooley's anaemia), and the heterozygous β-thalassaemia

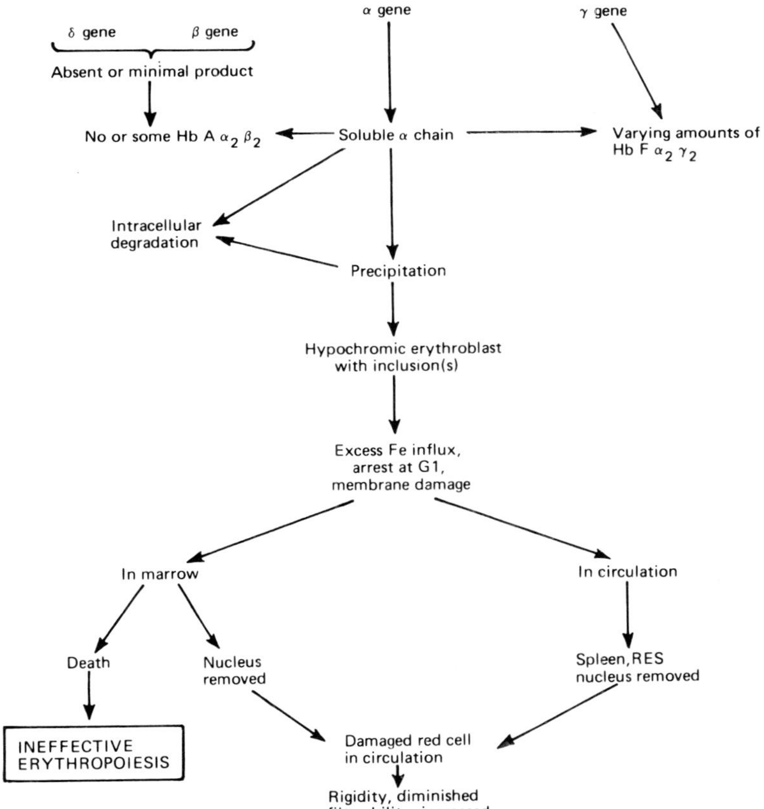

Figure 9.5 Pathogenesis of the anaemia in severe β thalassaemia. Modified from reference [36]

minor or trait. Disorders of intermediate severity may be due to homozygosity of lesser defects of β-chain synthesis or by the interaction of different types of thalassaemia defect. Of considerable influence is whether chain synthesis is absent, β^0 or $(\delta\beta^0)$, or present to a varying degree, β^+ or $(\delta\beta^+)$, and the amount of Hb F present in the form of 'F' cells (erythrocytes containing Hb F). The high Hb F level in β^0 and β^+ thalassaemias are probably due to an expanded population of F cells accompanied by selective destruction of 'non-F' cells. In δβ thalassaemia and the hereditary persistence of fetal haemoglobin (HPFH) syndromes the presence of Hb F is due to primary-gene expression.

Classification on the basis of haemoglobin electrophoresis shows four major patterns:

1. High A_2 β thalassaemia with a normal or slightly elevated Hb F.
2. δβ thalassaemia or F-thalassaemia with a normal or slightly decreased A_2 and Hb F levels between 5 and 20%.
3. δβ thalassaemia with normal levels of Hb A_2 and Hb F. This is difficult to distinguish from α-thalassaemia trait and is almost a 'silent' gene. Recognition is by globin-synthesis studies, DNA analysis or by finding β thalassaemia in offspring.
4. Hb Lepore trait with normal or low Hb A_2 levels, a slight increase in Hb F values and 5–15% Hb Lepore.

Additional causes of excess α chains are over-production of α chains with normal β-chain synthesis[37] which is associated with inclusion bodies, increased Hb A_2 and an intermediate degree of severity in the heterozygotes. Hb K Woolwich is an abnormal haemoglobin due to amino-acid substitution in the β chain which was reported to result in reduced β-chain synthesis and consequent excess of α chains, thus simulating β thalassaemia[38]. Although this has not been confirmed[39], other variants are documented[40] (*Table 9.4*).

Laboratory findings of β thalassaemias

Heterozygous states

β^0 and β^+ thalassaemia

The characteristic finding is a low MCV, usually less than 75 fl, with a normal or high-normal red-cell count. The discriminant function (DF'; *see* page 247) gives a negative value in at least 90% of cases. The blood film is characteristically uniformly microcytic and hypochromic with some target cells. Basophilic stippling has long been considered a feature of β-thalassaemia trait in contrast to iron deficiency though this has been disputed. Red-cell osmotic fragility is always reduced. Studies of red-cell life span show that survival is slightly reduced. Plasma iron clearance is rapid but incorporation into red cells is slightly less than normal. Serum iron concentration and iron-binding capacity is usually normal, though iron deficiency may complicate the picture, particularly during pregnancy.

The ratio of α-chain to β-chain production in reticulocytes ranges from 1.5 to 2.2:1 indicating the excess α-chain production.

On occasions children with apparent homozygous β thalassaemia are seen when one parent has typical β-thalassaemia trait and the other has minimal or no changes in the blood picture and normal Hb A_2 level. Chain synthesis studies nevertheless show reduced β-chain synthesis and these subjects are probable examples of 'silent' β (or δβ)-thalassaemia trait.

Table 9.4 A classification of the β thalassaemias, modified from reference [41]. Further heterogeneity of the β-thalassaemia syndromes is found due to double heterozygosity of the various β-thalassaemia defects

Type of thalassaemia	*Homozygote*	*Heterozygote*	*Molecular defect*
β^+ (type 1)	Thal major, A + A_2 + > 80% F	Thalassaemia minor, raised A_2, slight increase in F in ≈ 50% of cases	Severe reduction in β-chain mRNA
β^+-Negro (type 2)	Thal intermedia, A + A_2 + 30–50% F	Thalassaemia minor, raised A_2	Moderate reduction in β-chain mRNA
β^+-high F (type 3)	A + A_2 + 15–30% F	Thalassaemia minor, 5–12% F raised A_2	?
β^0	Thal major, ≈98% F + A_2	Thalassaemia minor raised A_2	Types 1, 2 and 3. Absent, present or non-functional β mRNA
β^0 (Ferrara)	Thal major, ≈98% F + A_2	Thalassaemia minor raised A_2	β mRNA in nucleus but not in cytoplasm. Chain synthesis can be induced in an *in vitro* system
$(\delta\beta)^0$	Thal major, F only	Thalassaemia minor, 5–15% F, normal A_2	Absent δβ mRNA due to gene deletion. Two forms, ${}^G\gamma\,{}^A\gamma$ and ${}^G\gamma$, dependent on activity of γ genes
$(\delta\beta)^+$	?	Minimal blood changes. Normal F and A_2	?
Hb Lepore ((δβ)-Lepore)	Thal major, F + 70% 30% Lepore	Thalassaemia minor, A, low A_2, increased F, 5–8% Lepore	δβ fusion gene, unstable δβ mRNA
Excess α chain	Not described	Thalassaemia intermedia + inclusion bodies. Raised A_2	Gene duplication
β^0 thalassaemia/β-chain variant	Similar to homozygous chain variant, e.g. S/S C/C, etc.	No A, variant and raised F+ A_2	No βA-chain synthesis, as for β^0 thalassaemia
β^+ thalassaemia/β-chain variant	Similar to homozygote but milder	Variant ≈70%, A ≈20%, increased F and A_2	Variable reduction in βA mRNA
$(\delta\beta)^0$ thalassaemia/β-chain variant	Similar to homozygote but milder	No A. Variant + F but reduced A_2	No βA-chain synthesis

Haemoglobin pattern: (1) Hb A_2. With the exception of certain unstable haemoglobins due to amino-acid substitutions, an elevated Hb A_2 may be considered specific for β thalassaemia trait. The mean Hb A_2 level is approximately 5%, with a range of 3.6–7%. The increased Hb A_2 level is due to increased activity at both chain loci. Though there is no correlation between Hb A_2 levels and Hb concentration, PCV, red-cell abnormalities or Hb F level there is evidence that genetic factors are concerned with the final level of Hb A_2. It must be emphasized that iron deficiency causes a fall in Hb A_2 levels. Thus β-thalassaemia trait complicated by iron deficiency may have a Hb A_2 level in the normal range.

(2) Hb F. About half the cases of β-thalassaemia trait have a slight increase in Hb F values, in the range 1–5%, with a mean value of 2.1%. Only a small number of cases have levels greater than 5%. The distribution of the Hb F is heterogeneous as shown by the Kleihauer technique and is of the intermediate type in that the cells contain both Hb A and Hb F.

δβ thalassaemia trait
The blood picture is similar to that of β-thalassaemia trait. The *haemoglobin pattern* is Hb A + Hb F + Hb A_2. The Hb A_2 is usually normal in contrast to β thalassaemia. Hb F is increased (hence the synonym of F thalassaemia) with values between 5 and 20% and a mean of about 10%. The Hb F is heterogeneously distributed, an important distinction from the typical HPFH syndromes. Heterogeneity of δβ thalassaemia has been shown by demonstrating that the Hb F may consist of $^{G}\gamma$ $^{A}\gamma$ or $^{G}\gamma$ alone which represents deletion of the $^{A}\gamma$ gene along with δ- and β-globin gene deletion.

Hb Lepore trait
The occurrence of the abnormal δβ fusion genes characterized by Hb Lepore may be considered a form of δβ thalassaemia in that the abnormal chain is synthesized at a reduced rate due to unstable δβ mRNA. The blood picture is similar to that of β-thalassaemia trait. The *haemoglobin pattern* is Hb A + Hb F + Hb A_2 + Hb Lepore. Hb F value is usually elevated to between 1 and 5%. Hb A_2 level is normal or slightly low. Hb Lepore is present to about 5–15% of the total haemoglobin and is identified by electrophoresis.

Heterozygous αβ thalassaemia
This pattern of inheritance results in haematological changes no more severe than might be expected by either abnormality alone. Indeed it has been found [42] that normal red-cell parameters may occur although the Hb A_2 level would be increased. The measurement of Hb A_2 would therefore be a primary investigation in screening programmes for β thalassaemia where α thalassaemia is also prevalent.

Homozygous and doubly heterozygous states

β^0 and β^+ thalassaemia
Severe microcytic, hypochromic anaemia is usual in the first year of life though the intermediate forms of severity may not be recognized until childhood or even later. Red-cell abnormalities include marked anisopoikilocytosis with variable numbers of larger cells; basophilic stippling is usually prominent with a variable reticulocytosis (*Figure 9.6*). Nucleated red cells are always found. A leucocytosis is common. Platelets are usually normal though as splenomegaly increases thrombocytopenia may develop. The appearances after splenectomy are even more abnormal with many erythroblasts and increased reticulocytosis. The post-splenectomy picture includes the presence of inclusion bodies in the erythroblasts and reticulocytes which are demonstrable by phase-contrast microscopy or after supravital staining with methyl violet. They probably represent denatured α chains.

Bone-marrow appearances There is gross erythroid hyperplasia with a predominance of basophilic and early polychromatic forms. The cytoplasm shows defective haemoglobinization and many contain PAS-positive material. Prussian blue staining shows increased intracellular iron granules but 'ringed sideroblasts' are not a feature of thalassaemia. Extra-erythroblastic iron is increased and after many transfusions reflects a degree of tissue siderosis which contributes to the severe consequences of the disease. Inclusion bodies are present in the erythroblasts whether or not splenectomy has been performed. The chronic haemolysis results in an increased demand for folate and megaloblastic changes may be superimposed.

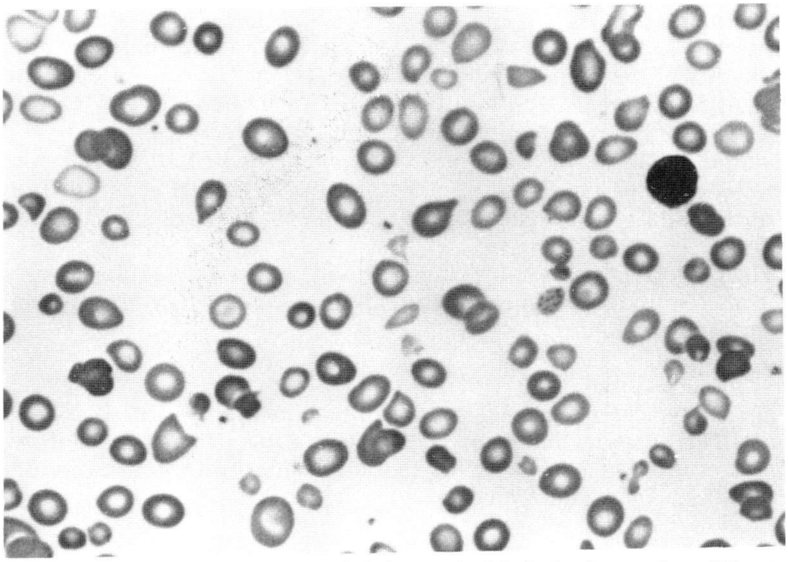

Figure 9.6 Blood film. Homozygous β thalassaemia. Marked anisocytosis, poikilocytosis, hypochromasia and a stippled cell are shown. ×550

Erythrokinetics Red-cell survival studies always show a shortened life span with evidence of two red-cell populations; a short-lived population, which probably contains Hb A, and cells containing Hb F which survive longer. Ferrokinetic studies show that iron is cleared rapidly from the plasma to the bone marrow but incorporation into the red cells is markedly reduced indicating marked ineffective erythropoiesis. This is confirmed by the techniques of [^{3}H]thymidine labelling and quantitation of DNA which show a marked maturation arrest in the early normoblasts which results in intramedullary erythroblast destruction.

Haemoglobin constitution β-thalassaemia major is characterized by a high, though variable, Hb F level with a low, normal or elevated Hb A_2 concentration when expressed as a percentage of total haemoglobin. Hb A is present or absent depending on whether the β^+ or β^0 defect is responsible. It should be noted that the detection of Hb A should be based on sensitive electrophoretic methods or by chain-synthesis studies rather than by subtracting Hb F levels obtained by alkali denaturation techniques which are known to be unreliable in measuring high concentrations of Hb F.

Hb A_2 Levels expressed as a percentage of total haemoglobin are of limited diagnostic value in homozygous thalassaemia and must be interpreted with caution. Several workers have reported that only a minority of cases of homozygous β thalassaemia show elevated Hb A_2 levels. A low Hb A_2 level should not be interpreted as evidence for the inheritance of δβ thalassaemia with β thalassaemia. If Hb A_2 levels are related to the concentration of Hb A (if any) the ratio Hb A:Hb A_2 may be 10:1 or less compared with the normal 40:1 ratio. Those cases with the highest levels of Hb F usually have the lowest levels of Hb A_2.

Hb F When determined by alkali denaturation techniques levels range from 10 to 90%. However, as Hb A_2 levels are rarely greater than 5% there must be some doubt as to the validity of the higher levels particularly when Hb A is absent. The Hb F is identical with that of normal fetal haemoglobin though the $^G\gamma$ $^A\gamma$ ratio shows variation between different families suggesting genetic control.

The intracellular distribution of Hb F is heterogeneous when studied by the acid-elution technique as distinct from the homogeneous distribution of Hb F in most examples of hereditary persistence of Hb F (HPFH) (*see* page 246).

Free α chains Haemolysates prepared freshly without the use of organic solvents may contain a trace component which migrates more slowly than Hb A_2 and probably represents free α chains.

δβ thalassaemia (F thalassaemia)
The blood findings are typical of thalassaemia major with marked anisopoikilocytosis and target cells. The haemoglobin consists entirely of Hb F; no Hb A or Hb A_2 is present. Analysis of the $^G\gamma$ $^A\gamma$ forms of the Hb F indicates heterogeneity in that two patterns are found: $^G\gamma$ $^A\gamma$ and $^G\gamma$ alone.

δβ Lepore thalassaemia
Blood changes are those of thalassaemia major. The haemoglobin pattern is Hb F + Hb Lepore. No Hb A or Hb A_2 is present. Hb Lepore is the minor component, constituting about 20% of the total haemoglobin; the remainder is Hb F.

β thalassaemia intermedia
The distinction between classical homozygous β thalassaemia and β thalassaemia intermedia is essentially based on whether survival is dependent or independent of blood transfusion therapy which in turn is dependent upon the degree of imbalance of globin chain production. The imbalance is less severe in the β^+ form of homozygous thalassaemia and is also ameliorated by the co-inheritance of α thalassaemia or more efficient γ-chain production.

In β thalassaemia heterozygotes who have also inherited the triplicated α-chain complement, the consequent additional α-chain production can result in sufficient αβ imbalance to produce the intermedia form [43,44].

Other rarer forms of thalassaemia

Homozygous α/β thalassaemia
An example of homozygous α thalassaemia + homozygous β thalassaemia has been reported with gross microcytosis, compensatory erythrocytosis and a mild clinical picture without haemolysis which further emphasizes the role of imbalanced chain synthesis in the pathophysiology of classic homozygous thalassaemia [45].

δ thalassaemia
As δ chains are only associated with the presence of the minor fraction Hb A_2, no clinical effect would be expected by suppressed δ-chain formation. However, the occurrence of δ thalassaemia is relevant in that, apart from an appreciation that low or absent Hb A_2 levels may occur in other than δβ thalassaemia, the double heterozygote δ/β would result in a normal Hb A_2 level thus masking the effect of the β-thalassaemia gene.

γ thalassaemia

Deletion of one or both of the γ-chain loci or suppression of their products may be expected to occur but would only be relevant in the fetal or neonatal period and only then if the $^G\gamma$ locus was involved as this gene is responsible for the major component of γ-chain production. An affected infant might be expected to have a hypochromic anaemia at birth which would be self-limiting due to the switch to β-chain synthesis. Lower than usual levels of Hb F in cord blood would be expected. A probable example of γ thalassaemia has been described[46].

γδβ thalassaemia

Adult heterozygotes have blood changes similar to those of β-thalassaemia trait but have a normal Hb A_2 level. The condition is said to be associated with jaundice and haemolytic anaemia in the newborn.

Interaction of the thalassaemia defects and the association of thalassaemia with globin-chain variants

It will be obvious from the preceding descriptions that many possible genotypes are possible in the 'thalassaemia syndromes' and further description is beyond the aims and scope of this book. Many of the possible combinations may only be resolved by family studies and only then if the family is sufficiently large and the techniques of measuring globin-chain synthesis and DNA analysis are available. The geographical distribution of the thalassaemias is often matched by a high incidence of haemoglobin variants due to amino-acid substitutions in one of the globin chains. Increased clinical severity is associated with the interactions of α thalassaemia with α-chain variants or β thalassaemia with β-chain variants. Again family studies are an essential aspect of the investigation.

Prenatal and neonatal diagnosis of thalassaemia

The disastrous medical, social and economic effects of thalassaemia major are obvious.

The accurate recognition of the heterozygotes for the α and β thalassaemias permits more effective genetic counselling to reduce the incidence of β-thalassaemia major and intermedia and also Hb H disease. However, as the chance of parents each with β-thalassaemia trait having a child with the homozygous disease are only one in four, parents may wish to ignore the risk. Social and religious attitudes may also prejudice an effective prevention programme.

Progress in the molecular pathology of thalassaemias, methods for analysis of DNA, and sampling fetal tissue, now allow prenatal diagnosis in the great majority of cases within the first trimester of gestation. The classical method of fetal blood sampling is now limited to those couples in whom the mutation has not been defined, in those presenting too late to allow molecular characterization of the defect and in those in whom linkage analysis with polymorphic sites is not applicable[47].

Fetal DNA for analysis is obtained from either cells from amniotic fluid or from chorionic villi, both procedures having a lower risk of fetal mortality than fetal blood sampling. Those thalassaemias caused by gross structural changes in DNA such as deletions or inversions may be directly detected by restriction endonuclease analysis and hybridization with globin gene probes. This group includes the majority of α and δβ thalassaemias, the γδβ and a few β-thalassaemia defects. In contrast the vast majority of β thalassaemias are caused by single nucleotide substitution, deletion or by addition of a few nucleotides. A few mutations alter a recognition site for a restriction enzyme and can be detected directly by Southern blot analysis. The remainder can be directly detected by complementary oligonucleotide probes.

Linkage to polymorphic restriction sites within the β-globin gene may also be used in defined situations. Diagnosis by DNA analysis requires that the gene or genes involved must be identified by family or population studies. In those situations, now rare, where this has not been possible, fetal blood sampling and measurement of *in vitro* globin-chain synthesis may still be used. An alternative method is the detection of β-chain synthesis by labelled monoclonal antibodies [48].

Neonatal diagnosis of thalassaemia

As α chains represent the major component of globin synthesis *in utero* it might be expected that the α-thalassaemia syndromes can be identified from studies of cord blood. In the two (α-1) and three (Hb H disease) gene deletional forms diagnosis can be made by the presence of Hb Barts and an MCV < 94 fl [49]. In α thalassaemia-2 (one gene deletion) diagnosis is unreliable.

At present there is little advantage in identifying at birth infants homozygous for β thalassaemia, which is fortunate as the findings are far from conclusive by routine haematological methods. Red-cell parameters will probably be within the normal ranges and Hb A_2 levels will not have reached maximum. Hb F levels will not be helpful except in β^0 or $(\delta\beta^0)$ thalassaemia when no Hb A or Hb A_2 will be present. Erythroblast inclusion bodies have been reported in new-born infants with β-thalassaemia major. It is not possible to identify heterozygotes for β thalassaemia.

Hereditary persistence of fetal haemoglobin (HPFH)

This group of conditions describes the persistence of Hb F synthesis into adult life without any major haematological abnormality except in the rare homozygous states in which the blood findings resemble β-thalassaemia trait.

HPFH can be classified using the Kleihauer acid elution technique as 'pancellular' in which the Hb F is found in all red cells or 'heterocellular' when the Hb F is heterogeneously distributed. Each form is in turn extremely heterogeneous in respect of the genetic defect responsible and whether the persistent Hb F consists of $^G\gamma$ $^A\gamma$ or $^G\gamma$ or $^A\gamma$ alone. The commonest, first defined or 'Negro type HPFH' shows pancellular distribution of Hb F consisting of both $^G\gamma$ and $^A\gamma$ chains associated with deletion of the δβ genes. The condition can therefore be regarded as a form of δβ thalassaemia almost totally compensated by Hb F levels of 15–30%, and may be written as $^G\gamma$ $^A\gamma$ $(\delta\beta^0)$. The Greek form is also pancellular having about 15% Hb F which is of $^A\gamma$ type. The heterocellular forms generally have lower levels of Hb F in the 1–5% range, the most studied form being known as 'Swiss' type HPFH.

The persistence of Hb F in adults may result in difficulties in the interpretation of laboratory tests, e.g. in the acid elution test in pregnancy and because the interaction of HPFH with β thalassaemia may result in unusually high levels of Hb F and, indeed, may modify the clinical course of homozygous thalassaemia. The inheritance of the different forms of HPFH and thalassaemia can result in haemoglobin patterns that may be resolved only by extensive family study or DNA analysis [50,51].

Investigation of microcytic anaemias

The laboratory investigation of microcytic anaemia can follow a logical sequence:

1. Recognition by routine blood count and MCV or MCH measurement.
2. Evaluation of blood-film appearances (*see* Chapter 5).
3. Use of discriminant function (DF′) analysis, other formulae or parameters as an aid in differentiating iron depletion and the heterozygous thalassaemia syndromes.
4. Determination of iron status.
5. Bone-marrow biopsy to determine the amount and distribution of tissue and erythroblast iron (*see* Chapter 6).
6. Measurement (as indicated by (1)–(5)) of the minor components of haemoglobin, red-cell enzymes and the intermediate products of haem synthesis.
7. Additional special investigations indicated by (1)–(6).

Table 9.5 summarizes the typical findings in microcytic anaemias due to various causes.

Table 9.5 Summary of laboratory findings in the microcytic anaemias

Variable	*Iron depletion*	*Chronic disorders*	*Sideroblastic anaemias*	*Thalassaemia syndromes*
Tissue iron	Reduced	Increased	Normal or raised	Raised
Erythroblast iron	Reduced	Reduced	Increased with ringed forms	Increased, very few ringed forms
Serum iron	Reduced	Reduced	Normal or raised	Raised
TIBC	Increased	Reduced	Normal	Normal
Serum ferritin	Reduced	Normal	Normal or raised	Raised
Erythrocyte protoporphyrin	Increased	Increased	Increased	
ALA-dehydratase	Normal	Increased	Reduced in secondary types	?
Hb A_2	Reduced or normal	Normal	Reduced	Increased, normal or reduced

Techniques for investigating microcytic anaemias

Analysis of red-cell data

Several formulae have been proposed for differentiating iron deficiency from thalassaemia trait. Their application and value depends on the population to be studied. In a population-screening programme which demands that all subjects with possible thalassaemia trait be identified, further investigation could be undertaken of all subjects with an MCV less than 80 fl. This approach would detect the vast majority of patients with β-thalassaemia trait but would also include most patients with iron deficiency. On the other hand, microcytic anaemia in the UK is most often due to iron deficiency and clearly a more effective discriminant is required that would identify iron deficiency with reasonable certainty at the risk of misclassifying a small proportion of thalassaemia traits. If a population with a high incidence of thalassaemia trait is to be studied, a discriminant can be modified accordingly to include all thalassaemias at the expense of unnecessary investigation of a small proportion of iron deficiencies.

Suggested formulae

1. Pearson *et al.* [52]. *MCV less than 79 fl*. For population screening there is little doubt that this simple decision will detect almost all cases of β-thalassaemia trait but will also include iron-deficient subjects.
2. England and Fraser [53]. *MCV – ((5 × Hb) – RBC – k)* where k is a constant determined by the method of calibrating the blood analyser. Using the Coulter counter and an MCV related to the PCV of an uncorrected haematocrit, k has a value of 8.4; when the PCV is corrected for trapped plasma, k = 3.4. In the case of the Technicon H1, k also = 8.4. A positive value indicates iron deficiency and a negative value β-thalassaemia trait. This discriminant function (DF′) misclassifies about 10% of cases of β-thalassaemia trait and approximately 7% of cases of iron deficiency [54].
3. Mentzner [55]. *MCV/RBC*; values less than 13 indicate β-thalassaemia trait. This ratio results in a similar error in thalassaemia trait as the DF′ but misclassifies about 20% of iron deficiencies.
4. Srivastava [56]. *MCH/RBC*. Over 4.4 = iron depletion, under 4.4 = thalassaemia trait. As MCH is a function of MCV the results might be expected to be similar to the MCV/RBC ratio of Mentzner.
5. Shine and Lal [57]. $(MCV)^2 \times MCH/100$; values less than 1530 = thalassaemia trait. Though effective in detecting with certainty β-thalassaemia trait the product also includes virtually all iron deficiencies and is therefore similar to the simple decision of MCV less than 79 fl.
6. Red-cell count: less than 5.0×10^{12}/l = iron deficiency; greater than 5.0×10^{12}/l = thalassaemia trait.

Any formulae or decision should be applied only to adult patients who have not received transfusions or treatment with iron. Though originally derived from a study of iron deficiency and β-thalassaemia trait, the DF′ will detect α-1 thalassaemia trait, Hb H disease and heterozygotes for the Lepore haemoglobins [58]. α-2 thalassaemia is not identified nor is Hb Constant Spring trait.

Negative values may be found in iron deficiency associated with polycythaemia vera and have been observed in a family with hereditary sideroblastic anaemia. False results may occur in the third trimester of pregnancy and in partially treated iron deficiency. The coexistence of thalassaemia trait with iron deficiency will produce a negative value if the iron deficiency is mild and a positive value in severe deficiency. The platelet count has been suggested as an additional discriminant. Counts above 400×10^9/l are associated with iron deficiency and below 400×10^9/l with thalassaemia trait [59]. Hb E trait may be misdiagnosed as thalassaemia trait by the use of the DF′ alone [60].

An alternative approach is to measure the CV of the red-cell volumes, i.e. the degree of anisocytosis [61]. Histograms of red-cell volume are produced by most automated instruments. Analysis of CV indicates that in subjects with iron deficiency and an MCV less than 70 fl the CV is over 14%, whilst in 90% of patients with β-thalassaemia trait and an MCV under 70 fl the CV is under 14%.

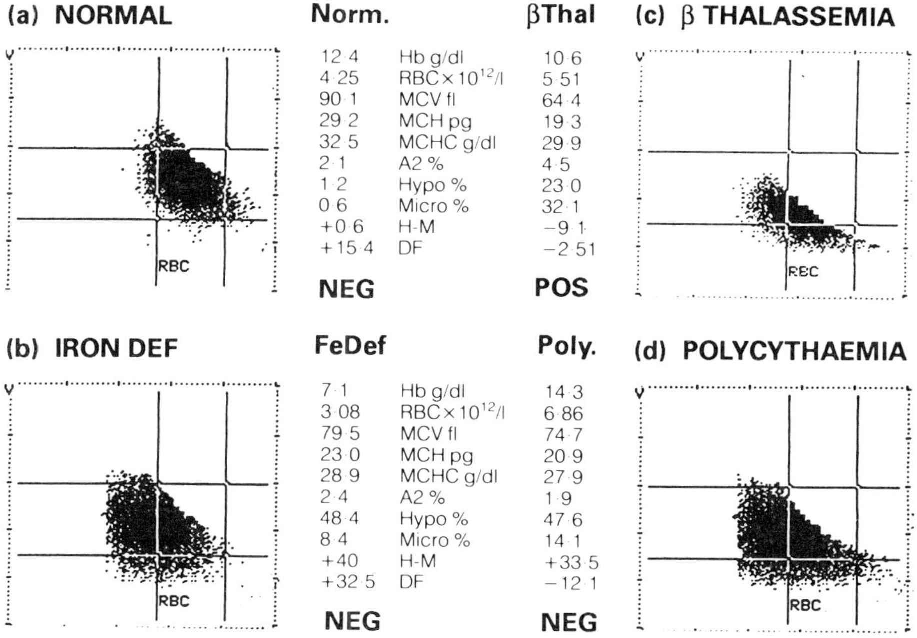

Figure 9.7 *a–d*. Eyrthrograms of red cell populations analysed by the Technion H1. Cell volumes are plotted on the ordinate and cell densities on the abscissa in each example. H-M = % hypochromic cells − % microcytic cells; DF = England and Fraser discriminant function. The characteristic shape of the erythrogram of β-thalassaemia trait – 'Cooley's Comma' (7c), can be compared to the appearances of normal red cells (7a), those of iron deficiency (7b) and the microcytosis of primary polycythaemia (7d). Slightly modified from reference [62]

Unfortunately, patients with thalassaemia trait with an MCV in the range of 70–80 fl are not uncommon, and the CV in these patients may not allow differentiation from iron deficiency.

The Technicon H1 analyser measures red-cell volume and density by light diffraction (*see* Chapter 8) and presents the data as an 'erythrogram' by plotting volume against density. A characteristic pattern is found in β-thalassaemia trait (*Figure 9.7*). The pattern has been nicknamed 'Cooley's Comma' [62] and has been reported to predict β-thalassaemia trait in 97% of cases. Additionally, if the percentage of microcytic cells <60 fl (M) is subtracted from the percentage of hypochromic cells <28 g/dl (H), then H–M gives a positive value in 87% of iron deficiencies and a negative value in 84% of β-thalassaemia traits. It may be concluded that none of the formulae allow *diagnosis* of iron deficiency or thalassaemia trait but the best discriminants are helpful in planning further investigation.

Measurement of serum iron

The method is that recommended by the ICSH (EP7/1978) [63].

Principle

Ferrous iron produces a stable colour on reaction with the chromogen disodium 4,7-diphenyl-1,10-phenanthroline disulphonate.

Materials and reagents
Sample containers and test tubes Contamination of glass and plastic equipment by iron is a major source of error. 'Iron-free' plastic containers are available commercially but each batch should be tested for contamination. Glassware should be immersed in 2 mol/l HCl for 6 hours to remove iron contamination.

Water containing less than 0.3 μmol/l (1.1 μg/dl) of iron. Glass distilled water may be satisfactory or may be further purified by deionization and charcoal absorption. *Reagent grade HCl*, iron content <5 μmol/l (28 μg/dl). *Trichloroacetic acid*, iron content <5 μmol/kg (280 μg/kg). *Sodium acetate*, iron content <0.5 μmol/mol (200 μg/kg).

Solution A Protein precipitant: aqueous solution containing 0.6 mol/l trichloroacetic acid (98 g/l), 0.4 mol/l thioglycollic acid (27 ml/l) and 1 mol/l HCl. Stable for 2 months at 4°C in a brown bottle.

Solution B Chromogen solution: sodium acetate 1.5 mol/l containing disodium 4,7-diphenyl-1,10-phenanthroline disulphonate 0.5 mmol/l (0.27 g/l).

Solution C Iron standard solution. Stock solution – 2 mmol (0.112 g) polished iron wire (not less than 99.5%) dissolved in 2 ml HCl (7 mol/l) by boiling. Cool and make up to 250 ml with iron-free water. Working standard – 5 ml of stock iron solution made up to 1000 ml with HCl (5 mmol/l). Final iron content, 40 μmol/l (2.24 μg/ml).

Method
Test 2 ml of Solution A is added to 2 ml of serum and mixed forcibly for 1 minute in an iron-free test tube. The mixture is covered and heated for 15 minutes at 56°C. Centrifuge until optically clear. To 2 ml of supernatant is added 2 ml of Solution B. The mixture is allowed to stand for at least 5 minutes.

Standard 2 ml of Solution C is treated as for the serum.

Reagent blank 2 ml of iron-free water is treated as for the serum.

The absorbance of the chromogen-treated solutions are read against a distilled-water blank in a spectrophotometer at 535 nm in 1 cm cells.

$$\text{Serum iron } (\mu\text{mol/l}) = \frac{A_{\text{serum}} - A_{\text{blank}}}{A_{\text{standard}} - A_{\text{blank}}} \times 40$$

The absorbance of the reagent blank should not exceed 0.015. Normal range: 9.0–27 μmol/l (50–150 μg/dl), higher in males.

Notes
1. Diurnal variation with higher values in the morning.
2. Higher normal range for males.
3. Haemolysis does not interfere with the assay.
4. The iron-chromogen is stable.
5. The volumes stated may be scaled down at the risk of loss of precision.
6. The method may be automated.
7. A method for manufacturing a serum iron reference preparation is described [63].

Measurement of TIBC of serum

The ICSH recommend the magnesium-carbonate absorption method for the determination of TIBC[64] (EP7/1978).

Principle

Serum transferrin is saturated with iron by the addition of ferric chloride. Excess iron is removed by absorption with magnesium carbonate and the total iron content measured by the method recommended for serum iron.

Materials and reagents

Water and glassware As specified for serum iron estimation.

Stock ferric chloride solution 1 mmol/l in HCl 50 mmol/l. 0.27 g Analar ferric chloride ($FeCl_3.6H_2O$) dissolved in 50 ml HCl, 1 mol/l and diluted to 1 litre with water.

Working ferric chloride solution 100 μmol/l in HCl 5 mmol/l (dilute stock solution 1 in 10 with water).

Light magnesium carbonate $3MgCO_3\ Mg(OH)_2.3H_2O$ (*see* note 1).

Protein-precipitating solution (Solution A), *chromogen reagent* (Solution B), and *iron standard* (Solution C), as described for serum iron determination.

Method

Add 2 ml of working ferric chloride solution to 2 ml serum in a 125 × 15 mm iron-free tube, mix and leave at room temperature for 15 minutes. Using a previously calibrated 8 mm diameter tube add about 0.4 mg magnesium carbonate. Close the tube with a stopper covered with Parafilm and mix mechanically for 30 minutes. Centrifuge at over 1000 *g* for 15 minutes and pipette off the supernatant without disturbing the sediment. Re-centrifuge the supernatant. The supernatant, a blank and standard is treated in the same manner as described for serum iron.

Calculation

$$\text{TIBC } (\mu\text{mol/l Fe}) = \frac{A_{\text{serum}} - A_{\text{blank}}}{A_{\text{standard}} - A_{\text{blank}}} \times 80$$

Normal range: 45–73 μmol/l (250–410 μg/dl). Percentage saturation, 33%.

Notes

1. Light magnesium carbonate is available in two forms which differ in their ability to remove unbound iron and the degree of packing after centrifugation. Type A is most suitable but more importantly a single source of supply should be adhered to.
2. The calibration of the tube for transferring the magnesium carbonate will depend on the type and source of reagent.
3. This method for TIBC does not fulfil the criteria for a reference method.

Unsaturated iron-binding capacity in serum

This value is rarely quoted or requested and may be deduced from serum iron and TIBC measurement. It may be measured directly by adding $^{59}FeCl_3$ to serum, removing the excess with magnesium carbonate, counting the retained radioactivity and relating the activity to the iron content of the added radioactive $FeCl_3$[64].

Immunological determination of serum transferrin level as a measure of TIBC

Serum transferrin levels are sufficient to allow quantitation by radial immunodiffusion or by quantitative immunoelectrophoresis (Laurell). These techniques may be preferred to chemical determination, though functional and immunological levels may differ particularly after freezing or lyophilization of serum. Anti-transferrin serum is commercially available, as are prepared gels and standards for immunodiffusion.

Demonstration and quantitation of fetal haemoglobin

The structural properties of Hb F allow various approaches to its demonstration and quantitation. Quantitative methods can be based on its resistance to denaturation at alkaline pH, by ultraviolet spectrophotometry, electrophoretic or chromatographic mobility and by immunological techniques. Demonstration of Hb F in individual red cells depends on the resistance of Hb F to subunit dissociation at acid pH. Alternatively, an immunological method may be used.

Demonstration in individual red cells. 1. Acid elution technique (after Betke and Kleihauer)

Principle
When dry blood films are exposed to mild fixation followed by immersion in isotonic buffer of suitable pH, dissociation of the Hb A molecule occurs followed by elution, leaving red-cell ghosts. Hb F is more resistant to dissociation and is retained in the red cell. Cells containing Hb F may be recognized by light microscopy with or without staining. Each stage – drying (strictly dehydration), the fixative and time of fixation, pH of the eluting buffer and the duration of elution – influences the results. The interacting influences of these factors has been described in detail[65].

Reagents
Fixative 80% ethanol (500 ml 95% ethanol + 95 ml water).

Eluting buffer, pH 3.3 Solution A, 0.1 mol/l citric acid (21.01 g citric acid in 1 litre distilled water). Solution B, 0.2 mol/l $Na_2HPO_4.2H_2O$ (35.60 g in 1 litre water). Working buffer: Solution A, 73.4 ml, Solution B, 26.6 ml. *Check pH* and adjust if necessary. The working buffer should be prepared each week.

Stains (i) Erlich's acid haematoxylin. (ii) 1 g/l erythrosin or 25 g/l eosin.

Method
Thin films are made from fresh or anticoagulated blood. Blood in EDTA is suitable even after storage for several days. To obtain thinner films dilute the blood one in three in isotonic NaCl. Films are allowed to dry for 10 minutes and fixed for 5 minutes at room temperature. Rinse with tap water and immerse in the citrate phosphate buffer for 5 minutes at 37°C (elution may be carried out at room temperature for a longer period which must be determined by experiment). Rinse with tap water and air dry. Do not blot. Films may be examined at this stage if desired. If staining is preferred, immerse in haematoxylin for 3 minutes, rinse and counter-stain with erythrosin or eosin. Rinse and air dry. Do not blot.

Examination and results

Whether unstained or stained, films are examined with a 'dry' objective; with oil-immersion lenses the eluted ghost cells are difficult to see. In unstained preparations red cells that contained Hb A are seen as ghosts. Cells containing Hb F are refractile and clearly visible. However, confusion may be caused by nucleated red cells, reticulocytes and lymphocytes. Haematoxylin staining will clearly identify normoblasts and lymphoblasts. With eosin counter-staining cells containing Hb F appear pink; intermediate concentrations of Hb F will show lesser staining. Inclusion bodies may be seen in eluted cells and the technique has a particular application in such circumstances[66].

The number of 'F'-containing cells may be crudely expressed as 'number per low-power field' or as a proportion of total cells by counting 'F' cells and ghost cells. For a more accurate determination of Hb F distribution, a photodensitometric method may be used[67].

Modifications

The substitution of pure methanol as fixative with elution at pH 3.9[65] or a combined staining and eluting solution containing haematoxylin, ferric chloride and HCl at a pH of 1.5[68] also give satisfactory results.

Interpretation and application

By the acid elution technique the blood of normal adults may contain an occasional F-cell. Heterogeneous distribution of F-cells is found in the β-thalassaemia syndromes and in some homozygous abnormal haemoglobins, notably S/S. In HPFH, Hb F is classically homogeneous though variants with heterogeneous distribution are now recognized. Re-appearance of heterogeneous Hb F distribution is found in juvenile chronic granulocytic leukaemia, Fanconi's anaemia, acute and chronic leukaemias, myelofibrosis, aplastic anaemia, refractory anaemia and PNH[69]. The test is also widely used for detecting and quantitating fetal cells in the maternal circulation and may also be used for identifying fetal cells in blood from ante-partum haemorrhage or in neonatal gastric contents.

Demonstration in individual red cells. 2. Immunofluorescent technique

As Hb A and Hb F are immunologically distinct, antibodies specific for Hb F can be produced by immunizing animals with purified Hb F, and after labelling with fluorescein the antibodies can be used to demonstrate red cells containing Hb F. In normal adults 0.5–7% of red cells may show fluorescence[70]. Clearly, the sensitivity of the technique is far greater than the acid elution and is therefore unsuitable for detecting fetomaternal bleeding. The major application is in the study of hereditary and acquired conditions associated with elevated Hb F levels.

Quantitation of Hb F by alkali denaturation

The characteristic resistance of Hb F to denaturation by alkali is due to its having only one side chain at the αβ contact ionizable at pH 12, instead of the three side chains of Hb A which when ionized cause dissociation into subunits[71].

The original technique of Singer comprises adding alkali to an oxyhaemoglobin solution and after 1 minute of denaturation the process is halted by neutralization and precipitation of the denatured Hb A. After filtration the resistant haemoglobin is measured spectrophotometrically at 540 nm by reference to the original haemoglobin solution suitably diluted in water. Methods using denaturation of haemoglobin in its oxyhaemoglobin form are suspect because of spontaneous methaemoglobin formation which is not resistant to alkali.

The ICSH recommend the technique of Betke *et al.* [72], in which haemoglobin and its derivatives are converted to HiCN, denatured with alkali for 2 minutes, precipitated by ammonium sulphate at a final concentration of 40%, filtered and read in a spectrophotometer at 540 nm.

Preparation of haemolysate

Red-cell lysates are prepared from anticoagulated whole blood. Wash the cells three times with isotonic sodium chloride and lyse the packed cells with 1–2 volumes of distilled water and a half volume of carbon tetrachloride. Shake vigorously for 5 minutes and centrifuge at 1200 *g* for 30 minutes. The supernatant should be clear but if not a further volume of carbon tetrachloride is added and the procedure repeated. The final haemoglobin concentration should be adjusted to 10 g/dl. This is important.

Reagents

1.2 mol/l NaOH freshly prepared. Saturated ammonium sulphate. Drabkin's solution (KCN, 0.05 g; $K_3Fe(CN)_6$ 0.20 g; distilled water, 1000 ml).

Method

Prepare a solution of HiCN (approximately 0.5 g/dl) by diluting the lysate 1 in 20 in Drabkin's solution. To 2.8 ml HiCN solution, add 0.2 ml of 1.2 mol/l NaOH. Mix by inversion and after exactly 2 minutes add 2.0 ml of saturated ammonium sulphate with vigorous mixing. Allow to stand for 5 minutes and filter through a double layer of Whatman No. 6 filter paper. For a standard, mix 1.6 ml distilled water, 1.4 ml HiCN solution and 2.0 ml ammonium sulphate. Absorbance is read at 540 nm.

Calculation

$$\text{Percentage Hb F} = \frac{A_{540}\ \text{test} \times 100}{A_{540}\ \text{standard} \times 2}$$

A widely used modification of the ICSH-recommended technique is to read at 415 nm to improve sensitivity [73]. The choice of wavelength is difficult to justify as the A_{max} of the Soret band of HiCN is 421 nm. If reading in the Soret band the standard should be further diluted 1 in 10.

Normal range

With A_{540} = 0.2–0.8%. With A_{415} = 0.15–0.9%.

Notes

1. The rate of denaturation is influenced by temperature. Ideally 20°C should be maintained but room temperature (18–26°C) is acceptable. All reagents must be equilibrated to room temperature.
2. Modified or neutral Drabkin's solution as used for routine haemoglobinometry must not be used because of its buffering capacity and the presence of a 'wetting' agent.

3. The choice of filter paper is important. It must not allow denatured material to enter the filtrate but must not remove resistant haemoglobin by absorption which will result in falsely low values. Each batch of paper should be tested by accurate measurement of the absorbance of a dilute HiCN solution before and after filtration.
4. The method is considered to be suitable only for levels of Hb F below 40%. For higher concentrations the method of Jonxis and Visser is suggested[74].
5. A procedure for preparing a Hb F reference preparation has been described[75].

Estimation of high concentrations of Hb F [74]

Principle
Denaturation of Hb F proceeds as a monomolecular reaction. The log % of undenatured haemoglobin at various times will show a straight line when plotted against time. By extrapolation to zero time, the percentage of Hb F originally present can be calculated.

Haemolysate This is prepared as described above.

Reagents 10% NH_4OH; 0.06 mol/l NaOH.

Procedure 0.1 ml haemolysate to 10 ml water. Add two drops of 10% NH_4OH and measure $A_{576}(A_B)$. 0.1 ml haemolysate is added to 10 ml 0.06 mol/l NaOH. Add two drops 10% NH_4OH. Measure A_{576} at 1-minute intervals (A_T) until a plateau is reached. Finally, place in a water bath at 37°C for 15 minutes and measure A_{576} (A_E). Percentage undenatured haemoglobin at each time is calculated by: $(A_T - A_E) \times 100/A_B - A_E$. Plot percentage undenatured Hb on log scale against time of denaturation on an arithmetic scale. Extrapolate to zero time for percentage Hb F in the haemolysate.

Note Chromatography may be the method of choice for measuring high concentrations of Hb F.

Immunological measurement of Hb F

The preparation of specific antisera to Hb F has permitted quantitative immunological methods to be applied to the measurement of Hb F. The technique of radial immunodiffusion[76] does not appear to be sufficiently sensitive to detect Hb F in normal adults though the Laurell technique should be better. Radioimmunoassay has been described[77,78] and is recommended by the ICSH for values of Hb F less than 2%.

Electrophoretic demonstration of Hb F

Hb F may be identified by electrophoresis using support media such as starch gel and cellulose acetate at pH 8.6 or 8.9, citrate agar at pH 6.0 and by isoelectric focusing. The identification of Hb F is important in electrophoretic studies of haemoglobin mixtures and in particular the separation of small amounts of Hb A from Hb F. Electrophoresis is rarely used for quantitation of Hb F.

Estimation of Hb A_2

Accurate quantitation of Hb A_2 is an essential investigation in the differentiation of microcytic anaemias. Demonstration of an elevated A_2 level is the most practical method of recognizing carriers of β thalassaemia. Electrophoresis and microcolumn chromatography are suitable techniques and are the methods recommended by the ICSH[79].

Electrophoretic determination of Hb A_2

The original recognition of the importance of the Hb A_2 fraction was by visual examination of separations on paper and in starch gel. Visual assessment of the amount of A_2 has been shown to be inaccurate and a quantitative technique is necessary. Starch-block electrophoresis followed by elution has been used but starch has been superseded by cellulose acetate as a support medium. Isoelectric focusing gives good separation but is relatively expensive. Elution from cellulose acetate membranes followed by spectrophotometric measurement has been shown to be superior to scanning densitometry.

Cellulose acetate elution method[79]

Buffer 0.13 mol/l Tris buffer, pH 9.1, 82.5 g Tris (hydroxymethyl) methylamine, 7.8 g EDTA, 4.6 g boric acid. Dissolve in distilled water to make 5 litres.

Preparation of sample As described for Hb F determination.

Electrophoresis Equilibrate the strips of cellulose acetate in buffer for at least 10 minutes. Allow the lightly blotted strips to equilibrate in the tank for a further 10 minutes. Apply 10 µl of the lysate to each of two strips (i.e. 20 µl of each sample) as a streak slightly to the cathode side of the centre line, leaving a 0.5 cm margin at each side. Electrophorese for 100 minutes at 200 V (or 0.4 mA per cm strip-width) or until good separation is achieved.

Measurement Cut the strips midway between the areas of haemoglobin. Place the Hb A_2 fraction in 4.0 ml buffer and the Hb A fraction in 20 ml of buffer. Elute for 30 minutes and mix at intervals. Determine the absorbance of the eluates at 413 nm using 1 cm cells.

Calculation Percentage Hb $A_2 = A^{A2} \times 100/(A^{A} \times 5) + A^{A2}$.

Normal range 1.5–3.2%.

Notes

1. A within-run CV of 3.6% can be attained.
2. At the risk of loss of precision two applications can be made on a single 5 cm wide strip.
3. To prevent spontaneous methaemoglobin formation a drop of 3% KCN may be added to the haemolysate. Alternatively the haemoglobin fractions may be eluted in Drabkin's solutions and read at 421 nm.
4. If a single sample is to be tested a normal control sample or reference preparation should be run at the same time.

5. The measurement of Hb A_2 in the presence of Hb S is less accurate due to the closer proximity of the haemoglobin bands.
6. Hb A_2 cannot be estimated in the presence of Hb C.
7. The presence of Hb E cannot be confused with Hb A_2. Hb A_2 is always less than 8% while Hb E is always greater than 15% (except perhaps in cord blood).
8. Hb A_2 levels are raised in the presence of unstable β-chain variants and, inconsistently, in megaloblastosis.
9. Low levels are found in δβ thalassaemia, δ thalassaemia, iron deficiency and sideroblastic anaemias. Thus a 'false' normal Hb A_2 level may be found in β-thalassaemia trait complicated by iron deficiency.

Determination of Hb A_2 by microcolumn chromatography [80]

Buffers

Buffer A: 0.05 mol/l Tris containing 100 mg/l KCN adjusted to pH 8.5 with HCl.
Buffer B: buffer A adjusted to pH 8.3 with HCl.
Buffer C: buffer A adjusted to pH 7.0 with HCl.

Microcolumns

DE-52 cellulose is swollen in buffer A, washed and decanted to remove the fine particles and again equilibrated with buffer A for 24 hours. Prepare a slurry of one volume of settled resin and one volume of buffer A. Lightly plug the constriction of a Pasteur pipette with moistened cotton wool and fill with slurry to prepare a 6 cm column. Flexible tubing may be attached to the fine end of the pipette.

Sample

Haemolysate is prepared as for Hb F determination.

Procedure

Dilute one drop of lysate with five or six drops of distilled water and apply to the top of the column. Develop the column with buffer B and collect about 9 ml in a 10 ml measuring cylinder or volumetric flask. The Hb A_2 elutes at about 6 ml. Elute the remaining haemoglobin with buffer C and collect 10 ml into a measuring cylinder or volumetric flask graduated at 25 ml. Make up the volumes to 10 ml and 25 ml, respectively, and determine their absorption at 413 nm.

Calculation

Percentage Hb A_2 = $A^{A2} \times 100/A^{A2} + (2.5 \times A^{A})$.

Normal range

1.4–3%.

Notes

1. A CV of 2.5% is attainable.
2. Microcolumn technique is said to give results about 0.2% lower than the cellulose acetate elution method.
3. The microcolumn method is probably best for testing large numbers of samples.
4. Chromatography in the presence of haemoglobin components other than Hb A may cause problems requiring adjustment of the pH, the molarity of the developers or both.

Hb A_2 reference preparations
A method for preparing a Hb A_2 reference preparation that is stable for many months has been described[79].

Immunological measurement of Hb A_2

The level of Hb A_2 present in lysates of normal and pathological blood samples of between 50 and 250 mg/dl should be readily detectable by radial immunodiffusion, quantitative immunoelectrophoresis and radioimmunochemical methods. An obvious advantage of an immunological quantitation would be the ability to measure Hb A_2 in the presence of Hb C and Hb E[77]. However, since the original description of the immunological measurement of Hb A_2 in 1976, commercial sources of anti-Hb A_2 have not become available; therefore the possibility of producing specific anti-A_2 must be questioned.

Demonstration of Hb Barts, Hb H and Hb Constant Spring

The demonstration of Hb Barts, Hb H and Hb Constant Spring is important in the recognition and differentiation of the α-thalassaemia syndromes. Though starch gel electrophoresis is the method of choice, cellulose acetate and Tris-EDTA-borate buffer, pH 9.0, as used for the quantitation of Hb A_2, may be used to recognize the 'fast' minor components of Hb Barts and Hb H in thalassaemia traits. The minor components separate from Hb A quickly and the strip should be examined at 15 and 30 minutes. Quantitation can be performed by elution and measurement as practised for Hb A_2.

The small number of red cells exhibiting Hb H inclusions in α_1-thalassaemia trait makes diagnosis tedious and uncertain and in α_2-thalassaemia trait inclusions are not seen. The production of an antibody to Hb Barts and demonstration of the haemoglobin by precipitation tests appears to be a simple and sensitive method of detecting α-thalassaemia traits[81]. Again, the fact that commercial sources of anti-Hb Barts have not become available despite a certain market, makes consideration of immunological measurement hypothetical.

Microscopical demonstration of Hb H

Principle
Anticoagulated whole blood is incubated with a redox dye. Films are prepared and, without further staining, are examined for the presence of precipitated Hb H.

Method
Equal volumes of blood and a solution of 10 g/l Brilliant Cresyl Blue (BCB) in 9 g/l NaCl are incubated at 37°C for 1–2 hours. Films are made of the supravitally stained cells and examined by light microscopy at a magnification of approximately ×500.

Results
Hb H-containing cells have multiple inclusions of similar size of precipitated Hb H and show a typical 'golf ball' appearance (*Figure 9.4*). In Hb H disease the majority of red cells show precipitates. In α_1-thalassaemia trait cells containing Hb H are usually very scanty and careful examination of at least 10 000 cells is recommended.

Note
New Methylene Blue (NMB) may be substituted for BCB and therefore standard reticulocyte stain may be used. It has been pointed out[82] that some batches of NMB and BCB may be of dubious identity. Alternative dyes such as Methylene Blue produce coarser precipitates of unequal size.

Assay of erythrocyte protoporphyrin [83]

The level of erythrocyte porphyrins, predominantly protoporphyrin, is increased in microcytic hypochromic anaemia, whatever the cause. In populations other than those with a high incidence of thalassaemia the estimation of erythrocyte protoporphyrin may be the most sensitive indicator of iron depletion.

Principle
Blood is stirred with acetone–ethyl acetate and the porphyrins extracted with formic acid–ether. They are further extracted into HCl and measured spectrophotometrically at three wavelengths to allow corrected absorbance to be calculated.

Materials

Reagents Reagent-grade acetone, ethyl acetate, formic acid (98–100%) and diethyl ether. Solvent mixtures prepared in 1:9 v/v acetone:ethyl acetate and formic acid:diethyl ether. 1.5 mol/l HCl.

Apparatus Graduated 15 ml polypropylene centrifuge tubes with friction-fitting polypropylene stoppers. Spectrophotometer, preferably with double-beam optics. Centrifuge capable of firmly packing the precipitated protein.

Samples EDTA anticoagulated blood. The PCV is determined. The sample may be stored frozen after the pH has been adjusted to about 5.0 with a few drops of glacial acetic acid to stabilize the protoporphyrin.

Procedure Pipette 2 ml of whole blood into a centrifuge tube and add 2 ml of acetone:ethyl acetate solution. Stir the mixture vigorously with a glass rod for 1 minute. Add 4 ml of formic acid:ether solution and stir vigorously for 1 minute. Centrifuge to pack the precipitated protein solidly. Decant the supernatant into a second centrifuge tube. Re-extract the precipitate with a second volume of formic acid:ether solution, centrifuge and combine the two supernatants. 2 ml of 1.5 mol/l HCl is added, the tube stopped and shaken vigorously for 30 s. The volume (X ml) of the lower HCl layer is recorded. Transfer the HCl layer to a small test tube using a Pasteur pipette. The absorbance is measured against a HCl blank at 380, 407 and 430 nm.

Calculation

$$\text{Protoporphyrin } \mu\text{g/dl RBC} = \frac{[2(A_{407}) - (A_{380} + A_{430})] \times 1.28 \text{ `}X\text{ ml' HCl} \times 100}{\text{PCV (l/l)} \times \text{ml whole blood}}$$

where A_{407} is the Soret band for protoporphyrin. The factor 1.28 is the absorbance of pure protoporphyrin in this solvent system.

Normal range Up to 100 μg/dl (mean 86 μg/dl).

Notes
1. Thorough stirring is essential for maximum recovery.
2. Protoporphyrin is light sensitive. Keep out of direct sunlight.
3. The use of a double-beam spectrophotometer is convenient as the instrument can be zeroed at 407 nm and the other wavelengths can be read while the samples and blank remain in the cuvette.
4. Coproporphyrin and uroporphyrin are also measured but contribute only slightly to the result though in lead poisoning their contribution will be greater.

Assay of plasma ferritin

Ferritin is present in μg/l quantities in plasma and can be detected only by reaction with specific antibodies. The antigen/antibody reaction can be measured by radioassays or by enzyme-linked immunosorbent assay (ELISA).

Radioimmunoassay (RIA) uses antiferritin serum as the reagent and the product (ferritin–antiferritin complex) is measured indirectly by the amount of radioactive ferritin bound in conditions in which unlabelled ferritin (in serum) and labelled ferritin (added to the reaction) compete for binding with a limited amount of antiferritin, i.e. a competitive binding assay. There are theoretical and practical objections to this approach in that all the ferritin in the serum sample is not reacted, resulting in loss of sensitivity, and that the amount of free or bound labelled ferritin is measured against an unnecessarily high 'background' [84].

RIA of plasma ferritin has been largely replaced by immunoradiometric assays (IRMA) using radiolabelled antibodies as distinct from using labelled ferritin in RIA. Two methods have been described. In one the serum ferritin is reacted with soluble radioactive antiferritin and any antibody not complexed is removed by a second reaction with a solid-phase antigen [85]. Alternatively the serum ferritin is insolubilized using solid-phase antibody followed by reaction with soluble labelled antibody. The labelled complex is insoluble, and the unreacted labelled antibody is washed away. This technique is the two-site IRMA and is claimed to be superior to IRMA [86,87]. Both methods are suitable for automation [88,89]. The specificity of the solid phase and labelled antiferritin antibodies affect the sensitivity of the technique and the use of antibodies raised against different tissue ferritins has been recommended [90]. A possible disadvantage of the two-site IRMA is the fall in radioactivity in the dose–response curve associated with high levels of ferritin, the so-called 'high-dose hook effect'. This can result in falsely normal values unless the serum is further diluted for testing.

Several ELISA methods have been recommended using either coated tubes or microplate wells and either peroxidase or alkaline phosphatase as the enzyme label of the anti-ferritin [91,92].

The ICSH have published recommendations for the preparation and storage of a human ferritin standard for use in assays [93,94].

The preparation of the reagents for ferritin estimation by RIA, IRMA and two-site IRMA is lengthy, detailed and complex and most laboratories other than those involved in developing the techniques use commercially available preparations, often in kit form. Precise details of reagent preparation are given in the references quoted.

Notes

1. Blood samples. Serum or plasma from EDTA or heparin anticoagulated blood is suitable. Haemolysis does not affect the results. Samples may be stored at 4°C for several days. Longer storage should be at −20°C under which conditions ferritin is stable for months. Some techniques specify the use of serum.
2. Patients with iron overload, hepatitis, cirrhosis, inflammation, leukaemia, Hodgkin's disease, carcinoma, etc. may have levels over 200 μg/l and serum should be further diluted if the two-stage IRMA method is used.
3. In patients who have recently received iron supplements, particularly children, the serum ferritin value rises and can mask depleted iron stores.
4. The higher levels associated with inflammation and neoplastic disease can also mask concurrent iron depletion.

References

1. Hill, R. S., Pettit, J. E., Tattersall, M. H. N., Kiley, N. and Lewis, S. M. (1972) Iron deficiency and dyserythropoiesis. *Br. J. Haematol.,* **23**, 507–12
2. Das, K. C., Herbert, V., Colman, N. and Longo, D. L. (1978) Unmasking covert folate deficiency in iron-deficient subjects with neutrophil hypersegmentation: dU suppression tests on lymphocytes and bone marrow. *Br. J. Haematol.,* **39**, 357–75
3. Campbell, B. C., Meredith, P. A., Moore, M. R. and Goldberg, A. (1978) Erythrocyte delta-amino laevulinic acid dehydratase activity and changes in delta-amino laevulinic acid concentration in various forms of anaemia. *Br. J. Haematol.,* **40**, 397–400
4. Langer, E. E., Haining, R. G., Labbe, P., Jacobs, P., Crosby, E. F. and Finch, C. A. (1972) Erythrocyte protoporphyrin. *Blood,* **40**, 112–28
5. Walford, D. M. and Deacon, R. (1980) Globin chain synthesis in iron deficiency. *Br. J. Haematol.,* **44**, 201–9
6. Ben-Bassat, I., Mozel, M. and Ramot, B. (1974) Globin synthesis in iron deficiency anaemia. *Blood,* **44**, 551–5
7. Adams, J. G., Coleman, M. B., Morrison, W. T. and Steinberg, M. H. (1985) Modulation of fetal haemoglobin synthesis by iron deficiency. *N. Engl. J. Med.,* **313**, 1402–5
8. Dawkins, S., Cavill, I., Ricketts, C. and Worwood, M. (1979) Variability of serum ferritin concentration in normal subjects. *Clin. Lab. Haematol.,* **1**, 41–6
9. Cazzola, M. and Ascari, E. (1986) Red cell ferritin as a diagnostic tool. *Br. J. Haematol.,* **62**, 209–13
10. Cartwright, G. E. and Lee, G. R. (1971) The anaemia of chronic disorders. *Br. J. Haematol.,* **21**, 147–52
11. Haurani, F. I., Young, K. and Tocantins, L. M. (1963) Reutilisation of iron in anaemia complicating malignant neoplasms. *Blood,* **22**, 73–81
12. Beamish, M. R., Davies, A. G., Eakins, J. D., Jacobs, A. and Trevett, D. (1971) The measurement of reticulo-endothelial iron release using iron-dextran. *Br. J. Haematol.,* **21**, 617–22
13. Konijn, A. M. and Hershko, C. (1977) Ferritin synthesis in inflammation. *Br. J. Haematol.,* **37**, 7–16
14. Lukl, P., Wiedermann, B. and Barbŏrík, M. (1958) Hereditäre leptocyten – Anämie bei Männerin mit Haemochromatose. *Folia Haematol.,* **3**, 17–45
15. Losowsky, M. S. and Hall, R. (1965) Hereditary sideroblastic anaemia. *Br. J. Haematol.,* **11**, 70–85
16. Konopka, L. and Hoffbrand, A. V. (1979) Haem synthesis in sideroblastic anaemia. *Br. J. Haematol.,* **42**, 73–83
17. White, J. M. and Ali, M. A. M. (1973) Globin synthesis in sideroblastic anaemia. II The effect of pyridoxine, delta amino laevulinic acid and haem *in vitro*. *Br. J. Haematol.,* **24**, 481–9
18. Wickramasinghe, S. M., Fulker, M. J., Losowsky, M. S. and Hall, R. (1971) Microspectrophotometric and electron microscopic studies of bone marrow in hereditary sideroblastic anaemia. *Acta Haematol.,* **45**, 236–44

19. White, J. M., Brain, M. C. and Ali, M. A. M. (1971) Globin chain synthesis in sideroblastic anaemia, I. alpha and beta peptide chain synthesis. *Br. J. Haematol.,* **20**, 263–75
20. Hall, R. and Losowsky, M. S. (1966) The distribution of erythroblast iron in sideroblastic anaemia. *Br. J. Haematol.,* **12**, 334–40
21. Mollin, D. L. (1965) Sideroblasts and sideroblastic anaemia. *Br. J. Haematol.,* **11**, 41–8
22. Cartwright, G. E. and Deiss, A. (1975) Sideroblasts, siderocytes and sideroblastic anaemia. *N. Engl. J. Med.,* **292**, 185–93
23. Ritchey, A. K., Hoffman, R., Dainaik, N., McIntosh, S., Weininger, R. and Pearson, H. A. (1979) Antibody mediated acquired sideroblastic anaemia: response to cytotoxic therapy. *Blood,* **54**, 734–41
24. Hershko, C., Konijn, A. M., Link, G., Moreb, J., Graver, F. and Weissenberg, E. (1985) Combined use of zinc protoporphyrin (ZPP), mean corpuscular volume and haemoglobin measurement for classifying microcytic RBC disorders in children and young adults. *Clin. Lab. Haematol.,* **7**, 259–69
25. White, J. M. and Harvey, D. R. (1972) Defective synthesis of alpha- and beta-globin chains in lead poisoning. *Nature* (*Lond.*), **236**, 71–3
26. Paglia, D. E., Valentine, W. N. and Fink, K. (1977) Lead poisoning. Further observations on erythrocyte pyrimidine nucleotidase deficiency and intracellular accumulation of pyrimidine nucleotides. *J. Clin. Invest.,* **60**, 1362–6
27. Valentine, W. N., Paglia, D. E., Fink, K. and Madakoro, G. (1976) Lead poisoning. Association with haemolytic anaemia, basophilic stippling, erythrocyte pyrimidine-5-nucleotidase and intra-erythrocytic accumulation of pyrimidines. *J. Clin. Invest.,* **58**, 926–32
28. Lachant, N. A., Tomoda, A. and Tanaka, K. R. (1984) Inhibition of the pentose phosphate shunt by lead: a potential mechanism for hemolysis in lead poisoning. *Blood,* **63**, 518–24
29. Honig, G. R., Shamsuddin, M., Mason, G. *et al.* (1980) Hemoglobin Nigeria (α-81 Ser→Cys): a new variant asociated with α-thalassaemia. *Blood,* **55**, 131
30. Wasi, P., Na-Nakorn, S. and Pootraku, S. N. (1974) The alpha thalassaemias. *Clin. Haematol.,* **3**, 383–411
31. Simpkins, H., Hill, A. V. S., Derry, S., Clegg, J. B. and Weatherall, D. J. (1986) Interaction of five globin gene abnormalities in a Cambodian family. *Br. J. Haematol.,* **63**, 7–15
32. Hedge, U. M., White, J. M., Hart, G. H. and Marsh, G. W. (1977) Diagnosis of alpha thalassaemia trait from Coulter counter 'S' indices. *J. Clin. Pathol.,* **30,** 884–9
33. Fucharoen, S., Thong Lairuam, V. and Winichagoon, P. (1988) Hematologic changes in α-thalassaemia. *Am. J. Clin. Pathol.,* **89**, 193–6
34. Lie-Injo, L. E., Solai, A., Alejandro, R. *et al.* (1982) Hb Barts level in cord blood and deletions of alpha-globin genes. *Blood,* **59**, 370–6
35. O'Brien, R. T. (1973) The effect of iron deficiency on the expression of haemoglobin H. *Blood,* **41**, 853–6
36. Fessas, P. and Loukopoulos, D. (1974) The beta thalassaemias. *Clin. Haematol.,* **3**, 411–35
37. Weatherall, D. J., Clegg, J. B., Knox-Macaulay, H. H. M., Bunch, C., Hopkins, C. R. and Temperley, I. J. (1973) A genetically determined disorder with features both of thalassaemia and congenital dyserythropoietic anaemia. *Br. J. Haematol.,* **24**, 681–702
38. Lang, A., Lehmann, H. and King-Lewis, P. A. (1974) Hb K Woolwich: The cause of a thalassaemia. *Nature (Lond.),* **249**, 467–9
39. Zago, M. A., Costa, F. F., Greene, L. J. and Bottura, C. (1986) Balanced globin synthesis by Hb K Woolwich heterozygotes. *Br. J. Haematol.,* **64**, 187–94
40. Kobayashi, Y., Fukumaki, Y., Komatsu, N., Miyaji, T. and Miura, Y. (1987) A novel globin structural mutant, Showa-Yakushigi (β110 Leu → Pro) causing a β-thalassaemia phenotype. *Blood,* **70**, 1688–91
41. Weatherall, D. J. and Clegg, J. B. (1979) Recent developments in the molecular genetics of human haemoglobin. *Cell,* **16**, 467–79
42. Melis, M. A., Pirastu, M., Galanello, R., Furbetta, M., Tuveri, T. and Cao, A. (1983) Phenotypic effect of heterozygotous α and β^0-thalassaemia interaction. *Blood,* **62,** 226–9
43. Kanavakis, E., Metaxotou-Mavromati, A., Kattamis, C., Wainscoat, J. S. and Wood, W. G. (1987) The triplicated α gene locus and β-thalassaemia. *Br. J. Haematol.,* **66**, 109–12

44. Kulozik, A. E., Thein, S. L., Wainscoat, J. S. *et al.* (1987) Thalassaemia intermedia: interaction of the triple α-globin gene arrangement and heterozygous β-thalassaemia. *Br. J. Haematol.,* **66**, 109–12
45. Loukopoulos, D., Loutradi, A. and Fessas, P. (1978) A unique thalassaemia syndrome: homozygous alpha thalassaemia + homozygous beta thalassaemia. *Br. J. Haematol.,* **391**, 377–89
46. Kan, Y. W., Forget, B. G. and Nathan, D. G. (1972) Gamma-beta thalassaemia. A cause of haemolytic disease of the newborn. *N. Engl. J. Med.,* **286**, 129–34
47. Cao, A., Piratso, M. and Rosatelli, C. (1986) The prenatal diagnosis of thalassaemia. *Br. J. Haematol.,* **63**, 215–20
48. Allen, C., Weeratne, H., Gale, R., Beverley, P. C. L. and Huehns, E. R. (1987) The use of monoclonal antibodies UCH β and UCH γ for the antenatal diagnosis of β-thalassaemia. *Br. J. Haematol.,* **65**, 199–203
49. Hall, F. W. and Lundgrin, D. B. (1987) Screening for alpha-thalassaemia in neonates. *Am. J. Clin. Pathol.,* **87**, 389–91
50. Weatherall, D. J. and Clegg, J. B. (1981) *The Thalassaemia Syndromes*, 3rd edn. Oxford: Blackwell
51. Thein, S. L. and Weatherall, D. (1988) The thalassaemias. In *Recent Advances in Haematology*, No. 5 (ed. A. V. Hoffbrand), pp. 43–74. Edinburgh: Churchill Livingstone
52. Pearson, H. A., O'Brien, R. T. and McIntosh, S. (1973) Screening for thalassaemia trait by electronic measurement of mean corpuscular volume. *N. Engl. J. Med.,* **288,** 351–3
53. England, J. M. and Fraser, P. M. (1973) Differentiation of iron deficiency from beta-thalassaemia trait by routine blood count. *Lancet,* **i**, 449–52
54. England, J. M., Bain, B. J. and Fraser, P. M. (1973) Differentiation of iron deficiency from thalassaemia trait. *Lancet,* **i**, 1514
55. Mentzner, W. C. (1973) Differentiation of iron deficiency from thalassaemia trait. *Lancet,* **i**, 882
56. Srivastava, P. C. (1973) Differentiation of thalassaemia minor from iron deficiency. *Lancet,* **ii**, 154–5
57. Shrine, I. and Lal, S. (1977) A strategy to detect beta-thalassaemia minor. *Lancet,* **i**, 692–4
58. England, J. M. and Fraser, P. M. (1979) Discrimination between iron deficiency and heterozygous thalassaemia syndromes in differential diagnosis of microcytosis. *Lancet,* **i**, 145
59. Seigneurin, D. (1978) Diagnosing thalassaemia trait from platelet count and England's discriminant function. *J. Clin. Pathol.,* **31**, 500–1
60. Fairbanks, V. F., Gilchrist, G. S., Brimhall, B., Jereb, J. A. and Goldston, E. C. (1979) Haemoglobin E trait re-examined; a cause of microcytosis and erythrocytosis. *Blood,* **53**, 109–15
61. Bessman, J. D. and Feinstein, D. I. (1979) Quantitative anisocytosis as a discriminant between iron deficiency and thalassaemia minor. *Blood,* **53**, 288–93
62. Mead, S. (1987) Cooley's Comma. *Autoanalyst*, October, Technicon Instruments Co. Ltd, UK
63. International Committee for Standardisation in Haematology (1978) Recommendations for measurement of serum in human blood. *Br. J. Haematol.,* **38**, 291–4
64. International Committee for Standardisation in Haematology (1978) The measurement of total and unsaturated iron-binding capacity in serum. *Br. J. Haematol.,* **38**, 281–90
65. Raper, A. B. (1964) Notes on the acid elution test for detecting foetal erythrocytes. *Med. Lab. Technol.,* **21**, 287–92
66. Kleihauer, E. and Kohne, E. (1975) Application of the acid elution technique for the detection of inclusion bodies. In *Abnormal Haemoglobins and Thalassaemia: Diagnostic Aspects* (ed. R. M. Schmidt), pp. 149–59. London: Academic Press
67. Shepherd, M. K., Weatherall, D. J. and Conley, C. L. (1962) Semiquantitative estimation of the distribution of foetal haemoglobin in red cell population. *Bull. John Hopkins Hosp.,* **110**, 292–310
68. Nierhaus, K. and Betke, K. (1968) Eine vereinfachte Modifikation der sauren Elution für die cytologische Darstellung von fetalem Hämoglobin. *Klin. Wschr.,* **46**, 47
69. Weatherall, D. J., Fembrey, M. E. and Pritchard, J. (1974) Fetal haemoglobin. *Clin. Haematol.,* **3**, 467–508
70. Wood, W. G., Stamatoyannopoulos, G., Lim, G. and Nute, P. E. (1975) F-cells in the adult; normal values and levels in individuals with hereditary and acquired elevations of Hb F. *Blood,* **46**, 671–82
71. Perutz, M. F. (1974) Mechanism of denaturation of haemoglobin by alkali. *Nature (Lond.),* **247**, 341–4

72. Betke, K., Marti, H. R. and Schlicht, I. (1959) Estimation of small percentages of foetal haemoglobin. *Nature (Lond.),* **184**, 1877–8
73. Pembrey, M. E., McWade, P. and Weatherall, D. J. (1972) Reliable routine estimation of small amounts of foetal haemoglobin by alkali denaturation. *J. Clin. Pathol.,* **25**, 738–40
74. Jonxis, J. H. P. and Visser, H. K. A. (1956) Determination of low percentages of foetal haemoglobin in blood of normal children. *J. Dis. Child.,* **92**, 588–9
75. International Committee for Standardisation in Haematology (1979) Recommendation for foetal haemoglobin preparation and foetal haemoglobin determination by the alkali denaturation method. *Br. J. Haematol.,* **42**, 133–6
76. Kohn, J. and Payne, B. V. (1972) An immunological method for the detection and estimation of foetal haemoglobin. *J. Clin. Pathol.,* **25**, 830–1
77. Garver, F. A., Jones, C. S., Baker, M. M. *et al.* (1976) Specific radioimmunochemical identification of haemoglobin A2 and F. *Am. J. Haematol.,* **1**, 459–69
78. Rutland, P. C., Pembrey, M. E. and Davies, T. (1983) The estimation of fetal haemoglobin in healthy adults by radioimmunoassay. *Br. J. Haematol.,* **53**, 673–82
79. International Committee for Standardisation in Haematology (1978) Recommendations for selected methods for quantitative estimation of Hb A2 and for Hb A2 reference preparation. *Br. J. Haematol.,* **38**, 573–8
80. Efremov, G. D. and Huisman, T. H. J. (1974) The laboratory diagnosis of the haemoglobinopathies. *Clin. Haematol.,* **3**, 542–3
81. Wasi, P. and Pravatmuang, P. (1973) Immunologic diagnosis of α thalassaemia. *J. Med. Assoc. Thailand,* **56**, 654–7
82. Gadson, D., Hughes, M., Dean, A. and Wickramasinghe, S. M. (1986) Morphology of redox-dye treated Hb H-containing red cells: confusion caused by wrongly identified dyes. *Clin. Lab. Haematol.,* **8**, 365–70
83. Heller, S. R., Labbe, R. F. and Nutter, J. A. (1971) Simplified assay for porphyrins in whole blood. *Clin. Chem.,* **17**, 525–8
84. Miles, I. E. M. and Hales, C. N. (1968) Labelled antibodies and immunological assay systems. *Nature (Lond),* **219**, 186–9
85. Addison, G. M., Beamish, M. R., Hales, C. N., Hodgkins, M., Jacobs, A. and Llewellyn, P. (1972) An immunoradiometric assay for ferritin in the serum of normal subjects and patients with iron deficiency and iron overload. *J. Clin. Pathol.,* **25**, 326–9
86. Miles, L. E. M., Lipschitz, D. A., Bieber, C. P. and Cook, J. D. (1974) Measurement of serum ferritin by a 2-site immunoradiometric assay. *Anal. Biochem.,* **61**, 209–24
87. Worwood, M. (1988) Serum ferritin. In *Methods in Haematology*, Vol. 1 (ed. J. D. Cook), pp. 59–89. New York: Churchill Livingstone
88. Jones, B. M. and Worwood, M. (1975) An automated immunoradiometric assay for ferritin. *J. Clin. Pathol.,* **28**, 540–2
89. Harries, H., Shankland, D. and Henley, R. (1985) An automated assay for serum ferritin. *Med. Lab. Sci.,* **42**, 230–2
90. Cowan, S. I., Stagg, B. H. and Niemann, E. (1978) The effect of variations in the specificities of the antibody components on a 2-site immunoradiometric assay for ferritin. In *Radioimmunoassay and Related Procedures in Medicine*, Vol. 1, pp. 347–59. International Atomic Energy Authority
91. Zuyderhoudt, F. M. J., Boers, W., Linthorst, C., Jorning, G. G. A. and Hengeveld, P. (1978) An enzyme-linked immunoassay for ferritin in human serum and rat plasma and the influence of the iron in serum ferritin on serum iron measurement, during acute hepatitis. *Clin. Chim. Acta,* **88**, 37–44
92. Theriault, L. and Page, M. (1977) A solid-phase enzyme immunoassay for serum ferritin. *Clin. Chem.,* **23**, 2142–4
93. International Committee for Standardisation in Haematology (1984) Preparation, characterization and storage of human ferritin for use as a standard for the assay of serum ferritin. *Clin. Lab. Haematol.,* **6**, 177–91
94. International Committee for Standardisation in Haematology (1985) Proposed international standard of human ferritin for the serum ferritin assay. *Br. J. Haematol.,* **61**, 61–3

Chapter 10

Anaemias. II. Macrocytosis and megaloblastic anaemias

The term macrocytosis may be applied to increased red-cell diameters as seen by examination of the stained blood film, or to an increased MCV as determined by calculation from the PCV and RBC or by instrumentation.

Macrocytosis in the blood film is not necessarily associated with an increased MCV; e.g. the macrocytic target-cell picture of obstructive liver disease is often associated with red cells of normal volume that have an increased diameter but are abnormally thin. Conversely, any slight increase in cell thickness can result in an increased MCV, with the cells maintaining a normal diameter.

The advent of accurate red-cell counting and sizing has resulted in a switch of emphasis from the subjective assessment of macrocytosis by red-cell diameter in the blood film to the measurement of macrocytosis as represented by the MCV. Though the measurement of MCV is not without error or artefact, its use in defining the presence of macrocytosis is logical and inevitable and subsequent discussion of macrocytosis and its significance is based on an increased MCV. Alternatively, the MCH may be used as it is proportional to the MCV. Unlike microcytosis, which although having varied causes is mainly due to diminished haemoglobin synthesis, macrocytosis can be caused by widely differing mechanisms affecting erythropoiesis or by modification of the red-cell volume in the circulation.

Macrocytosis is defined as an MCV greater than 95 fl when the value is derived from an instrument calibrated for a PCV corrected for trapped plasma. This value is the upper 2SD limit of a normal range with a mean of 88 fl. It is important to recognize that a continuation of the normal distribution to include +3SD, i.e. up to 99 fl, will include five normal samples with an MCV between 95 and 99 fl in every 200 normal samples tested. The problems arising from the recognition and further investigation of small increases in the MCV have been emphasized [1], and for this reason some laboratories adopt 100 fl as the upper limit of normal. However, increases in MCV below 100 fl can undoubtedly be significant and should not be ignored. The importance of blood-film appearances in the interpretation of MCV values cannot be over-emphasized. In particular, the presence of polychromasia, anisocytosis, poikilocytosis, ovalocytosis, target cells and hypersegmented neutrophils are collectively or independently of importance. Analysis of the distribution of red-cell volumes are of value in interpreting small increases in MCV [1].

Causes of macrocytosis

Established causes of macrocytosis are as follows:

1. Physiological:
   (a) neonates;
   (b) familial;
   (c) pregnancy.
2. Dyserythropoiesis:
   (a) megaloblastic change;
   (b) aplasia;
   (c) myelodysplastic syndrome.
3. Reticulocytosis:
   (a) response to haemolysis;
   (b) response to haemorrhage;
   (c) response to treatment with haematinics.
4. Liver disease.
5. Alcohol abuse.
6. Cytotoxic-drug therapy.
7. Hypothyroidism.
8. Neoplastic disease.
9. Chronic hypoxia.

The frequency of macrocytosis in routine haematological practice has been studied[2–4]. The results of such studies depend on the method of instrument calibration, the MCV value chosen and the population tested.

In a study of 6524 patients, 200 blood samples had an MCV of over 100 fl[1]. Drug therapy, liver disease (including alcoholism), neoplasia and primary disorders of erythropoiesis were established clinical associations. In 22% no satisfactory explanation was found, though investigation was incomplete. Macrocytosis in the blood film was reported in only 65% of patients. In another study of 100 consecutive patients with an MCV of over 115 fl[3], 50% had cobalamin or folate deficiency, 26% had liver disease or alcoholism and the remaining 24% had a variety of causes, prominent among which were neoplasia and cytotoxic therapy, together with other widely varying disorders. Chanarin, England and Hoffbrand[4] recommend further investigation only when the MCV is consistently above 96 fl, a value based on a ±2SD range of 80–90 fl.

Clearly, the high frequency of primary haematological disorders associated with macrocytosis makes further appraisal and investigation essential. As macrocytosis may result from normoblastic or megaloblastic erythropoiesis a bone-marrow aspiration is an important part of the investigation though the practical implications of the presence of macrocytosis in almost 4% of samples, even with a high 'cut-off' of 100 fl[2], indicates the importance of haematological profile, blood-film appearances and clinical findings in determining the investigative approach.

Pregnancy The proportion of macrocytes increases in normal pregnancy in the majority of cases and can result in an increased MCV[5,6]. The increase is most evident in the last trimester. The macrocytosis is not usually apparent from examination of the blood film, i.e. *volumetric macrocytosis* without increase in diameter. It is independent of folate status though iron stores appear to be a limiting factor.

Dyserythropoiesis Disordered erythropoiesis resulting in macrocytosis is usually associated with anisocytosis and poikilocytosis. Although 'non-specific' poikilocytosis may be seen, of particular significance are oval macrocytes. When associated with neutrophil hypersegmentation the appearances indicate megaloblastic change.

Liver disease The macrocytosis of liver disease is not usually poikilocytic though target cells are often a feature, particularly when there is an obstructive element. Acanthocytes may be seen in severe hepatic failure.

Alcohol Macrocytosis due to alcohol abuse is common. It is usually independent of cobalamin or folate status although in severe alcoholism megaloblastic change due to folate deficiency may be an additional factor. Of particular significance is the presence of stomatocytes and the combination of macrocytosis with stomatocytes points to alcohol abuse[7] (*see Figure 5.18*). A quantitative parameter, helpful in screening, is the HDW (haemoglobin distribution width) of the Technicon H1 analyser (*see* Chapter 8). A low HDW (<2.1) is found in association with alcohol-induced macrocytosis with stomatocytes (unpublished data).

Cytotoxic drugs Many agents modify or inhibit DNA synthesis and dyserythropoiesis can be expected with associated changes in red-cell morphology. Studies of patients treated with the S-phase inhibitor hydroxyurea[8] indicate that volumetric macrocytes are produced which have an increased volume but are of normal diameter. Nevertheless, hydroxyurea and similar agents can produce macrocytosis in the blood film.

Hypothyroidism This is consistently associated with macrocytosis and the MCV falls following treatment with thyroxine. Irregular red cells (rhytiocytes) are often seen before treatment (*see Figure 5.15*).

Megaloblastic anaemias

The term 'megaloblast' was originally applied to the abnormal erythroblasts of untreated pernicious anaemia but is now applied also to the abnormal morphology due to other causes of disordered DNA synthesis. Impaired DNA chain elongation results in arrest at the G_2 stage of interphase, intramedullary cell death (ineffective erythropoiesis), macrocytosis, giant metamyelocytes and neutrophil hypersegmentation[9]. The evidence that megaloblastosis is due to faulty DNA synthesis has been summarized[9].

1. *De novo* synthesis of the DNA precursor thymidine monophosphate (dTMP) is defective in cobalamin and folate deficiency; the salvage pathway of thymidine to dTMP is more active; the anaemia responds to infusion of thymidine.
2. Drugs that cause megaloblastosis in the absence of cobalamin or folate deficiency, inhibit biochemical reactions in the formation of purine and pyrimidine precursors.
3. Inherited biochemical defects not affecting cobalamin and folate metabolism can affect one or other of the reactions in DNA synthesis.

Classically, megaloblastosis is caused by deranged DNA synthesis due to defective conversion of deoxyuridylate (dUMP) to deoxythymidylate (dTMP) as a result of a reduced activity of 5–10-methylene THF (THF = tetrahydrofolate), the co-enzyme of thymidylate synthetase. 5–10-methylene THF is derived from THF by its role as a one-carbon acceptor in the conversion of serine to glycine. Thus the activity of 5–10-methylene THF depends upon the availability of THF. THF is formed by the reduction, by dihydrofolate reductase (DHFR), of dihydrofolate (DHF) produced from 5–10-methylene THF during the conversion of dUMP to dTMP. Inhibition or deficiency of DHFR will result in reduced levels of THF. A further and important source of THF is from the catalysation, by 5-methyl THF, of the methylation of homocysteine to methionine which also requires methylcobalamin as co-factor; the methyl group of 5-methyl THF transfers to the cobalamin and then to the homocysteine (*Figure 10.1*). In the absence of cobalamin, folate accumulates in the 5-methyl THF form, the so-called 'methyl folate trap'. The methyl folate trap hypothesis was widely but not entirely accepted as an explanation of the defect by which cobalamin deficiency induces megaloblastosis.

The observation that prolonged administration of nitrous oxide induces megaloblastosis and the recognition that it is due to cobalamin inactivation rather than folate 'deficiency' provided an experimental model for further study of

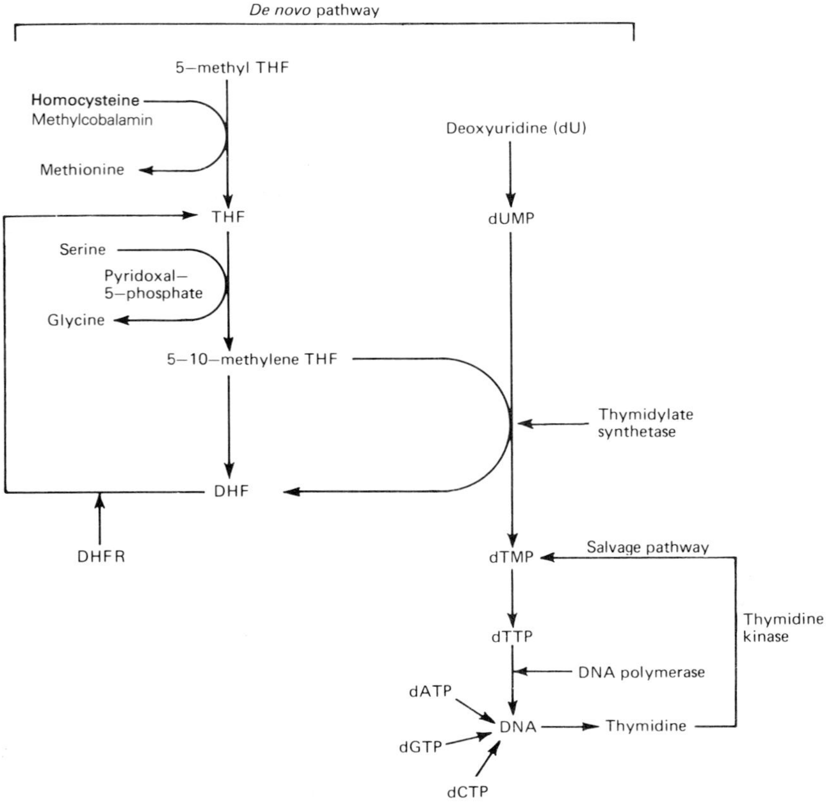

Figure 10.1 Intracellular DNA synthesis. Deoxyuridine is not a natural substrate for *de novo* synthesis of thymidylate but influences dTMP synthesis when added *in vitro*. See text for explanation

cobalamin–folate interrelationships. Such studies have produced evidence that the homocysteine to methionine reaction, which requires both cobalamin and 5-methyl THF as co-factors, is impaired and that the failure in the supply of methionine leads to a reduced availability of single carbon units for the synthesis of formate, formyl THF and folate polyglutamate which is the active co-enzyme [10–12] – the 'formate starvation hypothesis'.

The experimental studies using nitrous oxide exposure of animals and the effect on erythropoiesis are followed by the deoxyuridine suppression test. Animal species vary in their response to nitrous oxide. Whether the animal studies can be directly related to humans is arguable. However, defective methionine synthesis is the important rate-limiting step in folate biosynthesis.

Mechanism of anaemia in megaloblastosis

The anaemia is due to ineffective erythropoiesis associated with a shortened red-cell survival; those red cells that reach the circulation are destroyed in a random manner. When red cells from a patient with untreated pernicious anaemia are transfused to a normal recipient their survival is reduced, indicating an intracellular defect. However, when normal red cells are transfused to a patient with untreated pernicious anaemia their survival is also shortened, indicating an extracorpuscular mechanism which disappears about 10 days after cobalamin therapy. Similar mechanisms probably occur in folate deficiency. When the anaemia is severe as much as 60% of erythropoiesis may be ineffective and the mean life span of the red cells as short as 30 days.

The nature of the red-cell defect is not clear. Abnormally high levels of many red-cell enzymes have been demonstrated, a feature of other dyserythropoietic anaemias. A frequent finding is a positive direct antiglobulin test due to components of complement on the red-cell membrane, but the association, if any, to the shortened red-cell survival is not clear.

Blood and bone marrow in megaloblastic anaemia

Typically the morphological changes in the red cells are macroanisocytosis, slight ovalocytosis and, in severe anaemia, irregular poikilocytosis (*Figure 10.2*). Howell–Jolly bodies may be seen and the few reticulocytes present may stain unusually blue. Hypersegmentation of the neutrophils is almost always present and is associated with leucopenia when the anaemia is marked. Thrombocytopenia may be severe. The percentage of reticulocytes may be slightly increased but is typically low, reflecting not only the ineffective erythropoiesis but also the asynchrony of megaloblastic maturation by which the cytoplasm of the late megaloblasts is mature, fully haemoglobinized and without ribosomes. The blood changes can precede anaemia and are clearly recognizable when the haemoglobin is within the normal range.

Although it is not usually possible to differentiate between the appearances due to lack of cobalamin or folate, the aetiology of the development of these deficiency states influences the blood appearances. Cobalamin deficiency develops slowly over months or even years and the red-cell appearances are often typical when anaemia is slight or even absent. Folate deficiency may also develop slowly in which case the blood picture is indistinguishable from that of cobalamin deficiency. However, folate stores can be depleted in a matter of weeks, well within the life

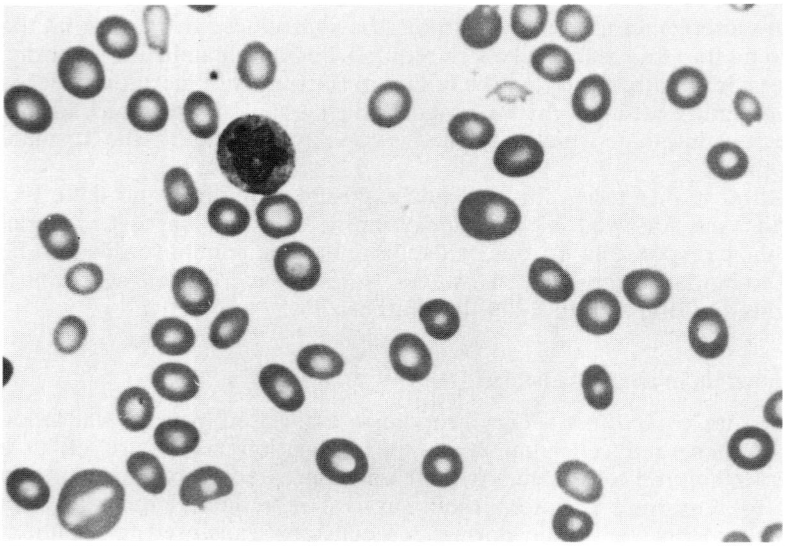

Figure 10.2 Blood film in megaloblastic anaemia, showing oval macroanisocytosis, poikilocytic cells and a hypersegmented neutrophil. ×550

span of the circulating red cells. Thus erythropoiesis may be megaloblastic but the 'megalocytic' red cells are mixed with cells produced when erythropoiesis was normoblastic and consequently the picture may not be typical. In severely ill patients, particularly after major surgery, those on artificial feeding, those with infection and where there is renal insufficiency, acute megaloblastosis can develop with bone-marrow failure; the red-cell picture is not typical, hypersegmentation may be minimal and the only indication may be the development of severe thrombocytopenia in the absence of disordered blood coagulation. A similar situation can develop by oxidation of cobalamin during extended exposure to nitrous oxide [13].

If megaloblastic change develops as a complication of an existing anaemia the blood-film appearances may be bizarre. When the anaemia is severe, megaloblasts may be seen in the blood film and even when scanty can be demonstrated in 'buffy-layer' preparations. Whether the demonstration of circulating megaloblasts obviates the need for bone-marrow aspiration is debatable.

With the exception of the acute megaloblastic states described above, concurrent iron deficiency or thalassaemia trait, the MCV is typically increased. A progressive increase in MCV, even within the normal range, in the absence of significant reticulocytosis, suggests megaloblastic development. The greater the MCV the more likely is it due to megaloblastosis and values as high as 140 fl may be found. In some cases with severe anaemia the MCV may be only in the 100–110 fl range due to gross anisopoikilocytosis.

When iron deficiency and megaloblastic change coexist, the blood picture is typically microcytic and hypochromic. After iron therapy, a dimorphic picture is characteristic with the normochromic population being oval and macrocytic. The converse may also occur when a megaloblastic anaemia is treated and iron deficiency develops; the 'new' population is microcytic and hypochromic in contrast to the original macrocytic, normochromic cells.

Megaloblastic erythropoiesis

The criteria differentiating megaloblastic from normoblastic erythropoiesis are based on nuclear structure, asynchrony between nuclear and cytoplasmic maturation and increased size. The appearances are illustrated in *Figure 10.3*. The megaloblast nuclear chromatin is fine and less dense than that of the normoblast

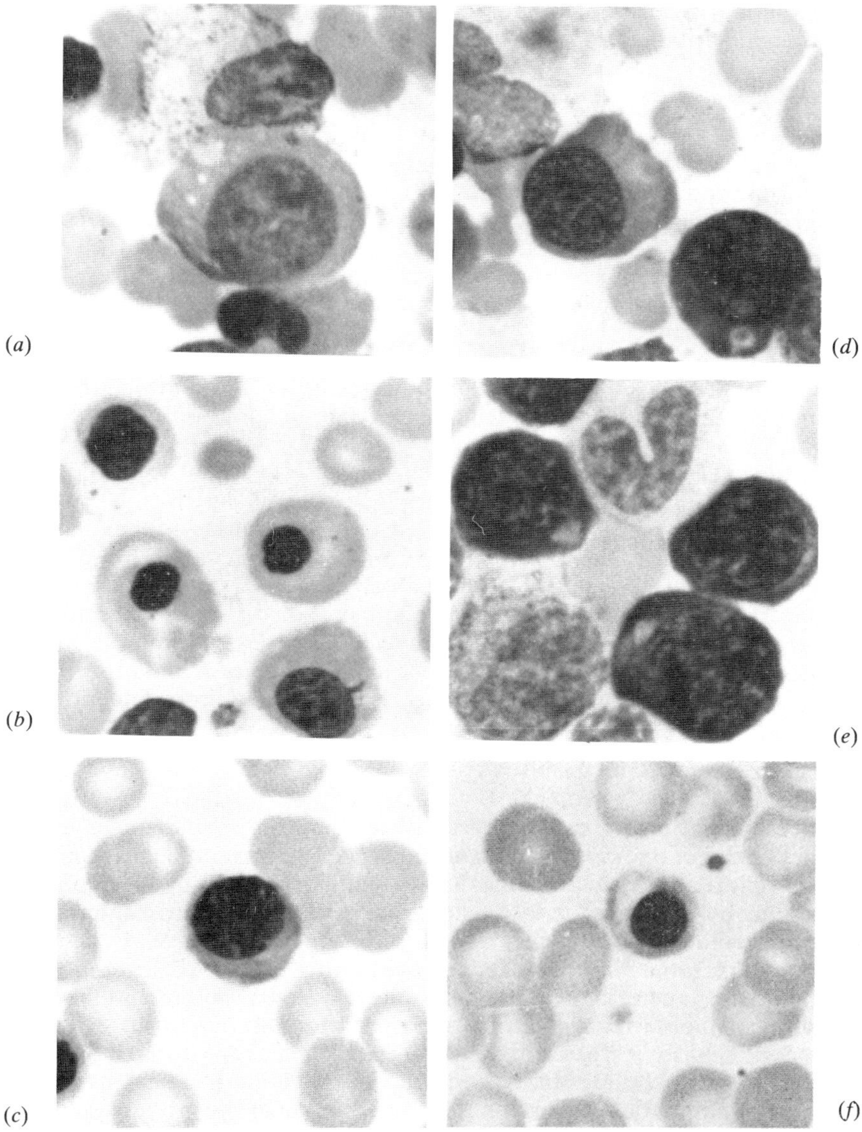

Figure 10.3 Bone-marrow preparations. ×825. (*a*) promegaloblast; (*b*) late megaloblasts; (*c*) intermediate normoblast. (*d*) early and intermediate megaloblast; (*e*) pronormoblasts and a basophilic or early normoblast; (*f*) late or pyknotic normoblast

and has an open, lacy appearance. Nuclear maturation is delayed resulting in 'out of phase' nuclear/cytoplasmic development with the intermediate forms showing advanced haemoglobinization and the late megaloblasts having a completely normochromic cytoplasm with no trace of polychromasia. The reticulocyte stage is therefore not a feature of megaloblastic erythropoiesis. Early or 'transitional' megaloblastic change is best recognized by the slightly 'open' nuclear structure of the intermediate forms and by the fully haemoglobinized late erythroblasts. Although megaloblasts are typically larger than normoblasts, diameter is not a sensitive or specific criterion.

The bone marrow in megaloblastic anaemia

The bone-marrow changes determine the blood findings; when marrow changes are minor there is little or no anaemia. As the megaloblastic process becomes more severe the anaemia and morphological changes become progressively more marked until in severe anaemia the marrow is hyperplastic and often with a reduced myeloid:erythroid ratio, though on occasion megaloblasts are scanty. Gross megaloblastic change is often associated with an apparent maturation arrest at the early polychromatic cell level which reflects the intramedullary destruction of the cells arrested in interphase.

Other cell lines are affected, notably the granulocytes. The characteristic abnormality is the presence of giant metamyelocytes up to 25 μm in diameter. In contrast with normal metamyelocytes which are a non-dividing cell class with 2n DNA content, the giant forms occur in all stages of interphase (2n–4n) and represent ineffective granulopoiesis with cell death. The giant cells do not, however, mature to the hypersegmented neutrophils [14]. Cell destruction probably occurs during thrombocytopoiesis and contributes to the thrombocytopenia found in severe megaloblastosis. Mitoses are usually more frequent and chromosome studies show a variety of non-specific abnormalities.

Intracellular iron granules are increased in number and size and a small number of ringed sideroblasts may be seen in the late megaloblasts. Extracellular iron level is typically increased, though latent iron depletion may be present and reflected by reduced iron stores. Megaloblastic change may be masked by iron depletion but becomes evident after iron therapy.

Biochemical changes

Megaloblastic anaemia results in marked and varied biochemical changes due to complex metabolic disturbances. As the anaemia is due to increased destruction of circulating red cells together with intramedullary death of developing megaloblasts, biochemical changes associated with increased cell destruction and haemoglobin catabolism are present.

Unconjugated plasma bilirubin is increased with increased excretion of urobilinogen in faeces and urine. Haptoglobins are reduced or absent and in severe anaemia methaemalbumin can often be demonstrated. Serum iron levels are usually normal or slightly increased in uncomplicated megaloblastosis.

Elevated activities of the plasma enzymes normally found in red cells can be demonstrated, notably lactic dehydrogenase (LDH) and hydroxybutyrate dehydrogenase, the activities being related to the severity of the megaloblastic process. Studies of the isoenzyme pattern of the increased LDH indicate that the enzymes are derived from the destruction of megaloblasts in the marrow.

Lysozyme levels are increased in plasma and urine and probably originate from granulocyte destruction in the marrow.

Intermediate products of the metabolic pathways requiring cobalamin or folate as co-enzymes are excreted in increased amounts in urine. The conversion of histidine to glutamic acid requires the transfer of the formimino group for formiminoglutamic acid (Figlu) to tetrahydrofolate; when tetrahydrofolate is deficient Figlu excretion is increased. The isomerization of methylmalonyl co-enzyme A to succinyl co-enzyme A depends upon the deoxyadenosyl form of cobalamin, a deficiency that results in increased urinary excretion of methylmalonic acid. Aminoimidazole carboxamide ribotide (AICAR), an intermediate of purine synthesis, is excreted in increased amounts in both folate and cobalamin deficiency. Cobalamin and folate levels in plasma and red cells are considered in detail in a later section.

In severe megaloblastic anaemia elevated levels of Hb F and Hb A_2 are found. The increase in Hb A_2 level probably reflects asynchrony of α/β polypeptide chain synthesis. The re-emergence of Hb F is of considerable interest, not only in megaloblastic anaemia but also in other disorders.

Causes of megaloblastic anaemia

Megaloblastic anaemia is usually caused by a reduced availability of folate or cobalamin due to depletion of body stores. Other causes include thiamine deficiency, drugs, inborn errors of metabolism and the vitamins being in metabolically inactive forms; it may occur in association with disorders such as myelodysplastic syndrome, erythroleukaemia, myeloma, etc.

Folate deficiency

Causes of folate deficiency are:

1. Nutritional deficiency.
2. Malabsorption.
3. Increased requirement for folate.
4. Drugs inhibiting folate.
5. Congenital defects of folate metabolism.

Nutritional deficiency

Inadequate folate intake is the commonest cause of folate depletion. Failure to supply the daily requirement of 100–200 μg of folate may be due to the type of diet or loss of folate during storage of food or more usually due to loss during cooking. Elderly subjects and low-income families are particularly likely to have inadequate folate intake. Infants fed entirely on goats' milk, which contains very little folate, risk developing megaloblastic anaemia. Patients in hospital are commonly in negative folate balance. Severely ill patients having intravenous nutrition readily develop significant folate deficiency unless folate supplements are given. Alcoholics are often folate deficient, probably due to an inadequate diet exacerbated by alcohol-induced malabsorption. Experimental folate deficiency in an adult resulted in rapid fall in serum folate within 3 weeks, hypersegmentation by 7 weeks and low red-cell folate by 4 months followed rapidly by macrocytosis, megaloblastic change and anaemia[15]. The rapid fall in serum folate level represents the negative folate balance rather than depletion of folate stores.

Malabsorption of folate

As absorption of folate takes place in the small bowel, functional disorders of the jejunum or ileum commonly result in folate malabsorption. Of particular importance are coeliac disease (gluten sensitivity), tropical sprue, Crohn's disease, small-bowel resection and the presence of diffuse malignant infiltration of the small-bowel mucosa. The association between folate deficiency and anticonvulsant drugs is due, at least in part, to impaired absorption of folate. Other drugs that reduce absorption are sulphasalazine (salazopyrine) and paraminosalicylic acid. A rare congenital disorder of folate absorption has been described that is possibly due to abnormal transport of folate across the intestinal barrier[16]. The malabsorption of folate in alcoholism is probably due to a combination of the effects of nutritional folate deficiency on the small bowel, malnutrition and alcohol itself.

Increased folate requirement

Increased cell growth or turnover increases the demand for folate. Pregnancy is the commonest example, in which the daily requirement due to the growing fetus increases to about 250 μg. Haematological disorders associated with increased cell turnover, notably the chronic haemolytic anaemias, may develop megaloblastic changes due to depletion of folate stores by increased utilization. A similar mechanism probably occurs in malignant proliferative diseases. However, other factors may be involved, particularly the presence of intercurrent infection. Folate is lost during renal dialysis and supplements are therefore required by patients on long-term dialysis.

Drugs

Drugs that directly inhibit intracellular folate metabolism and consequently DNA synthesis are used in the treatment of malignant disease, malaria, bacterial infection and for stimulating diuresis. They act as dihydrofolate reductase (DHFR) inhibitors and consequently the reduction of folate monoglutamates and dihydrofolate is impaired with a resulting lack of tetrahydrofolate. The drug with the greatest affinity for DHFR inhibition is methotrexate which also inhibits folate uptake by cells. Methotrexate will consistently produce megaloblastic change in therapeutic doses even when folate stores are normal. Other drugs such as the antimalarial pyrimethamine, the diuretic triamterene and the antibiotic trimethoprim have less affinity for DHFR and in normal dosage will probably only induce megaloblastosis when folate stores are already low. Anti-tuberculous therapy using isoniazid and cycloserine has reportedly been associated with low serum folate and megaloblastosis. It may be significant that isoniazid is an antagonist of pyridoxal-5-phosphate which is the co-enzyme in the folate-dependent conversion of serine to glycine.

Congenital defects of folate metabolism

Rare defects of folate metabolism have been reported, some being associated with megaloblastic anaemia developing soon after birth. The reliability of the identification of the enzyme defects in some cases has been reviewed and criteria for suspecting an inborn error of folate metabolism have been suggested[17].

Vitamin B_{12} (cobalamin) deficiency

Lack of cobalamin may be due to:

1. Malabsorption:
   (a) Lack of intrinsic factor – (i) gastric atrophy (pernicious anaemia); (ii) post-gastrectomy; (iii) congenital absence of intrinsic factor.
   (b) Congenital abnormality of intrinsic factor.
   (c) Intestinal abnormality – (i) congenital cobalamin malabsorption (Immerslund–Gräsbeck syndrome); (ii) coeliac disease; (iii) tropical sprue; (iv) Crohn's disease; (v) anatomical abnormalities, e.g. blind loop, ileal resection, diverticulosis.
   (d) Fish tapeworm (*Diphyllobothrium latum*).
   (e) Drugs – PAS, neomycin, colchicine, potassium chloride.
2. Nutritional deficiency – vegans.
3. Transport – transcobalamin II deficiency.
4. Defective conversion to active co-enzymes associated with methylmalonicaciduria and homocysteinuria.
5. Drugs – oxidation of cobalamin by nitrous oxide.
6. Congenital deficiency due to maternal deficiency.

Pernicious anaemia (PA)
This is the classic example of megaloblastic anaemia due to B_{12} deficiency. It is due to gastric atrophy resulting in absent intrinsic factor (IF) secretion by gastric parietal cells. Hydrochloric acid secretion is also absent. Any residual IF activity may be neutralized by antibody in gastric juice directed against IF (*see* below). In the absence of IF, dietary B_{12} cannot be absorbed through the mucosa of the terminal ileum (*see* page 37).

PA is usually a disorder of the elderly and there is often a familial incidence. In subjects over 60 years the incidence of PA approaches 1%, with women being affected more often than men. The development of the anaemia is usually insidious because of the relatively high body stores of cobalamin undergoing gradual depletion over a number of years.

Autoimmune aspects of PA Antibody against gastric parietal cells is present in the serum of 85–90% of patients with PA and in the gastric juice in 75%, as demonstrated by immunofluorescent techniques against normal human gastric mucosa. Antibodies against IF are of two types. The 'blocking' or type I antibody prevents the binding of vitamin B_{12} to IF. The 'binding' or type II antibody reacts with IF or IF–B_{12} complex and inhibits the absorption of the complex. The type I antibodies are present in serum in about 60% of patients with PA, while type II antibodies have been demonstrated in about 50% but only in association with type I antibody. The antibodies are predominantly of IgG type, though IgA antibody may be present. There are, however, ethnic differences, possibly due to genetic influences. IF antibodies in gastric juice can be demonstrated in about 50% of patients with PA and the incidence of IgA antibody is higher than in serum.

Significance of parietal cell and IF antibodies The finding of parietal cell antibody in patients with megaloblastic anaemia is not diagnostic of PA; they are found in subjects without PA but who probably have atrophic gastritis. The incidence may be as high as 20% in the elderly. The association with PA of autoimmune disease such as thyroid disease, adrenal atrophy, diabetes and immune deficiency is reflected by a high incidence of parietal-cell antibody in these groups – 30% in thyroid disease, 20% in adrenal atrophy. About one third of healthy relatives of patients with PA have parietal-cell antibodies. Thus, though parietal-cell antibodies are found in most cases of PA and probably have a causative role in producing the gastric lesion, their presence is clearly not diagnostic. In contrast the association of circulating IF antibodies with megaloblastic anaemia and low serum B_{12} is virtually diagnostic of PA. In addition to their diagnostic association, the presence of IF antibodies in gastric juice can influence the results of B_{12} absorption studies in the presence of added IF. Evidence of cell-mediated immunity against IF has been demonstrated in 40% of patients with PA. Of particular interest is that in those patients without humoral antibody, cell-mediated immunity may be demonstrated and it may be a significant mechanism in the pathogenesis of the gastric lesion.

Post-gastrectomy

Total gastrectomy removes the source of IF. It follows that B_{12} absorption is inevitably reduced and that body stores will become depleted. Though serum B_{12} levels fall to low values in about 6 months, megaloblastic anaemia will develop on average only after an interval of about 5 years though it may be as short as 2 or as long as 10 years.

The incidence of megaloblastic anaemia after partial gastrectomy depends on how much of the stomach is removed and in the method of reconstruction with the small bowel. A low B_{12} level may be found in as many as 30% of patients 10 years after the operation, though the incidence of megaloblastic anaemia is in the order of 5%. Iron deficiency commonly follows gastric surgery and may mask megaloblastic change. Findings are further confused by the influence of iron deficiency in producing a low serum B_{12} level. Splenectomy is commonly performed with gastrectomy and the typical 'post-splenectomy' blood picture is grossly exaggerated when megaloblastosis is present. About 20% of cases of megaloblastic anaemia after partial gastrectomy are due to folate deficiency.

Congenital absence or abnormality of IF

There are many reports of children with normal gastric mucosa who fail to absorb B_{12} due to an apparent lack of IF. Though absence of IF may occur, it is more likely that an abnormal IF molecule is produced which binds B_{12} but is incapable of promoting absorption, or fails to bind B_{12}[18]. Megaloblastic change is not present during the first year of life and may take years to develop depending on whether there is any absorption-promoting activity. This delay in inducing megaloblastic change is an important distinction from the congenital folate disorders.

Malabsorption due to intestinal abnormalities

Disordered intestinal transport of IF–B_{12} (Immerslund–Gräsbeck syndrome) is a congenital defect in transport across the wall of the intestinal cell and results in megaloblastic changes developing during the second year of life. Several hundred cases have been reported. As the syndrome includes the presence of proteinuria it is suggested that the defect is 'transmembrane translocation of large molecules'[19].

Coeliac disease (*idiopathic steatorrhoea*) is due to sensitivity to gluten which produces an abnormal small-bowel mucosa with resulting malabsorption of B_{12} in about one third of cases. However, as folate malabsorption is abnormal in the majority of patients with untreated coeliac disease it is difficult to ascribe the presence of megaloblastic anaemia to B_{12} deficiency alone.

Tropical sprue is a form of intestinal malabsorption of unknown aetiology in which B_{12} malabsorption is almost always present, resulting in depletion of B_{12} stores and the development of megaloblastic anaemia. Again folate malabsorption is usual and combined deficiency of B_{12} and folate is commonly found.

Regional enteritis (*Crohn's disease*) typically affects the terminal ileum where B_{12} absorption normally occurs and thus predisposes to B_{12} deficiency and megaloblastic anaemia. When the disease involves other areas of the small bowel, folate absorption may be abnormal and again megaloblastosis may be due to combined or single deficiencies. Many patients undergo surgical resection of the terminal ileum which inevitably results in B_{12} malabsorption.

Anatomical abnormalities due to surgery, particularly when resection of the small bowel is performed, can obviously cause malabsorption of B_{12} (and/or folate). A further consequence of surgery is the production of a 'blind-loop' after partial gastrectomy by the Polya technique which involves anastomosis of the remaining stomach to the jejunum; the duodenum thereby becomes a cul-de-sac into which bile and pancreatic secretions are emptied. Normally the small bowel is sterile. In the 'blind-loop syndrome' significant bacterial growth can occur with associated B_{12} malabsorption.

Diverticulitis of the small bowel is usually associated with B_{12} malabsorption and often megaloblastic anaemia. Again abnormal bacterial flora are the cause. Abnormal bacterial flora in the small bowel are not associated with folate malabsorption.

Fish tapeworm The fish tapeworm *Diphyllobothrium latum* is a parasite of man acquired by consuming raw or partially cooked fish infected with tapeworm larvae. Megaloblastic anaemia due to *D. latum* is virtually confined to Finland where, although the infestation is very common, the incidence of megaloblastic anaemia is low. Nevertheless, low serum B_{12} levels are usual. The worm has a remarkable ability to absorb B_{12} in amounts similar to that in the diet, particularly if the head is situated in the jejunum. Increased intake of B_{12} allows some to be absorbed by the host. Expulsion of the worm corrects the B_{12} malabsorption.

Drugs that have been shown to impair absorption of B_{12} are paraminosalicylic acid, neomycin, colchicine and potassium chloride. As body stores of B_{12} are sufficient to maintain haemopoiesis for several years, megaloblastic anaemia would be unlikely to result from drug therapy even in the long term. Nevertheless, an established B_{12} malabsorption could be aggravated by drug treatment.

Nutritional B_{12} deficiency

Deficiency causing megaloblastic change is not common. Any diet containing animal protein will contribute sufficient B_{12} to maintain normoblastic erythropoiesis. A strict vegetarian diet, excluding milk and eggs, has a very low B_{12} content, yet contamination with soil, B_{12} in water etc., provides sufficient B_{12} to prevent megaloblastic change. Nevertheless the serum cobalamin levels of vegans are usually subnormal and often in the megaloblastic range.

In patients with megaloblastic anaemia that is suspected to be nutritional, other causes must be excluded and the haemopoietic response to oral administration of physiological amounts of B_{12} monitored. An important consideration is that PA can occur in vegans[20].

Defective transport of B_{12}

Transcobalamin II (TCII) deficiency can be found as a rare congenital disorder which is severe and potentially lethal. Megaloblastic anaemia appears in the first few weeks after birth in contrast to the congenital defects of absorption. The protein is absent rather than abnormal. Serum B_{12} levels are normal or raised indicating adequate transcobalamin I (TCI) levels and B_{12} body stores. Acquired deficiency of TCII has been described in association with increased TCI levels[21]. An example of megaloblastic anaemia due to an abnormal TCII capable of binding cobalamin but being unable to deliver the vitamin to cells has been described[22].

Defective conversion to active co-enzyme

Conversion of exogenous B_{12} to the active co-enzymes methyl- and deoxyadenosyl B_{12} is an intracellular process apparently requiring a binding protein which has been designated 'intracellular cobalamin binding protein' (ICB)[23]. The protein is probably an enzyme rather than a carrier protein. Rare instances of children with normal serum levels of B_{12}, low tissue levels and with methymalonic acid and homocysteine in the urine have been described. Megaloblastic anaemia has not been present in all cases for reasons which are not clear[24].

Exposure to nitrous oxide

The active co-enzymes of B_{12} contain cobalt in the reduced state. Oxidation of cobalt converts B_{12} to a non-functional form. Administration of nitrous oxide for periods of 24 hours induces megaloblastic changes with kinetic effects similar to those produced by 'S' phase cytotoxic drugs. Withdrawal of nitrous oxide results in prompt reversal of the changes[13].

Congenital deficiency due to maternal deficiency

Vitamin B_{12} stores in the neonate are derived by transfer from the mother during development *in utero*. Though pregnancy is unusual in the presence of B_{12} deficiency, when it occurs the infant is also B_{12} deficient and megaloblastic anaemia may develop[25]. In racial groups with vegetarian diets, for example in Hindus, megaloblastic anaemia in pregnancy is more common, particularly when chronic tropical sprue may be present, and because a younger female age group is involved.

Causes of megaloblastosis other than B_{12} or folate defects

Megaloblastic anaemia is due to deranged DNA synthesis due to inadequate supply of deoxyribonucleoside precursors of DNA, or by inhibition of DNA polymerase. Although megaloblastic anaemia is usually due to decreased availability of dTTP due to defective conversion of dUMP to dTMP caused by lack of 5-10-methylene THF due to B_{12} or folate deficiency, it is clear that any defect in the synthesis of dTTP or one of the other precursors of DNA may produce megaloblastosis. Of particular importance are cytotoxic drugs which act by inhibiting DNA synthesis.

Cytotoxic drugs

Drugs acting as pyrimidine antagonists consistently produce megaloblastic change. The purine antagonists, while all reported as being capable of inducing megaloblastosis, do so less consistently and frequently. *Table 10.1* lists the drugs and their mode of action.

Table 10.1 Inhibition of DNA synthesis

Antagonists	*Mechanism of action*
Pyrimidine antagonists:	
5-Fluorouracil	Inhibition of thymidylate synthesis
Cytosine arabinoside	Inhibits DNA polymerase and ribonucleotide reductase
Hydroxyurea	Inhibits ribonucleotide reductase
6-Azauridine	Inhibits orotidylate decarboxylase
Purine antagonists:	
6-Mercaptopurine	Inhibition at several stages
6-Thioguanine	
Azathioprine	

Orotic aciduria

Megaloblastic anaemia in infants associated with excretion of orotic acid in the urine has been reported on several occasions. The anaemia is unresponsive to folate, B_{12} or pyridoxine but does respond to large doses of uridine. The disorder is due to an inherited defect in the conversion of orotidylate to uridylate, caused by a deficiency of either or both orotidylate pyrophosphorylase and orotidylate decarboxylase. The latter is the enzyme inhibited by the cytotoxic agent azauridine and, significantly, results in the same morphological changes.

Association with primary haematological disorders

Megaloblasts may be found in the bone marrow in a variety of haematological disorders. In some instances, e.g. chronic haemolysis, myelofibrosis, the changes are due to folate deficiency. More difficult to explain is the presence of megaloblasts in myelodysplasia, acute leukaemia, myeloma and erythroleukaemia.

In sideroblastic anaemia, megaloblastic change is common and is often associated with evidence of folate depletion. The association of sideroblastic anaemia with disturbed pyridoxine metabolism and the requirement of pyridoxal-5-phosphate as a co-enzyme in the conversion of serine to glycine suggest a fundamental association in the occurrence of megaloblasts in sideroblastic anaemia.

The appearances of the abnormal erythroblasts in erythroleukaemia are often indistinguishable from the megaloblasts in B_{12} and folate deficiency. In such cases there is usually no evidence of B_{12} or folate deficiency and the disorder is refractory to B_{12} and folate therapy.

Investigation of megaloblastic anaemia

The causes of megaloblastic anaemia detailed in the previous section indicate that the great majority of cases are due to tissue depletion of B_{12} or folate or both. The investigation of megaloblastic anaemia, particularly in the adult, is therefore directed to the assessment of B_{12} and folate status.

Vitamin B_{12} status

Serum B_{12}

With certain exceptions the assay of cobalamin in serum is a reliable indication of tissue B_{12} stores. The exceptions are – the falling B_{12} level in late normal pregnancy, the low levels associated with a vegetarian diet, in severe iron deficiency, following acute blood loss, in about one-third of patients with megaloblastic anaemia due to folate deficiency but with normal B_{12} absorption after partial gastrectomy, in treated epileptics and the very rare deficiency of TCI. Additional rare causes of a normal serum cobalamin when the patient is deficient are prolonged nitrous oxide inhalation, TCII deficiency, inborn errors of cobalamin metabolism and B_{12} deficiency masked by B_{12} bound to TCI associated with granulocyte proliferation. Nevertheless, despite what appears at first sight to be a formidable list of exceptions, *in the investigation of megaloblastic anaemia* careful assay of cobalamin in serum will provide valuable information in the great majority of cases. Different methods of assay give differing normal ranges but these are well recognized and the levels associated with megaloblastic anaemia due to B_{12} deficiency are well defined.

Red-cell B_{12} content

This is normally about half the serum level and falls to low levels in B_{12} deficiency. As B_{12} does not enter the red cell after the reticulocyte stage, estimation of red-cell B_{12} can be helpful in distinguishing low serum B_{12} levels due to redistribution of B_{12} and those due to tissue depletion. The red-cell B_{12} level is usually normal in vegans who have low serum B_{12} levels. Low red-cell B_{12} levels are, however, found in folate deficiency in the presence of a normal serum B_{12} value.

Urinary excretion of methylmalonic acid (MMA)

This is increased in moderate to severe megaloblastic anaemia due to B_{12} deficiency, though when the anaemia is mild there is not a good correlation even after a loading dose of valine. The lack of a relatively simple and reliable technique for estimating MMA is also a drawback to its use in the routine assessment of B_{12} status. However, MMA in urine is specific for deficiency of deoxyadenosyl B_{12} or its apoenzyme methylmalonyl CoA mutase and therefore has a definite role in the investigation of certain rare causes of megaloblastic anaemia.

The use of the deoxyuridine suppression test in determining B_{12} status is discussed on page 282.

Folate status

Serum folate

The level of folate in serum is a sensitive indication of folate balance; a negative balance is reflected by a rapid fall in the serum level which will obviously precede depletion of body stores. Low serum folate levels are found in a high proportion of hospital patients and reflect a reduced folate intake due to loss of appetite, illness, infection or possible loss of folate from food by prolonged heating. A low serum folate value does not therefore necessarily indicate depletion of tissue folate. Nevertheless a very low serum folate level *associated with a megaloblastic anaemia* indicates that folate deficiency is wholly or partly responsible, as megaloblastic anaemia due to B_{12} deficiency is usually associated with normal, high-normal or even elevated levels of serum folate due to the accumulation of 5-methyl THF.

An objection to serum folate assay as a reliable indication of folate status is on the basis that fluctuations in serum folate level occur in relation to dietary intake of folate. Though this occurs in folate-replete subjects, the clearance of folate from the plasma of deficient subjects is so rapid that the amount of folate present in a meal is very unlikely to transform a low serum folate to a normal value. It can therefore be reasonably re-stated that a low serum folate *in megaloblastic anaemia* indicates folate deficiency.

Red-cell folate

This is unaffected by day-to-day variation in folate intake and is a more reliable reflection of tissue folate stores. An objection to the red-cell folate as an indication of folate status is the 'lag' between the development of folate deficiency and the time taken to replace with folate-deficient red cells the circulating red cells produced when folate stores were adequate. Interpretation of red-cell folate levels may also be difficult in the presence of a haemolytic anaemia, because of the higher folate content in reticulocytes. However, in patients with megaloblastic anaemia due to folate deficiency that has developed over more than 2–3 months, red-cell folate levels will be low. In patients who have recently been treated with folic acid – in whom the serum folate level will be meaningless – the red-cell folate will still indicate folate status as it was 2–3 months or more before treatment. In the differential diagnosis of the cause of a megaloblastic anaemia red-cell folate is of limited value, as low levels are found both in folate and in B_{12} deficiency. The low red-cell folate level in B_{12} deficiency is due to reduced levels of folate polyglutamates due to reduced availability of THF and is regarded as reflecting a cellular folate deficiency secondary to the B_{12} deficiency.

Excretion of formiminoglutamic acid in urine

Demonstration or measurement of increased formiminoglutamic acid (Figlu) in urine, usually after a loading dose of histidine, has been used as an indication of folate status. Unfortunately, increased Figlu excretion reflects a negative folate balance, as does the serum folate, and its usefulness is therefore limited. Furthermore, increased amounts of Figlu are excreted in B_{12} deficiency and reflect the low red-cell folate described above. Figlu measurement is therefore rarely used nowadays as an indication of folate status.

Table 10.2 summarizes folate and B_{12} levels in megaloblastic anaemia due to B_{12} and folate deficiencies.

Table 10.2 Vitamin B_{12} and folate levels in megaloblastic anaemias due to B_{12} deficiency and in chronic and acute folate deficiency

	Assay			
	Serum B_{12}	*Red-cell B_{12}*	*Serum folate*	*Red-cell folate*
B_{12} deficiency	Low	Low	Normal to raised	Low
Folate deficiency (chronic)	Normal or low	Low	Low	Low
Folate deficiency (acute)	Normal	Normal	Low	Normal or ±low

Studies of vitamin B_{12} absorption in megaloblastic anaemia

As the great majority of megaloblastic anaemias due to B_{12} deficiency are caused by malabsorption due to lack of intrinsic factor (IF), small-bowel disease or, more rarely, nutritional deficiency, studies of B_{12} absorption are of value in the investigation of B_{12} deficiency.

When radioactive B_{12} is administered orally the amount of B_{12} absorbed can be measured by a variety of methods. The most commonly used is the *Schilling test* in which an intramuscular 'flushing' dose of non-radioactive B_{12} is given and the radioactivity excreted in the urine measured. In the normal subject over 14% of the oral dose is excreted in the urine in 24 hours. Values below 10% are found in B_{12} malabsorption and are often less than 2% when IF is absent. The test can be repeated with added IF; partial or complete correction indicates lack of IF and no correction is found when the cause of the malabsorption is an abnormality of the small intestine. Failure of correction will also be found when IF antibodies, which inhibit the action of the added IF, are present in the gastric juice. Poor correction may also be found in classic PA without IF antibodies and is probably due to small-bowel changes secondary to the B_{12} deficiency. Similarly, small-bowel changes due to folate deficiency may result in impaired B_{12} absorption. A problem with the Schilling test is the requirement that a full urine collection must be obtained, a notoriously difficult exercise in a general ward. The additional measurement of plasma radioactivity can help in the interpretation of results[12,26]. Typical examples of the results of the Schilling test in a variety of B_{12}-deficient states are shown in *Table 10.3*.

Table 10.3 Typical results of Schilling tests with and without added intrinsic factor (IF) in a variety of conditions associated with vitamin-B_{12}-deficient megaloblastic anaemia

	B_{12} excretion	
Condition	*Without IF*	*With IF*
Pernicious anaemia	Low	Corrected
Pernicious anaemia with IF antibody in gastric juice	Low	Partial or no correction
Post-gastrectomy	Low	Corrected
'Blind-loop', jejunal diverticulosis	Low	No correction
Crohn's disease	Low	No correction
Nutritional B_{12} deficiency	Normal	–

The standard Schilling test has been criticized as being non-physiological in that aqueous B_{12} is given whereas dietary B_{12} is usually protein bound[27]. The absorption of protein-bound vitamin B_{12} may be measured by administering the radioactive B_{12} bound to chicken serum[28], though the value of the modification has been questioned[12].

The deoxyuridine suppression test

In the absence of *de novo* synthesis of thymidylate, normal erythroblasts utilize thymidine (dTdR) derived from the salvage pathway of DNA catabolism. When deoxyuridine (dU) is present less than 10% of added [^{3}H]dTdR is incorporated into DNA, i.e. incorporation is suppressed by addition of deoxyuridine. This forms the basis of the 'deoxyuridine suppression test'. In megaloblastic anaemia due to B_{12} or folate deficiency the addition of dU to short-term bone-marrow cultures does not suppress the incorporation of [^{3}H]TdR, as the conversion of dU to thymidine monophosphate (dTMP) is defective. The test has been used extensively to investigate the interrelationships of B_{12} and folate in a megaloblastic anaemia.

The addition of B_{12} to bone-marrow cultures of B_{12}-deficient subjects results in partial correction of the failure of suppression but has no effect on dTdR incorporation in cultures from folate-deficient subjects. The addition of folic acid will correct the failure of suppression in cultures from both folate- and B_{12}-deficient patients. The test therefore provides a rapid method of establishing whether B_{12} or folate deficiency is present and is claimed to be of particular value in diagnosing folate deficiency when the red-cell folate is normal. The method can be applied to phytohaemagglutinin-stimulated lymphocytes which, because of their long survival, can reflect the B_{12} and folate status of several months before.

Response to therapy as a means of investigation

An optimal response to specific replacement therapy can be recognized in patients who are sufficiently anaemic by:

1. A maximum reticulocyte response within 8 days.
2. A peak reticulocyte response in proportion to the severity of the anaemia as judged by the red-cell count.
3. A rise in red-cell count to over 3.0×10^{12}/l by the 15th day of treatment.

Physiological doses should be used, as pharmacological amounts of B_{12} will elicit a reticulocyte response, albeit suboptimal, in folate deficiency and vice versa. An oral dose of 2 μg of B_{12} daily will produce a response only in nutritional B_{12} deficiency. Daily intramuscular injections of 2 μg of B_{12} will produce maximum haematological response in the other, commoner, B_{12} deficiencies. Administration of 200 μg of folic acid each day by injection will produce an optimum response in folate deficiency. Oral folate can only be used when it is certain that there is no folate malabsorption.

In addition to the reticulocytosis and increase in red-cell count other less specific parameters may be followed such as a fall in serum iron level, the fall in serum folate value with a rising red-cell folate value in treated B_{12} deficiency, and the rise in serum B_{12} in folate deficiency.

Other investigations

The full diagnostic picture of pernicious anaemia will include the demonstration of the absence of IF by the Schilling test and the possible presence of IF antibodies in serum and gastric juice. The demonstration of parietal cell antibodies is of little diagnostic value because of their occurrence in subjects without PA. Studies of small-bowel function are often indicated in folate deficiency.

This section has concentrated on the investigation of megaloblastic anaemia as an acquired disorder in the adult. Congenital defects producing megaloblastosis require a special investigative approach and much of what applies to megaloblastic anaemia in the adult is not necessarily relevant to megaloblastic anaemia in infancy.

Techniques in the investigation of megaloblastic anaemia

Assay of vitamin B_{12} in serum

Microbiological assays of vitamin B_{12} were used for many years and the great bulk of data relating to serum levels in health and disease had been obtained by these methods. In the investigation of megaloblastic anaemia the assay of B_{12} in serum is an established method for demonstrating B_{12} deficiency. The criterion of a satisfactory assay procedure is that it must reliably separate B_{12}-deficient sera from those of a control, non-deficient group. B_{12} assay procedures in general have been criticized as being insensitive and non-specific[29]. The very rare clinical conditions in which the test may be insensitive, i.e. produce normal results when the patient is deficient, are well recognized and low serum B_{12} values when the patient is not deficient (non-specific) are known to occur in association with certain clinical situations and assay results would be interpreted accordingly. It is recognized, however, that for various reasons incorrect results may be obtained due to fundamental defects in methods, inadequate technique and interference or inhibition in the assay.

The introduction of radioisotope dilution methods and their availability from commercial sources has resulted in their widespread adoption but also raised questions regarding their sensitivity and specificity[30].

Microbiological assay

General principle

An organism that requires vitamin B_{12} for its growth is inoculated into a series of tubes of culture medium containing all growth requirements other than B_{12} which is supplied by the serum under assay. After incubation the growth of the organism is measured and related to that of a series of cultures containing graded amounts of B_{12}.

Choice of test organism

The most widely used organisms were *Euglena gracilis*[31] and *Lactobacillus leichmanii*[32]. More rarely *Ochromonas malhamensis* and a mutant strain of *Escherichia coli* have been used. An improved method using *E. coli* has been described[33] which gave very similar results to the *E. gracilis* method.

E. gracilis is generally accepted as being more specific and sensitive than *L. leichmanii*. Addition of B_{12} to serum can be totally recovered. There is limited interference of growth by antibiotics or other drugs and the values obtained in megaloblastic anaemia due to vitamin B_{12} deficiency are, in the great majority of cases, clearly separated from those of normal subjects and non-B_{12}-deficient haematological disorders. For the above reasons the Euglena assay is widely accepted as the reference method.

Present status of microbiological assays

Although the various assays give similar results they are tedious to perform and fastidious technique is necessary to maintain the test organism and to exclude contaminating B_{12} from the test system. National quality assessment surveys also demonstrated that the results from laboratories showed unacceptably different results using the same sera.

The development of radioisotope dilution (RID) methods and their subsequent commercial availability has resulted in their widespread adoption, despite the fact that the results did not necessarily compare well with microbiological methods. Recent modifications have improved the reliability of RID assays and microbiological methods are performed routinely in very few diagnostic laboratories. They are therefore, in practice, obsolete and detailed descriptions of the methods have been deleted.

Radioisotopic assay of vitamin B_{12}

The principle of radioisotope dilution assay (RIDA) or saturation analysis assay has been applied to the measurement of serum B_{12} since 1963. During the first 12 years over 50 assay protocols were published which indicates the many possible variations in method, reagents and techniques.

The principle of RIDA is straightforward. B_{12} in serum is freed from its protein carrier and mixed with radiolabelled B_{12}. A 'binder' is added to the mixture of non-radioactive (endogenous, serum) B_{12} and radioactive B_{12}. Remaining 'free' B_{12} is separated from the 'bound' B_{12} and the activity of the mixture of the labelled and unlabelled B_{12} is measured. The radioactivity reflects the relative concentrations of unlabelled (serum) and labelled (added) B_{12}. Thus when the serum B_{12} is low the amount of labelled B_{12} will be high and vice versa. Therefore the radioactivity of the B_{12} mixture attached to the binder is inversely proportional to the serum B_{12} concentration.

The multiplicity of published methods and the variety available in commercial kit form reflect the major differences between methods – (1) the method of freeing the serum B_{12} from its carrier proteins; (2) the binding agent and the type of solid phase; (3) the technique of separating free from bound B_{12}; (4) the possible addition of B_{12}-free serum or albumin; (5) buffer pH. The position has been further complicated by the introduction of dual isotope methods for assaying B_{12} and folate in the same system.

The RID assays generally showed higher values than the microbiological methods and frankly incorrect results can be obtained [34,35]. Much attention has been given to the presence of cobalamin analogues in serum combining with 'R-binders' in serum or other binders. The term 'R-binders' refers to cobalamin-binding proteins, lacking in intrinsic factor activity, but present in human gastric juice and other body fluids which have a rapid (R) electrophoretic mobility. Some methods have attempted to 'block' the action of R-binders by adding cobalamin analogue to the assay system, an approach which we have not found entirely satisfactory. The preparation of purified human intrinsic factor, free from R-binder, and the use of charcoal or polyacrylamide beads to provide solid phase separation have resulted in assay values closely comparable to those obtained by microbiological assay and should have eliminated the problem of normal results from deficient sera.

Nevertheless the main criteria of a satisfactory assay is that it must reliably differentiate between normal sera and those deficient in B_{12}. In the course of a multi-laboratory study to develop a vitamin B_{12} serum standard [36] using both microbiological and radioisotope assays, a variety of binders were used including human saliva, CGL serum, chicken serum, dog stomach binder and TC I. Each of these gave results much higher than those using either *Euglena* or *Lactobacillus* assays, yet identified deficient serum when related to the reference range for the particular method.

The intensive investigations of Muir and Chanarin [37,38,39] have provided sensitive, highly specific and robust assays using either R-binder or purified human intrinsic factor. The method using human intrinsic factor shows clear separation of normal and deficient sera and provides sufficient practical detail for 'in-house' development.

All assays should benefit from the production and availability of serum standards for B_{12} assay [36,40].

Assay of folate in serum and red cells

Assessment of folate status by microbiological assay has a history almost as long as that for vitamin B_{12}. Although the major transport form of folate, 5-methyl tetrahydrofolate (MTHF), does not support the growth of *Streptococcus faecalis,* folate status can be deduced using this organism by the rate of clearance from plasma of an intravenous injection of pterylglutamic acid (PGA); depleted subjects show more rapid clearance curves than those of folate-replete subjects. *Pediococcus cerevisiae* (formerly *Leuconostoc citrovorum*) responds to tetrahydrofolates other than the 5-methyl forms. The introduction of *Lactobacillus casei* allows assay of MTHF in serum and red cells, and in its original or modified forms the *L. casei* assay is the accepted microbiological method for demonstrating folate deficiency.

Radioisotopic assay of folate has a more recent history than the corresponding B_{12} assays. Early RID assays using [^{3}H]– or [^{14}C]PGA or THF with milk as a binder were not widely used due to restricted availability of liquid scintillation counters. The introduction of the γ-emitting labels [^{75}Se]selenofolate and [^{125}I]PGA allowed wide adoption of RIDA for serum and red-cell folate.

Microbiological assay

The basic principle of the *L. casei* assay is that described for microbiological assays in general (*see* page 284). Early *L. casei* assays involved heating to coagulate the serum proteins, with the addition of ascorbate to protect the labile folate, followed by autoclaving of the prepared standard and test tubes before inoculation. The procedure is therefore lengthy.

An 'aseptic addition' method has been described in which the test standard and blank tubes containing medium and ascorbate are pre-sterilized with the subsequent addition of serum followed by inoculation. This method eliminates the protein precipitation stage and while requiring good aseptic technique, the growth of the *L. casei* overwhelms any contaminating organisms. This modification is clearly simpler.

Adaptation of a strain of *L. casei* to grow in the presence of chloramphenicol [41] eliminates the need for strict aseptic technique and allows the use of automatic pipettes and even full automation [42]. The chloramphenicol-resistant *L. casei* method has been widely accepted though alteration of the growth requirements of the strain may be a problem [43]. The last reference described a 'direct' assay of serum using a routine strain of *L. casei* without heat extraction or subsequent sterilization and depends on the rapid growth of the *L. casei* to overcome any contaminants. Assay of red-cell folate is less satisfactory due to turbidity and bacterial contamination in the presence of haemolysis. The method described in detail below is widely used and is readily adaptable to automatic pipetting or full automation.

Assay of folate using chloramphenicol-resistant L. casei

Collection and preparation of samples

Serum Blood samples are collected into unused plain glass tubes and allowed to clot. Serum is separated within 2 hours. Ascorbic acid, 5 mg/ml, may be added at this stage but the samples would not then be suitable for assay of B_{12} by microbiological or radioisotopic assay. The samples can be stored in the dark at −20°C for up to 2 months. Haemolysed samples are unsuitable due to the release of folate from the red cells.

Haemolysates for red-cell folate assay Blood collected into EDTA is diluted 1 in 10 in water containing 10 g/l ascorbic acid. The PCV of the whole-blood sample is determined and recorded. The whole-blood sample may be stored at 4°C for 1 week before processing, provided that the PCV is determined on the fresh sample. Haemolysates may be stored at −20°C for at least 2 months. For accurate estimation of red-cell folate a sample for serum folate assay must be collected at the same time as the whole blood.

Materials

Glassware Scrupulously clean glassware, free from detergents, inhibiting substances or folate contamination must be used. New glassware is usually satisfactory which if re-used should be soaked in suitable detergent, rinsed at least six times with tap water and twice with distilled water. Metal caps (Oxoid) are used as closures.

Organism Chloramphenicol-resistant *L. casei* NCIB 1 0463 (National Collection of Industrial Bacteria, Torrey Research Station, Aberdeen, UK).

Chloramphenicol solutions 300 mg of chloramphenicol (Parke Davis) are dissolved in 1 ml absolute ethanol and the volume made up to 100 ml with water to a give a 3 g/l solution. A solution of 1 g/l is prepared by diluting the 3 g/l solution 1 in 3 with water.

Maintenance culture Bacto Lactobacilli Broth AOAC (Difco Code 0901); 19 g are added to 500 ml distilled water and boiled for 2 minutes to dissolve. The culture is distributed in 9 ml amounts in screw-capped bottles and autoclaved at 121°C (15 p.s.i., 103.4 kPa) for 15 minutes and stored in the dark to prevent deterioration. The dried culture is transferred to the maintenance medium with 1 ml of 3 g/l chloramphenicol solution to give a final concentration of 300 μg/ml and incubated at 37°C for 48 hours. The stock culture is stored at 4°C and 1 ml sub-cultured into maintenance medium every 2 weeks. Maintenance of the strain as a dried culture or in liquid nitrogen is also recommended.

Preparation of inoculum The day before the assay 1 ml of the stock culture is transferred to 9 ml of maintenance medium containing 100 μg/ml chloramphenicol (1 ml of 1 g/l chloramphenicol) and incubated at 37°C for 24 hours. The culture is centrifuged at 1200 *g* for 5 minutes, washed twice with 10 ml of assay medium, resuspended in 10 ml of assay medium and 1 ml diluted with 99 ml of assay medium.

Assay medium Bacto-Folic Acid Casei medium (Difco Code 0822). Suspend 9.4 g in 100 ml distilled water and add 50 mg ascorbic acid and 1 ml of 1 g/l chloramphenicol. Dissolve by boiling for 1–2 minutes.

Standards
A stock solution containing 150 mg/l PGA (Sigma) in alkaline solution is stored at 4°C in a dark bottle. This solution is stable for 6 months. A working solution of 150 μg/l is made by diluting 1 ml of the stock solution to 1 litre with distilled water. A range of standards is prepared as in *Table 10.4.*

Table 10.4 Standards used in folate assay with chloramphenicol-resistant *L. casei*

Tube	*1*	*2*	*3*	*4*	*5*	*6*	*7*	*8*
PGA 150 μg/l (ml)	0.5	1.0	2.0	4.0	6.0	8.0	10.0	12.0
Distilled water	←			to 100 ml				→
PGA concentration (μg/l)	0.75	1.5	3.0	6.0	9.0	12.0	15.0	18.0

These standards may be stored in small volumes at −20°C

Procedure
Three 150 × 19 mm tubes are used for each standard, serum and haemolysate with three additional tubes containing only medium as blanks. Standards are set up in triplicate and tests in duplicate, each with an additional tube which serves as a sample blank. 6 ml of media and 0.05 ml of standard, serum or haemolysate are added to each tube. One drop of inoculum is added to all tubes except the test blanks and mixed by vortexing. The tubes are incubated at 37°C for 18–24 hours.

Reading of results Turbidity is read in a nephelometer, in a 1 cm cell in a spectrophotometer at 620 nm, or a photometer with a red filter. The readings of the inoculated blanks are deducted from all standard and test reading. The uninoculated standard and test blanks are deducted from each standard and test reading as appropriate.

Calculation of results The average turbidity readings for each standard are plotted against concentration on arithmetic graph paper. The values for serum folate are read as μg/l direct from the graph. Values for whole-blood folate are multiplied by 10 to allow for the dilution in preparing the haemolysate and red-cell folate (RCF) calculated from:

$$\text{RCF } (\mu g/l) = \frac{\text{whole-blood folate} - (\text{serum folate} \times (1 - \text{PCV}))}{\text{PCV } (l/l)}$$

Normal ranges Hospital patients, serum folate 3.0–12.0 μg/l; red-cell folate 160–320 μg/l.

Notes
If the inoculum is added to bulk culture, increasing turbidity of the mixture may be a problem due to crystal formation. Fast mixing of the medium during setting up and warming the incubated tubes at 56°C for 10 minutes before reading has been recommended.

Radioisotope assay of folate

The radioisotopic assay of serum and red-cell folate is based on the principle of radioisotope dilution (saturation analysis, competitive protein binding assay) as described for the RIDA of vitamin B_{12}.

The development of the radioassay of folate was hampered by certain practical difficulties which were overcome mainly by the extraction of a suitable binder from milk [44]. The early methods used [^{3}H]PGA as the labelled form of folate which have been superseded by the availability of [^{125}I]-labelled folate compounds. The preparation and standardization of the reagents for the assay of folate is complex and time consuming and the widespread adoption of radioassay techniques is largely due to the availability of the reagents in kit form from commercial sources, the majority of which follow the same general procedure. Variation in the performance of different kits has been found by comparative evaluations. This description of the radioassay of folate will be confined to a brief description of the major practical aspects. A more detailed review of the assay and its development is available [45].

Folate binder Folate will bind non-specifically to positively charged macromolecules. A specific binder with a high equilibrium constant is essential in a satisfactory RIDA. The recognition of the folate binder in milk, which has a high equilibrium constant and from which folate cannot be removed by charcoal, has provided the binding reagent used in folate assay kits. The binder has been identified as a β-lactoglobulin. At pH 7.4 the binder from cows' milk shows different affinities for different forms of folate, e.g. PGA and MTHF, but at pH 9.3 binding with both compounds is almost identical. This is important in the choice of labelled compound, which need not be the same as the compound to be assayed but must have the same affinity for the binder. The normal folate binding capacity of serum can interfere with the assay and therefore the binder must be extracted from the serum, a 'serum blank' assayed, or, more usually, the binder destroyed by boiling.

Standards A fundamental requirement of competitive binding assays is that the unlabelled standard is identical with the substance being assayed, which in the case of folate is MTHF. This form of folate is very unstable and although it is used in some kits, the majority use PGA and perform the assay at pH 9.3.

Separation of free from bound folate This is achieved with dextran-coated charcoal which is incapable of dissociating the milk-folate binding.

Protection of labile folate This is important during the assay and for folate in serum is achieved with dithiothreitol as reducing agent rather than ascorbic acid which would destroy vitamin B_{12} and make simultaneous radioassay of folate and B_{12} impossible. As folate is sensitive to light, samples must be stored in the dark and protected from light during the assay.

Assay of red-cell folate Folate in red cells is in the form of polyglutamates which are more reactive with milk binder than the monoglutamate commonly used as the standard. Lysis of the red cells at acid pH in the presence of ascorbic acid allows progressive conversion of polyglutamates to monoglutamates by endogenous (red-cell) conjugase and is complete in 90 minutes at room temperature.

Choice of assay It would be exceptional for any particular assay to satisfy all requirements such as precision (both between and within batches), recovery of added folate, accuracy (which is difficult to evaluate in the absence of validated reference preparations), simplicity, cost-effectiveness, etc. The ultimate objective is the ability of the assay to separate deficient samples reliably from those from a control population. To help achieve this aim each laboratory should establish its reference range using the chosen assay method.

Comprehensive assessment of the value of RID assays of serum and red-cell folate are few. A study which compared red-cell folate results with folate status [46] determined by the deoxyuridine suppression test showed that while sensitivity was satisfactory, 12% of patients unlikely to be either folate or B_{12}-deficient had low values.

Vitamin B_{12} absorption – the Schilling test

Principle

A physiological dose of 1 μg of vitamin B_{12} labelled with ^{57}Co with a specific activity of about 1 μCi (37 kBq) is administered by mouth after an overnight fast. In normal subjects the absorbed vitamin appears in the blood 2–3 hours after administration and the maximum level in the liver is reached after 24 hours. The amount of B_{12} absorbed may be measured by residual excretion in the faeces, surface counting over the liver, whole-body counting, by measuring urinary excretion (the Schilling test) and by measuring radioactivity of the plasma. Only the last two methods are widely used and will be described.

Method

The patient is fasted overnight (water is permitted). The bladder is emptied and urine discarded. Approximately 1 μg of labelled B_{12} is given by mouth and is followed within 2 hours by the intramuscular injection of 1 mg of non-radioactive B_{12} (flushing dose) to saturate the transcobalamins and allow excretion of absorbed B_{12} in the urine. Food may be eaten 2 hours after the oral dose. Urine is collected for 24 hours following the test dose. The radioactivity of the whole sample is calculated and expressed as a percentage of the activity of the dose administered by reference to the activity of a 'standard' representing the test dose. If an aliquot of the urine is to be counted the 24-hour volume is measured, an aliquot counted and compared with a similar aliquot of the standard diluted 1 in 100.

Example of calculations

1. Whole sample counted:

$$\text{Percentage excretion} = \frac{\text{counts per min of 24-hour sample}}{\text{counts per min of test dose}} \times 100$$

2. Aliquot counted:

$$\text{Percentage excretion} = \frac{\text{counts per min/ml of urine} \times \text{24-hour vol}}{\text{counts per min/ml of test dose} \times 100\ \text{(dilution)}} \times 100$$

Results

Normal subjects and hospital control subjects given an oral dose of 1 μg of B_{12} excrete 10% or more in 24 hours. Patients with PA excrete less than 5% and usually less than 2% of the dose. Gastric surgery or intestinal malabsorption of B_{12} may produce results in the PA range but results between 5 and 10% are more usual.

Notes

Falsely low results
Incomplete urine collection is a common cause of false low results. Urine collection in incontinent, uncatheterized patients is clearly unsatisfactory. Incomplete urine collection may be suggested by a 24-hour urine volume of less than 750 ml.

Impaired renal function will delay excretion, and collection should be extended to 48 hours or even 72 hours. The administration of a second 'flushing dose' at 24 hours has been recommended but this may cause problems in interpretation as additional activity is excreted in normal subjects following a second flushing dose. An alternative is to apply a correction factor obtained by the ratio of normal creatinine clearance to the patient's creatinine clearance. The possibility of falsely low values being reported is diminished by combining the Schilling method with the measurement of plasma radioactivity[26].

Falsely high values are unusual but may possibly occur due to contamination with faeces during bedpan urine collection. Other radioactive tracer studies may result in urine radioactivity which will invalidate the results of the Schilling test.

Absorption with added intrinsic factor (IF) (Part II test)

Subnormal excretion may be due to lack of IF or due to malabsorption. After an interval of at least 48 hours the test may be repeated with the simultaneous administration of IF and the percentage excretion determined as for the standard test. Impaired absorption due to lack of IF will be corrected significantly by the added IF. No correction occurs in the presence of B_{12} malabsorption.

Notes

1. The IF is best dissolved in water rather than be given in capsule form.
2. IF antibodies in gastric juice may result in failure to correct absorption by blocking the formation of IF–B_{12} complexes or by binding to complexes and preventing absorption.
3. It is actually appropriate to perform the Part II test first. If there is low excretion in the presence of IF there is little point in performing the test without IF.

Combined test using free and IF-bound B_{12}

A combined test using a dual-isotope modification of the Schilling test can be used[47]. Free [^{58}Co]B_{12} and [^{57}Co]B_{12} bound to IF are given simultaneously, the procedure otherwise being identical with the standard test. The differing energies of the γ emissions of ^{58}Co and ^{57}Co allow the amounts of free and bound B_{12} excreted to be calculated by reference to ^{57}Co and ^{58}Co standards.

Results
In normal subjects equal and normal amounts of each isotope are excreted and if a full 24-hour urine collection has been obtained the results may be expressed as for

the standard tests. In patients with intestinal malabsorption due to causes other than lack of IF, equal but reduced amounts of the isotopes are excreted. In malabsorption due to lack of IF a reduced amount of the free tracer and a normal amount of the bound tracer are excreted.

The normal range of the ratio of bound to unbound tracer is quoted as 0.8–1.3 and in the absence of IF greater than 2.0[48], but these data have been questioned and a ratio of 1.4 has been suggested as providing the best discriminant between the PA and non-PA groups[49] whilst another study suggests a ratio of 1.7[50].

Notes

1. Apart from the saving in time, the advantage claimed for the dual-isotope method is that if urine collection is incomplete or in the presence of renal disease, the ratio of bound to unbound tracer can be used to identify lack of IF.
2. Differences have been pointed out between the excretion levels with the dual-isotope test and those obtained by the standard Schilling test followed by repeat testing with IF[51]. Some exchange of free and bound isotope may occur and a modification in which the bound B_{12} is given 2 hours after the free B_{12} may reduce this effect and thus obtain better separation of PA and non-PA groups[51].

Plasma radioactivity method

The level of radioactivity in plasma during the standard Schilling test reaches a peak 6–14 hours after the oral dose and in normal subjects is usually greater than 0.6% of the oral dose per litre of plasma.

Method

A 20 ml blood sample is taken into dry anticoagulant 8 hours after the oral dose of labelled B_{12}, the plasma separated, the radioactivity compared with that of a 'standard' representing the oral dose and expressed as a percentage of oral dose per litre of plasma. In patients with PA the value is usually less than 0.1%.

Notes

The value of the test is simplicity, its possible use in incontinent patients and particularly as a supplement to the standard Schilling test in the detection of incomplete urine collection or unsuspected renal disease. In one series[26] 21% of Schilling tests revealed a discrepancy between urinary excretion and plasma radioactivity. Incomplete urine collection or renal disease were incriminated in approximately 95% of the discrepant results.

The deoxyuridine suppression test

Principle

The *de novo* synthesis of thymidine triphosphate (dTTP) from deoxyuridine monophosphate (dUMP) via thymidine monophosphate (dTMP) requires 5-10-methylene THF. When *de novo* synthesis is reduced, thymine is available for DNA synthesis from a salvage pathway by the conversion of thymidine deoxyriboside (TdR) to dTMP. The activity of the salvage pathway can be determined by the addition of radioactive TdR ($[^3H]$TdR) and measuring the radioactivity of the resulting DNA.

The addition of deoxyuridine (dU) to cultures of bone-marrow cells in autologous serum in the presence of adequate 5-10-methylene THF will *suppress* the incorporation of [^{3}H]TdR into DNA. Thus normal levels of 5-10-methylene THF will result in low DNA radioactivity, while reduced availability of 5-10-methylene THF due to B_{12} or folate deficiency will give high DNA radioactivity, i.e. 'high suppressed values'. The addition of cobalamins and folate compounds to additional separate cultures has been used to differentiate high suppressed values due to B_{12} or folate deficiency.

Method[52]

Bone marrow is aspirated inhto 5 ml Hanks' solution containing 500 units of preservative-free heparin and a single cell suspension of nucleated marrow cells is prepared by passing the marrow suspension through a 50-mesh, 0.003-inch gauze wire screen or by forcing the suspension once through a 21-gauge and twice through a 25-gauge needle. The cell suspension is centrifuged at 1100 *g* for 5 minutes and the buffy layer re-suspended to produce a nucleated cell count of 5–10 × 10^9/l of Hanks' solution. Marrow cultures with and without dU are set up in duplicate or triplicate by mixing 1 ml of the marrow suspension with 0.5 ml autologous serum, 0.2 ml Hank's solution and 0.2 ml Hank's solution with and without 1 μmol 2-deoxyuridine per ml. The cultures are incubated in a shaking water bath at 37°C for 1 hour after which 0.1 ml of a solution containing 5 μCi (185 kBq) [6-^{3}H]thymidine per ml (specific activity 25 Ci/mmol (825 GBq/mmol)) is added to each culture and the cultures incubated for a further hour. The cells are washed three times in ice-cold isotonic NaCl and resuspended in about 2 ml isotonic NaCl.

The number of nucleated cells in each washed cell suspension is determined by visual counting and two 0.1 ml aliquots of each suspension are delivered on to individual Whatman paper discs (1.9 cm diameter, 3 MM grade). The discs are dried, immersed in ice-cold 10% trichloroacetic acid for 20 minutes, washed in two changes of absolute ethanol (10 minutes each), rinsed briefly in acetone and finally dried and counted in standard scintillation fluid in a β-counter. The amount of [^{3}H]TdR incorporated into the DNA of 10^6 nucleated cells is calculated from the average counts per minute per disc and the total number of cells on each disc. The uptake of [^{3}H]TdR after pre-incubation with dU is expressed as a percentage of the uptake without pre-incubation with dU. This percentage is called the dU-suppressed value. With the technique described it is possible to aspirate a sample of marrow in the morning and obtain a result in the afternoon of the same day.

Results

Normal range of the dU-suppressed value is 1.4–8.6% with a modal mean of 3.5%. Values greater than 9.0% indicate B_{12} or folate deficiency irrespective of other haematological parameters. The dU-suppressed values obtained in a variety of disorders have been reported[53,54].

Applications

The test has been proved to be a sensitive and relatively simple method of diagnosing B_{12} or folate deficiency and is particularly useful when:

1. There is little or no anaemia.
2. Bone-marrow morphology is equivocal.
3. In the presence of coexistent iron deficiency.
4. When serum B_{12} and red-cell folate are within the normal range.

Application of the test has been limited by:

1. The need to use bone-marrow cells.
2. The test must be performed on the same day of marrow aspiration.
3. The time taken in the performance of the test.
4. The need for a β counter.

Some of these limitations may be overcome by the use of [^{125}I]dU instead of [^{3}H]TdR, and the use of lymphocyte suspensions or whole blood instead of bone-marrow cells[55–57].

The addition of cobalamins and folate compounds in the differentiation of B_{12} and folate deficiency

The high dU-suppressed values of B_{12}-deficient marrow cells are partially corrected by the addition of cyanocobalamin while the values of folate-deficient marrow are not. The addition of folate compounds corrects the high dU-suppressed values of folate-deficient marrow but may also correct the high values of B_{12}-deficient marrow. There is conflicting information on the best form of additive and its final concentration to obtain clear differentiation of B_{12} and folate deficiency[58]. The cobalamin derivative may not be important but 5-methyl THF appears to be more specific for folate deficiency than PGA or folinic acid. A protocol for the dU suppression test with the addition of additives has been described that includes additional control tubes[59] but the necessity for additional controls when testing human bone marrow has been questioned[60].

Detection of antibodies to intrinsic factor

The demonstration of antibodies to intrinsic factor (IFab) in megaloblastic anaemia with a low serum B_{12} is virtually diagnostic of pernicious anaemia[61] and can obviate the need to perform Schilling tests.

The most widely used methods are based on the method of Gottlieb *et al.* [62] which detect Type I (blocking) IFab. The method involves adding ^{57}Co-labelled B_{12} to gastric juice in the presence of test serum. If antibodies are present the binding of B_{12} to the IF in the gastric juice is prevented. Free isotope is separated from bound isotope by albumin- or haemoglobin-coated charcoal. Using this approach IFab in serum can be demonstrated in only 50–60% of patients with pernicious anaemia and therefore is of limited sensitivity. By increasing the ratio of serum to IF a detection rate of 78% has been claimed[63].

A limitation of the Gottlieb and similar methods is the unsaturated binding capacity of the endogenous binding proteins (transcobalamins) in the test serum. To overcome this problem, the binding capacity of the serum can be saturated with non-radioactive cobalamin or the binding protein (transcobalamin II, TCII) can be absorbed out by a microfine precipitate of silica (QUSO).

An alternative approach which has been adopted in commercially available kits is to immobilize purified IF on a solid-phase binder such as micro-crystalline cellulose and incubate with serum. IF, if present, will interact with the IF reducing the number of available B_{12} binding sites. The solid phase is then separated by centrifugation, discarding the supernatant containing the endogenous TCII, and resuspending in the presence of ^{57}Co-labelled B_{12} which binds to sites still available.

A possible problem in all the above methods is the presence of free B_{12} in serum, particularly from patients treated by B_{12} injections; at least 7 days should elapse from the last treatment. Free B_{12} due to bacterial contamination of the sample must be avoided. Thus a positive IFab result in the presence of a high serum B_{12} value should be interpreted with caution. Alternatively, a high level of IFab may interfere with some B_{12} radioassays causing spuriously high results.

Conn [64] has described a cheap, rapid and reproducible assay which relies on the binding of IFab to ^{125}I-labelled purified IF and the subsequent precipitation of the antigen/antibody complex with polyethylene glycol. The sensitivity of the assay is similar to previously published series using charcoal absorption. The method has been expanded to demonstrate Type II (binding) IFab [65].

Quantitation of IFab has been approached by making serial dilutions of IFab-positive sera. There is clearly a need for an IF reference preparation if quantitation can be shown to be of value.

Quantitation of transcobalamins

The absence of TCII causes severe B_{12}-deficient megaloblastic anaemia and therefore its measurement can be important, albeit rarely. The quantitation of TCI and TCIII can be of value in the investigation of liver disease and myeloproliferative disorders.

Measurement of TC levels in serum are higher than those using plasma. This is due to the release of TCI and TCIII from granulocytes. Although it is generally assumed that TCII is derived from the liver, some arise from granulocytes. Plasma from blood collected into EDTA with added NaF is to be preferred [66].

TCII is selectively absorbed by microfine precipitated silica (QUSO). TCI and TCIII are absorbed by diethylaminoethyl (DEAE) and the absorbed TCIII can be selectively released by washing the DEAE in 0.06 M phosphate buffer. By combining separation techniques with measurement of unsaturated B_{12} binding capacity (UBBC) of each fraction, the amount of each TC can be determined [66].

References

1. Proctor, S. J., Cox, J. R. and Sheridan, T. J. (1976) Anisocytosis and the C-1000 Channelyser in macrocytic anaemia. *J. Clin. Pathol.*, **29**, 719–23
2. Davidson, R. J. L. and Hamilton, P. J. (1978) High mean red-cell volume: its incidence and significance in routine haematology. *J. Clin. Pathol.*, **31**, 493–8
3. McPhedean, P., Barnes, M. G., Weinstein, J. S. and Robertson, J. S. (1973) Interpretation of electronically determined macrocytosis. *Ann. Intern. Med.*, **78**, 677–83
4. Chanarin, I., England, J. M. and Hoffbrand, A. V. (1973) Significance of large blood cells. *Br. J. Haematol.*, **23**, 351–8
5. Chanarin, I., McFadyen, I. R. and Kyle, R. (1977) The physiological macrocytosis of pregnancy. *Br. J. Obstet. Gynaecol.*, **84**, 504–8

6. Cauchi, M. N. and Smith, M. B. (1982) Quantitative aspects of red cell size variation in pregnancy. *Clin. Lab. Haematol.,* **4**, 149–54
7. Wisloff, F. and Boman, D. (1979) Acquired stomatocytosis in alcoholic liver disease. *Scand. J. Haematol.,* **23**, 43–50
8. Burns, E. R., Reed, L. J. and Wenz, B. (1986) Volumetric erythrocyte macrocytosis induced by hydroxyurea. *Am. J. Clin. Pathol.,* **85**, 337–41
9. Hoffbrand, A. V., Ganeshagaru, K., Hooton, J. W. I. and Tripp, E. (1976) Megaloblastic anaemia: initiation of DNA synthesis in excess of DNA chain elongation as the underlying mechanism. *Clin. Haematol.,* **5**, 727–45
10. Chanarin, I., Deacon, R., Lumb, M. and Perry, J. (1980) Vitamin B_{12} regulates folate metabolism by the supply of formate. *Lancet,* **ii**, 505–8
11. Chanarin, I., Deacon, R., Lumb, M., Muir, M. and Perry, J. (1985) Cobalamin–folate interrelationships: a critical review. *Blood,* **66**, 479–89
12. Chanarin, I. (1987) Megaloblastic anaemia, cobalamin and folate. *J. Clin. Pathol.,* **40**, 978–84
13. Cullen, M. H., Rees, G. M., Nancekievill, D. G. and Amess, J. A. L. (1979) The effect of nitrous oxide on the cell cycle in human bone marrow. *Br. J. Haematol.,* **42**, 527–34
14. Wickramasinghe, S. N. and Bush, V. (1977) An investigation into the development and fate of neutrophil giant metamyelocytes using the techniques of electron microscopy and high resolution autoradiography. *Br. J. Haematol.,* **35**, 659–64
15. Herbert, V. (1962) Experimental nutritional folate deficiency in man. *Trans. Assoc. Am. Phys.,* **75**, 307–20
16. Lankowsky, P. (1970) Congenital malabsorption of folate. *Am. J. Med.,* **48**, 580–3
17. Erbe, R. W. (1975) Inborn errors of folate metabolism (part 2). *N. Engl. J. Med.,* **293**, 807–12
18. Katz, M., Lee, S. K. and Cooper, B. A. (1972) Vitamin B_{12} malabsorption due to a biologically inert intrinsic factor. *N. Engl. J. Med.,* **287**, 425–9
19. Grasbeck, R. (1972) Familial selective vitamin B_{12} malabsorption. *N. Engl. J. Med.,* **287**, 358
20. Mathews, J. H. and Wood, J. K. (1984) Megaloblastic anaemia in vegetarian Asians. *Clin. Lab. Haematol.,* **6**, 1–7
21. Nex, E., Olesen, H., Norredam, K. and Schwartz, M. (1975) A rare cause of megaloblastic anaemia caused by disturbance in the plasma cobalamin binding proteins in a patient with hepatocellular carcinoma. *Scand. J. Haematol.,* **14**, 320–7
22. Haurani, F. I., Hall, C. A. and Rubin, R. (1979) Megaloblastic anaemia due to abnormal transcobalamin II (Cardeza). *J. Clin. Invest.,* **64**, 1253–9
23. Rosenberg, L. E. and Patel, L. (1975) Absence of a cobalamin binding protein in cultured fibroblasts from patients with defective cobalamin coenzyme synthesis. *Clin. Res.,* **23**, 399A
24. Carmel, R., Bedros, A. A., Mace, J. W. and Goodman, S. I. (1980) Congenital methylmalonic aciduria–homocysteinuria with megaloblastic anaemia. Observations on response to hydroxycobalamin and on the effect of homocysteine and methionine on the deoxyuridine suppression test. *Blood,* **55**, 570–9
25. Lampkin, B. C., Shore, N. A. and Chadwick, D. (1966) Megaloblastic anaemia of infancy secondary to maternal pernicious anaemia. *N. Engl. J. Med.,* **274**, 1168–71
26. Chanarin, I. and Waters, D. A. W. (1974) Failed Schilling tests. *Scand. J. Haematol.,* **12**, 245–8
27. Streeter, A. M., Bathur, F. A., Arnold, B. J., Crane, G. G. and Pheils, M. T. (1981) Limitations of the Schilling test. *Lancet,* **i**, 39–40
28. Gozzard, D. I., Dawson, D. W. and Lewis, M. J. (1987) Experience with dual protein bound aqueous vitamin B_{12} absorption test in subjects with low serum vitamin B_{12} concentration. *J. Clin. Pathol.,* **40**, 633–7
29. England, J. M. and Linnell, J. C. (1980) Problems with the serum B_{12} assay. *Lancet,* **ii**, 1072–4
30. Linnell, J. C. (1981) The value of radioisotopic assays for 'serum B_{12}' in the diagnosis of cobalamin deficiency disorders. *Clin. Lab. Haematol.,* **3**, 99–106
31. Anderson, B. (1964) Investigations into the Euglena method for the assay of vitamin B_{12} in serum. *J. Clin. Pathol.,* **17**, 14–26
32. Dacie, J. V. and Lewis, S. M. (1975) *Practical Haematology*, 5th edn., pp. 478–80. London: Churchill Livingstone

33. Sourial, N. A. (1981) Use of an improved *E. coli* method for the measurement of cobalamin in serum: comparison with the *E. gracilis* assay results. *J. Clin. Pathol.*, **34**, 351–6
34. Kolhouse, J. F., Kondo, H., Allen, N. C., Podell, E. and Allen, R. H. (1978) Cobalamin analogues are present in human plasma and can mask cobalamin deficiency because current radioisotope dilution assays are not specific for true cobalamins. *N. Engl. J. Med.*, **299**, 785–92
35. Cooper, B. A. and Whitehead, V. M. (1978) Evidence that some patients with pernicious anaemia are not recognised by radiodilution assay for cobalamins in serum. *N. Engl. J. Med.*, **299**, 816–18
36. International Committee for Standardisation in Haematology (1986) Proposed serum standard for human serum vitamin B_{12} assay. *Br. J. Haematol.*, **64**, 809–11
37. Chanarin, I. and Muir, M. (1982) Demonstration of vitamin B_{12} analogues in human serum not detected by microbiological assay. *Br. J. Haematol.*, **51**, 171–3
38. Muir, M. and Chanarin, I. (1983) Solid-phase vitamin B_{12} assays using polyacrylamide-bound intrinsic factor and polyacrylamide-bound R-binder. *Br. J. Haematol.*, **53**, 423–35
39. Muir, M. and Chanarin, I. (1983) Separation of cobalamin analogues in human serum binding to intrinsic factor and to R-type vitamin B_{12} binders. *Br. J. Haematol.*, **54**, 613–21
40. Curtis, A. D., Mussett, M. V. and Kennedy, D. A. (1986) British Standard for human serum vitamin B_{12}. *Clin. Lab. Haematol.*, **8**, 135–47
41. Davis, R. E., Nicol, D. J. and Kelly, A. (1970) An automated method for the measurement of folate activity. *J. Clin. Pathol.*, **23**, 47–53
42. Millbank, L., Davis, R. E., Rawlins, M. and Waters, A. H. (1970) Automation of the assay of folate in serum and whole blood. *J. Clin. Pathol.*, **23**, 54–9
43. Cooper, B. A. (1973) Superiority of simplified assay for folate with *Lactobacillus casei* ATCC 7469 over assay with chloramphenicol-adapted strain. *J. Clin. Pathol.*, **26**, 963–7
44. Waxman, S. and Schreiber, C. (1973) Measurement of serum folate levels and serum folic acid-binding protein by ^{3}HPGA radioassay. *Blood*, **42**, 281–90
45. Rothenberg, S. P. and Da Costa, M. (1976) Folate binding proteins and radioassay for folate. *Clin. Haematol.*, **5**, 569–87
46. Bain, B. J., Wickramasinghe, S. N., Broom, G. N., Litwinczuk, R. A. and Sima, J. (1984) Assessment of the value of a competitive protein binding radioassay of folic acid in the detection of folic acid deficiency. *J. Clin. Pathol.*, **37**, 388–94
47. Bell, T. K., Bridges, J. M. and Nelson, M. G. (1965) Simultaneous free and and bound radioactive vitamin B_{12} urinary excretion test. *J. Clin. Pathol.*, **18**, 611–13
48. Amersham International. Dicopac. Company literature
49. Pathy, M. S., Kirkman, S. and Molloy, M. J. (1979) An evaluation of simultaneously administered free and intrinsic factor bound radioactive cyanocobalamin in the diagnosis of pernicious anaemia in the elderly. *J. Clin. Pathol.*, **32**, 244–50
50. Domstad, P. A., Young, C. C., Edmund, K. E. and Deland, F. H. (1981) Reliability of the dual-isotope Schilling test for the diagnosis of pernicious anaemia or malabsorption syndrome. *Am. J. Clin. Pathol.*, **75**, 723–6
51. Briedis, D., McIntyre, P. A., Judisch, J. and Wagner, H. N. (1973) An evaluation of a dual isotope method for the measurement of vitamin B_{12} absorption. *J. Nucl. Med.*, **14**, 135–41
52. Wickramasinghe, S. N. and Longland, J. E. (1974) Assessment of deoxyuridine suppression test in diagnosis of vitamin B_{12} or folate deficiency. *Br. Med. J.*, **ii**, 148–50
53. Wickramasinghe, S. N. and Saunders, J. E. (1977) Results of three years experience with the deoxyuridine suppression test. *Acta Haematol.*, **58**, 193–206
54. Wickramasinghe, S. N. (1981) The deoxyuridine suppression test: a review of its clinical and research applications. *Clin. Lab. Haematol.*, **3**, 1–18
55. Herbert, V., Tisman, G., Le-Teng-Go and Brenner, L. (1973) The dU-suppression test using ^{125}I-UdR to define biochemical megaloblastosis. *Br. J. Haematol.*, **24**, 713–23
56. Das, K. C. and Hoffbrand, A. V. (1970) Lymphocyte transformation in megaloblastic anaemia: morphology and DNA synthesis. *Br. J. Haematol.*, **19**, 459–68
57. Das, K. C., Manusselis, C. and Herbert, V. (1980) Simplifying lymphocyte culture and the deoxyuridine suppression test by using whole blood (0.1 ml) instead of separated lymphocytes. *Clin. Chem.*, **26**, 72–7

58. Ganeshagaru, K. and Hoffbrand, A. V. (1978) The effect of deoxyuridine, vitamin B_{12}, folate and alcohol on the uptake of thymidine and on the deoxynucleoside triphosphate concentration in normal and megaloblastic cells. *Br. J. Haematol.*, **40**, 29–41
59. Wickramasinghe, S. N. and Saunders, J. E. (1979) A fault in the design of the deoxyuridine suppression test. *Clin. Lab. Haematol.*, **1**, 69–71
60. Deacon, R., Chanarin, I., Perry, J. and Lumb, M. (1981) The effect of folate analogues on thymidine utilisation by human and rat marrow cells and the effect on the deoxyuridine suppression test. *Postgrad. Med. J.*, **57**, 611–16
61. Lindenbaum, J. (1983) Status of laboratory testing in the diagnosis of megaloblastic anaemia. *Blood,* **61**, 624–7
62. Gottlieb, C., Lau, K. S., Wasserman, L. R. and Herbert, V. (1965) Rapid charcoal assay for intrinsic factor (IF), gastric juice unsaturated B_{12} binding capacity, antibody to IF and serum unsaturated B_{12} binding capacity. *Blood,* **25**, 875–84
63. Nimo, R. E. and Carmel, R. (1987) Increased sensitivity of detection of the blocking (Type I) anti-intrinsic factor antibody. *Am. J. Clin. Pathol.*, **88,** 729–33
64. Conn, D. A. (1986) Intrinsic factor antibody detection and quantitation. *Med. Lab. Sci.*, **43**, 48–52
65. Conn, D. A. (1986) Detection of Type I and Type II antibodies to intrinsic factor. *Med. Lab. Sci.*, **43**, 148–51
66. Jacob, E., Wong, K.-T. J. and Herbert, V. (1977) A simple method for the separate measurement of transcobalamins I, II and III: normal range in serum and plasma in men and women. *J. Lab. Clin. Med.*, **89**, 1145–52

Chapter 11

Anaemias. III. Haemolytic anaemias

Haemolytic anaemias are characterized by a reduced red-cell life span. The fundamental reason for a reduced red-cell life span, excluding that due to bleeding, is damage or loss of integrity of the red-cell membrane.

Mechanisms leading to reduced red-cell survival

The mechanisms may be classified as follows:

1. Changes in membrane permeability:
   (a) Increased cation permeability.
   (b) Macromolecular permeability (haemolysis).
2. Fragmentation:
   (a) By extracellular mechanisms.
   (b) Due to intracellular defects.
   (c) Phagocytic fragmentation.
3. Erythrophagocytosis.

Most of these mechanisms are probably extensions of the physiological processes involved in the removal of ageing normal red cells, notably cation permeability, fragmentation and erythrophagocytosis.

Increased cation permeability

The high potassium and low sodium content of the normal red cell is maintained by a cation pump requiring ATP generated by the Embden–Meyerhof pathway. The control of cation transport may be put under stress by either reduced ATP activity, passive cation diffusion across the cell membrane or a combination of these factors. Maintenance of red-cell flexibility also depends on a low membrane calcium content and studies in haemolytic states, particularly sickle-cell anaemia, indicate that cation permeability with an increase in red-cell calcium is associated with increased cell rigidity, which contributes significantly to reduced cell survival.

Macromolecular permeability (loss of haemoglobin, haemolysis)

Loss of haemoglobin through the cell membrane will only occur if the membrane is modified by the action of chemicals, bacterial toxins, venoms or by activation of the complement pathway. Chemicals such as soaps, detergents and saponin when introduced accidentally into the circulation can cause massive haemolysis due to gross disruption of the lipid structure of the red-cell membrane. Bacterial exotoxins may have a powerful lytic action, as for example the α-toxin of *Clostridium perfringens* which by virtue of its lecithinase activity produces haemolytic lysolecithin. Several snake venoms are powerful haemolysins, a property that has been used in laboratory tests.

Complement may be adsorbed on to the cell membrane by association with antibodies directed against antigens on the membrane or by direct adsorption on to the membrane. Whatever the method of adsorption, activation of the complement pathway leads to membrane damage and haemolysis.

Fragmentation by extrinsic mechanisms

Thermal injury

In vitro studies suggest that the critical temperature above which red-cell damage occurs is 47–48°C. In severely burned patients extreme microspherocytosis apparently due to 'budding' of red cells and schistocytosis (*Figure 11.1*) may be accompanied by acute transient haemolysis with haemoglobinuria. The shortened survival of heat-damaged red cells has been applied to the study of spleen size and function (*see* page 490).

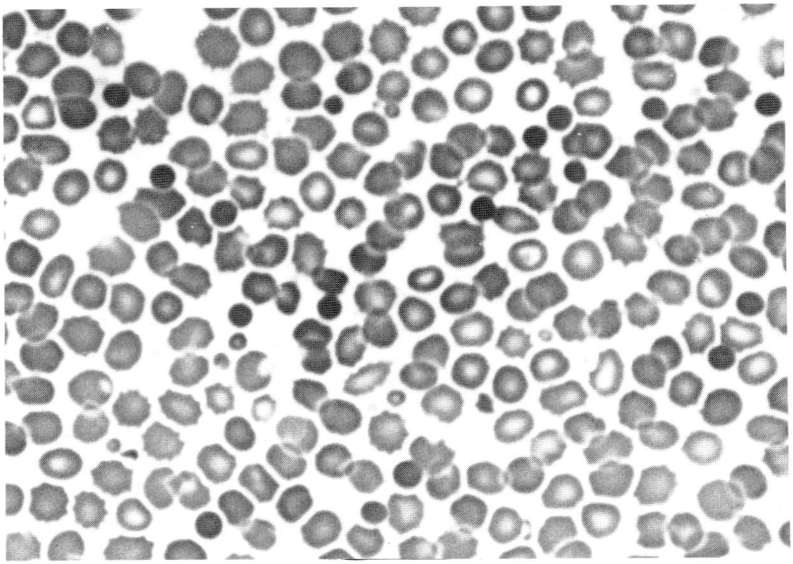

Figure 11.1 Blood film. Heat-damaged red cells due to burns. Extreme fragmentation and microspherocyte formation. ×550

Intravascular fragmentation by shearing

Fragmentation of a different appearance (*Figure 11.2*) has been reported in a wide variety of disorders such as carcinomatosis, thrombotic thrombocytopenic purpura, malignant hypertension, haemolytic-uraemic syndrome, etc. Two possible

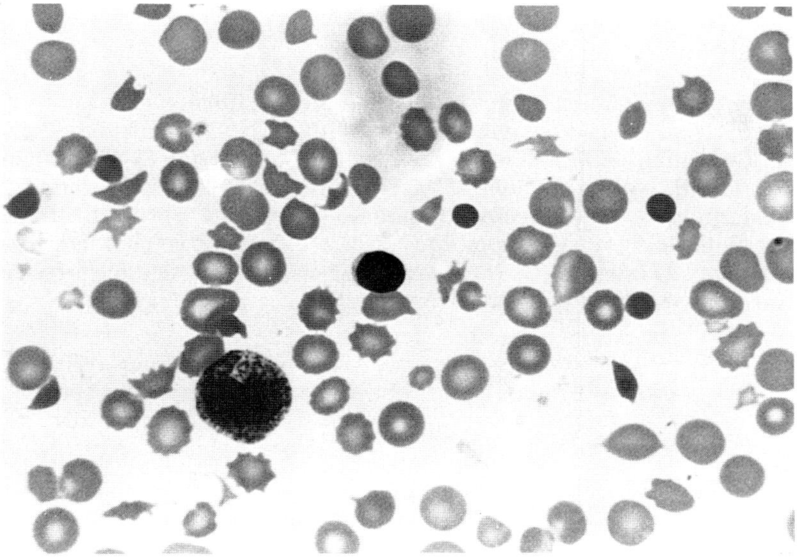

Figure 11.2 Blood film. Microangiopathic haemolytic anaemia. Markedly distorted red cells and some fragments. Note the angular irregularities and spherocyte formation. ×550

mechanisms have been suggested each supported by *in vitro* experiments and by observations in man and animals. (1) Fragmentation due to formation of fibrin strands within blood vessels; blood flowing through such strands results in shearing and the formation of the typical red-cell shapes. (2) Fragmentation by red cells adhering to and being extruded between damaged endothelial cells thus causing fragmentation which is indistinguishable from that due to fibrin formation. However, an alternative mechanism is probable in haemolytic-uraemic syndrome.

Cardiac surgery

Red-cell fragmentation probably indistinguishable from that described above has been commonly observed in patients after cardiac surgery for repair of septal defects or more commonly after the implantation of prosthetic heart valves. The mechanism of fragmentation has been ascribed to cells striking non-physiological surfaces such as implanted Teflon or due to turbulence and extreme shear rates in the artificial valves.

'March' haemoglobinuria

The occurrence of haemoglobinuria in certain athletes after extended running is probably due to the regular and continuous compression of the vessels of the feet, causing red-cell fragmentation. Haemoglobinuria has also been observed in exponents of Karate and in bongo-drum players. It is not usually possible to demonstrate red-cell changes in the blood during or immediately following such episodes. Gross disintegration of the red cells under such stress is a likely mechanism, though a structural protein abnormality has been suggested which would explain why the majority of athletes do not experience haemoglobinuria [1].

Fragmentation due to intracellular abnormalities

Heinz-body formation

The denaturation of haemoglobin – whether due to inherent molecular instability, diminished reductive potential or overwhelming oxidative stress – results in Heinz-body formation. Oxidation of –SH– groups, polymer formation via –S–S– bridges and attachment to the –SH– groups of the membrane results in reduced deformability, retention in the reticuloendothelial system and extrusion of the inclusion bodies with loss of cell membrane which produces a characteristic 'bitten-out' appearance (*Figure 11.3*). If the oxidative challenge is severe, massive intravascular lysis may occur with haemoglobinuria.

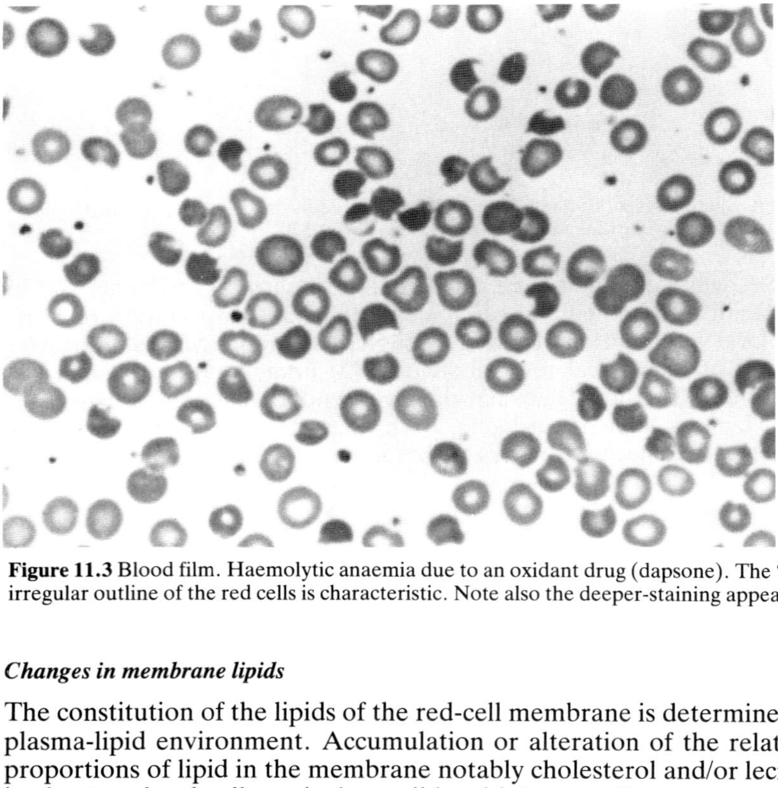

Figure 11.3 Blood film. Haemolytic anaemia due to an oxidant drug (dapsone). The 'bitten-out', irregular outline of the red cells is characteristic. Note also the deeper-staining appearance. ×550

Changes in membrane lipids

The constitution of the lipids of the red-cell membrane is determined largely by the plasma-lipid environment. Accumulation or alteration of the relative or absolute proportions of lipid in the membrane notably cholesterol and/or lecithin may result in shortened red-cell survival, possibly with 'spur-cell' or acanthocyte formation.

Progression to spherocytosis occurs probably due to progressive loss of cell membrane by fragmentation.

Abnormality in cytoskeletal proteins

The phosphorylation of spectrin by both cyclic-nucleotide (cAMP) dependent and independent protein kinases, interaction with actin, band 4.1, ankyrin and the role of calcium in maintaining red-cell integrity is generally accepted. Abnormalities of cytoskeletal proteins are recognized in hereditary spherocytosis, elliptocytosis, stomatocytosis and pyropoikilocytosis. Increased heat sensitivity of red cells producing fragmentation is found in hereditary pyropoikilocytosis and is due to an abnormal spectrin.

Phagocytic fragmentation

Complement activation

The adsorption of complement components on to red cells, classically in association with complement-binding antibodies, results in activation to the C1423 stage. Macrophages of the reticuloendothelial system have specific receptors for the C3 component C3b. Attachment of red cells to the macrophages via the specific receptors results in partial membrane phagocytosis and leads to membrane loss and spherocyte formation.

Adsorption of non-complement-binding IgG

Monocytes and lymphocytes have specific receptors for red cells sensitized with non-complement binding IgG antibodies (notably IgG_1 and IgG_3 subclasses). The Fc fragment of the IgG molecule carries the site for the receptors of the phagocytic cells. Again, partial red-cell fragmentation occurs, sometimes associated with characteristic distortion.

Erythrophagocytosis

Erythrophagocytosis is probably a normal physiological process, and can be seen in sections of normal lymph nodes. However, in lymphoreticular proliferations, erythrophagocytosis may be greatly increased. Similarly, bone-marrow histology in haemolytic disorders may display obvious erythrophagocytosis. In haemolytic anaemias due to complement-binding antibodies of the Donath–Landsteiner type (*see* page 329), erythrophagocytosis by monocytes is often a feature and probably represents a significant mechanism in the removal of the complement-coated red cells.

Classification of haemolytic anaemias

From an investigative aspect the most suitable approach to classification of haemolytic anaemias is by separating those due to fundamental defects of the red cell (intracorpuscular defects) from those due to extracorpuscular mechanisms. This classification has a firm pathophysiological basis which can usually be clearly demonstrated by cross-transfusion experiments. Some haemolytic anaemias, however, have features of both intra- and extracorpuscular mechanisms, e.g. the reduced red-cell survival in untreated megaloblastic anaemia. The main causes of haemolysis, classified on the above basis, are as follows:

1. Intracorpuscular abnormalities:
   (a) Primary disorders of the red-cell membrane:
   (i) hereditary spherocytosis; (ii) hereditary elliptocytosis; (iii) hereditary stomatocytosis; (iv) hereditary xerocytosis; (v) hereditary pyropoikilocytosis.

(b) Disordered red-cell enzymes:
(i) defects in the hexose monophosphate pathway (HMP); (ii) defects in the Embden–Myerhof pathway (EMP); (iii) abnormal nucleotide metabolism.
(c) Inherited abnormalities of the haemoglobin molecule:
(i) abnormalities due to amino-acid substitutions or deletions;
(ii) thalassaemia syndromes (*see* Chapter 9).
(d) Paroxysmal nocturnal haemoglobinuria.
(e) Disordered erythropoiesis:
(i) megaloblastosis (*see* Chapter 10); (ii) erythroleukaemia (*see* Chapter 13); (iii) primary acquired sideroblastic anaemia (*see* Chapter 12).

2. Extracorpuscular defects:
(a) Due to red-cell antibodies:
(i) autoantibodies; (ii) drug-associated antibodies; (iii) passively acquired antibodies; (iv) isoantibodies reacting with transfused red cells.
(b) Direct action of drugs, chemicals, toxins or venoms.
(c) Direct mechanism or physical trauma to red cells.
(d) Due to abnormal membrane lipids secondary to plasma abnormalities:
(i) acanthocytosis; (ii) lecithin:cholesterol acyl transferase (LCAT) deficiency; (iii) abetalipoproteinaemia; (iv) other lipid disturbances.

Primary disorders of the red-cell membrane

Hereditary spherocytosis (HS)

This disorder is predominantly and classically inherited as an autosomal dominant though the gene effect is very variable even within the same family and is reflected by less than the expected number of affected siblings and by some affected persons being clinically and haematologically normal as judged by red-cell morphology, osmotic fragility had haemoglobin turnover. A rare autosomal recessive type has been described. A linkage between HS and chromosome 8p has been described[2]. The incidence of HS is about 1 in 5000 in North Europeans.

The red-cell membrane is abnormal and allows an increased influx of sodium though the intracellular sodium level is maintained at a normal value by an increased sodium efflux under the control of the ATP-dependent sodium pump. This results in an increase in ATP breakdown which stimulates increased red-cell glycolysis with an inevitable increased requirement for glucose. Membrane lipid content is decreased and the loss of cholesterol and phospholipid is proportional which suggests an actual loss of membrane resulting in a reduced surface area and consequent sphering. Scanning electron microscopy can show that only a small proportion of the cells are in fact true spherocytes, the majority being stomatospherocytes. Although it has been suggested that the increased sodium efflux results in the loss of membrane there is no direct link with the increased activity of the sodium pump; in hereditary stomatocytosis the sodium pump is more active than in HS yet membrane lipid is not lost.

It is now clear that the primary molecular defect in HS is in the structure of the cytoskeleton. Studies have shown that membranes from all types of HS are partially deficient in spectrin[3, 4] due to either reduced spectrin synthesis, unstable forms or impaired binding to the membrane. Spectrin defects may be of α or β subunits and defective spectrin band 4.1 binding has been described. Abnormal phosphorylation appears unlikely to be a primary defect but rather that the function of phosphorylated protein is defective. The association of membrane calcium with spectrin phosphorylation and the role of increased calcium levels in reducing cell deformability is probably relevant. Reticulocytes are normal in shape, the spherocytosis being a progressive change associated with cell ageing. The rigidity or lack of deformability of spherocytes is of great significance in the passage of the cells through the spleen. Stagnation of red cells in the splenic cords is a feature in HS. Splenic trapping may be detrimental to metabolism, membrane structure or result in phagocytic damage. Decreased pO_2 and pH in the spleen may exaggerate the lack of deformability. Reduced availability of glucose, and consequent reduced glycolysis with lowered ATP production, may be a factor in splenic haemolysis though repeated 'passes' through the spleen are required to cause metabolic deprivation. Direct phagocytosis may be observed and oxidant radicals produced by activated phagocytic cells may induce haemolysis.

It is therefore clear that the spleen plays a paramount role in the pathogenesis of the anaemia in HS and judging by red-cell sequestration studies and response to splenectomy the spleen is the major site of red-cell destruction. Splenectomy results in the red-cell life span returning to near normal. The spherocytosis is, however, *not* improved and indeed as the red cells survive longer the spherocytosis increases as evidenced by red-cell morphology and osmotic fragility studies. The anaemia of HS varies considerably between affected subjects and even within the same family though only rarely is the haemoglobin value less than 7 g/dl. Compensated haemolysis is not unusual, a normal haemoglobin value being maintained by a reticulocytosis over 5%. The blood film in non-splenectomized cases shows regular spherocytes which contrast with the larger non-spherocytic polychromatic cells. In mildly affected cases the degree of spherocytosis in the film may be slight but nevertheless is probably a more sensitive indication than the standard osmotic fragility test. The MCV is normal or perhaps in the lower range of normal and the MCHC lies in the upper normal range and may be above 36 g/dl.

The red-cell life span varies from about 6 to 20 days, and ^{51}Cr labelling shows marked accumulation of radioactivity in the spleen. Normal cells survive normally in the patients' circulation proving the intracorpuscular nature of the disorder. The direct antiglobulin test is negative and is an important test in the differentiation of HS from spherocytic haemolytic states due to other causes, notably that due to immune mechanisms. The occurrence of parvovirus infection in patients with HS can result in a precipitate fall in haemoglobin level due to a halt in red-cell production which is reflected by a reduction or absence of reticulocytes. The bone marrow may show red-cell hypoplasia or marked maturation arrest at the early erythroblast stage. Mild, compensated examples of HS, or indeed any chronic haemolytic process, may be first recognized by acute, severe anaemia due to the red-cell 'aplasia' following infection by parvovirus [5]. The crisis is usually self-limiting. Megaloblastic change due to folate deficiency may occur, particularly during pregnancy.

A frequent additional clinical finding is the presence of pigment stones in the biliary tract due to the increased haemoglobin catabolism. Blood films should be examined from patients with biliary stone, particularly in young persons. Splenectomy corrects the haemolytic process and results in 'the post-splenectomy red-cell picture' though additional red-cell shape changes may be found. Spherocytosis is present at birth and is a cause of neonatal jaundice. HS must therefore be considered in the differential diagnosis of hyperbilirubinaemia in the newborn and in particular be differentiated from the spherocytic red-cell picture associated with ABO haemolytic disease.

Hereditary elliptocytosis and related disorders

Hereditary elliptocytosis (HE) is a heterogeneous group of disorders which differ in red-cell morphology, clinical expression and molecular pathology. The majority are inherited as an autosomal dominant and in North Europeans the incidence is about 1 in 3000. However, the incidence of haemolysis is much less and is variously reported as being as low as 12% and as high as 50%. It is clear that data are influenced by the populations studied and whether indirect evidence of haemolysis is sought or red-cell survival studies performed. In the UK the figure of 12% is certainly nearer the true incidence but is still probably an overestimate. Although the majority of examples of HE do not show haemolysis, the abnormality has been the subject of intensive study because of the wide range of clinical expression and has resulted in the definition of the molecular defects in relation to clinical severity.

Classification of HE

On the basis of elliptocyte morphology HE can be divided into three major categories [6] – biconcave (common) HE (CHE), spherocytic HE and stomatocytic HE. On the basis of clinical severity CHE can be further divided into nine subgroups ranging from non-haemolytic to severe homozygous HE and hereditary pyropoikolocytosis (HPP). Spherocytic HE exhibits heterozygous (mild) and homozygous (severe) forms while stomatocytic HE shows mild or no haemolysis [7]. An asymptomatic carrier type with normal red-cell morphology is also recognized. A molecular approach to classification can be made but does not necessarily correlate with the morphological appearances or clinical severity.

The most common defect, found in a subpopulation of CHE and in all HPP patients, is the spectrin dimer (SpD) self-association defect in which the abnormality is localized in the αI domain of spectrin which is the SpD–SpD contact site [8]. Three major variants of the αI domain have been detected: $Sp\alpha^{I/74}$, $Sp\alpha^{I/46}$ and $Sp\alpha^{I/65}$. Briefly, the nomenclature is that of reference [2]: Sp = spectrin; $\alpha = \alpha$ chain; I = the domain obtained by tryptic digestion I–V; superscript number refers to the molecular weight (kd) of a peptide replacing the normal 80 kd peptide of αI. β subunit variants have also been described. Partial or complete deficiencies of protein 4.1 are associated with mild and severe haemolysis respectively. The gene for protein 4.1 is located on the short arm of chromosome 1 (1*p*32→1*p*ter) which is the location of the Rhesus blood group locus and which explains the linkage expressed by some families of HE and the Rh phenotype. Defective spectrin–ankyrin (2.1) binding and ankyrin–protein 3 interaction have also been described in HE. Further molecular defects continue to be identified [9–12] and the nomenclature has now incorporated geographical locations to identify variants, e.g. spectrin Tunis ($\alpha^{I/78}$) [10].

Blood findings

In CHE elliptocytes comprise 20–100% of red cells though normal morphology does not exclude a structural defect. Evidence for haemolysis includes anisocytosis (or increased RDW), additional poikilocytic changes and polychromasia. Spherocytes may be a feature. Of particular relevance is the striking poikilocytosis and microcytosis of 'HE with infantile poikilocytosis' predominantly seen in Negroes and which reverts to mild CHE after the first year of life [13].

Hereditary pyropoikilocytosis (HPP) is associated with gross micro-poikilocytosis, micro-spherocytes and few elliptocytes. Unlike most forms of CHE and HS the disorder has autosomal recessive inheritance and occurs mainly in Negroes [7]. The disorder is characterized by marked thermal instability of red cells at a temperature as low as 46°C (cf. normal red cells >49°C). The thermal instability reflects instability of abnormal spectrin. It is emphasized, however, that red-cell thermal instability is found in other forms of HE due to spectrin defects.

Stomatocytic HE is common in Melanesians (about 30%) and may reflect selective protection from malarial infection of the red cells.

The mechanism of haemolysis in HE is unclear. Normal red cells can adopt reversible elliptical shapes under shear stress. *In vitro* evidence suggests that in HE deformability is reduced and the red cells are more susceptible to stress fragmentation. Instability of the cytoskeleton can also be demonstrated. Unlike HS, haemolytic HE is not fully corrected by splenectomy. Only HPP shows a marked improvement in the degree of anaemia.

Hereditary stomatocytosis

Stomatocytes show a well-defined slit-like area across the cell. They are a well-described phenomenon in association with alcoholic liver disease [14] and less consistently with a variety of other unrelated disorders. Stomatocytosis is seen as bowl-shaped red cells in wet preparations. Hereditary stomatocytosis is characterized by increased cell water and the term *hydrocytosis* has been used as an alternative to stomatocytosis [15]. Active transport of Na^+ and K^+ is increased more than tenfold. Passive fluxes of Na^+ and K^+ are markedly increased to 25–50 times normal and the pump is unable to maintain the cell impermeable to Na^+ and, consequently, water. This results in swelling, increased osmotic fragility and splenic trapping. Consequently, splenectomy results in improvement of the degree of anaemia. Total lipid is increased in keeping with the increased membrane surface area but is otherwise normal. A consistent finding in hereditary stomatocytosis appears to be the absence of a 28 kd integral protein in band 7 in SDS gels [16]. The defect is inherited as an autosomal dominant and the first report [17] was in a mother and daughter. A study of the cells of five unrelated patients [18] showed that the number of cation pumps was increased and the total lipid was increased in four cases. The cholesterol:phospholipid ratio was normal but phosphatidylcholine was in increased proportion producing a greater surface area. The heterogeneity of hereditary stomatocytosis was attributed to variability in the increase in surface area and also in the cell water content. A further form of stomatocyte associated with a shortened life span is that associated with the Rh^{null} phenotype [19] but see below.

Hereditary xerocytosis

In contrast to stomatocytosis, xerocytosis is characterized by dehydrated, thin, flat cells which are osmotically resistant and consistently low in total cations due to a passive potassium leakage [20]. It is inherited as an autosomal dominant. On metabolic depletion, haemolysis occurs with the development of myelin figure formation and increased release of lipid vesicles containing glycoprotein and acetylcholinesterase. The cells are more sensitive than normal to *in vitro* hydrogen peroxide.

Red-cell morphology is classically associated with 'puddling' of the haemoglobin at the cell periphery. However, and confusingly, stomatocytes are usually found together with target cells and Rh^{null} disease referred to above was almost certainly due to xerocytosis rather than hydrocytosis.

Disorders of red-cell enzymes

Inherited deficiency of specific enzymes involved in essential metabolic steps can result in haemolysis. They form a heterogeneous group of haemolytic anaemias which are typically 'non-spherocytic'. The defects can be divided into three categories – abnormalities of the Embden–Meyerhof pathway, of the hexose-monophosphate pathway and disorders of nucleotide metabolism.

Disorders of the Embden–Meyerhof path (*Table 11.1*)

The glycolytic enzymes associated with haemolysis are shown in *Table 11.1* in the sequential order of their involvement in the pathway. Theoretically a deficiency of any enzyme involved in glycolysis, if severe enough, could produce a haemolytic anaemia. However, deficiencies of glyceraldehyde phosphate dehydrogenase, phosphoglycerate mutase, enolase and lactate dehydrogenase have not yet been observed to produce haemolysis.

Table 11.1 Enzymes of the Embden–Meyerhof pathway that if deficient have been proved to cause haemolytic anaemia

Enzyme	*Inheritance*	*Order of frequency*
Hexokinase	AR	Rare
Glucose phosphate isomerase	AR	2
Phosphofructose kinase	AR	3
Triose phosphate isomerase	AR	4
Aldolase	AR	Very rare
Phosphoglycerate kinase	SLR	Very rare
2,3-Diphosphoglycerate kinase	AR	Very rare
Pyruvate kinase	AR	1

AR = Autosomal recessive; SLR = sex-linked recessive.

Clinical tolerance of a defect will be influenced by whether the defect is before or after the 2,3 DPG pathway. An increase in 2,3 DPG decreases the oxygen affinity of haemoglobin with increased release of oxygen to the tissues and *vice versa*. Thus a defect before the 2,3 DPG step such as is found in hexokinase deficiency will result in a low 2,3 DPG value as well as ATP concentration and the patient tolerates the anaemia poorly, while a defect after the 2,3 DPG step as in pyruvate kinase (PK) deficiency will result in an accumulation of 2,3 DPG and possible improved tolerance to the anaemia.

An important consideration in the investigation of possible enzyme deficiency is whether the defect is due to true deficiency or due to a structural alteration of the enzyme molecule. Structurally altered enzymes may simply show a lowered maximum reaction rate (decreased V_{max}) or may result in an altered affinity for its substrate, a K_m mutant.

These latter variants may not be detected under the test conditions used for V_{max} assay which are carried out with substrate and co-factor in excess. It is necessary to carry out the assay with reducing amounts of substrate and co-factor. The relatively common PK deficiency may exhibit this problem. An alternative approach is to assay first the levels of the intermediates in the glycolytic pathway, notably 2,3 DPG, in an attempt to localize a possible deficiency.

The 'non-spherocytic' haemolytic anaemias were divided into two groups, type I and type II, by the ability of added glucose to reduce haemolysis in the autohaemolysis test. The haemolysis in type I defects was reduced by the addition of glucose but not in the type II disorders. It was suggested that the majority of type II anaemias are due to PK deficiency and the type I variety due to hexokinase and glucose phosphate isomerase (GPI). The introduction of screening tests and assays for enzymes and intermediates has replaced the autohaemolysis test and the type I and II classification[21].

PK deficiency

The commonest deficiency in the Embden–Meyerhof pathway and the first to be identified is PK.

Anaemia is mild to moderate and is associated with splenomegaly. Reticulocytosis is inevitably present resulting in a regenerative, non-spherocytic blood picture. In some cases contracted red cells (pyknocytes) may be present. Neonatal jaundice is common and may require exchange transfusion. Infection may result in exacerbation of the anaemia. As the disorder is inherited as an autosomal recessive, anaemic subjects are homozygous or double heterozygotes for a defect; the levels of PK activity found in the heterozygote are able to support normal red-cell survival. Although PK is required for all tissues using the pathway, haemolysis is the only clinical abnormality as isoenzymes of PK are found in other tissues. Of particular significance to the laboratory is the isoenzyme found in leucocytes which can contaminate and invalidate the red-cell assay.

PK deficiency is due to a number of variant enzymes produced by mutant genes and most affected subjects are doubly heterozygous for two different mutant genes. It is accepted that the result of PK deficiency is a failure in energy metabolism due to depletion of ATP. Acquired defects of PK have been described in certain dyserythropoietic anaemias due to diminished or abnormal production of the enzyme or due to post-translational interference.

GPI deficiency

This enzyme is inherited as an autosomal recessive and does not have any characteristic haematological or clinical features to distinguish it from other red-cell enzymopathies. It is probably the second most frequent disorder of the Embden–Meyerhof pathway. As in the case of PK there is phenotypic heterogeneity. Inhibition of hexokinase is a possible mechanism leading to haemolysis. The level of reduced glutathione is lowered. *In utero* haemolysis may result in hydrops fetalis.

Phosphofructokinase deficiency

In addition to haemolytic anaemia a myopathy develops and a minority of cases have features of glycogen storage disease.

Triose phosphate isomerase deficiency

This enzyme is involved in many tissues other than red cells and is inherited as an autosomal recessive. The homozygotes not only have a severe haemolytic process but also usually succumb to neuromuscular disease in childhood.

Hexokinase (HK) deficiency

HK activity is very dependent on cell age and is several fold higher in young red-cell populations. HK deficiency is inherited as an autosomal recessive. As with other red-cell enzyme deficiencies the presentation is of neonatal jaundice due to haemolysis.

The conversion of glucose to glucose-6-phosphate is the major rate-limiting step in glycolysis and as this stage is before the 2,3 DPG pathway low levels of the intermediate are found with a left shift in the oxygen dissociation curve, i.e. haemoglobin has a higher affinity for oxygen. Reduced ATP level leads to haemolysis.

Other deficiencies

Very rare examples of other enzyme defects have been reported.

Adolase deficiency: only two kindreds have been reported. One had haemolysis alone, the other was associated with mental and growth retardation.

2,3 diphosphoglycerate mutase deficiency may be associated with mesobilifuchsin in urine and Heinz-body formation.

Phosphoglycerate kinase deficiency has been described with X-linked inheritance, haemolysis and neurological disturbance. In the female heterozygote red-cell mosaicism is found, one population being normal and the other deficient.

Other enzyme deficiencies said to cause haemolysis have been reported and include ATPase, enolase and glyceraldehyde phosphate dehydrogenase but their causal relationship has been questioned[22].

Disorders of the hexose-monophosphate pathway

The major antioxidant in red cells is reduced glutathione (GSH) which is maintained by the production of NADPH from the conversion of G6P to 6PG, a step catalysed by G6PD. A reduced level of GSH will be found when G6PD is deficient or more rarely when GSSG formation is defective due to deficiency of glutathione synthetase or γ-glutamyl-cysteine synthetase. Reports of haemolysis due to deficiency of other enzymes of the pathway – e.g. 6PGD, glutathione reductase and glutathione peroxidase – apparently cannot be substantiated[23]. Partial glutathione reductase deficiency reflects riboflavin nutrition and is not associated with haemolysis. Lower levels of glutathione peroxidase and 6PGD apparently represent genetic polymorphism and again are not associated with haemolysis.

G6PD deficiency [24]

Estimates of incidence vary but have been put as high as 1% of the world population though there are marked racial differences; about 13% of American Negroes are deficient and as the defect has a sex-linked inheritance about 20% of Negro women are heterozygous carriers and about 2% homozygotes. Because of X-chromatin inactivation heterozygotes have two red-cell populations, one being normal and one that is deficient. In male hemizygotes the entire red-cell population is deficient.

G6PD shows marked heterogeneity; over 250 variants have been distinguished on the basis of physicochemical properties. This heterogeneity produces different clinical manifestations:

1. Drug sensitivity.
2. Favism.
3. Haemolysis associated with infections.
4. Chronic non-spherocytic haemolysis with anaemia.
5. Neonatal jaundice.

The haematological effects of G6PD variants are summarized in *Table 11.2.*

Table 11.2 Haematological effects of glucose-6-phosphate dehydrogenase variants

Variant	*Enzyme activity* (%)	*Disorder*
Gd^{B} 'usual'	100	None
Gd^{A} Negro variant	100	None
Gd^{A-} Negro	10–20	Neonatal jaundice, drug-induced haemolysis
$Gd^{Mediterranean}$	0–5	Favism, neonatal jaundice
Gd^{Canton} Chinese	4–24	Drug-induced haemolysis, favism, neonatal jaundice
$Gd^{various}$, widely distributed	0–25	CNSHA
$Gd^{Mahidol}$ Thai	5–15	Drug-induced haemolysis, neonatal jaundice

CNSHA = Chronic non-spherocytic haemolytic anaemia.

Drug-induced haemolysis By far the most common effect of G6PD deficiency is drug-induced haemolysis and the list of agents reported as being capable of inducing haemolysis is formidable. Certainly many do not consistently cause haemolysis and are more likely to have been incriminated by their use to treat infection which in itself can induce haemolysis. Drugs that can truly be implicated are oxidants:

1. Antimalarials – primaquine and structurally related compounds.
2. Nitrofurantoin and related drugs.
3. Sulphonamides.
4. Diaminodiphenylsulphone (dapsone) and other sulphones.
5. Phenacetin.

6. Antihelminths.
7. Menadione derivatives.

Oxidant drugs produce hydrogen peroxide or superoxide. In order to handle the hydrogen peroxide the red cell uses the glutathione peroxidase system which requires reduced glutathione which in turn is dependent on NADPH which is inadequate when G6PD activity is blocked. Thus SH groups of haemoglobin and membrane proteins are oxidized and an observable phenomenon is the formation of unstable haemoglobin and Heinz-body formation with attachment to the red-cell membrane. Such cells are rapidly eliminated from the circulation. The relationship between drug dosage and haemolysis in normal and G6PD-deficient subjects has been reviewed[25].

Favism occurs mainly in Mediterranean races and in the Chinese and is due to eating the broad bean *Vicia fava* or by inhaling the pollen. There is often massive haemolysis with haemoglobinuria and Heinz bodies are found during the acute phase. The causative agent may be the glucoside divicine or its aglycone isouramil. The amount of divicine depends on how the beans are treated or cooked but haemolysis is commonest when eaten fresh and raw. The procalpaine-calpaine protease system may be an important defence against oxidant-induced Heinz bodies in favism.

Infection can cause haemolysis in G6PD deficiency irrespective of the drugs used for treatment. Many of the agents said to precipitate haemolysis have probably been used for treating infection and their role in causing haemolysis is possibly incidental. A possible explanation of the haemolysis associated with infection is that red cells have receptors for activated complement. In combination with immune complexes and in the presence of phagocytes this can lead to oxidative stress and damage in G6PD-deficient red cells.

Chronic non-spherocytic haemolytic anaemia (CNSHA) due to G6PD deficiency is an extremely heterogeneous group involving many different mutant enzymes of world-wide distribution without any particular racial prevalence[24,26]. The degree of haemolysis varies from a mild compensated form to moderately severe. Haemolytic anaemia is found only in males or homozygous females.

Neonatal jaundice due to G6PD deficiency may be expected. In the series of CNSHA mentioned above[24] about 70% of affected infants had jaundice. The other forms of G6PD deficiency are the single commonest cause of neonatal jaundice. Nevertheless, it is often difficult to ascribe the jaundice to a deficiency unless there is evidence of precipitating factors, and the jaundice may not be haemolytic but hepatic.

The high incidence of G6PD deficiency in areas where malaria is or was endemic is mentioned in Chapter 14.

Glutathione deficiency

This very rare deficiency has been reported in four families; in two instances the level of reduced glutathione was less than 10% of normal. The disorder is apparently due to a deficiency of either γ-glutamyl cysteine synthetase or of glutathione synthetase which catalyses γ-glutamyl cysteine and glycine into glutathione[27–29].

An unusual CNSHA with dominant inheritance associated with increased glutathione has been reported[30].

Abnormalities of nucleotide metabolism

Pyrimidine-5′-nucleotidase deficiency

This deficiency was originally described as a hereditary haemolytic anaemia with basophilic stippling, increased glutathione and adenine phosphates associated with a deficiency of ribosephosphate pyrophosphokinase. Further study showed that the increased nucleotides were pyrimidine nucleotides whose catabolism and excretion from red cells is blocked by a deficiency of pyrimidine-5′-nucleotidase. The unwanted and increased nucleotides can compete for ATP and ADP binding sites on enzymes normally occupied by ADP and ATP[31]. Alternatively uridine triphosphate or cytidine triphosphate may replace ATP as a substrate for ATPase[32]. The incidence of the deficiency is relatively high, possibly the third most common after G6PD and PK deficiencies. The relationship between pyrimidine-5′-nucelotidase activity and lead poisoning has been referred to previously (*see* page 232). It is suggested that the basophilic stippling seen in each disorder reflects the excess pyrimidine nucleotides.

Adenosine deaminase (ADA) over-production

An excess of enzyme activity can lead to haemolytic anaemia. ADA converts adenosine to inosine and three families have been described with haemolysis in which the affected members have ADA levels some 45–70 times the normal activity. As non-nucleated red cells cannot synthesize adenine the availability of adenine phosphates depends upon the salvage pathway and thus increased ADA activity results in diminished ATP activity and loss of red-cell viability[33].

Adenylate kinase deficiency

Haemolysis due to deficiency of this enzyme is due to reduced conversion of AMP to ADP and consequent limitation of conversion of ADP to ATP. Three families have been recorded.

Amino-acid substitutions or deletions in the globin chains of haemoglobin

Mutations resulting in structurally abnormal polypeptide chains can cause a haemolytic anaemia. Most mutations differ from the corresponding normal haemoglobin by a single amino-acid substitution in one of the two types of polypeptide chain. These substitutions generally reflect the exchange of a base in a DNA triplet. More rarely, variants occur as a result of two amino-acid substitutions in the same chain due to a second point-mutation in an existing variant, or by cross-over during meiosis. A few variants are due to one or more amino acids being absent, probably due to loss of DNA by unequal crossing over during meiosis. Fusion chain variants are due to unequal, non-homologous, meiotic crossing of closely linked genes. The chain termination and fusion chain abnormalities produce thalassaemia-like defects and are considered in Chapter 9.

Over 500 variants have now been described and the original identification by alphabet – A, F, S, C, D, E, etc. – has long been inadequate. The present approach is identification by geographical origin even down to districts within towns or cities.

The prevalence of a particular city or country in this scheme does not necessarily imply a higher frequency of variants but rather the interest, enthusiasm and possibly resources of investigators in that area.

Variants that cause haemolytic anaemia alter the stability of the haemoglobin molecule and may be manifest in two ways – reduced solubility, as typified by Hb S and C, and a form of instability which results in denaturation within the red cell and in Heinz-body formation. This latter group is known as the 'unstable haemoglobins'.

Abnormal haemoglobins are inherited as automosomal co-dominants and therefore produce heterozygous and homozygous states. Unstable haemoglobins cause haemolysis in the heterozygous state (homozygosity is probably incompatible with life) while the variants with reduced solubility show no haemolysis in the heterozygote and only result in haemolysis in homozygotes – e.g. S/S, C/C, etc. – or in double heterozygotes – e.g. S/C, S/β thalassaemia.

Haemoglobin with reduced solubility

Sickle haemoglobin (Hb S)

By far the most serious abnormal haemoglobin in terms of frequency and clinical effect is that due to the substitution of valine for glutamic acid at position 6 of the β chain (Hb S = β6(A3) glu→val) which, in the deoxygenated state results in insolubility, crystallization, polymer formation and gelation and consequent cell distortion and loss of deformability [34]. Deoxygenated Hb S forms unidirectional crystals consisting of double strands of molecules; the polymer is made up of seven double strands of Hb S with a slight helical twist. Reoxygenation results in rapid reversal of polymer formation indicating weak physicochemical forces such as hydrogen and hydrophobic bonds and Van der Waals forces. Reversion to normal cell shape does not necessarily follow.

Sickling depends not only on the degree of deoxygenation but also on the concentration of Hb S within a red cell; the higher the concentration the greater the propensity to sickle. Thus the presence of 60–70% Hb A in the red cells of A/S heterozygotes is protective and *in vivo* sickling occurs only when there is oxygen deprivation, e.g. during induction of anaesthesia, at altitude or by severe physical exertion. Of particular importance in the homozygote (S/S) is the persistence of Hb F into childhood and adult life. When Hb F levels are greater than 20% clinical effects are minor as is seen in S/HPFH and in certain Arab groups. Not all haemoglobins have this protective effect and a 50:50 mixture of S and C gels at almost the same concentration as S alone (26 g/dl).

The sickle–unsickle process is associated with accumulation of calcium and loss of cell water resulting in an increased concentration of Hb S. Thus a cell that is sickled is more likely to sickle again and will eventually assume a permanent sickle shape, an irreversible sickle cell (ISC), even when oxygenated and when the Hb S is not crystalline. This indicates permanent red-cell damage and rigidity. Irreversibly altered cells may be elliptical, 'oat' shaped or crescents. They do not show the finely pointed projections seen in wet preparations. However, there is *in vitro* evidence that sickle haemoglobin binds to the inner aspect of the cell membrane and contributes to reduced deformability.

The proportion of ISCs reflects *in vivo* sickling. Sickle cells *in vivo* have reduced deformability and ability to negotiate the microcirculation, and a tendency to form aggregates resulting in circulatory stasis and local infarction with painful crises.

This circulatory trapping is almost certainly a mechanism of haemolysis either by intravenous destruction or by trapping in splenic sinusoids. The denaturation of sickle haemoglobin is accompanied by generation of oxygen radicals and haemochromes and, ultimately, in the formation of micro-Heinz bodies. The release of haemin during degradation may have a significant role in the haemolytic mechanism by oxidation of proteins and lipids and by induced conformational changes in skeletal proteins[35]. Repeated splenic infarction results in loss of splenic function and the appearance of 'post-splenectomy' red-cell changes (*Figure 11.4*).

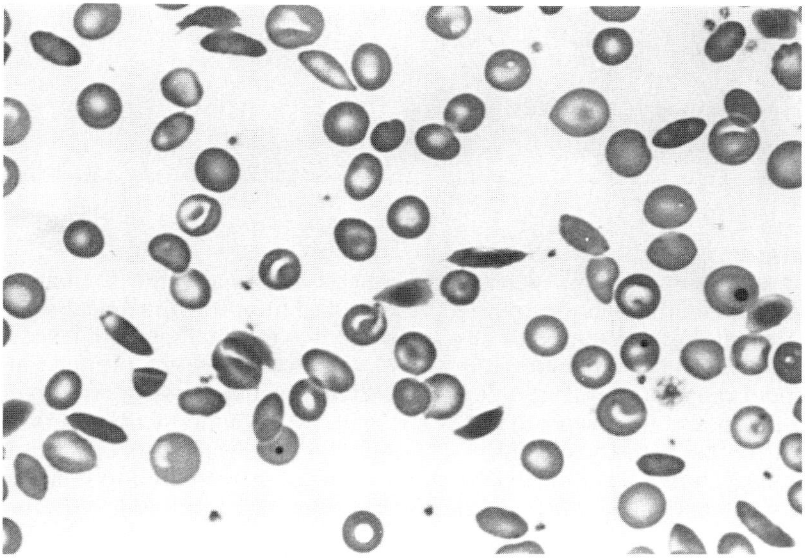

Figure 11.4 Blood film. Sickle-cell anaemia (Hb S/S). Fully sickled shapes are not shown but 'boat'- and 'oat'-shaped cells are numerous and reflect irreversible cell damage. Three red cells containing single Howell–Jolly bodies indicate the loss of splenic function due to repeated splenic infarction. ×550

Incidence and severity of the sickle-cell syndromes

The incidence of the Hb S gene is highest in Negro races. In Africa the incidence varies greatly between regions and can be as high as 45%. In the American Negro the overall incidence is about 8.5%. Other races of high incidence are the Veddoids of south India and southern Arabia and the Eti-Turks, and in certain areas of Greece the incidence may be as high as 20–30%. The reason for the high incidence of the potentially lethal mutation is almost certainly due to the protection awarded to the heterozygotes from falciparum malaria (*see* Chapter 14). As the geographical distribution of Hb S is similar to that of certain other haemoglobin substitutions – notably Hbs C, D and E – and the thalassaemia defects, the spectrum of sickling disorders is wide. The term 'sickle-cell anaemia' is reserved for the homozygous S/S state, and 'sickle-cell disease' for those conditions where Hb S is associated with another haemoglobin variant or thalassaemia gene producing clinical abnormality. A limited summary is shown in *Table 11.3*.

Table 11.3 Summary of sickle-cell syndromes

Disorder	*Hb constitution*	*Clinical expression*
Sickle-cell anaemia	S, F (1–15%), A_2	Severe
Sickle-cell anaemia with high Hb F	S, F (10–35%), A_2	Mild
Hb S/C	S, C, A_2	Moderate to mild
Hb S/D	S, D, A_2	Moderate
Hb S/E	S, E, A_2	Moderate to severe
Hb S/O Arab	S, O, A_2	Severe
S/β thal^0	S, F, ↑ A_2	Moderate to severe
S/β thal$^+$	S, F, A (6–10%), ↑ A_2	Moderate 'Mediterranean type'
S/β thal$^+$	S, F, A (18–25%), ↑ A_2	Moderate to mild 'Negro type'
S/α thal	A, S (less than 30%), A_2	Asymptomatic, microcytic
S/HPHF	S, F (18–25%), ↓ A_2	Asymptomatic
S trait	A, S, A_2	Asymptomatic
C^{Harlem} trait	A, C^{Harlem}, F	Asymptomatic
Sickle-cell anaemia + α-chain substitution, e.g. Hb G Philadelphia	S, S/G, F, A_2, $A_2G^{Philadelphia}$	Severe

Sickle-cell anaemia

The signs and symptoms develop when the synthesis of the affected β chain is established and anaemia may be recognized by the third month with clinical signs by 6 months. Except during haemolytic and aplastic crises the haemoglobin level is usually about 7 g/dl with a reticulocytosis of 5–15% which tends to produce an MCV in the upper range of normal (90–96 fl). Blood films show anisocytosis, target cells, polychromasia and the presence of ISCs is considered by many observers to be found only in the homozygous form (*Figure 11.4*). Normoblasts are often present, particularly when splenic atrophy due to repeated splenic infarction has occurred. Red-cell survival is shortened and the pattern of destruction indicates intravascular lysis.

Survival is greatly influenced by environment and degree of supportive medical care. Even with good medical support the mortality from sickle-cell disease of all types in children less than 2 years old can be as high as 13% [36]. The major hazards are: overwhelming infection due to functional asplenia, acute splenic sequestration, cerebrovascular accidents and aplastic crises associated with human parvovirus infection. Neonates from 'at risk' communities must be screened *at birth* for sickle-cell disease [37].

Some groups of patients attain adult life with minimal clinical complications. They represent distinct, genetically determined, sub-populations of sickle-cell anaemia and are associated with high levels of heterogeneously distributed Hb F. In addition to the more benign clinical course, there is less haemolysis and higher haemoglobin levels are maintained.

The co-existence of α thalassaemia with sickle-cell anaemia also results in less severe haematological findings and a milder clinical pattern. Improved rheological features have been demonstrated.

Laboratory diagnosis

Blood-film appearances, demonstration of sickling, haemoglobin electrophoresis, Hb F and A_2 quantitation and solubility testing, perhaps supported by a family study will establish the diagnosis in most instances. Sickle-cell anaemia must be differentiated from S/β thalassaemia (particularly the β^0 variant) and the double heterozygote S/D which will show a single electrophoretic component. On preliminary laboratory testing S/HPFH can simulate the benign (high F) form of sickle-cell anaemia.

Haemoglobin S/C disease

All the clinical complications of sickle-cell anaemia may be seen in S/C disease though splenic atrophy is probably less common. The anaemia is milder, and haemolysis and the consequent reticulocytosis less marked. The predominant feature of the blood film are target cells, and ISCs are not seen though 'boat-shaped' cells may be seen together with a few spherocytes. A few cells may contain elongated crystals. Because of the limited geographical origins of Hb C, S/C disease is virtually confined to Negroes and in Ghana is as common as sickle-cell anaemia. Laboratory diagnosis is based on the demonstration of sickling, electrophoretic demonstration of the two haemoglobin components with solubility tests showing approximately 50% insoluble haemoglobin. The much rarer sickling disorders S/C Harlem and S/S together with the α-chain variant Hb G Philadelphia show very similar electrophoretic patterns to S/C disease but the blood picture and severity of the anaemia should indicate that further studies are necessary.

Haemoglobin S/D Punjab disease

This rare combination results in a clinical course and anaemia very similar to sickle-cell anaemia with a single haemoglobin band on electrophoresis migrating in the S position. Differentiation is by demonstration that not all the haemoglobin is insoluble and by electrophoretic separation at acid pH.

Haemoglobin S/E disease

The differing racial distribution of Hb S and Hb E make this an uncommon disorder with a mild to moderate microcytic anaemia. Unlike Hb D and Hb O Arab, Hb E does not interact in the sickling phenomenon and the clinical signs of sickle-cell anaemia are not seen. Laboratory diagnosis is by electrophoresis. Although on racial grounds Hb C and Hb E are unlikely to be confused, differentiation should be performed. The identical mobilities of Hb E and Hb A_2 is not a problem; Hb A_2 is never greater than 8% and in the adult heterozygote Hb E will be greater than 20% even in association with α thalassaemia.

Hb S/β thalassaemia

This doubly heterozygous condition is of particular importance clinically because of its frequency in certain populations and in its laboratory investigation.

The clinical signs may be as severe as sickle-cell anaemia or follow a milder course. An important difference is that splenomegaly rather than splenic atrophy is usual. The differing severity is related to the populations affected. In Caucasian races such as Greeks and Italians β thalassaemia is often of the β^0 type and thus S/β^0 thalassaemia is not associated with Hb A production and consequently a severe disorder results. In the Negro, β thalassaemia is less severe and up to 30% Hb A may be found and symptoms are less severe.

The laboratory findings are a mild to moderate anaemia, depending on the type of β thalassaemia, microcytosis and target cells. In the β^+ form ISCs are not seen. Haemoglobin studies show two patterns: S + F + A_2 in the β^0 type with a single major component in the S position on electrophoresis, or S + F + A + A_2 in the β^+ type. It is important to differentiate the β^0 type from sickle-cell anaemia as the prognosis is better and a family study is the easiest approach when the parents are available. Small amounts of Hb A may be demonstrated more readily by electrophoresis in agar at acid pH or by isoelectric focusing.

Hb S/HPFH

This combination produces minimal clinical signs of sickling with only slight blood-film changes which include target cells and hypochromia. Haemoglobin studies, however, show a pattern very similar to the benign 'high F' form of sickle-cell anaemia (*see* above). About 80% is Hb S and the remainder Hb F which is *homogeneously* distributed throughout all the red cells. Hb A_2 level is normal or reduced. The presence of Hb F in all red cells inhibits *in vivo* sickling.

Hb S trait

The heterozygote with the haemoglobin genotype A/S is relatively benign, without anaemia, and with minimal blood-film changes though some target cells may be seen. If exposed to severe hypoxia, as may occur during the induction of anaesthesia, sickling episodes can occur with tissue infarction. Haematuria is not uncommon. Between 25 and 45% of haemoglobin is S with a bimodal distribution. Lower levels of Hb S are associated with the presence of α-thalassaemia trait and are also found in iron deficiency. Fixed sickle cells are never seen and *in vitro* sickling induced by reducing agents occurs more slowly, with 'intermediate' sickled forms often of 'holly-leaf' appearance.

Hb C–β6(A3) glu→lys

This mutation occurs with a frequency of about 20% in Ghana and in about 2% of American Negroes. The haemoglobin has a lower solubility, resulting in a crystalline structure and producing increased red-cell rigidity. In the homozygote, intracellular tetragonal crystals may be seen in routinely prepared and stained blood films, particularly after splenectomy. Mild haemolytic anaemia is present in the homozygote and the blood film is somewhat characteristic with many target cells and a proportion of spherocytes (*Figure 11.5*). Almost all the haemoglobin is C with a small amount of Hb F. In Hb C trait there is no anaemia or reticulocytosis though frequent target cells are found.

About 40% of total haemoglobin is C but as is the case in other β-chain substitutions, when associated with α thalassaemia or iron deficiency, lower levels are found.

The association of Hb C with the HPFH gene results in a picture very similar to Hb C disease with target cells and spherocytes but with about 25% Hb F. Hb C/β thalassaemia may show a similar picture with microcytosis but the level of Hb F is lower. Again family studies are a convenient approach to differentiation.

Hb C Harlem–β6(A3) glu→val; β73(E17) asp→asn is a rare but interesting double β-chain substitution with an electrophoretic mobility of the much commoner Hb C. The substitution of valine for glutamic acid at position 6, as is present in Hb S, induces the sickling phenomenon and the double heterozygote Hb S/C Harlem produces severe sickle-cell disease with ISCs but has the electrophoretic pattern of S/C disease. A similar pattern is found in sickle-cell

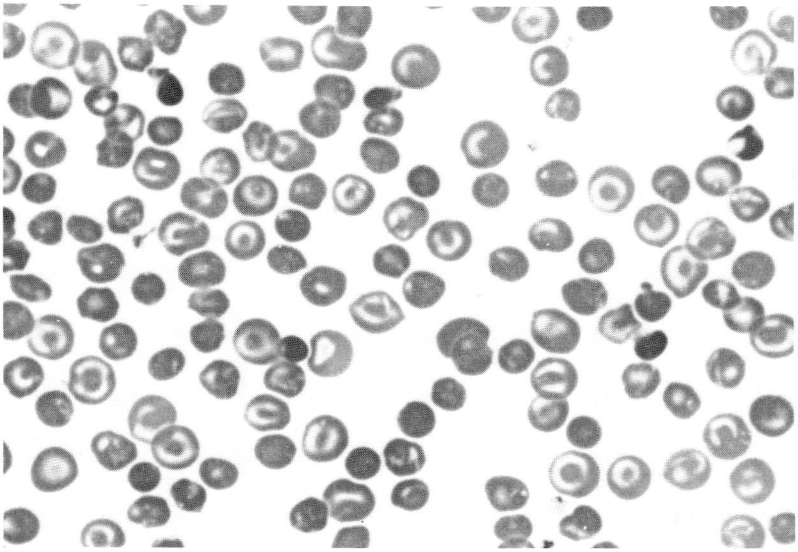

Figure 11.5 Blood film. Homozygous Hb C disease. The target cell, microspherocytic picture is typical. Note the tendency for the haemoglobin to 'puddle' at one side of the cell. ×550

anaemia in association with Hb G Philadelphia (α 68(E17) asn→lys), with the hybrid molecule S/G Philadelphia having a mobility similar to Hb C. Because of the differing prognosis proper identification is important.

Other common substitutions

Hb D

This designation includes a number of variants with similar electrophoretic mobility which is identical with Hb S. The variant with the highest frequency is Hb D Punjab (β121 (GH4) glu→gln) which in its relatively rare homozygous form produces a mild haemolytic anaemia with numerous target cells and on electrophoresis a single haemoglobin component in the S position. It is obviously important to differentiate the disorder from sickle-cell anaemia or S/β thalassaemia by the absence of sickling and normal solubility. The possibility of S/D disease or D/β thalassaemia must also be considered, the latter differentiation being again most readily approached by family studies. The reason for the shortened cell survival in D/D disease is not clear.

Hb E–β26(B8) glu→lys

This substitution is particularly common in South-east Asia and in Thailand has a frequency of 13.6% though a higher incidence is found in malarial areas suggesting that Hb E heterozygotes may be at an advantage. Homozygous Hb E disease results in a mild haemolytic anaemia with many target cells which are also strikingly microcytic and associated with a compensatory erythrocytosis. Heterozygotes also show microcytosis and the red-cell parameters simulate thalassaemia trait (*see* page

248). This is particularly important in an area where the incidence of thalassaemia is high and the many combinations between Hb E, the thalassaemia defects and other haemoglobin substitutions has been referred to earlier (*see* page 236). The mechanism of increased red-cell destruction is not clear.

The inclusion of Hbs D and E in the same section as Hbs S and C is on rather tenuous grounds. The mechanism(s) of haemolysis is not fully understood but they are not 'unstable variants'. As they are substitutions of relatively high incidence their occurrence with Hb S is well described in the literature and the laboratory differentiation of Hb S from Hb D and Hb C from Hb E etc. is sufficient reason for consideration in this chapter.

The unstable haemoglobins

The unstable haemoglobins are structural variants that undergo denaturation within the red cell and precipitate to form Heinz bodies. Their presence results in a disorder formerly called congenital Heinz body haemolytic anaemia (CHBHA) which is now designated 'unstable haemoglobin disease'. The unstable haemoglobins comprise a large well-defined group of over 100 variants and the associated haemolysis covers a wide spectrum from extremely severe to extremely mild. About one third have no clinical haemolysis. The severity of haemolysis associated with each variant can be explained by the nature and position of the amino-acid defect [38]. Unstable variants often have altered oxygen affinity. It should be noted that although other haemoglobins such as Hb S and Hb H are unstable under certain conditions, they are not considered in this group.

The concept of haemoglobin instability was developed from the observation that in patients with CHBHA part of the haemoglobin was precipitated by heating to 50°C for 60 minutes [39].

The stability of the haemoglobin tetramer depends on the collective forces of four factors – a large α-helical content of each chain, the firm binding of the haem group, the internal siting of non-polar amino acids and the stability of the $\alpha_1\beta_1$ contacts holding the four chains together. Instability can result if amino-acid abnormalities interfere with one or more of the above factors and can occur in one of six processes.

Replacement of haem-contact amino acids

This abnormality usually results in a very unstable molecule, and the first unstable haemoglobin variant identified, Hb Koln (β 98(FG5) val→meth), has an abnormality of this type. The large methionine side chain distorts the FG segment, breaking several haem-contact amino acids. In Hb Hammersmith (β 42(CD1) phe→ser) the loss of the long side chain with its strong bond and replacement with a small, slightly hydrophilic side chain results in weakened binding of the haem and also in the tendency for water to enter the haem pocket.

Replacement of non-polar by polar residues

This type of substitution may have very variable effects depending on whether the polar side chain has to be neutralized internally. In Hb Bristol (β 67(E11) val→asp) the side chain of aspartic acid has to be neutralized internally resulting in distortion of the haem pocket, high instability and severe haemolysis.

Deletions or insertions
At least nine examples of amino-acid deletion, either single or multiple, have been reported and all involve the β chain with haematological symptoms ranging from severe haemolysis to none. In Hb Freiburg (β 23(B5) missing), the first described deletion, there is a mild haemolytic anaemia, while in Hb Niteroi (β 42–44 or 43–45(CD1–3, CD2–4) missing) haemolysis is severe.

Replacement by proline
The substitution of an amino acid in a helical portion by the iminoacid proline which is normally found in the non-helical sections may cause marked instability as is seen in Hb Santa Ana (β 88(F4) leu→prol).

Replacement at subunit contacts
If a substitution on the $\alpha_1\beta_1$ contact weakens the bonds at the contact, dissociation into dimers and monomers can occur which are less stable. Hb Philly (β 35(E1) tyr→phen) is an example which results in a moderate degree of instability.

Replacement of glycine by amino acids with large side chains
In areas of the haemoglobin molecule where atoms are very closely packed, substitution of glycine by amino acids with larger side chains may produce marked changes in stability, e.g. Hb Savannah (β 24(B6) gly→val).

The majority (approximately 85%) of unstable variants are due to β chain abnormalities; the remainder are α substitutions with one γ chain abnormality (Hb Poole γ 130(H8) trp→gly).

Genetics of unstable haemoglobins

All reported cases of unstable haemoglobins have been heterozygotes (examples of double heterozygotes with thalassaemia variants have been described). No homozygotes have been described, possibly because the defect would be lethal. The combination of a β chain variant with β^0-thalassaemia results in features of a homozygous state – a single haemoglobin component. Although inherited as autosomal dominant genes, some highly unstable haemoglobins have arisen as a single mutation within a family. It has been suggested that such variants are incapable of transmission through several generations. Therefore, the absence of significant family history or the presence of normal laboratory findings in the parents of a patient suspected of having an unstable haemoglobin should not preclude further investigation.

Laboratory findings

As mentioned, haematological effects range from none to severe haemolysis. In non-splenectomized subjects blood-film changes are not characteristic: polychromasia, slight hypochromia, slight anisopoikilocytosis and perhaps occasional contracted cells. Basophilic stippling may be a feature. Heinz bodies are not a feature of the blood film though they can be induced by incubation with brilliant cresyl blue as in reticulocyte preparations. Following oxidative challenge, however, the picture may alter markedly with many contracted cells and spherocytes.

In a splenectomized case, Heinz bodies are a constant feature and may be seen in Romanowsky-stained blood films as whitish or pale blue inclusions and in methyl violet preparations may be found in over 50% of cells. Electrophoresis is not particularly useful as about two-thirds of the unstable mutations show no change in the net charge of the molecule. When an abnormal band is found, as for example in Hb Koln, it is often present as a minor fraction together possibly with a haem-depleted band in a position similar to Hb S. The reason for the small amount of the unstable variant is precipitation and selective removal together with intraerythroblast destruction of denatured chains. Of particular interest is that elevated Hb A_2 levels are often found in the presence of unstable β-chain mutants. Increased levels of met- and sulphaemoglobin may be found in fresh blood samples and incubation at 37°C for 24 hours readily induces further abnormal pigment production and Heinz body formation.

The definitive tests for the presence of unstable variants are the denaturation tests, either by heating at 50°C, by isopropanol precipitation at 37°C or by precipitation with *p*-chlormercuribenzoate (PCMB) or *p*-hydroxymercuribenzoate (PMB).

Mechanisms of haemolysis

Heinz-body formation is undoubtedly the cause of the reduced red-cell survival. An early concept was that the precipitated globin chains were bound to the red-cell membrane by disulphide linkages with altered permeability of the membrane to allow potassium and calcium influx. Further evidence, however, indicates that red-cell damage is due to the formation of Heinz bodies *per se* which are removed from the cells together with membrane in the microcirculation. This leads to sphering and destruction. The mechanism of Heinz-body formation has also undergone re-appraisal, i.e. the role of superoxide ions as oxidizing agents leading to oxidation of haemoglobin *and* the unsaturated phospholipids of the red-cell membrane [40] and the formation of hemichromes.

Paroxysmal nocturnal haemoglobinuria

Paroxysmal nocturnal haemoglobinuria (PNH) is a unique chronic haemolytic anaemia with an acquired defect of the red-cell membrane due to the presence of an abnormal erythroblast population. The disorder is characterized by the presence of haemoglobinuria after sleep, lysis of the red cells *in vitro* when incubated in acidified normal serum and an association with bone-marrow hypoplasia or aplasia. The haemolytic component of the disorder is caused by an undue susceptibility of the abnormal red cells to lysis by complement.

Pathogenesis

Although the cause of red-cell defect is unknown, the association with aplasia (whether congenital, idiopathic or due to drugs) and a less frequent though significant evolution into other marrow disorders such as acute leukaemia, erythroleukaemia and myelofibrosis suggests that PNH is associated with bone-marrow damage or 'insult' producing an abnormal clone of stem cells from which an abnormal red-cell population is produced. This concept is confirmed by the observation that in a female patient with two G6PD variants the PNH defect was confined to cells with one enzyme variant, and that in a case with erythroleukaemia and PNH the defect was associated with the neoplastic cells.

Granulocytes and platelets have a similar defect to the red cells and two granulocyte populations differing in sensitivity to complement lysis have been demonstrated[41–43]. In most patients two (sometimes three) red-cell populations are present with up to a 20-fold difference in sensitivity to complement lysis[44].

The basic abnormality is a defect in membrane protein rather than membrane lipid. This was suggested by the observations that normal red cells may be converted to PNH-like cells by certain proteolytic enzymes and perhaps more significantly by some sulphydryl compounds. Further evidence is provided by polyacrylamide gel electrophoresis of PNH membranes which shows an abnormal protein component. A reduced activity of membrane-associated inhibitors of complement activation has been suggested as the defect[45]. More recently[46], studies of a membrane protein, decay-accelerating factor (DAF) which has complement regulatory activity, has shown partial or complete deficiency in PNH erythrocytes. DAF inhibits the assembly and accelerates the natural decay of the classical and alternate pathway C3 convertase.

The haemolytic mechanism

The degree of haemolysis is related to the proportion of C-sensitive red cells which, when in large numbers, results in haemoglobinuria. Intravascular lysis is, however, continuous and results in the more constant finding of haemosiderinuria.

The C-sensitive cells are prone to lysis irrespective of the mechanism of C′ activation – the 'classical' pathway involving C1 activation after antibody absorption or the 'alternative' pathway of C3 activation not requiring antibody. The latter mechanism is the usual *in vivo* mechanism and is the basis for most of the *in vitro* lysis tests other than the sucrose lysis test (*see* page 377). The episodic haemolysis associated with sleep has not been adequately explained and variation in pH, cortisol level, magnesium concentration and C′ level have not been proved causes. Reticulocyte-rich red-cell fractions have a higher proportion of sensitive cells and release of reticulocytes from the marrow during sleep has also been suggested as an explanation. Exacerbations of haemolysis occur and important causes are infection, blood transfusion and iron therapy. Infection and transfused blood products probably result in C′ activation and although iron is a catalyst in lipid peroxidation its administration is likely to cause increased erythropoiesis and consequently a higher proportion of sensitive cells. Intravascular lysis is a possible cause of the tendency to venous thrombosis, but the abnormal platelet population is a more likely explanation. Venous thrombosis in unusual sites, e.g. hepatic vein (Budd-Chiari) is an indication to consider PNH as a possible cause.

Laboratory findings

Anaemia may be mild or severe and the red-cell picture depends on the degree of reticulocytosis and whether iron depletion has developed. A leucopenia of less than 2.5×10^9/l is common and thrombocytopenia less than 50×10^9/l is found in 40% of cases. The PNH defect should therefore be considered in all patients presenting with pancytopenia. Intravascular haemolysis is present with haemosiderinuria the most constant feature.

Red-cell survival studies typically show a two-component destruction curve, a very rapid loss due to the C-sensitive cells and a slower or normal destruction of the less sensitive or normal populations.

Diagnosis requires the demonstration of lysis in a properly controlled acidified serum test which is described and discussed together with other methods on page 376.

Additional laboratory findings are the presence of a low red-cell acetylcholinesterase (AChE) activity; the more sensitive the cells to C′ lysis the lower the enzyme activity. It is not suggested that the low AChE activity is the cause of the defect but rather that it is a secondary manifestation of the disorder. Granulocyte function has been shown to be impaired and neutrophil alkaline phosphatase activity is often low or absent.

For a fuller account and for clinical, prognostic and therapeutic aspects the reader is referred to the reviews by Sirchia and Lewis[47] and Rosse[48].

Extracorpuscular mechanisms of haemolysis

Immune haemolytic anaemia

The presence of antibodies capable of causing sensitization of red cells will usually result in a shortened red-cell survival due to phagocytosis by macrophages, lymphocyte-mediated cytotoxicity, sequestration or by intravascular lysis. The fate of the sensitized red cell will depend on the characteristics of the antibody involved, i.e. specificity, immunoglobulin class, ability to activate complement and the optimum temperature for binding to the red cells. Immune haemolytic anaemia may be caused in four ways:

1. Passively acquired antibody:
   (a) By maternal antibodies crossing the placenta to react with the fetal red cells – haemolytic disease of the new-born (HDNB). Despite the successful programme for preventing HDNB due to anti-D, HDNB remains the most frequent cause of immune haemolysis and is due to IgG antibodies of the Rhesus or other major blood group systems and, in particular, fetomaternal ABO incompatibility.
   (b) The rare occurrence of an antibody in donor blood transfused to a recipient having the corresponding red-cell antigen. The administration of blood components containing anti-A or anti-B may react with recipients of groups A, B or AB as appropriate.
2. The presence or development of antibody against transfused donor red cells – a haemolytic transfusion reaction whether immediate or delayed.
3. The action of antibodies formed against drugs or drug–protein complexes. Three mechanisms are recognized – drug adsorption, immune complex and drug-induced autoantibodies[49,50].
4. The presence of autoantibodies other than due to drugs – autoimmune haemolytic anaemia (AIHA).

Drug adsorption mechanism

This mechanism is typified by the production of antibodies against penicillin. Treatment with high doses of the drug causes coating of the red cells and the anti-penicillin antibodies react with the drug-coated cells. Haemolysis characteristically appears only in patients having high dose therapy, i.e. 10 mega units daily and then only after an interval of several days. Red cells are sensitized with IgG and free antibody is present in the serum, often with a titre of over 1000. Occasionally complement sensitization may also be detected and may be associated with high antibody titres to produce immune complexes. Cephalosporins also bind to red-cell membrane and have occasionally caused immune haemolysis. A more common effect of cephalosporins is their ability to modify the red-cell membrane allowing adsorption of non-immunological proteins. In such instances there will be no antibody in the serum and the red-cell eluate will be non-reactive.

Immune complex mechanism

The concept of a drug–protein complex acting as an immunogen with the consequent production of an anti-drug antibody which complexes with the drug and then adsorbs on to the cell membrane was first considered as a mechanism of drug-induced thrombocytopenia and has been subsequently shown to apply to drug-associated immune haemolysis. The adsorption of immune complex results in complement activation and haemolysis.

As immunization does not require conjugation of drug and cell and as the antibodies do not have specificity for red-cell antigens, the sequence leading to immune haemolysis has been referred to as 'the innocent bystander mechanism'.

The pattern of haemolysis is of an acute onset with normal or small doses of the drug in contrast to the immune adsorption mechanism of penicillin. Usually only complement components can be demonstrated on the red cells by the direct antiglobulin test (DAT). To demonstrate the drug–antibody interaction *in vitro* the presence of the drug is required.

Both in this mechanism and in the drug adsorption mechanism antibody is directed against a drug and not the patients' red cells and therefore are not autoimmune in nature.

Drug-induced autoimmune haemolytic anaemia

Frequently patients treated with α-methyldopa develop a positive DAT and some have overt haemolysis. The antibody in the serum reacts directly with normal red cells *in vitro* in the absence of the drug. Eluate from sensitized red cells will also coat normal red cells in the absence of the drug. This pattern of reaction is that found in 'idiopathic' warm AIHA and is appropriately termed 'drug-induced AIHA'. The antibody is IgG and does not bind complement. A positive DAT persists for some months after ceasing therapy.

The following drugs are associated with immune haemolysis:

1. *Group A – acting by the adsorption mechanism:* Penicillin, cephalosporins, tolbutamide, erythromycin, cisplatin, tetracycline.
2. *Group B – acting by the immune complex mechanism:* Acetaminophen (paracetamol), aminopyrine, *p*-amino-salicylic acid, antazoline, antihistamines, carbimazole, chlorinated hydrocarbon insecticides, chlorpromazine, chlorpropamide, dipyrone, hydralazine, hydrochlorothiazide, 9-hydroxymethylellipticinium, insulin, isoniazid, melphalan, methotrexate, nomifensine, phenacetin, probenecid, quinidine, quinine, rifampicin, stibophen, streptomycin, sulphonamides, teniposide (VM-26), thiopentone, triamterene.
3. *Group C – acting by inducing autoantibody formation:* Ibuprofen, levodopa, α-methyldopa, mefenamic acid, procainamide, phenacetin, chlorpromazine,

The presence of autoantibodies (other than drug-induced) – autoimmune haemolytic anaemia (AIHA)

Overt AIHA is not a common disorder: a general hospital serving a population of 250 000 may expect to see 3–5 cases each year but the observed incidence depends greatly on the awareness and interests of the haematology staff.

Classification of AIHA can be based on whether it is idiopathic or secondary with further subdivision of the secondary types. However, from a laboratory and clinical standpoint a serological separation into 'warm' and 'cold' types related to whether the autoantibodies react optimally at 37°C or 4°C is an accepted approach. Further division into idiopathic or secondary AIHA may then be made.

Warm AIHA is more common than cold AIHA in a ratio of about 4:1 though in some series which include a large number of drug-associated cases the proportion may be different. The proportion of idiopathic to secondary warm AIHA shows much greater variation though secondary types are more common. In cold AIHA idiopathic and secondary forms are of approximately equal frequency. Inevitably, in both warm and cold types initially classed as idiopathic, there may be an underlying cause which is revealed later, even after some months or even years. Several large series have been published[51,52] and *Table 11.4* illustrates the types and associations of AIHA.

Table 11.4 Classification of 323 patients with autoimmune haemolytic anaemia (AIHA)*

Type of condition	*Males*	*Females*	*Total*	
Warm AIHA				
Idiopathic	43	62	105	59
Secondary:				
Lymphoma	13	15	28	
SLE	0	16	16	
Other AI disease	11	18	29	
Miscellaneous	6	3	9	
Drugs	26	46	72	
Cold AIHA				
CHAD:				
Acute (mycoplasma, infectious mononucleosis, other viruses)	5	15	20	64
Chronic	19	17	36	
PCH:				
Acute (virus infection)	5	2	7	
Chronic, syphilis (very rare), idiopathic	1	0	1	
Grand total	129	194	323	

*Taken from reference [51].
AI = Autoimmune; CHAD = cold haemagglutinin disease (or cold agglutinin syndrome, CAS); PCH = paroxysmal cold haemoglobinuria; SLE = systemic lupus erythematosus.

The secondary forms due to warm antibodies can be seen to be particularly associated with other autoimmune diseases, lymphoproliferative disorders and in association with drugs. Secondary forms of cold AIHA are clearly associated with infections with viruses or mycoplasma[53]. Paroxysmal cold haemoglobinuria (PCH) associated with syphilis is now very rare.

Red-cell destruction in AIHA

Autoantibody mediated red-cell destruction is due to the presence of immunoglobulin and/or complement on the cell membrane. Using specific antisera in the direct antiglobulin test three general patterns are found – IgG only, C3 only and a mixed pattern of IgG + C3. In addition, published series[51,52] of warm AIHA have included cases with IgA alone or IgA + C3 or IgM + C3. Antiglobulin reagents in routine use have no requirement for activity against either IgA or IgM but if these immunoglobulins are present on red cells, it is in association with IgG and/or C3. A summary of three published series[54] of warm AIHA indicates that 35% were IgG without C3, 56% IgG + C3 and 9% C3 without IgG.

The strength of positivity of the direct antiglobulin test shows poor correlation with the severity of haemolysis which, though in part is due to technical factors, is also influenced by the Ig class, Ig subclass, the ability to activate complement and the number of immunoglobulin molecules on each cell. The number of antigen sites and the phagocytic activity of the RES are additional factors.

Warm AIHA

IgG is demonstrable alone or in association with C3 by the DAT in over 90% of cases, the remainder being mainly C3 only. The antibodies are primarily IgG_1 and IgG_3 subclasses, occasionally IgG_2 and very rarely IgG_4. The phagocytic cells of the RES have receptors for the Fc component of the heavy chain of subclasses IgG_1 and IgG_3 but lack receptors for subclasses IgG_2 and IgG_4. This correlates with the finding that IgG_2 and IgG_4 are not associated with haemolysis. The immune adherence of phagocytes and IgG-coated cells results in red-cell damage at the site of adherence with loss of surface, deformation, sphering and erythrophagocytosis. The additional presence of C3 components augments erythrophagocytosis. Thus the destruction of IgG-coated cells is usually ‘extravascular’ and occurs mainly in the spleen. The ability to bind complement depends on the class of immunoglobulin; one molecule of IgM will activate one complement molecule whereas two molecules of IgG are necessary. Subclasses IgG_1 and IgG_3 activate complement and IgG_4 does not. The two IgG molecules must be closely situated on the membrane and therefore the antigen density or distribution is important. Rh antigens are widely spaced and are not associated with complement fixation.

A small number, less than 5%, of patients with warm AIHA fail to show a positive DAT. It is clear that the number of IgG molecules bound to the red cell necessary to produce a positive DAT (>120) is more than required to induce immune-mediated cell destruction (>35). More sensitive techniques are available based on either enhancement of serological procedures or by mononuclear phagocytic assay.

Cold AIHA

Cold antibodies do not usually bind to red-cell membranes at 37°C. This is thought to be due to membrane alteration in the cold rather than conformational changes of the antibody. Most of the cold-reactive antibodies are IgM cold agglutinins, the notable exception being the IgG autoantibody of PCH. IgM antibodies readily fix complement and then elute from the red cell. When the full complement sequence is activated, intravascular lysis occurs but when sub-lytic amounts are present the presence of C3 components allows reaction with phagocytes. Incompletely phagocytosed cells are coated with C3d and tend to be spherocytic. Despite the element of phagocytic haemolysis, the destruction in cold AIHA is characteristically intravascular with haemosiderinuria and in severe cases, haemoglobinuria.

The degree of haemolysis in cold AIHA is highly variable and does not correlate well with agglutinin titres in saline at 4°C or 30°C. A far better correlation with haemolysis is found if titration and determination of thermal amplitude is performed in the presence of bovine albumin [55]. Another factor is that the presence of inactive complement components on the cell membrane can inhibit antibody fixation [56].

Paroxysmal cold haemoglobinuria (PCH) is associated with the bi-phasic IgG Donath–Landsteiner antibody. Red cells are sensitized in the cold and complement-dependent lysis occurs on warming to 37°C. If the DAT is performed at 4°C IgG will be detected, otherwise only C3 will be found.

Specificity of antibodies in AIHA

Warm AIHA

Almost all cases of warm AIHA have a positive DAT due to IgG and/or complement on the red cells. Early studies of the antibodies suggested that they were 'non-specific' in that they appeared to react with all normal red cells. The demonstration of an anti-e autoantibody was followed by reports of other specificities within the Rh system, e.g. C, c, D, E. In most instances the specific autoantibody was associated with other 'non-specific' antibodies which could be absorbed using cells of selected Rh phenotype to reveal the specific antibody. Free autoantibody may be found in the serum only when the cells are maximally coated and if present may not represent the antibodies on the red cells. Specificity studies must therefore be performed using red-cell eluate.

By using red cells lacking basic Rh determinants, i.e. D deletion (–D–/, partially deleted, pdl) and Rh_{null} (– – –/, deleted, dl) three classes of 'non-specific' autoantibody can be identified: (1) those that react with cells of normal Rh phenotype (anti-nl); (2) those that react with pdl cells but not dl-cells (anti-pdl); and (3) those that react with all three cell types (anti-dl). Absorption studies of anti-nl, -pdl and -dl have shown that many contain antibodies of 'simple' Rh specificity. Some auto anti-dl antibodies have been shown to have anti-Wr^b or anti-En^a specificities. Other anti-pdl and anti-dl autoantibodies have been shown to contain anti-U or anti-LW. Specificities have also been shown within the MN, Kell, Kidd and Xg systems. A further complication in determining specificity is that specific antibodies may be eluted from red cells lacking the corresponding antigen: for example, an anti-E that can be absorbed and eluted from E-negative red cells. Such an antibody is termed 'mimicking anti-E' [54,57]. If transfusion is unavoidable in the management of the patient, cells lacking the antigens to specific or mimicking antibodies should be selected.

Cold AIHA

Cold agglutinins are IgM antibodies which are usually directed against the I or related antigens. Normal or pathological cold autoagglutinins are assigned I specificity when they react more strongly with the red cells of adults than with those of infants, and conversely i specificity when they react more strongly with fetal cord cells than with adult cells. Many normal sera contain low-titre anti-I with a low thermal amplitude. In contrast auto anti-I capable of causing haemolysis is usually present in high titre (often over 1000) with a thermal amplitude allowing reaction at temperatures which are found *in vivo* (28–30°C). The majority of cold autoantibodies are anti-I, a smaller number are anti-i and more rarely examples of 'non-Ii' antibodies, which react equally well with adult and cord cells are found and have been designated anti-Sp_1 (species) which also differ in that their reaction is diminished by enzyme treatment of the red cells in contrast to anti-Ii which is enhanced. In cold AIHA induced by infection, the IgM is usually polyclonal in contrast to the anti-I of cold haemagglutin disease (CHAD) which is almost always monoclonal with κ light chains whilst anti-i usually have λ light chains. The association of anti-i with infectious mononucleosis and the rare occurrence of haemolysis is discussed on page 510.

Donath–Landsteiner (DL) antibody In contrast to the IgM cold agglutinins, the biphasic DL antibody is an IgG which was considered to be non-specific, until haemolysis with P_1 and P_2 but not P_1^K, P_2^K or p cells was demonstrated, i.e. anti-P specificity. Other specificities such as anti-I have been reported but may be due to the additional presence of CHAD.

Drugs, chemicals, bacterial toxins and animal venoms

Drugs and chemicals

The susceptibility of red cells to drug or chemically induced haemolysis, other than that associated with immune mechanisms, can occur in several ways: (1) as a result of the drug being potentially dangerous even at normal dosage; (2) by accidental or deliberate over-dosage; or (3) as a result of hypersensitivity to drugs which in normal dosage do not cause damage (considered previously in relation to G6PD deficiency and the unstable haemoglobins).

Although some inorganic compounds can cause haemolysis (e.g. arsine, nitrites, potassium and sodium chlorate), organic chemicals and drugs are usually responsible and the haemolysis is due to oxidative stress. Red-cell changes due to oxidation include lipid peroxidation, oxidation of reduced sulphydryl groups of the membrane and oxidation of haemoglobin with the formation of met- or sulphaemoglobin during which there is rearrangement of the globin moiety and Heinz-body formation (*Figure 11.6*).

The effect of oxidative compounds depends on their oxidizing potential, dosage, absorption and excretion. The clinical manifestations range from methaemoglobin formation without overt haemolysis, to acute intravascular haemolysis with intravascular coagulation and renal failure. Many of the drugs listed as causing haemolysis in G6PD deficiency will, in higher dosage, cause haemolysis of normal cells. Probably the most commonly encountered are dapsone, used in the treatment of dermatitis herpetiformis, and salazosulphapyridine (Salazopyrin, sulphasalazine) commonly used in the treatment of inflammatory bowel disorders. As functional hyposplenism occurs in both disorders the number of Heinz bodies in circulating red cells may be considerable. Aspects of oxidative haemolysis have been reviewed, with a list of drugs and dosage in relation to haemolysis [25].

Acute haemolysis due to accidental or self-poisoning can be caused by a wide variety of compounds.

Bacterial toxins and animal venoms

The anaemia associated with infection is undoubtedly multifactorial and only rarely is there overt haemolysis. It may be anticipated that a septicaemia due to bacteria

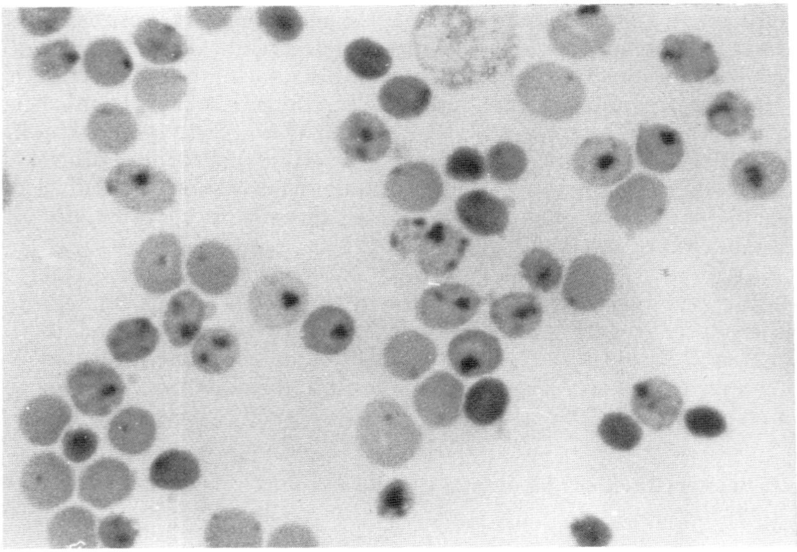

Figure 11.6 Methyl violet supravital preparation of blood. Gross Heinz-body formation due to poisoning with sodium chlorate. ×825

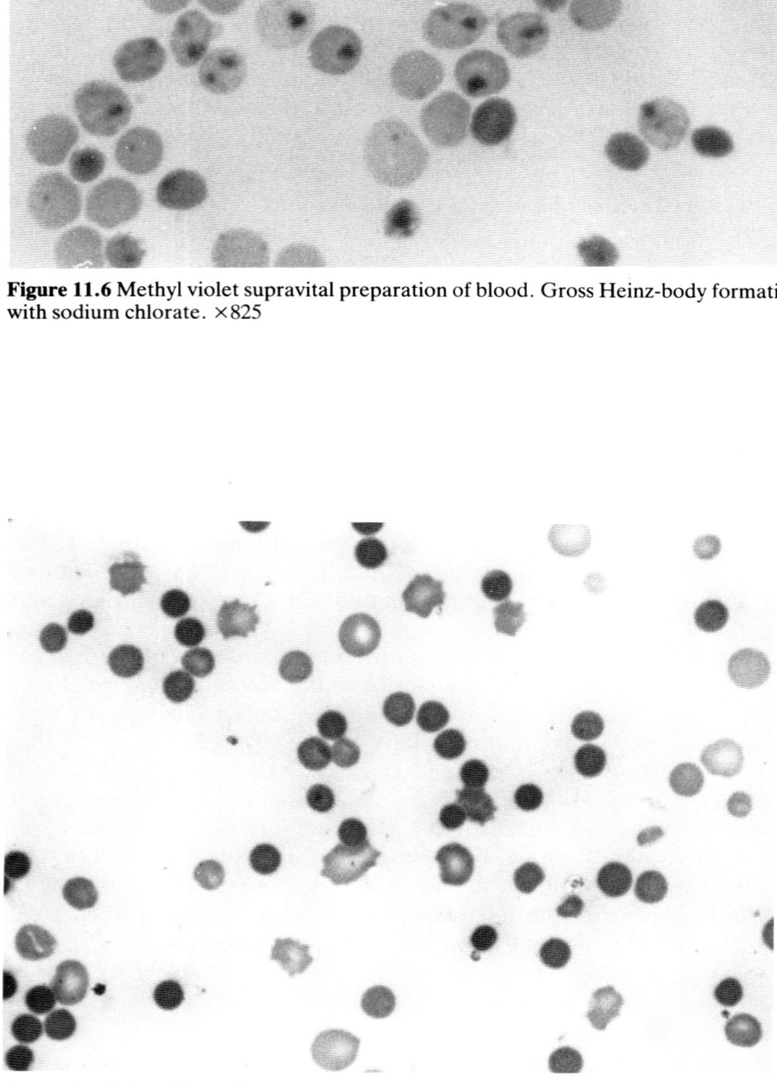

Figure 11.7 Blood film. *Clostridium perfringens* (*welchii*) septicaemia. Grossly spherocytic red cells; the hazy background is due to the staining of free haemoglobin in the plasma. ×550

which produce haemolysis in culture will also result in a shortened red-cell survival. The classic example is *Clostridium perfringens* septicaemia which is associated with acute haemolysis, marked spherocytosis (*Figure 11.7*) and all the evidence of severe intravascular haemolysis. Meningococcal infection is associated with a fragmenting red-cell picture. Other mechanisms which may rarely be involved in haemolysis are non-specific absorption by red cells of bacterial polysaccharides which then react with the anti-bacterial antibodies produced by the patient, and the exposure of T-antigen determinants which react with the anti-T present in normal serum, i.e. polyagglutinability.

Snake, bee and spider venoms may produce acute intravascular haemolysis.

Direct physical or mechanical red-cell damage

Microangiopathic haemolytic anaemia (MHA)

The blood changes in MHA are characteristic. Fragmented and distorted red cells often of triangular or 'pincered' shape indicate the 'tearing' or 'shearing' mechanism responsible. Microspherocytes are commonly present and thrombocytopenia is usual. The haemolysis is intravascular and in chronic or severe cases haemosiderinuria and even haemoglobinuria may be found. MHA is associated with a variety of disorders which have in common the deposition of fibrin in small blood vessels, or an abnormal vascular endothelium:

1. Thrombotic thrombocytopenic purpura.
2. Haemolytic uraemia syndrome.
3. Polyarteritis nodosa.
4. Malignant hypertension.
5. Rejection of renal transplant.
6. Eclampsia.
7. Mucin-secreting adenocarcinomatosis.
8. Haemangioma.

Cardiac abnormalities

Red-cell changes associated with intravascular haemolysis and probably indistinguishable from those of MHA are associated with valvular disease, earlier patterns of prosthetic heart valves and implants of synthetic materials. Correction of the valve defects or replacement of prostheses results in cessation of haemolysis.

Physical factors

The effect of high temperature on red-cell integrity and the mechanical damage found in exertional haemoglobinuria has been referred to on pages 300 and 301.

Parasitization of red cells

Protozoal or bacterial parasitization of erythrocytes results in direct lysis of the cells either by mechanical disruption in the case of malaria and babesiosis, or by the liberation of toxins as probably occurs in bartonellosis. The subject is dealt with further in Chapter 14.

Abnormalities of membrane lipids secondary to plasma abnormalities

Although sometimes classified as intracellular defects these disorders must be included with the extracellular mechanisms as the influence of plasma lipids on the membrane and shape of the red cell is well recognized[58]. Changes in plasma lipids, particularly cholesterol, lecithin and sphingomyelin, have a notable effect with target cells and acanthocytes being characteristic appearances.

Acanthocytosis

Hereditary acanthocytosis Although rare, this has been described many times and is due to an inherited deficiency of the low-density β lipoproteins, i.e. abetalipoproteinaemia. Plasma phospholipids are reduced with an inverted sphingomyelin:lecithin ratio, a pattern that is reflected in the red-cell membrane. Haemolysis is apparently intermittent and it has been suggested that the cells are unduly susceptible to peroxidation.

Acquired acanthocytosis This is particularly associated with the haemolytic anaemia in hepatic cirrhosis ('spur-cell anaemia'). Incubation of normal red cells in a patient's plasma induces 'spur-cell' formation while conversely the patient's cells in normal plasma revert to normal shape. The cholesterol:phospholipid ratio is considerably increased.

LCAT deficiency

This rare inherited (and acquired) deficiency is associated with an absence of esterified cholesterol in the plasma which is reflected by a marked accumulation of membrane cholesterol resulting in target cells, but for some reason spur cells are not a feature. Haemolysis is mild.

Other lipid abnormalities

It is already clear that acanthocytosis, spur cells and target cells are due to a variety of lipid abnormalities perhaps associated with variation in the antioxidant levels of α-tocopherol (vitamin E).

A complex pathophysiology probably exists in the haemolytic anaemia of alcoholic liver disease (Zieve's syndrome) which is characterized by haemolytic anaemia, elevated cholesterol and triglycerides. Membrane changes include elevated cholesterol and polyunsaturated fatty acids which, in association with red-cell vitamin E deficiency, may result in oxidation of reduced glutathione thus producing enzyme instability[59]. Reduced ATP levels due to hypophosphataemia may also be an important mechanism.

A single case of haemolytic anaemia with stomatocytes in hereditary analphalipoproteinaemia has been described[60].

Investigation of haemolytic anaemias

The variety of mechanisms producing haemolytic anaemia demands a multiplicity of techniques for their investigation and the problem of which techniques to apply can appear formidable. A logical sequence of investigation can, however, be devised which will establish all but the rarest causes.

Laboratory investigation can be divided into those tests that demonstrate increased haemolysis and those used to identify the cause. A schematic approach to investigation is shown in *Figure 11.8* which we have used, with up-dating as required, for over 30 years. It is not suggested that the scheme be followed rigidly; the patient's history and clinical presentation often indicates a specific test or series of tests. For example, haemoglobinuria in a Negro after treatment of malaria with primaquine clearly indicates the probability of G6PD deficiency, whereas haemoglobinuria in a child after measles would suggest an autoimmune mechanism.

The scheme depends upon first establishing that increased haemolysis is present. Although a reduced red-cell survival is the criterion of a haemolytic state the measurement of mean red-cell life is usually confined to those cases in which haemolysis is in doubt, to determine whether a defect is intra- or extracellular, to study the effect of treatment or as a research procedure. Morphological evidence of red-cell damage and erythroid regeneration are usually the initial indications, supported by evidence of increased haemoglobin release and catabolism. The autohaemolysis test, though not now widely used in the differentiation of CNSHA, is a sensitive, though non-specific, test but demands strict technique. Whether the DAT should be regarded as an indication of increased haemolysis or used to separate immune mechanisms from the remainder is debatable but the majority of haemolytic anaemias do not have an immune basis nor does a positive DAT necessarily equate with increased haemolysis. In this scheme, therefore, the DAT is not used as evidence of haemolysis.

Although a corrected reticulocyte count (*see* page 100) is an indication of erythropoietic activity and, in the steady state, an indication of the rate of red-cell destruction, in mild to moderate haemolysis the reticulocyte count may not be a sufficiently sensitive index. Red-cell constituents which vary in amount or activity according to cell age have been used as indicators of the severity of haemolysis. The red-cell creatine levels appear to be a reliable index of cell age [61], and since it is an easily measured stable component unaffected by contamination with leucocytes or platelets it could be of value in the study of haemolytic states.

Glycosylation of haemoglobin depends not only on blood glucose level but also on red-cell life span. In haemolytic anaemias levels of glycosylated Hb are significantly lower than in healthy controls and the lowered levels correlate with the reduced red-cell life span [62].

Determination of red-cell survival

Prior to the availability of radioisotopes, red-cell survival was determined by the Ashby technique of transfusing up to a litre of compatible though antigenically distinct red cells, e.g. group O to a group A recipient, MN to an N or M recipient or Rh negative to a Rh-positive recipient. The proportion of transfused cells in the resulting red-cell mixture is determined *in vitro* by differential agglutination using

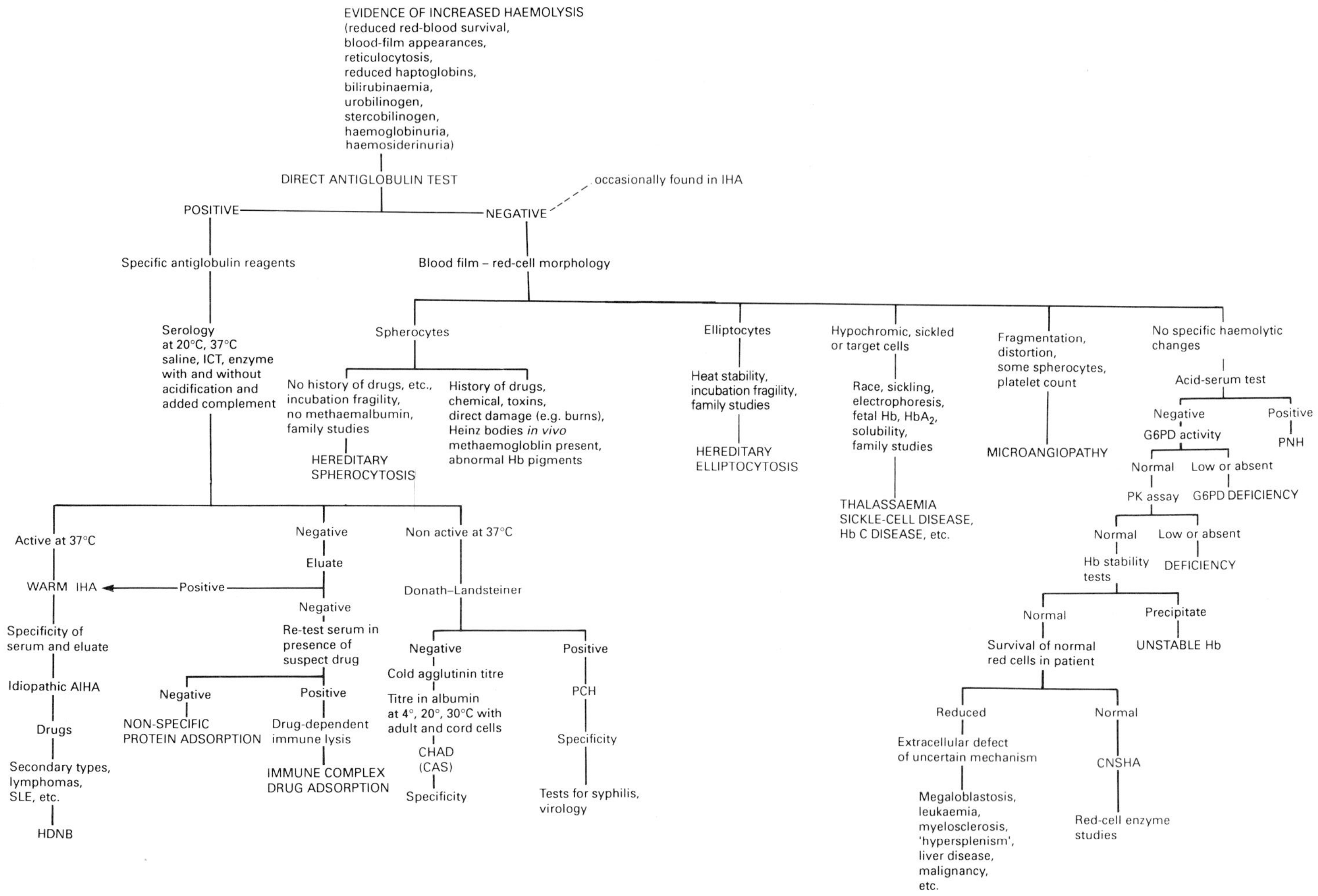

Figure 11.8 A schematic approach to the investigation of suspected haemolytic anaemia. AIHA = autoimmune haemolytic anaemia; CAS = cold agglutinin syndrome; CHAD = cold haemagglutinin disease; CNSHA = chronic non-spherocytic haemolytic anaemia; G6PD = glucose-6-phosphate dehydrogenase; HDNB = haemolytic disease of the new-born; ICT = indirect Coombs' test; IHA = immune haemolytic anaemia; PCH = paroxysmal cold haemoglobinuria;

an appropriate high avidity, specific anti-serum, e.g. anti-A, anti-N or anti-D. Despite the inherent errors of the technique, the normal red-cell survival of 120 days and the evaluation and development of anticoagulants for blood donations and the criteria for storage were established. Modifications to improve the technique have been developed, particularly the use of an autoanalyser for the differential agglutination stage and by counting free cells using a cell-counting instrument. Although perhaps still having some applications, the use of the technique in the study of haemolytic anaemias is limited to following the survival of normal cells in the patient's circulation and therefore no information regarding an intrinsic red-cell defect can be obtained as the infusion of patient's cells to a normal subject must be considered unethical. Study of the survival of the patient's cells in the patient's circulation is now the recognized procedure and is made possible by radioisotopic red-cell labelling.

The most widely used radioisotope method is the labelling of a population of red cells of all ages, i.e. random labelling. The commonly used isotopes are ^{51}Cr as hexavalent sodium chromate ($Na_2{}^{51}CrO_4$) and ^{32}P as di-isopropylphosphofluoridate ($DF^{32}P$). For patients in whom radioisotope studies are contraindicated, e.g. children and in pregnancy, random labelling with non-radioactive ^{50}Cr followed by *in vitro* neutron activation analysis has been recommended[63].

Red cells may also be labelled as a cohort (a population of cells produced during a relatively limited period) by the incorporation of isotopes such as ^{59}Fe or ^{14}C-labelled glycine into haemoglobin. This technique has been considered to be essentially a research method but ^{59}Fe labelling during the course of ferrokinetic studies has been shown to give results comparable with random labelling using ^{51}Cr[64] and in some instances may be superior[65].

The relative merits of $DF^{32}P$ and ^{51}Cr for random labelling are summarized in *Table 11.5*.

Table 11.5 Relative merits of $DF^{32}P$ and ^{51}Cr for random labelling

$DF^{32}P$	*^{51}Cr*
In vivo or *in vitro* labelling	*In vitro* labelling only
Minimal elution after the first 24 hours	Continuing elution but usually predictable
No reutilization	No reutilization
No damage to red cells	May damage unduly susceptible cells possibly resulting in early loss
β emitter, surface counting not possible	γ emission permits surface counting
β counting equipment less widely available	Solid scintillation counting widely available
Labels membrane via acetylcholinesterase (but *see* reference [66])	Labels β-globin chain

Although $DF^{32}P$ is claimed to be the most accurate method due to the absence of continuing elution, ^{51}Cr is usually considered to be the most suitable when all aspects are considered and is recommended by the ICSH as the reference method[67].

ICSH method for red-cell survival study

To avoid the risk of alloimmunization and of transferring infectious disease, survival studies should be performed using the patient's own red cells.

Exceptionally donor red cells may be used to study compatibility or to determine whether a haemolytic state is due to an intrinsic defect of the patient's red cells or to a pathological process resulting in increased destruction of normal red cells. All solutions must be sterile and pyrogen-free and all procedures carried out using sterile technique. Regulations regarding the handling of radioisotope preparations for injection could limit the availability of red-cell survival studies.

Collection and labelling of red cells

Blood is obtained by venepuncture and 10 volumes of blood is added to 1.5 volumes 'NIH A' ACD solution (trisodium citrate dihydrate 22 g; citric acid 8 g; dextrose 25 g; water to 1 litre; sterilized by autoclaving at 126°C for 30 minutes; final pH 5.4). The mixture is centrifuged at 1000–1500 *g* for 5–10 minutes. The supernatant plasma is removed and discarded; care is taken not to remove any red cells. If the leucocyte count is greater than 25×10^9/l the buffy coat is removed and discarded.

[^{51}Cr]sodium chromate solution is added slowly and with continuous gentle swirling. The amount of ^{51}Cr added should be as low as possible while consistent with the equipment used to measure the radioactivity of the samples and in any case limited to 0.5 μCi/kg body weight (0.018 MBq). The specific activity of the ^{51}Cr should be such that less than 2 μg chromium is added per ml of packed cells. The added [^{51}Cr]sodium chromate should be in a volume of at least 0.2 ml, being diluted if necessary in isotonic sodium chloride. The cells should be kept at room temperature, or in a water bath at 37°C, for 15 minutes.

The cells are washed in 4–5 volumes isotonic sodium chloride. After the second wash there is generally less than 1% of the remaining radioactivity in the supernatant. The red cells are resuspended in a sufficient volume of isotonic saline to allow injection of 20 ml or a lesser amount in children. When osmotic fragility is greatly increased the red cells should be washed in 12 g/l sodium chloride. If red-cell volume or external blood loss is to be measured an aliquot of the labelled red-cell suspension should be set aside for preparation of appropriate standards.

The major portion of the labelled cell suspension is then injected. If red-cell volume is to be determined the actual amount must be known. Methods to determine this amount precisely are described in the section on blood volume determination (*see* page 483).

Sampling

At 10 minutes 5 ml of blood is collected into solid anticoagulant from a vein other than that used for injection. If it is suspected that mixing will be incomplete at 10 minutes a further sample is taken at 60 minutes. A further sample is taken at 24 hours, three samples between day 2 and day 7 and thereafter at least two further specimens per week for the duration of the study. The haemoglobin level or PCV is measured on a part of each specimen.

Sample preparation and radioactivity measurement

To each sample add a small amount of saponin powder and mix well for 5 minutes. Using pipettes of uniform type deliver an appropriate volume of each specimen into a counting tube. When blood is unusually viscous the blood should be pipetted before adding saponin. The volumes of blood should be known precisely and if necessary made up to the same volume in each tube. When possible replicate samples of each specimen should be prepared.

Measure the radioactivity in a γ-ray detection system. The coefficient of variation attributable to counting statistics should not exceed 2%. If there is a significant difference in counts (greater than 2%) between the 10 minutes and 60 minutes sample the latter should be used for subsequent calculation of red-cell survival.

Presentation and analysis of red-cell survival data

It is common to use ^{51}Cr survival data to determine the $T_{50}Cr$, that is, the time taken for the concentration of ^{51}Cr in the circulating blood to fall to 50% of its initial value after correction of the data for physical decay. Without additional information on the type of destruction (random or as a function of age) mean red-cell life span cannot be calculated from $T_{50}Cr$ and it is preferable to estimate mean red-cell life span as described below.

If the patient is in a 'steady state' the measurement of radioactivity in blood samples may be expressed as counting rate/g Hb, counting rate/ml red cells, or counting rate/ml whole blood. A steady state exists when the reticulocyte count and the haemoglobin concentration (or PCV) have not changed significantly during the previous 2 months and during the period of study, and therefore the rates of production and destruction of red cells have been constant ('destruction' includes loss of red cells by haemorrhage). In a non-steady state or when it has not been possible to establish a steady state, expression of radioactivity/ml whole blood enables mean red-cell life span to be estimated if it is assumed that the total blood volume remains constant.

^{51}Cr is eluted at an average rate of 1% per day which is of the same order as the normal rate of red-cell destruction. Variation in elution in different individuals may seriously affect the accuracy of estimates of mean red-cell life span when survival is normal or only slightly reduced. Elution is fairly constant in normal subjects and a correction factor can be applied. Though elution rates may vary when survival is severely reduced such variation becomes relatively unimportant.

All measurements are corrected for physical decay and further corrected for chromium elution using the correction factors in *Table 11.6*. The data are plotted as

Table 11.6 Correction factors to convert chromium survival into 'true' red-cell survival (ACD method)

Day	*Correction factor*	*Day*	*Correction factor*	*Day*	*Correction factor*
1	1.03	11	1.16	21	1.29
2	1.05	12	1.17	22	1.31
3	1.06	13	1.18	23	1.32
4	1.07	14	1.19	24	1.34
5	1.08	15	1.20	25	1.36
6	1.10	16	1.22	26	1.38
7	1.11	17	1.23	27	1.40
8	1.12	18	1.25	28	1.42
9	1.13	19	1.26	29	1.45
10	1.14	20	1.27	30	1.47

ACD = Acid–citrate–dextrose.

counting rate/ml whole blood against time on linear graph paper. If a straight line can be fitted to the data points a least-squares fitting procedure can be used to obtain the line and goodness of fit. A straight line indicates that red-cell destruction is largely the result of senescence (a function of red-cell age) and the mean red-cell life span can be derived as the reciprocal of the slope of the line or as the intercept obtained by extrapolating the line to zero activity.

If a straight line is not obtained on linear graph paper, the data are plotted on semi-logarithmic paper. If a straight line is then obtained, a least-squares fitting procedure is again used to determine the line and goodness of fit. A good fit indicates a random destruction mechanism and the mean red-cell life span can be derived as the time corresponding to 37% survival, or by multiplying the half time of the fitted line by 1.44. If neither procedure results in the data satisfactorily fitting

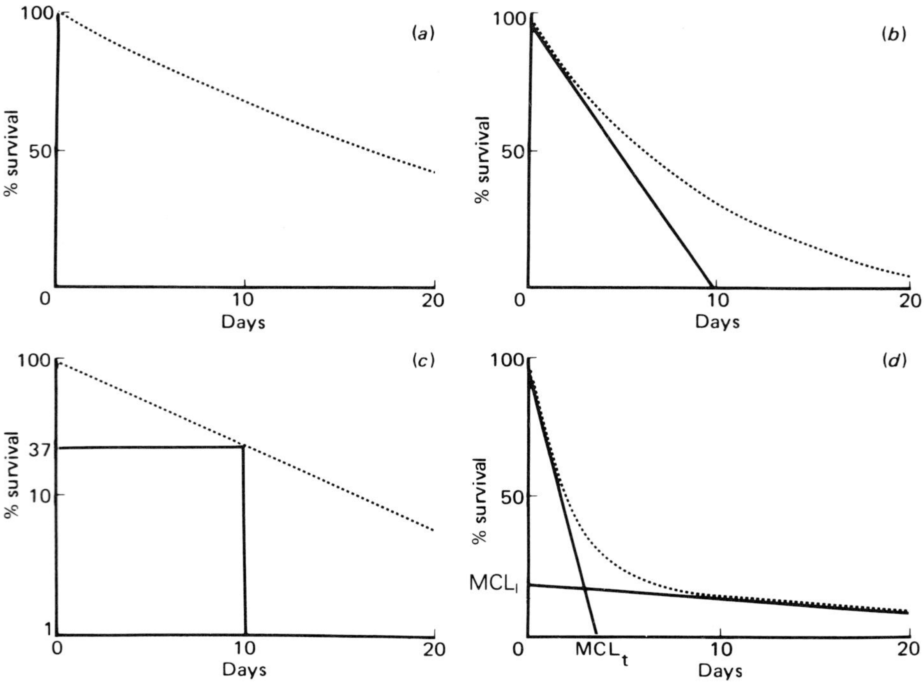

Figure 11.9 Red-cell survival plots. (*a*) Arithmetic graph paper; a near linear plot; mean cell life span (MCL) can be obtained by extrapolation to the abscissa. Linear plots indicate cell destruction to be a function of the age of the red cells. (*b*) Arithmetic graph paper; a near exponential survival curve typical of random red-cell destruction. MCL can be deduced by drawing a tangent to the early part of the curve and extrapolating to the abscissa. (*c*) The same data as in (*b*) plotted on semi-logarithmic paper to produce a linear plot. MCL is that time when 37% of the labelled red cells remain. (d) Arithmetic graph paper; a dual red-cell population with differing survival times. The MCL of the total population (MCL_t) is approximated by a tangent from the early part of the curve; the proportion of cells with longer survival is determined by extrapolation to the ordinate and the MCL (MCL_l) by extrapolation to the abscissa. The MCL of the short-lived population (MCL_s) can be calculated from:

$$MCL_s = \frac{S(\%)}{\dfrac{100}{MCL_t} - \dfrac{\%L}{MCL_l}}$$

where S = short-lived population; L = long-lived population

a straight line, the initial slope of the curve on the linear plot is obtained by drawing a straight line through the first few points only. A choice of functions can be used when computing facilities are available [67]. Examples of red-cell survival plots are shown in *Figure 11.9*.

Normal value for mean red-cell life span is taken as 120 days (SD 15 days). $T_{50}Cr$ is about 28 days. Red-cell survival studies may only be interpreted as being due to haemolysis if haemorrhage can be excluded or measured with reasonable certainty. Occult gastrointestinal blood loss is the major problem and if present can be quantitated by comparing the radioactivity in a series of 24-hour stool collections with the activity of measured blood samples taken on the corresponding days. True red-cell survival can be calculated as follows:

$$T = T_0 \frac{V}{(V - T_0 L)}$$

where T_0 = apparent mean red-cell life span (days); V = total red-cell volume (ml); and L = average rate loss of red cells (ml/day).

Demonstration of sites of red-cell destruction by external counting

In addition to the determination of red-cell survival the degree of destruction in the liver and spleen is of clinical value, particularly if splenectomy is being considered.

The ICSH has described a recommended method [68] using a single collimated scintillation detector by which qualitative information can be obtained. The activity over the heart, liver and spleen is followed during the period of the survival study. The heart count is used to predict the count rates that would be expected over the liver and spleen if their initial count rate fell at the same rate as the heart count. Any differences in activity are considered 'excess counts' and interpreted as accumulation of ^{51}Cr in that organ. Four general patterns may be found:

1. Little or no excess in the liver and spleen.
2. Excess accumulation in both organs.
3. Excess accumulation only in the spleen.
4. Excess accumulation only in the liver.

Splenectomy is considered if there is accumulation in the spleen only or perhaps both in liver and in spleen. Unfortunately, clinical benefit does not always correlate with the magnitude of the excess counts.

The variables responsible for this lack of correlation are, first, the volume of the organ scanned by the counter in relation to the total volume of the organ and other tissues in the field of counting; secondly the tissue thickness over the organ; and thirdly the loss of ^{51}Cr from the organ following red-cell destruction [69]. A further possible misleading aspect which does not appear to be generally considered is that it is the haemoglobin within the red cell that is labelled and if that haemoglobin is liberated intravascularly and cleared from the plasma by haemoglobin-binding proteins, accumulation in the liver would be expected. Although histological evidence of red-cell destruction by liver macrophages can be demonstrated, accumulation of ^{51}Cr in the liver may not necessarily reflect red-cell sequestration and destruction. It is perhaps significant that in some haemolytic processes characterized by intravascular haemolysis, e.g. sickle-cell anaemia, excess liver counts can usually be demonstrated.

In recent years the introduction of quantitative imaging equipment in radiology departments has made the relatively simple external scintillation counting procedure obsolete and has improved the correlation between spleen activity and the benefits of splenectomy mentioned above. For details of both external counting and quantitative imaging techniques see Bowring[69].

Techniques demonstrating increased release of haemoglobin

In haemolytic states significant amounts of haemoglobin are released into the plasma and are cleared by hepatocellular uptake and glomerular filtration. Circulating haemoglobin and haem are primarily transported by the plasma proteins haptoglobin (Hp), haemopexin (Hx) and albumin and, in the case of Hp and Hx, cleared by hepatic uptake. If haemolysis is rapid or severe, haemoglobinuria or haemosiderinuria will be present. The binding of Hb with Hp, Hx and albumin occurs as a consecutive sequence of iron salvage, each being activated when the previous one with a higher affinity and more rapid turnover is exhausted. Thus Hp depletion is, theoretically at least, the more sensitive index of increased haemoglobin turnover followed by Hx depletion and the presence of methaemalbumin, with haemoglobinuria only appearing when the binding proteins are depleted or saturated.

Determination of serum haptoglobin concentration

A variety of techniques have been developed to measure serum haptoglobin levels. Gelfiltration[70], colorimetric[71], electrophoretic[72] and immunological methods have been described. The choice of method depends mainly on the number of samples to be assayed, the requirement for a prompt result and perhaps economic considerations. Electrophoretic techniques are rapid, simple, cheap and can provide a result in 1–2 hours. For multiple samples when there is no urgency an immunological approach would be preferable.

Electrophoretic method [72]

Principle

By electrophoresis on paper or cellulose acetate membrane the Hps migrate with the α_2 globulin fraction, and when in complex with haemoglobin their mobility is slightly less though still in the α_2 band; free haemoglobin migrates in the β-globulin position. By adding varying amounts of haemoglobin the binding capacity of the serum can be determined by the appearance of the free haemoglobin band. Normal serum will bind 0.3–2.0 g/l of haemoglobin. The method described uses materials and apparatus for routine protein electrophoresis; the haemoglobin is demonstrated by its peroxidatic activity.

Materials

Serum is separated as soon as possible and must be free from haemolysis. It is stored at −20°C until tested.

Haemoglobin solutions A range of haemoglobin solutions is prepared from washed erythrocytes to contain 0.2–2.0 g/l in 0.2 g intervals. These solutions may be converted to carboxyhaemoglobin or HiCN and stored at −20°C.

Electrophoresis apparatus Cellulose acetate squares (10 × 10 cm) or two 10 × 5 cm strips are used. Any buffer suitable for routine protein electrophoresis may be used, with any tank designed for work with cellulose acetate.

Protein stain Ponceau S, 2 g in 1 litre of 30 g/l trichloracetic acid.

Differentiator 50 ml glacial acetic acid in 950 ml water.

Haemoglobin stain [73] Stock solution: 1 g tetramethylbenzidine (Sigma) in 90 ml glacial acetic acid made up to 100 ml with deionized water. Stable at 4°C in a dark bottle for up to 1 year. Working stain: prepare freshly. Stock solution 0.5 ml; glacial acetic acid 9.5 ml; hydrogen peroxide 100 volumes 20 μl; deionized water 10 ml.

Method
Into each of 10 tubes is placed 0.1 ml of the haemoglobin solution. To each tube is added 0.1 ml of serum and the mixture allowed to stand for 5 minutes. Smaller quantities may be used if desired. The cellulose acetate strip, previously impregnated in buffer and lightly blotted, is placed in position in the tank. About 3 μl of each of the serum-haemoglobin mixtures is applied as a spot or short streak towards the cathode end of the strip. A current of 0.4 mA/cm width of strip is applied and adequate separation is obtained in 1 hour. Without drying, the strip is placed in the protein stain for not more than 3 minutes and then washed in the acetic acid until all excess stain is removed followed by a rapid rinse with water. The haemoglobin stain is applied and the position of the haemoglobin band or bands can be clearly seen.

The Hp content is expressed as that level of haemoglobin immediately preceding the lowest concentration that shows a band of free haemoglobin in the β-globulin position. If no free haemoglobin band is present the serum may be diluted one in two or higher concentrations of haemoglobin may be used.

An additional advantage is that the technique is a sensitive indicator of methaemalbumin as shown by the blue staining of the albumin band.

Immunological methods

Antisera to human Hps are available commercially and therefore standard techniques for quantitating serum proteins such as radial immunodiffusion and quantitative immunoelectrophoresis (Laurell rocket technique) may be used. Agarose gels containing anti-haptoglobin can also be purchased together with reference sera of known haptoglobin content. The techniques are lengthy and relatively expensive and the necessity of preparing a calibration curve with each run or batch makes the immunological methods unsuitable for occasional or small numbers of measurements or when there is some degree of urgency for a result. On the other hand, for large numbers or when batching of tests is possible an immunological approach is probably the technique of choice.

Interpretation of Hp levels

The normal range of serum Hps is 0.3–2.0 g/l expressed as haemoglobin binding capacity, with a mean value of about 1.2 g/l. Levels are determined to some extent by Hp group. Depletion of Hps occurs when haemoglobin turnover exceeds twice normal, irrespective of whether the haemolysis is intra- or extravascular and therefore provides a sensitive index of haemolysis.

Interpretation is complicated by low levels due to diminished synthesis in hepatocellular disease and, as with other acute-phase proteins, Hps are increased in infections, tissue damage, malignancy etc. and in such conditions the presence of haptoglobins does not exclude haemolysis.

Demonstration of serum haemopexin (Hx)

Normal serum contains 0.5–1.0 g/l Hx which binds haem (free ferric protoporphyrin) but not haemoglobin. Unlike Hp, Hx is only rarely and minimally affected by non-specific stimuli and has therefore been suggested as a more reliable index of the severity of haemolysis. However, as Hx is synthesized exclusively in the liver, hepatocellular disease can be expected to be associated with reduced Hx levels. While probably a more reliable index of moderate to severe haemolysis, Hx levels must be less sensitive than Hp depletion in mild to moderate uncomplicated haemolytic states.

Serum Hx may be demonstrated by electrophoresis and quantitated by immunological techniques using anti-haemopexin antibody.

Demonstration of methaemalbumin

Haem has a greater affinity for Hx than for albumin and therefore methaemalbumin will only be formed when Hp and Hx are absent. Methaemalbumin is therefore an indication of severe haemolysis. Unlike Hb, Hp and haem–Hx complexes the turnover of albumin is not increased when complexed with haem and therefore methaemalbumin is the last haem pigment to disappear following intravascular haemolysis; the disappearance, in part at least, is due to transfer of haem to newly synthesized Hx. The presence of methaemalbumin imparts a reddish brown tinge to plasma and the absorption bands of the pigment may be demonstrated by direct vision or reversion spectroscopy. These methods are not very sensitive and the wide availability of spectrophotometers for the demonstration and measurement of the characteristic absorption spectrum has made direct spectroscopy virtually obsolete.

Methaemalbumin has a characteristic absorption band in the red part of the spectrum at 624 nm. Plasma or serum free from red cells is placed in a 1 cm cell in a spectrophotometer and the absorption spectrum recorded from 700 to 500 nm or alternatively repeated absorption measurements taken at 5 nm intervals. The peak at 624 nm may be slight and a more sensitive approach is to apply *Schumm's test*. The plasma or serum is covered with a layer of ether. A one-tenth volume of saturated yellow ammonium sulphide is added and mixed with the plasma. If methaemalbumin is present an intense absorption band can be demonstrated at 558 nm which represents the haemochromogen.

Differentiation of methaemoglobin, sulphaemoglobin and methaemalbumin

Methaemoglobin and sulphaemoglobin, though normally intracellular haemoglobin derivatives, may be found in plasma when associated with severe haemolysis and both have an absorption band close to that of methaemalbumin, methaemoglobin at 630 nm and sulphaemoglobin at 620 nm. The pigments may be differentiated by the separate addition of 5 mg sodium dithionite and one drop of ammonium hydroxide and observing the response of the band in the red as shown in *Table 11.7*.

Methaemalbumin may be quantitated by observing the change in absorption at 569 nm after the addition of sodium dithionite by reference to a calibration curve prepared by adding haemin to plasma[74]. Methaemalbumin may also be demonstrated by electrophoresis of serum and haemoglobin staining as described for haptoglobin measurement.

Table 11.7 Response of haem compounds to dithionite and ammonium hydroxide

Compound	*Dithionite*	*Ammonium hydroxide*
Methaemalbumin	Disappears	Disappears
Methaemoglobin	Disappears	Remains
Sulphaemoglobin	Remains	Remains

Demonstration of haemosiderin in urine

Haemosiderin in urine represents haemoglobin-iron released from the renal tubules following haemoglobin absorption and degradation. It therefore occurs after intravascular haemolysis associated with glomerular filtration of plasma haemoglobin.

Method 1 [75] 10 ml urine is centrifuged at 1200 *g* for 10–15 minutes. The deposit is transferred to a slide, spread out to occupy an area of 1–2 cm, allowed to dry in air and fixed in methanol for 20 minutes. The film is then stained by Perls' Prussian blue technique as for bone marrow or blood films. Haemosiderin appears in the form of isolated or grouped blue-staining granules from 1 to 3 μm in size. If present in small amounts and especially if distributed irregularly on the slide or if the findings are difficult to interpret, the test should be repeated on a fresh sample of urine collected into an iron-free container and centrifuged in an iron-free tube.

Method 2 10 ml of a fresh early-morning specimen of urine is centrifuged as above. The supernatant is decanted completely and 2 ml freshly prepared potassium ferrocyanide-HCl solution added and the deposit re-suspended. After incubation at 37°C for 15 minutes the mixture is re-centrifuged, the supernatant decanted and a drop of the deposit placed on a slide under a cover-slip. The preparation is examined with a dry ×40 objective for blue-staining granules or aggregates. Of particular importance is the observation of renal epithelial cells or casts which may contain haemosiderin granules thus proving it originated in the kidney.

Interpretation Haemosiderinuria is a valuable indication of chronic intravascular haemolysis as it will be present even when there is no haemoglobinuria. The granules are not seen at the onset of a haemolytic episode since absorption, degradation and excretion has to occur, but may persist for several weeks after a haemolytic episode.

Demonstration of haemoglobin or myoglobin in urine

Haemoglobinuria will be found only when the thresholds of the iron salvage proteins and renal tubular absorption have been overwhelmed, i.e. when haemolysis is rapid or severe. Gross haemoglobinuria appears red or even brown if conversion to methaemoglobin has occurred while the urine is in the bladder. True methaemoglobinuria may also be found due to lysis of red cells containing methaemoglobin as a result of haemolytic oxidant stress.

Apart from haemoglobin and its derivatives, non-protein pigments such as porphyrins or even vegetable colouring may be present and the possibility of myoglobinuria should also be considered. An ordered scheme of investigation should be followed to identify or exclude haemoglobin compounds.

The pigment can first be shown to be a protein by adding 3 ml of sulphosalicylic acid (30 g/l) to 1 ml of urine followed by centrifugation. If the pigment is a haem protein the supernatant will be of normal colour.

Myoglobin is differentiated from haemoglobin by dissolving 2.8 g ammonium sulphate in 5 ml of urine and centrifuging. Haemoglobin is found in the precipitate with the supernatant of a normal colour; myoglobin is not precipitated and the supernatant will be pigmented. Spectrophotometry of the urine may identify the haemoglobin pigment present.

Minor degrees of haemoglobinuria can be detected by scanning spectrophotometry particularly by studying the region of the Soret bands (405–425 nm). Haematuria must be excluded by examination of a centrifuged urine deposit. Myoglobinuria may also be minimal and differentiation from haemoglobin can be difficult as their absorption spectra are similar. In such instances an immunological approach using an antimyoglobin antibody is of value.

If the unknown pigment is in sufficient quantity or following concentration by dialysis, haemoglobin can be differentiated from myoglobin by electrophoresis at pH 8.6 under the conditions for haemoglobin electrophoresis (page 365). The urine is run alongside control samples. Myoglobin is more cathodic than haemoglobin – the relative mobility of myoglobin is that of Hb C compared with Hb A. Differentiation can also be made by centrifugation through a microconcentrator membrane with a 30 000 d cut-off. Myoglobin (16 500 d) will pass through while haemoglobin (64 000 d) will not.

Measurement of plasma haemoglobin level [76]

The plasma haemoglobin level may be increased in haemolytic anaemia when haemolysis is such that plasma Hp is fully saturated or absent. The highest levels are found when haemolysis is intravascular, i.e. in PNH, PCH and in mechanical haemolysis such as after surgery and in exertional haemoglobinuria.

Whether free haemoglobin is in fact found in normal circulating plasma is arguable as the procedures of specimen collection and subsequent handling can cause *in vitro* haemolysis. The published normal ranges of plasma haemoglobin include the effects of sampling procedures. The value of isolated estimations of plasma haemoglobin is limited and the method may be of most use when applied to serial measurements, for example in monitoring haemolysis after cardiac surgery when the other conventional indications of haemolysis will not immediately reflect fluctuations in red-cell destruction.

The peroxidase activity of haemoglobin is inhibited to varying extent by different plasmas and this is only partially due to the presence of haptoglobin. A method has been described for measuring haemoglobin at low concentrations which allows for the inhibitory action of plasma[77]. The normal range for plasma haemoglobin in specimens collected under the best conditions is probably less than 0.06 g/l.

Detection, identification and measurement of haemoglobin derivatives

Haemolysis may be associated with abnormal haemoglobin pigments or derivatives. The demonstration of methaemalbumin and its differentiation from methaemoglobin (Hi) and sulphaemoglobin (SHb) is described on page 342. Hi and SHb are essentially intracellular pigments and can be associated with haemolysis due to drugs or chemicals. Hi due to abnormal haemoglobin structure represents a separate category and is considered on page 347. Though artificially prepared solutions of Hi and SHb have characteristic absorption maxima throughout the visible spectrum, in pathological samples the intracellular pigments are always present as a minor component in the presence of normal haemoglobin and therefore cannot be easily detected or measured at those wavelengths associated with oxyhaemoglobin. Hi is present in small amounts (up to 3% of total haemoglobin) in normal blood; SHb is not normally present.

Qualitative demonstration of abnormal pigments

Blood is diluted 1 in 5 or 1 in 10 with water and centrifuged to remove the red-cell stroma. Such high concentrations will obliterate the spectrum other than in the red from 600 nm upwards. Both Hi and SHb have absorption bands in the red at 630 nm and 620 nm, respectively, which are too close for differentiation with a hand spectroscope. The behaviour of the band on the addition of a reducing agent such as sodium dithionite will differentiate between the pigments: the Hi band will disappear while that of SHb will persist.

With a well-calibrated reversion spectroscope the wavelength of the absorption bands can be measured or alternatively their identity confirmed by reference to Hi and SHb preparations. Hi can be prepared by adding a small quantity of potassium ferricyanide to a solution of Hb while SHb is prepared by the addition of a 100th volume of 1 g/l phenylhydrazine hydrochloride and a drop of water saturated with hydrogen sulphide, an unpleasant and essentially unnecessary procedure.

Recording sphectrophotometers have largely superseded direct vision or reversion spectroscopes and will readily differentiate the absorption maxima of the two pigments. For reference purposes the absorption maxima for haemoglobin pigments and derivatives are given in *Table 11.8*.

Whole blood can be used for preparing haemoglobin solutions as plasma pigments will not usually interfere at dilutions greater than 1 in 5. Exceptionally, however, gross methaemoglobinaemia such as occurs in sodium chlorate poisoning may be associated with Hi in the plasma, particularly in the presence of renal failure. If the presence of Hi in the red cells needs to be quantified in such circumstances then washed red cells should be used.

Quantitation of methaemoglobin

Principle When cyanide is added the absorption band at 630 nm disappears and the change in absorbance is proportional to the concentration of Hi. The total Hb in the sample is measured after complete conversion to HiCN by the addition of

Table 11.8 Absorption maxima of haemoglobin derivatives in pure solution (with the exception of sulphaemoglobin which is a mixture with oxyhaemoglobin). Myoglobin is included for comparison

Derivative	*Abbreviation*	*Position in spectrum*			
		Red	*Yellow-green*		*Violet*
Haemoglobin	Hb	–	–	555	431
Oxyhaemoglobin	HbO_2	–	577	542	415
Carboxyhaemoglobin	COHb	–	568	539	420
Methaemoglobin (pH 7–7.4)	Hi	630	–	500	406
Sulphaemoglobin	SHb	620	577	542	415
Cyanmethaemoglobin (hemiglobincyanide)	HiCN	–	–	540	421
Methaemalbumin	HiAlb	624	540	501	–
Myoglobin	MyoHb	–	560	–	434
Oxymyoglobin	$MyoHbO_2$	–	582	542	418

ferricyanide. The conversion is said not to include SHb but this is probably not a valid objection[78]. Turbidity of the haemolysate is overcome by the addition of a non-ionic detergent such as Nonidet P40.

Reagents Phosphate buffer 0.1 mol/l, pH 6.8; potassium cyanide 50 g/l; potassium ferricyanide 50 g/l; Nonidet P40 10 ml/l.

Method 0.2 ml of blood is lysed in a mixture of 4 ml buffer and 6 ml detergent and the lysate divided into equal parts (A and B). The absorbance of A is measured at 630 nm (D_1). One drop of KCN solution is added and the absorbance again measured (D_2). One drop of potassium ferricyanide is added to B and after 5 minutes the absorbance is measured at the same wavelength (D_3). One drop of potassium cyanide is then added to B and a final reading made (D_4). All measurements are made against a blank of buffer/detergent in the same proportions as used in the test.

Calculation Methaemoglobin (Hi) % $= \dfrac{(D_1 - D_2)}{(D_3 - D_4)} \times 100$

Notes Normally there is reconversion of Hi to haemoglobin in stored blood samples and the test should be carried out within 1 hour of collection. After dilution the buffered lysate may be stored for up to 24 hours at 2–4°C.

Significance and further investigation of methaemoglobinaemia

The normal range in adults is 1–3% with slightly higher levels in infants and heavy smokers. As little as 2 g/dl of Hi will produce clinical cyanosis. There are four mechanisms for the production of methaemoglobinaemia.

Acquired due to excessive formation of Hi by drugs or chemicals – toxic methaemoglobinaemia

Oxidative stress can result in Hi formation. Many drugs are potentially capable of inducing the formation of Hi, which in normal subjects is usually due to overdosage and may result in globin denaturation, Heinz-body formation and increased haemolysis, often with a characteristic blood picture (*see Figure 11.3*). In normal dosage certain drugs, e.g. dapsone and salazosulphopyridine, produce red-cell changes and haemolysis which is often compensated and may be considered an acceptable side effect. In subjects whose red cells have a reduced antioxidant potential due to low levels of reduced glutathione, the most frequent cause being G6PD deficiency, exposure to drugs at normal dosage can result in methaemoglobinaemia and haemolysis.

Environmental, accidental or suicidal exposure to chemicals such as nitrates and nitrites, nitro- or amino-derivatives of benzene or by chlorate poisoning can result in massive Hi formation and haemolysis.

Whatever the precipitating cause the Hi formed is 'normal', is capable of reconversion to haemoglobin *in vivo* or *in vitro*, has the characteristic absorption maximum at 630 nm and can be measured by the method described.

Hereditary due to diminished reconversion of Hi to haemoglobin

Each day about 1% of circulating haemoglobin is converted to Hi and by efficient protective mechanisms reconverted to haemoglobin. The major reconversion mechanism is by methaemoglobin reductase (MR) which requires NADH as co-enzyme (NADH-MR) and is also known as ferricyanide reductase and cytochrome b5 reductase. A method of assaying NADH-MR activity (cytochrome b5 reductase) is recommended by the ICSH[79] but a ferricyanide reductase assay has been suggested as being superior in its suitability for the detection of NADH-MR variants[80]. As hereditary methaemoglobinaemia due to NADH-MR deficiency is independent of haemoglobin composition it will be present at birth. Haemolysis is not a feature. The level of Hi in the acquired or hereditary (NADH-MR) types of methaemoglobinaemia may be reduced by stimulating the normally inactive NADPH-MR of the pentose-phosphate pathway by oral administration of ascorbate or a redox dye such as methylene blue. Riboflavin by mouth has been used with success as NADPH-MR is a flavin reductase, the reduced flavin converting Hi to haemoglobin non-enzymatically[81]. The Hi formed as a result of enzyme deficiency is of 'normal' type.

Hereditary – unstable haemoglobins

Instability of haemoglobin is frequently associated with methaemoglobinaemia and Heinz-body formation and may be exacerbated by oxidant drugs. The Hi has 'normal' absorption characteristics.

Hereditary due to a structural globin abnormality resulting in haem being permanently in the ferric state – the Hb Ms

Hb M can be readily differentiated from the other causes of methaemoglobinaemia in that the colour of the blood is unchanged by the addition of reducing agents. The Hi is due to an amino-acid substitution of the proximal or distal histidines of the α or β polypeptide chains or of an amino acid four residues distant, the presence of a negatively charged side chain interfering with haem-iron.

The location of the substitution in the α or β chain influences clinical presentation; cyanosis due to an α-chain Hb M will be present at birth as α chains are found in all neonatal haemoglobins while β-chain Hb M defects will not become manifest by cyanosis until the age of 2–3 months when β chains predominate over the γ chain of Hb F.

Hb M may be associated with mild anaemia suggesting slight instability and may show increased haemolysis in response to oxidant stress. As homozygous Hb M would be incompatible with life all cases of Hb M are heterozygotes for Hb M and Hb A and there is often abnormal oxygen affinity of the *normal* α- and β-chain haem due to interference in the configuration of the haemoglobin tetramer. The Hb Ms and their characteristics are shown in *Table 11.9.*

Table 11.9 The M haemoglobins

Name	*Chain*	*Substitution*		O_2 *affinity*
M Boston	α	58 E7	his→tyr	Low
M Iwate	α	87 F8	his→tyr	Low
M Saskatoon	β	63 E7	his→tyr	Nearly normal
M Hyde Park	β	92 F8	his→tyr	Nearly normal
M Milwaukee	β	67 E7	val→glu	Normal

Laboratory investigation of Hb M[82]

All samples containing Hb M will be a mixture of Hb A and Hb M with Hb A comprising 60–75% of total haemoglobin.

As methaemoglobin A is slightly cathodic to oxy-Hb A at alkaline pH due to the iron being in the ferric form, differences in electrophoretic mobility due to a *globin* abnormality can only be confirmed if the normal haemoglobin is converted to Hi. Potassium ferricyanide is therefore added to the haemolysate to convert oxy-Hb A to Hi-Hb A (add 0.1 ml 5% potassium ferricyanide to 1.0 ml haemolysate (10 g/dl)).

Electrophoresis Phosphate buffer pH 7.1 is preferred as at this pH the imidazole ring of histidine will carry a charge. Cellulose acetate, paper or starch gel may be used.

Buffer Disodium hydrogen phosphate $Na_2HPO_4.2H_2O$, 3.3 g; potassium dihydrogen phosphate KH_2PO_4, 1.08 g; distilled water to 1 litre. Immediately before use dilute 1 in 5 with distilled water.

Hb A and 'normal' Hb M will be cathodal, with Hb M due to the his→tyr substitution being slightly slower, i.e. all but Hb Milwaukee.

Spectrophotometry The absorption spectra of Hb Ms differ from that of 'normal' Hi and may be distinctive for the Hb M under investigation. As most of the sample will be Hb A much of the spectral characteristics of the Hb M will be blurred or hidden and for more precise spectrophotometry, separation of the Hb M by electrophoresis followed by elution is necessary. The pH influences the absorption spectrum and the data in *Table 11.10* were obtained at pH 7.0. The variable position of the band in the red must be considered when attempting to assay the Hb M.

Formation of cyanmethaemoglobin (HiCN) Hi will complex with cyanide to form HiCN. 'Normal' Hi, M Saskatoon and M Milwaukee react rapidly while M Hyde

Table 11.10 Absorption maxima of the M haemoglobins

Haemoglobin	*Maxima*		*(nm)*
Meth-A (normal)	630		502
M Boston	602		495
M Hyde Park	610	578	496
M Iwate	590		490
M Milwaukee	622		500
M Saskatoon	602		492

Park reacts less readily. M Boston reacts slowly and M Iwate particularly poorly. The rate of reaction can therefore be used as a means of differentiation. There are obvious implications in the determination of total haemoglobin concentration by the HiCN method.

Semi-quantitation of SHb [83]

Principle

Absorbance at 620 nm measures the sum of the absorbance of HbO_2 and SHb. The absorption band for SHb is unchanged by the addition of cyanide. The residual absorbance at 620 nm is therefore proportional to the concentration of SHb.

The absorbance of HbO_2 alone at 620 nm can be inferred from absorbance at 577 nm by using a conversion factor determined experimentally for each instrument by determining the ratio $A^{577}:A^{620}$ on a number of normal blood samples. The absorbance of the SHb is obtained by subtracting the absorbance of HbO_2 from that of the total Hb. Because complete conversion of Hb to SHb has not been achieved experimentally it is not yet possible to assess the reliability of the method but it may be regarded as adequate for clinical purposes.

Method

0.1 ml of blood is diluted in 10 ml of a 20 ml/l solution of Nonidet P40. The absorbance (A) at 620 nm is determined (total Hb). One drop of 50 g/l KCN is added, and after 5 minutes absorbance is recorded at 620 nm and at 577 nm.

Calculation

$$\text{SHb}\ \% = 2 \times \frac{A^{620}\ \text{SHb}}{A^{620}\ \text{HbO}_2} \quad \text{where}$$

$$A^{620}\ \text{HbO}_2 = \frac{\text{absorbance read at 578 nm}}{\text{conversion factor}} \quad \text{and}$$

$$A^{620}\ \text{SHb} = A^{620}\ \text{total Hb} - A^{620}\ \text{HbO}_2$$

Significance

Normal blood does not contain SHb but has been described after the ingestion of drugs such as phenacetin, acetanilid and sulphonamides. With these drugs the origin of the sulphur atom is said to be H_2S produced in and absorbed from the intestine. Glutathione is also a suggested source [84]. Elemental sulphur, sulphides and thiosulphates are known to produce SHb directly. SHb formation is not reversible *in vivo* and its disappearance depends on the elimination of the affected cells. Because the absorption of light in the red is greater than that of Hi, SHb is more effective in producing cyanosis and has been described in cases with as little as 0.5 g SHb/dl.

Direct antiglobulin test

Principle

Washed red cells having immunoglobulin or complement absorbed on their surface can be agglutinated by the addition of a suitable antiglobulin serum. If an antiglobulin serum reacts with more than one class of immunoglobulin or reacts with immunoglobulin and complement the reagent is said to be polyspecific or to have a 'broad spectrum' of activity. If activity is confined to one immunoglobulin class or component of complement it is a specific antiserum.

Antiglobulin reagents (AHG)

1. Antiserum containing anti-IgG and anti-C3d or anti-C3d + C3b(C3c) is essential.
2. Monospecific IgG and C3d antisera for further characterization of a positive DAT obtained with the broad-spectrum reagent.
3. Anti-IgA for use when negative results are found with IgG and C3d antisera.
4. Anti-IgM may be used but is not essential in that IgM, if present, is always accompanied by C3d.

Notes

1. Suitable polyspecific and monospecific anti-IgG and C3d standardized for use in the antiglobulin test are available commercially, though several surveys have shown that not all sources are satisfactory. Monoclonal antibodies are available.
2. Anti-IgA and anti-IgM sera suitable for the DAT are not widely available. Careful standardization using cells sensitized with IgG, IgA, IgM and C3 is essential.

Preparation of cells for testing

Blood is collected into EDTA which will prevent *in vitro* complement sensitization even if cooled. Red cells are washed four times in comparatively large volumes of saline (some workers recommend phosphate-buffered saline, pH 7.4, to reduce possible antibody dissociation during washing; normal saline often has a pH below 6.0). Saline at room temperature is usually satisfactory though an unexpected negative result may be found due to antibody dissociation which may be prevented by using saline at 4°C. Washed cells must be tested immediately to prevent further dissociation. The cells are re-suspended to 2–5% for testing by the tube technique or 10–20% for the tile method. Alternatively two drops of 2–5% cells may be washed in a series of tubes and are then ready for testing.

Control-sensitized cells

IgG-coated cells

RhD-positive cells sensitized with anti-D suitably diluted to give a 1 + (clumps of 20–40 cells) at the optimum dilution of antiglobulin serum.

IgA- and IgM-coated cells

As pure incomplete IgA and IgM antibodies are rare, passive sensitization is recommended.

Reagents A stock solution of 1% chromic chloride stored at 4°C in a dark bottle is diluted 1 in 20 in unbuffered saline for use. Purified IgA, 0.5–1 mg/ml, purified IgM, 2 mg/ml. Group O red cells (1–8 days old).

Procedure (1) Mix one volume IgA or IgM solution and one volume packed washed red cells in a glass container; (2) add one volume of diluted chromic chloride; (3) mix continuously for 5 minutes at room temperature; (4) wash cells four times in unbuffered saline, centrifuging for not longer than 30 seconds at 1000 *g*; (5) reconstitute to the required cell concentration.

C3d-coated cells

1. From a case of cold haemagglutinin disease; these cells can be stored in liquid nitrogen.
2. *In vitro* preparation.

Diluent Solution A: dissolve 23.1 g sucrose, 173 mg $NaH_2PO_4 . H_2O$ and 395 mg $Na_2EDTA . 2H_2O$ in water and make up to 250 ml in a volumetric flask. Solution B: dissolve 23.1 g sucrose, 178 mg Na_2HPO_4 and 395 mg $Na_2EDTA . 2H_2O$ in water and make up to 250 ml in a volumetric flask. Adjust solution A to pH 5.1 by addition of solution B (approximately 6.5 ml).

Procedure (1) Chill all reactants in ice-water. (2) Place 19 ml diluent in a small flask in an ice-bath on a magnetic stirrer in the cold-room. (3) While stirring add 1 ml ACD whole blood rapidly drop by drop. (4) *Immediately* add 0.1 ml of 0.4 mol/l $MgCl_2$ (810 mg $MgCl_2 . 6H_2O$ in 10 ml water). (5) Stir for 1 hour. (6) Wash cells four times with saline at 4°C. The cells are now coated with C3b. (7) Incubate equal volumes of packed, washed cells and 0.1% trypsin (pH 7.3) for 30 minutes. Non-complement sensitized cells should also be incubated with trypsin as a negative control. (8) Wash cells four times and re-suspend as required.

Positive controls

Monospecific AHG should be controlled by including appropriately sensitized cells as prepared above with each test or batch of tests. Polyspecific AHG need only be tested with IgG-sensitized cells as there is no evidence that selective deterioration of anti-C3d occurs.

Negative controls

1. Washed patient's cells plus saline should give a negative result.
2. Normal washed cells.

Method

Tube technique

To one drop of 2–5% washed red cells add one or two drops of AHG depending on the volumes used in the standardization procedure or according to the manufacturer's instructions. Centrifuge at 1000 *g* for 20 seconds. Examine immediately for agglutination and check all negative or doubtful results microscopically. If no agglutination is present, stand the tube at room temperature for 5–10 minutes, repeat the centrifugation and re-read. This further step is optimal for the detection of C3.

The strength of reaction does not necessarily correlate with the severity of haemolysis but a good estimate of the amount of protein molecules adsorbed on to the cells can be obtained by the 'semi-quantitative DAT' by testing against dilutions of AHG.

The choice of dilution depends on the source of the AHG. Commercial antisera are usually already diluted and doubling dilutions 1:1, 1:2, 1:4 and so on are recommended. Using undiluted or 'raw' antiserum, four-fold dilutions are appropriate: 1:4, 1:16, 1:64, etc. By this technique the amount of red-cell bound protein can be followed during treatment and different patterns obtained in haemolysis due to various causes. It is necessary to grade the agglutination and an established scheme is shown in *Table 11.11*[85]. A titration score is obtained by

Table 11.11 Agglutination grading and scores

Grading	*Appearance of red cells*	*Score*
4+	No unagglutinated cells	10
3+	Several large agglutinates, few free cells	8
2+	Large agglutinates in a sea of smaller clumps and free cells	6
1+	Many small agglutinates (approximately 20 cells)	4
(1+)	Scattered small agglutinates in a sea of free cells just visible macroscopically	3
½+	Small agglutinates only visible microscopically	1
0	No agglutinates seen	0

summing the agglutination score obtained at each dilution. The highest titration scores using anti-C3d are found in cold-agglutinin disease and C3d-coated cells not associated with haemolytic anaemia generally have low scores. Titres in the semi-quantitative DAT are also informative. Warm AIHA associated with methyldopa have anti-IgG titres over 1000 and about two-thirds over 2000, in contrast to warm AIHA not associated with methyldopa and negative for C3d where the titre is 2000 or more in only about 10% of patients[85].

Causes of positive direct antiglobulin tests

1. Autoantibodies against red-cell antigens resulting in immunoglobulin or complement sensitization.

2. Antibodies against drugs attached to the red-cell membrane, e.g. penicillin.
3. Immune-complex formation, e.g. anti-drug complex.
4. Non-specific uptake of protein on to an altered red-cell membrane, e.g. following treatment with cephalosporin.
5. Weak MN antigens.
6. Haemolytic disease of new-born.
7. Haemolytic transfusion reaction.
8. Polyagglutinable cells due to T antigen exposure and anti-T in the AHG.
9. Complement components on red cells in a variety of disorders and not associated with haemolytic anaemia (approximately 7% of hospital patients [86,87]).
10. Hypergammaglobulinaemia [88].
11. Chemical agents containing multiple reactive carbonyl groups [89].

Note

The presence of transferrin on reticulocytes is not considered to be a problem, due to its rapid dissociation during washing and the availability of specific antisera.

Causes of false-negative results

1. Poor technique:
   (a) Inadequate washing of red cells.
   (b) Inhibition of AHG activity due to contamination of saline or AHG with human globulin.
   (c) Failure to recognize weak agglutination.
   (d) Delay in testing or reading results thus allowing antibody dissociation.
2. AHG lacking appropriate antibody.
3. Antibody concentration on the red cells too low to allow detection. This is an accepted limitation of the standard DAT and as many as 1 in 20 cases of AIHA may have a negative DAT.

Other direct antiglobulin tests

Levels of immunoglobulins on red cells below the detection limit of the classical DAT may be demonstrated and quantitated by more sensitive methods. Enzyme-linked DATs, radio-labelled antiglobulin reagents, radio-labelled staphylococcal protein A and mononuclear phagocytic assays each have their proponents.

Detection of antibody in serum and red-cell eluates

Free autoantibody (or alloantibody) may be found in serum. This is the rule in cold-antibody AIHA but in warm AIHA incomplete antibody is only found when the haemolytic process is severe (an exception is warm AIHA due to methyldopa). If antibody is not present a red-cell eluate must be tested to characterize the antibody and even if free antibody is present in the serum an eluate should be examined as the antibodies on the cells may not be reflected by the antibody in the serum.

The characteristics of autoantibodies are varied in respect of being complete or incomplete, warm or cold and their thermal range, haemolytic or non-haemolytic with or without acidification, complement fixing or not and whether they react by indirect antiglobulin test (IAT) or only by enzymes. A preliminary screening protocol can be devised to cover all possibilities with the exception of those antibodies reacting only in the presence of drugs or with drug-sensitized cells and the characteristic bi-phasic lysis of the DL antibody.

Serum and eluate is therefore tested undiluted, diluted 1 in 2 with fresh normal serum both at normal pH and acidified, at 20°C and 37°C against a pool of group O cells both untreated and enzyme modified containing the common red-cell antigens.

Collection and preparation of samples

Serum is collected from clotted blood. Defibrinated blood has been recommended but a degree of haemolysis almost always results which is undesirable when testing for haemolysins. Except in the investigation of severe cold agglutinin disease it is not necessary to use warm syringes. Incubation at 37°C for 15 minutes to allow full coagulation and centrifugation at 37°C prevents *in vitro* sensitization, possible autoagglutination, loss of antibody by autoabsorption and possible haemolysis.

Preparation of eluates from red cells

Ether elution method[90]

Wash red cells six times in large volumes of saline (an aliquot of the last saline wash should be retained and tested with the eluate as a negative control to show that no residual antibody remains). To one volume of packed cells add one volume of saline and two volumes of diethyl ether. Stopper and invert repeatedly for 1 minute. Incubate at 37°C for 30 minutes and then centrifuge at 1200 *g* for 10 minutes. The eluate is the bottom of the three well-defined layers and is carefully removed with a pipette and placed at 37°C for 30 minutes to drive off residual ether. A more potent eluate may be obtained by removing the ether layer and heating the stroma and eluate at 56°C for 10 minutes with intermittent agitation, followed by centrifugation at 1200 *g* for 10 minutes. A disadvantage of this method is that the eluate is heavily stained with haemoglobin, an obvious disadvantage when looking for haemolysis.

A non-flammable method using chloroform has been described[91].

Digitonin – acid method[92]

This technique produces haemoglobin-free stroma which is then eluted in acid buffer to produce a clear eluate.

Reagents Digitonin solution, 5 mg/ml in saline (stable at 4°C). 0.1 mol/l glycine buffer pH 3.0, 3.574 g in 500 ml water. Adjust pH to 3.0 with 12 mol/l HCl (about 34 drops). 0.8 mol/l phosphate buffer: solution A, 113.57 g Na_2HPO_4 to 1 litre distilled water; solution B, 108.87 g KH_2PO_4 to 1 litre distilled water; working buffer, 9.65 ml solution A and 0.35 ml solution B. Stable at 4°C.

Method Re-suspend one volume of washed packed cells in nine volumes of saline and add 0.5 volumes of digitonin. Invert several times until haemolysate is clear. Centrifuge at 1000 *g* for 5 minutes and discard supernatant. Wash the stroma four times with saline or until free from haemoglobin. Elute by adding twice the original volume of glycine buffer. Invert repeatedly for 1 minute and centrifuge at 1000 *g* for 5 minutes. Remove the supernatant and add one-fifth volume of phosphate buffer. Mix and centrifuge for 2 minutes. The supernatant is the final eluate.

Note After washing of the stroma, ether, heat, or both may be used for elution.

Xylene method[93]

One volume of washed packed cells, one volume of saline and two volumes of analytical grade xylene are mixed in a stoppered tube for 1 minute and then incubated at 56°C for 10 minutes. The mixture is then centrifuged at 1000 *g* for 10 minutes. Three distinct layers are formed; the upper layer is xylene, the middle layer a fine film of stroma and the lower layer a deeply haemoglobin-stained eluate. The two upper layers are removed by vacuum aspiration together with an upper layer of the eluate. All xylene must be removed to prevent subsequent lysis of red cells. If any particulate stroma remains a second centrifugation is indicated. This simple method is claimed to produce eluates superior to either the ether or acid–digitonin methods from cells sensitized with auto- and passively acquired antibodies. Xylene is less dangerous to store and use than ether.

Method

A series of 75 × 10 mm tubes are set up as shown in *Table 11.12*. Volumes of patients' serum and normal serum with and without acidification are distributed as shown and two rows placed at 37°C and two rows at 20°C and the temperature allowed to equilibrate together with 10% suspensions of untreated and enzyme-modified cells. One drop or volume of appropriate cell suspension is delivered directly into the serum in each of the tubes; the cells must not be allowed to run down the inner surface of the tubes. The cells and serum are mixed and allowed to stand for 2 hours. Without disturbing the cells each tube is examined for

Table 11.12 Serological screening for autoimmune haemolytic anaemia

		Tube						
		1	*2*	*3*	*4*	*5*	*6*	
	Patient's serum (volumes)	10	10	5	5	0	0	
	Normal serum (volumes)	0	0	5	5	10	10	
	0.2 mol/l HCl (volumes)	0	1	0	1	0	1	
		In each of four rows of tubes:*						
Row 1	10% group O red cells	1	1	1	1	1	1	37°C
Row 2	10% enzyme-modified group O red cells	1	1	1	1	1	1	37°C
Row 3	10% group O red cells	1	1	1	1	1	1	4°C
Row 4	10% enzyme-modified group O red cells	1	1	1	1	1	1	4°C

*1. Normal serum = less than 24 hours at 4°C or less than 14 days at −20°C. 2. Group O red cells = a pool of not more than three samples containing all common red-cell antigens.

haemolysis and then gently tilted and any agglutination noted by examining over a concave mirror. The tubes with enzyme-treated cells are discarded and the cells in the remaining tubes washed four times with buffered saline at 20°C or 37°C as appropriate. Two drops of polyspecific AHG are added to each tube, centrifuged for 15 seconds at 1000 *g* and read for agglutination as described. Tubes 5 and 6 of each row should be negative throughout. Positive tests may usefully be repeated using specific anti-IgG and anti-C3d or, if indicated by the results of the DAT, with anti-IgA and anti-IgM. The specified strength of the cell suspension is for use only with the tube-spin technique.

Notes

1. Warm haemolysins are rare.
2. Cold antibodies are more lytic in acidified serum and with enzyme-treated cells.
3. If the patient's serum is depleted in complement, lysis may only be seen in those tubes with added complement.
4. Negative results may be observed in the IAT yet show agglutination with enzyme-treated cells.
5. Equivocal or negative results using the patient's serum *must* be followed by testing an eluate.
6. Red-cell eluates should be tested as for the serum.
7. Negative results with serum and eluate do not exclude immune haemolysis. The possibility of drug-associated immune lysis must be considered.
8. Antiglobulin tests positive only at 20°C with anti-C3d and possibly anti-IgG strongly suggest a Donath–Landsteiner-type antibody.

Techniques for detecting drug-associated antibodies other than those of methyldopa type

Preparation of penicillin-sensitized cells

To 1 ml of washed fresh group O cells add 10^6 units (approximately 600 mg) of potassium benzyl penicillin G dissolved in 15 ml of pH 9.6 barbitone buffer (sodium barbitone 20.6 g/l, adjusted to pH 9.6 with approximately 15 ml 0.1 mol/l HCl). Incubate for 1 hour at room temperature. Wash three times. Slight lysis may occur. The sensitized cells may be kept at 4°C for 7 days suspended in ACD.

Preparation of cephalosporin-sensitized cells

To 1 ml of washed fresh group O cells add 400 mg of cephalosporin dissolved in 10 ml of pH 9.6 barbitone-buffered saline (one part buffer and nine parts saline). Incubate at 37°C for 2 hours. Wash three times.

Indirect antiglobulin tests using drug-sensitized cells

Doubling dilutions of the patient's serum are made to 1 in 2048 and incubated with the sensitized cells for 1 hour at 37°C. After washing four times with saline the cells are tested against anti-IgG. In penicillin-induced haemolytic anaemia high-titre antibody is typically present [85]. In cephalosporin-associated haemolysis only titres greater than 1 in 20 are significant as non-specific protein absorption occurs, though

though the use of monospecific anti-IgG should eliminate this problem. In each instance undiluted eluates instead of patient's serum will give positive results.

Technique with other drugs possibly acting by the immune-complex mechanism

The protocol described for the testing of serum and eluates described on pages 354–6 should be followed but modified by the presence of the suspect drug. *In vivo* therapeutic levels of drugs are usually in the μg/ml range and therefore a useful starting concentration is 1 mg/ml in buffered saline or alternatively in a saturated solution. Preliminary studies can be performed to determine whether this drug concentration causes lysis of the normal cells and if so dilutions should be made until lysis no longer occurs. As the anti-drug antibody may be IgG or IgM and possibly capable of activating complement, a polyspecific antiglobulin serum should be used. If negative results are obtained extended incubation or attempts to pre-sensitize normal red cells are recommended [85].

Determination of cold agglutinin titre, thermal range and specificity

When agglutination is observed in the standard serum screen, the titre and thermal range of the antibody is determined against group OI adult cells, Oi cord cells and the patient's own cells which have been washed at 37°C.

'Master dilutions' of the patient's serum which has been separated at 37°C are prepared in saline from 1 in 2 to 1 in 16 000 in 0.5 ml amounts. To prevent 'carry over' a separate pipette must be used to transfer each 0.5 ml volume.

Three rows of 14 tubes are set up and starting at the highest dilution one drop is transferred into each of three tubes and the rack placed at 37°C. The red cells are washed and adjusted to a 2–5% suspension and allowed to warm to 37°C. Maintaining the cells and serum at 37°C, one drop of cells is added to each row as appropriate and incubated for 2 hours at 37°C and read for agglutination over a concave mirror. The tubes are then transferred to a 30°C water bath for 2 hours and again read for agglutination. The procedure is repeated at 20°C and 4°C. If time is limited the tubes may be left overnight at 4°C.

Interpretation

Cold haemolytic anaemia is associated with titres greater than 1 in 64 at 4°C and/or a thermal amplitude of 20°C or higher. Very high titres may be found requiring further serum dilutions. If a significant cold agglutinin is present it is recommended that the titrations be repeated in 30% albumin, as a better correlation between clinical haemolysis and albumin titre has been reported [94]. Specificity within the Ii system is, perhaps surprisingly, more evident at 20°C and 30°C than at 4°C. The inclusion of the patient's own cells in the study is recommended because if the antibody has i specificity, higher titres may be obtained with the patient's cells. Lack of specificity within the Ii system should be followed up by studying the reaction of the antibody with papain-treated cells; negative or weak reactions indicate specificity within the Pr system.

High-titre cold agglutinins are potentially lytic and lysis may be expected to be observed in the standard serum-testing protocol particularly in acidified serum and fresh normal serum and with enzyme-treated cells. Titration of cold haemolysins should be made by diluting in fresh normal serum with acidification and using enzyme-treated cells if indicated. Temperature equilibration is important and the cells must be added directly to the serum and not allowed to run down the tubes.

Donath–Landsteiner (DL) test

PCH, as the term implies, is typically associated with haemoglobinuria after exposure to cold, and the standard DAT reveals C3d (and possibly IgG) sensitization, negative serum screening (though the IAT at 20°C may be positive), a non-reactive eluate and a normal cold agglutinin titre, i.e. the condition can simulate the pattern associated with the immune-complex type of drug-associated haemolysis. Furthermore, at the time of blood sampling unless there has been recent exposure to cold, the DAT may be negative. The definitive test is to demonstrate the bi-phasic lytic nature of the IgG complement binding antibody by exposure of cells and serum to low temperature followed by warming to 37°C.

Screening test

Approximately 1 ml amounts of freshly taken non-anticoagulated blood are delivered into three tubes pre-warmed to 37°C. One tube is left undisturbed at 37°C, allowed to clot and incubated for 1 hour. The blood in the second tube is allowed to clot and placed at 4°C for 1 hour. The third tube is transferred to 4°C for 30 minutes and then re-warmed at 37°C for 1 hour and inspected for haemolysis which if present indicates a DL antibody provided that the tubes at 37°C and 4°C show no haemolysis thus excluding warm and cold haemolysins, respectively. A 'false' negative result due to complement depletion may be found if the test is performed after a recent episode of haemolysis.

Standard technique

Patient's blood is collected without cooling, allowed to clot at 37°C and separated at 37°C. Normal group O cells are washed and prepared as a 50% suspension. Fresh normal serum is required as a source of complement. Nine 75 × 10 mm tubes are set up and cell/serum mixtures prepared after equilibration at 37°C as shown in *Table 11.13*.

Tubes one, two and three are left at 37°C and tubes four, five and six are placed at 4°C, all for 1 hour. Tubes seven, eight and nine are placed at 4°C or in melting ice for 30 minutes and then incubated at 37°C for 30 minutes. If no haemolysis is found

Table 11.13 Standard Donath–Landsteiner test

	Tube								
	1	*2*	*3*	*4*	*5*	*6*	*7*	*8*	*9*
Patient's serum	10	5	–	10	5	–	10	5	–
Normal serum	–	5	10	–	5	10	–	5	10
50% normal cells	1	1	1	1	1	1	1	1	1
Temperature (°C)	37			4			37→4→37		

in tubes seven, eight or both the test is negative; no haemolysis should occur in tube nine. If haemolysis is present in tubes seven, eight or both the test is positive provided that no haemolysis is present in tubes 1–6. If the patient's serum already contains haemoglobin the observation of further haemolysis may not be obvious. In such instances examination of the button of remaining red cells may indicate whether further haemolysis has occurred. The indirect antiglobulin test with anti-IgG is more sensitive than the haemolysin test provided that the cells are not warmed after being at 4°C and are washed in ice-cold saline to reduce elution of the antibody. Titration of the DL antibody may be performed by diluting in normal serum and may be useful in clinical management as there is a direct correlation between titre and the degree of cooling necessary to induce *in vivo* lysis, i.e. higher titres will sensitize at higher temperatures.

An example of a very weak DL antibody has been studied in which a weak positive result was found only when the patient's cells were substituted for the normal cells, probably due to small amounts of residual IgG remaining on the patient's cells.

Red-cell osmotic fragility

Principle

Equal volumes of blood are added to a series of buffered hypotonic sodium chloride solutions, allowed to stand for 30 minutes at room temperature and the degree of haemolysis recorded photometrically and expressed as percentage lysis at each sodium chloride concentration.

Reagent

Stock solution of buffered sodium chloride osmotically equivalent to 100 g/l NaCl: NaCl 90 g, Na_2HPO_4 13.65 g, $NaH_2PO_4 . 2H_2O$ 2.43 g dissolved in water and made up to 1 litre. Stable for many months in a tightly closed container.

For preparing hypotonic solutions first dilute the stock solution to 10 g/l and prepare a range of equivalent concentrations from 1.0 to 10.0 g/l in 0.5 g intervals. 5 ml volumes are suitable but if a series of tests are to be performed larger volumes may be prepared and aliquots taken.

It is important to control the pH as each 0.1 reduction in pH is equivalent to a decrease of 0.1 g/l in tonicity.

Method

To 5 ml of each sodium chloride concentration is added 0.05 ml of blood, i.e. diluted about 1 in 100 (strictly 1 in 101). The proportions of blood to saline should not be less or the added plasma may influence the test. Although heparinized or defibrinated blood is usually specified, EDTA anticoagulated blood may be used as it can be calculated that the added EDTA in 0.05 ml of blood (0.05 mg) has a negligible effect on the final tonicity. The test should be performed within 2 hours of sample collection or up to 6 hours if the blood is kept at 4°C. The saline–cell suspensions are mixed and allowed to stand at room temperature which, within reasonable limits, is not critical (each 5°C reduction in temperature is equivalent to a 0.1 g/l fall in tonicity). After 30 minutes the tubes are again mixed and centrifuged to deposit the red cells. Lysis should be complete in the 1.0 g/l solution (no button of intact red cells) and optical density of the supernatant is determined in the photometer at 540 nm and taken as 100% lysis. The optical density of the supernatants in each tube is measured, compared with the 100% lysis tube and expressed as % lysis. The supernatant of the 10 g/l tube is used as a photometer blank; lysis in this tube would be exceptional.

Recording of results

Results may be presented in numerical form as percentage haemolysis at each NaCl concentration together with the concentration showing 50% haemolysis (mean corpuscular haemolysis, MCF). Alternatively or additionally the results may be expressed in graph form by plotting on arithmetic paper. Graphic presentation allows a ready comparison with normal osmotic fragility and perhaps allows more subtle interpretation of the pattern of lysis. The presence of cell populations with differing fragilities may be deduced by plotting incremental haemolysis on arithmetic paper against NaCl concentration or alternatively probability paper may be used. *Figure 11.10* shows osmotic fragility curves plotted on arithmetic graph paper together with normal ranges.

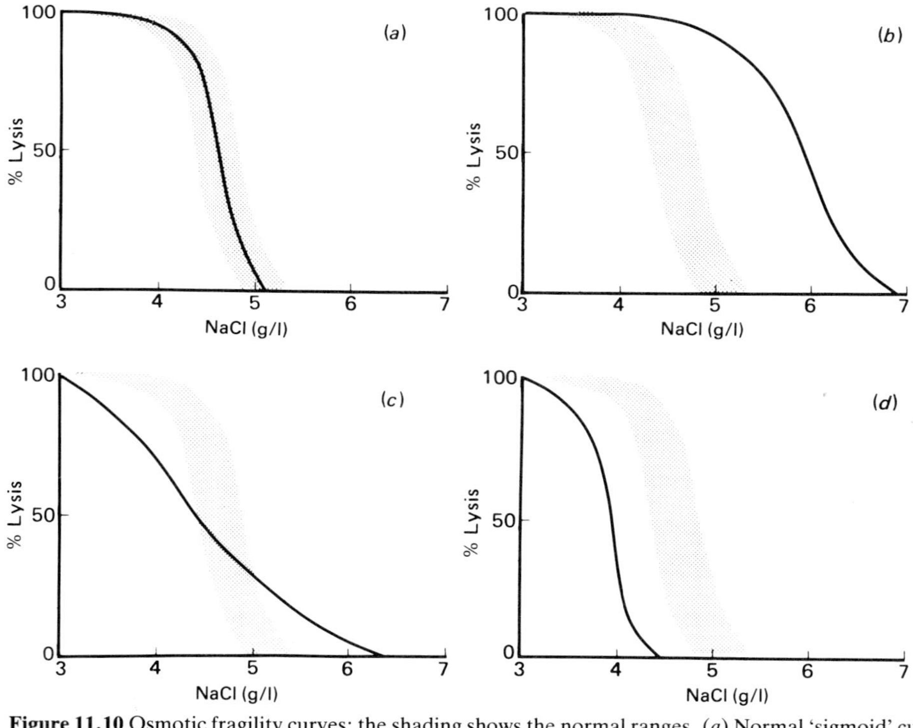

Figure 11.10 Osmotic fragility curves; the shading shows the normal ranges. (*a*) Normal 'sigmoid' curve. (*b*) Markedly increased fragility of almost the whole red-cell population due to spherocytosis. (*c*) A 'two-population' curve due to the presence of cells with reduced fragility (e.g. hypochromic, thin cells) and a population with increased fragility. (*d*) Reduced fragility; a typical result of microcytic, hypochromic red cells

Interpretation of osmotic fragility tests

The lysis of red cells in hypotonic solutions is usually a reflection of the surface area:volume ratio, i.e. spherocytes have an increased fragility and leptocytes (thin cells) have a decreased fragility. It is clear, however, that some cases of hereditary spherocytosis have normal or only marginally increased fragility and that the examination of a well-prepared and stained blood film by an experienced observer is more sensitive than the standard osmotic fragility test. Furthermore, if the proportion of spherocytic cells is small, the 'tail' of spherocytic cells in the osmotic fragility test is less sensitive than the demonstration of a small number of abnormal cells in the blood film.

A single-tube fragility test with a 4.0 g/l osmotic equivalent has been widely used as a screening test in population surveys for thalassaemia trait but has been largely supplemented by the measurement of MCV by electronic red-cell counters. A notable exception to the general rule that only spherocytic cells have an increased osmotic fragility is that some examples of hereditary stomatocytosis (hydrocytosis) have a markedly increased osmotic fragility despite there being no suggestion of spherocytosis in the blood film and indeed, in the presence of stomatocytes, a reduced fragility would be expected.

Modified osmotic fragility test

The limitations of the standard osmotic fragility test for the demonstration of spherocytosis have resulted in the *incubated osmotic fragility test* which is performed with an extended range of hypotonic solutions and after the blood has been incubated under sterile conditions for 24 hours at 37°C. There seems little doubt that the modified test is more sensitive in the detection of mild spherocytosis or elliptocytosis but it has not been demonstrated to be more sensitive than the examination of a blood film. Sterility must be maintained and heparinized or defibrinated blood must be used, as incubation of EDTA anticoagulated samples is known to produce shape change even with normal samples.

Other variations in technique are the addition of ATP or glucose during the incubation period as a means of differentiating different causes of spherocytosis. It is not clear how much pH differences during incubation are responsible for the apparent effect of the additives.

As the standard osmotic fragility test is usually used for demonstrating spherocytes and in particular hereditary spherocytosis the introduction of the acidified glycerol lysis test (AGLT) will probably replace the osmotic technique though it must be emphasized that the AGLT is not based on the same principle of lysis in hypotonic solutions and is not necessarily demonstrating spherocytosis *per se*.

Acidified glycerol lysis test for hereditary spherocytosis [95]

Principle

Red cells are suspended in slightly acidified phosphate buffered-sodium chloride–glycerol reagent and the time taken for 50% haemolysis to occur is measured ($AGLT_{50}$).

Reagent

1. Isotonic phosphate buffered saline (PBS) pH 6.85 ± 0.05 is prepared by adding nine volumes 0.15 mol/l NaCl to one volume 0.1 mol/l phosphate buffer (52.5 ml 14.39 g/l Na_2HPO_4, 47.5 ml 13.78 g/l KH_2PO_4).
2. 21.98 ml (27.62 g) reagent grade glycerol is added to 300 ml PBS and made up to 1 litre with distilled water.

Note

The pH is critical and the osmolality should be strictly controlled (290–300 mOs/kg).

Procedure

20 µl EDTA anticoagulated blood (1 mg/ml) 24 hours old are added to 5 ml PBS. The suspension is carefully and gently mixed and 1 ml is pipetted into a cuvette of a colorimeter or spectrophotometer at 625 nm preferably with a pen-recorder. Alternatively the change in transmission can be timed with a stop-watch. 2.0 ml of the glycerol reagent is added quickly. The volumes of red cell suspension and glycerol reagent are critical. The rate of haemolysis is followed by the fall in turbidity. Results are expressed as the time required for the optical density to fall to half the initial value ($AGLT_{50}$).

Interpretation

All cases of hereditary spherocytosis show shortened $AGLT_{50}$ times compared with normal controls and in the majority of cases where neither parent shows clinical or haematological evidence of spherocytosis, one parent has a shortened $AGLT_{50}$. Normal controls show values greater than 1800 seconds; the values for hereditary spherocytosis are 25–142 seconds. The test has been criticized[96] as being insufficiently sensitive and for giving abnormal results in normal subjects. The original method did not specify the time elapsed before testing; if the sample is left at room temperature for 24 hours, the test is positive in all cases of hereditary spherocytosis[97] and controlling the osmolality eliminates false positives in normal subjects. A modified technique, the 'Pink Test'[98], substitutes bis-tris buffer for phosphate buffer with a resulting pH of 6.66.

Although highly sensitive for hereditary spherocytosis, similar $AGLT_{50}$ times may be found not only in AIHA, which might be expected, but also in some cases of chronic renal failure, myeloproliferative disorders and, surprisingly, in a minority of women in late pregnancy. The test, therefore, is not specific for hereditary spherocytosis and is possibly demonstrating the abnormality of red-cell membrane rather than an alteration in surface-area:volume ratio.

Demonstration and identification of haemoglobin variants associated with haemolytic anaemia

Over 500 haemoglobin variants have been described but not all are associated with a shortened red-cell life span. The haemolytic variants may be broadly classified into those associated with intracellular haemoglobin degradation and precipitation, the unstable variants (*see* page 320) – which, although about 100 have been described, are relatively uncommon – and the smaller number of high-frequency variants, notably Hbs S, C, D.

Most of the clinically important haemoglobin variants are due to the substitution of an amino acid in either the α or β chain though one unstable γ-chain variant has been described. The amino-acid substitution often results in a change in the net charge of the haemoglobin molecule which alters its electrophoretic mobility relative to Hb A. Electrophoresis on solid support media is therefore a widely used technique for the demonstration and preliminary identification of variants and is particularly satisfactory for the identification of the high-frequency variants. Recognition of unstable variants by electrophoresis is less useful, many having a mobility similar to Hb A, and tests based on their instability are most suitable for their initial detection.

A variety of electrophoretic techniques using different support media have been used including paper, starch gel, starch block, cellulose acetate membrane, agar gel, polyacrylamide gel and the technique of isoelectric focusing has been shown to be capable of resolving different haemoglobins with similar isoelectric points. Cellulose acetate is recommended for routine screening, supplemented by citrate agar. Additional techniques demonstrating the insolubility of Hb S (sickling and solubility testing) can be used as confirmatory or as screening tests. The techniques of hybridization and the electrophoresis of dissociated globin chains are within the scope of a laboratory that is regularly involved in the detection of haemoglobin variants. 'Fingerprinting', by two-dimensional chromatography, of the tryptic digests of individual globin chains and the final identification of the precise amino-acid substitution(s) is better restricted to reference laboratories. Screening for Hb S is of prime importance because of its clinical significance and high incidence in certain ethnic groups and often influences the overall approach to the detection of abnormal haemoglobins. The problem may be approached in two ways: demonstration by electrophoresis of possible examples of Hb S (and other abnormal haemoglobins) and confirmation by solubility testing; or screening by a solubility test with confirmation and further study by electrophoresis.

Each approach has its adherents and choice is influenced by the population being studied and its purpose, e.g. healthy-population screening or hospital patients, and whether samples are from adults or neonates. Preliminary electrophoretic screening will identify Hb A/A samples which do not require further study and therefore the majority of specimens will require only one procedure. Solubility screening only identifies those samples containing Hb S and electrophoresis is still necessary to confirm its presence, to establish the Hb genotype and to detect other variants. With the exception, therefore, of those samples requiring an urgent report, an electrophoretic approach can be considered the most effective from both economic and practical standpoints, and for urgent requests certain electrophoretic systems can produce results in 30 minutes.

Neonatal haemoglobinopathy screening

Guidelines for haemoglobinopathy screening, particularly in respect of the sickle-cell and thalassaemia syndromes, have been published [99,100]. Of particular importance is neonatal screening. All babies from mothers who are heterozygotes, homozygotes or double heterozygotes for haemoglobins S, C, D, E and β^0 or β^+ thalassaemia should be tested at birth. Samples should be collected by heel prick or as cord blood by *venepuncture* of the umbilical vein to avoid contamination with maternal blood.

Each sample should be examined by electrophoresis on cellulose acetate at alkaline pH supplemented by citrate agar gel electrophoresis at acid pH if any abnormality is found. Of particular importance is the presence or absence of Hb A which differentiates between probable heterozygotes and homozygotes or double heterozygotes. Exceptions are homozygous β^+ thalassaemia and S β^+ thalassaemia. Contamination with maternal blood clearly invalidates the findings. If in doubt a fresh sample from the baby should be obtained.

In some communities it will be more practical to test *all* neonates rather than attempting to select those at risk which may result in some not being tested.

Electrophoretic techniques

Preparation of haemolysates

Several methods have been recommended for the preparation of haemolysates and the choice of technique depends on practical circumstances and the additional techniques to be applied to the haemolysate.

For routine screening a simple lysate of unwashed cells in an EDTA/KCN or saponin and KCN reagent is quite satisfactory and is particularly suitable for small samples or single drops of blood though subsequent solubility tests for Hb S are not satisfactory in the presence of the EDTA. A disadvantage of using unwashed cells is that protein staining of the separated components is confusing due to the presence of plasma proteins.

Techniques using extraction with organic solvents are commonly used but for large numbers of samples the method is time consuming and for initial screening is unnecessary. Furthermore, unstable haemoglobins may be degraded and 'lost' during the extraction procedure. The 'purest' method of preparation is that of lysis by water followed by high-speed centrifugation to remove red-cell debris. This is certainly the method of choice when an unstable haemoglobin is suspected.

The addition of KCN to a haemolysate not only prevents streaking by inhibiting Hi formation but also protects Hb F which is more susceptible to Hi formation in which form it is not resistant to alkali denaturation. The occurrence of false-positive results in the isopropanol precipitation test is also reduced by the addition of KCN.

The preparation of lysates can be avoided by the addition of saponin (1 g/l final concentration) to the buffer used for impregnating the cellulose acetate membrane; lysis of the whole-blood sample occurs after application to the strip.

A rapid method for preparing haemoglobin solutions which removes plasma proteins by using 30% sucrose plus detergent and with only a single centrifugation has also been described[101].

Rapid preparation of haemolysate for electrophoretic screening

EDTA/KCN method

1 g tetrasodium EDTA and 1 g potassium cyanide in 1 litre distilled water. Keep in a brown bottle and prepare freshly each week. Add one drop of whole blood to three drops of reagent and stand for 10 minutes. If blood has been collected on filter paper, add 0.3 ml of reagent to a punched-out 5 mm circle and agitate gently.

The haemolysate is not suitable for Hb S solubility studies. Protein staining should not be used.

Saponin haemolysis
1 g of white saponin dissolved in 1 litre of water and 0.5 g KCN added. One volume of red cells is added to three volumes of saponin reagent. The haemolysate is suitable for solubility studies. Protein staining should not be used.

Conventional extraction with organic solvent

Samples collected into EDTA or ACD are washed twice with isotonic saline and to one volume of packed cells is added one volume of water and 0.5 volumes toluene or carbon tetrachloride and shaken vigorously for 10 minutes followed by centrifugation at 3000 *g* for 30 minutes. The top layer (haemolysate) is removed by pipette and one drop of 50 g/l potassium cyanide added to each 1 ml of lysate. The haemoglobin concentration is adjusted to 10 g/dl and may be further diluted dependent upon the procedures to be adopted. Protein-staining methods may be applied. Unstable haemoglobins may be degraded during the extraction procedure.

High-speed centrifugation method

To one volume of washed packed cells is added two volumes of water and after standing for 10 minutes the solution is centrifuged at 18 000 *g* for 30 minutes at 4°C. Potassium cyanide is added as above.

Storage of haemolysates

Although freezing of lysates is widely practised, the stability of extracted lysates is satisfactory at 4°C if kept sterile and particularly if kept in a carbon monoxide atmosphere. Haemolysates may be lyophilized and should have a shelf life at room temperature of approximately 18 months but are possibly less stable than liquid samples stored at 4°C. Further details on the preservation of haemolysates are recommended by the ICSH [102].

Cellulose acetate electrophoresis

Cellulose acetate membrane (CAM) is available from several commercial sources, some being prepared specifically for use with purpose-designed tanks or chambers. Precise details of procedure will therefore depend on the source of the material and type of apparatus and only the general procedure will be described.

Equipment
As CAM is not inexpensive, an unnecessarily long strip should be avoided. As the maximum distance of separation between the fastest and the slowest migrating haemoglobins is no more than 4 cm, a bridge width of 8 cm is suitable and certainly should not exceed 10 cm. A power pack capable of providing 400 V or 50 mA, preferably with constant voltage and constant current facilities, is recommended.

CAM

The structure of CAM varies depending on the method of manufacture, though consistency of structure from batch to batch is more important. Material from different sources may be of different thicknesses and show differences in the sharpness of separations but they should not show any tendency to absorption as evidenced by 'trailing' of the separated fractions. The membranes are brittle when dry and should be handled with forceps. Strips of the required length can be cut with a sharp blade or scissors. Titan III Myler-backed plates (Helena Laboratories) are strongly recommended.

Buffer: Tris-EDTA-borate, pH 8.4 (TEB)

Tris (hydroxymethyl) methylamine 10.2 g, ethylenediamine tetracetic acid 0.6 g, boric acid 3.2 g, dissolved in distilled water to 1 litre. This formulation allows clear separation of Hbs A, F, S and C and also the 'fast' haemoglobins.

Procedure

CAM is floated on TEB buffer and allowed to soak before being submerged; this is essential to prevent trapping of air within the membrane. The membrane is then submerged and allowed to soak for 10 minutes before being removed and blotted between filter paper. The strip may then be positioned in the tank before applying the haemolysates or if the membrane is laid on a non-absorbent material the haemolysates may be applied before placing the membrane in position. Lysates are applied with a fine pipette as a thin streak using 2–3 μl of sample or by using a purpose-designed applicator. Samples should be applied at the centre of the strip or slightly to the anode side.

The voltage or current and length of run will depend on the apparatus, bridge width, size of strips, etc. Voltage should not be in excess of 350 V or if constant current is used, should be about 0.4 mA/cm strip width. Adequate separation should be achieved within 1 hour. Reference haemolysates should be included with each run and an absolute minimum would be Hb A/A and Hb A/S samples. Reference samples are available containing Hbs C, S, F and A.

Subsequent handling will depend largely on the purpose of the separation; if for routine screening then the strip may be examined directly without drying or staining and the position, number and intensity of the bands noted. A more permanent preparation is obtained by staining with Ponceau S (20 g/l in 30 g/l tricholoracetic acid) followed by differentiation in acetic acid (50 ml/l). Protein staining cannot be used if unwashed red cells were used for preparing the haemolysates as traces of plasma proteins will simulate haemoglobin fractions. More specific demonstration of haemoglobin fractions is obtained by staining for haemoglobin with tetramethylbenzidine reagent (page 341) but this is of doubtful necessity as bands comprising as little as 2% of total haemoglobin can be visualized without staining. However, if very dilute haemolysates are used or perhaps in the screening of cord blood samples where very small components may be present, haemoglobin staining is preferred to protein staining. If it is desired to quantitate the proportion of haemoglobin in each fraction, the haemoglobins may be eluted from the CAM after dividing the strip with scissors and the haemoglobin content read photometrically in the manner described for Hb A_2 quantitation on page 256. The mobilities of the individual commoner haemoglobin variants are shown in *Figure 11.11*.

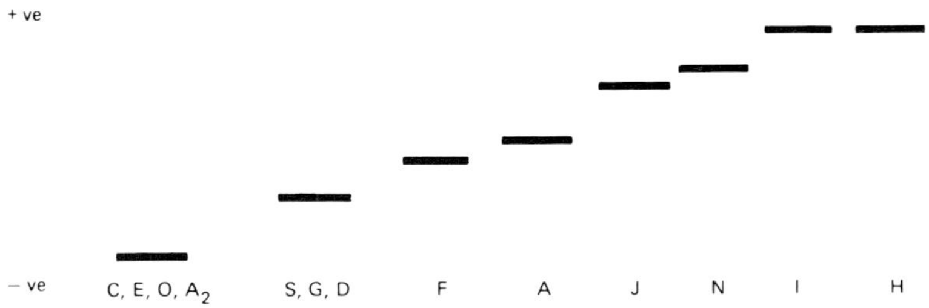

Figure 11.11 Relative mobilities of haemoglobins on cellulose acetate membrane in Tris-EDTA-borate buffer, pH 8.4

A systematic approach to the further study of abnormal components can be adopted. Haemolysates with a single component with the mobility of Hb A may be considered normal unless there is other evidence that an abnormal haemoglobin is likely to be present. All haemolysates showing a haemoglobin component migrating as Hb S are subjected to a solubility test (*see* page 374). 1 ml aliquots of 2.24 mol/l and 1.10 mol/l potassium phosphate buffer pH 6.5 are placed in small tubes. Three drops of lysate (not EDTA/KCN technique) are added to each tube together with a 'pinch' of sodium dithionite. If Hb S is present the 2.24 mol/l phosphate becomes cloudy within 5 minutes, the other tube remaining clear and acting as a control. Appropriate AA and AS controls are included with each batch.

All samples with an unequivocal AS electrophoretic pattern and a positive solubility can be reported as Hb AS without further testing. All other samples showing Hbs AF, SF, SS, SC, 'AS' etc. with negative solubility, or other patterns, are subjected to electrophoresis in citrate agar at acid pH.

Unusual haemoglobin patterns

Samples doubly heterozygous for α- and β-chain substitutions

Samples with more than two haemoglobin fractions (not including Hb A_2 and small amounts of Hb F) can be due to the interaction of α- and β-chain substitutions. The most frequent occurrence in Negro subjects is the occurrence of Hb S (β chain) and Hb G Philadelphia (α chain) resulting in the hybrid Hb S/G, as follows:

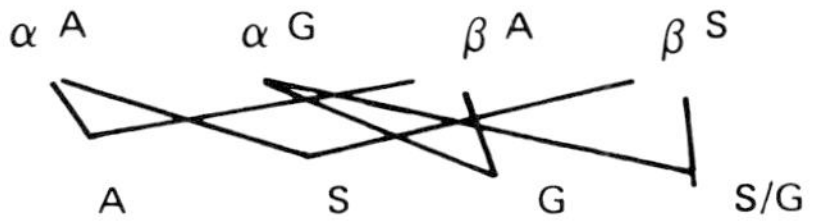

The electrophoretic separation will show three components – Hbs A, S and G which have similar mobilities, and the hybrid Hb S/G which will run in the position of Hb C due to the combined net change in charge of Hb S + Hb G.

Another, rarer, occurrence is the association of Hb C with Hb G Philadelphia, as follows:

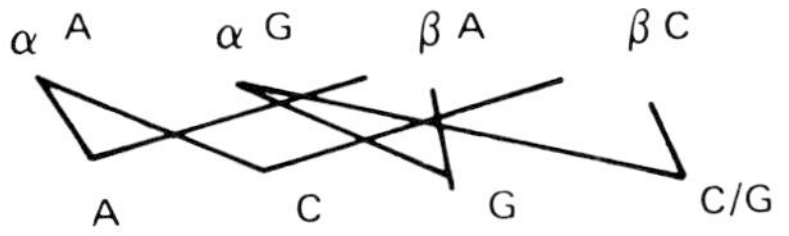

The separation will show four components – Hbs A, C, G and C/G – the first three with their usual mobilities and the hybrid C/G more cathodic than Hb C as the combined change in net charge is the sum of Hb C and Hb G.

β- or α-chain homozygotes with a substitution in the other chain
This occurrence must be rarer than the doubly heterozygous situations described above. The most common and of clinical and prognostic importance is that of sickle-cell anaemia (Hb S/S) together with heterozygosity for Hb G Philadelphia, as follows:

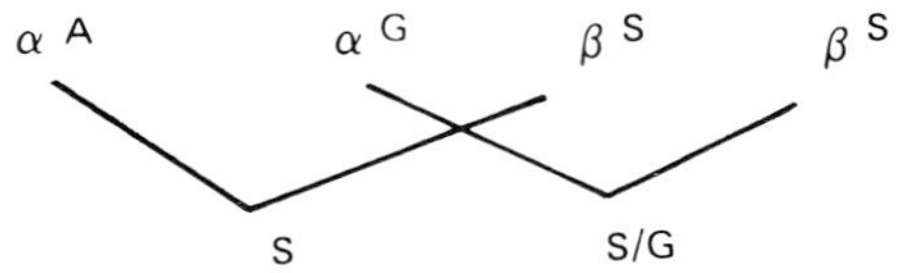

The pattern is therefore of two components with mobilities corresponding to Hb S and Hb C. The appearance therefore suggests Hb S/C disease though the blood-film changes and the clinical signs are those of sickle-cell anaemia. Another possible explanation of the haemoglobin pattern is the occurrence of Hb C Harlem with Hb S, again with the blood changes and clinical severity of sickle-cell anaemia. Hb S/O Arab should also be considered. Differentiation is readily accomplished by electrophoresis of separated globin chains.

Figure 11.12 illustrates the electrophoretic patterns of haemoglobin phenotypes and genotypes.

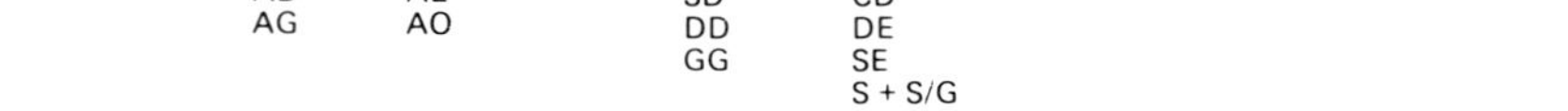

Figure 11.12 Examples of electrophoretic patterns of the commoner haemoglobin abnormalities

Citrate agar electrophoresis

The original technique of citrate agar electrophoresis was cumbersome and time consuming with an electrophoresis time of 16 hours. More recent techniques have recommended the use of commercial CAM plates impregnated with citrate agar[103] and an electrophoresis time of 30 minutes or a thin agar gel on glass slides with a separation time of 1 hour[104]. Though these techniques have been described for use with specific type of apparatus and accessories, the latter technique can be adapted for other equipment.

Preparation of haemolysate
One volume of once-washed and packed red cells is lysed by the addition of eight volumes of 1 g/l saponin containing 0.5 g KCN. The lysate is spun for 10 minutes at 1500 *g*. One drop of haemolysate is added to four drops of working citrate buffer (*see* below).

Citrate buffer 0.5 mol/l, pH 6.2
Stock buffer Dissolve 147 g trisodium citrate . $2H_2O$ and 4.3 g citric acid in 1 litre distilled water. Store at 4°C.

Working buffer Dilute stock buffer 1 in 10 with distilled water and adjust to pH 6.2 with 200 g/l citric acid. The pH is not critical within the range 6.0–6.4.

Agar
Use an unpurified agar such as Difco Bacto-agar. Refined agars do not give satisfactory results. Poor results are most likely to be the result of unsatisfactory agar. Agar for pre-coating the slides is made by boiling 1 g/l in distilled water. The agar-gel proper is prepared at 10 g/l and allowed to cool to 50°C before use.

Preparation of agar-coated slides
Glass slides of a size suitable for the electrophoresis tank are selected. For rapid separation a slide width of not more than 7.5 cm should be used. The slides are pre-coated by dipping them into the hot 1 g/l agar, allowed to drain and dried in an oven at 100°C for about 1 hour. The pre-coated slides are placed on a levelling tray and about 6 ml of 10 g/l agar is rapidly pipetted on to the slide and spread to all corners and margins. It is important that the gel is of even thickness. When set, the slides may be stored in wrapping film and kept at 4°C in a tightly closed box containing a small piece of cotton wool moistened with formaldehyde.

Electrophoresis
The chambers of the tank are filled with working buffer and the connections to the gel made with Whatman No 3 chromatography paper. A constant current of 40 mA is applied for each plate for 2–3 hours. If a cooled platten is supporting the plate then the run can be carried out at room temperature, otherwise the tank may have to be placed in a cold-room or refrigerator to prevent over-heating and uneven migration. Fresh buffer and wicks should be used for each run.

Staining
The gel may be examined without staining but if there is any possibility of minor fractions being present, because of the very dilute haemolysate, they may be missed and haemoglobin staining is therefore recommended. Tetramethylbenzidine reagent is prepared as described on page 341, applied for 30 s and washed off with copious volumes of 5% glacial acetic acid in deionized water.

Interpretation
Figure 11.13 illustrates the relative mobilities of selected haemoglobin variants. Of particular importance is that Hb F is cathodic to Hb A, Hb S is anodic to Hb A in contrast to Hbs D and G which run with Hb A, and that Hb C has the greatest anodic mobility in contrast to Hb E which runs with Hb A. Hb O Arab is slightly anodic to Hb A but less than Hb S, in contrast to Hbs C and E.

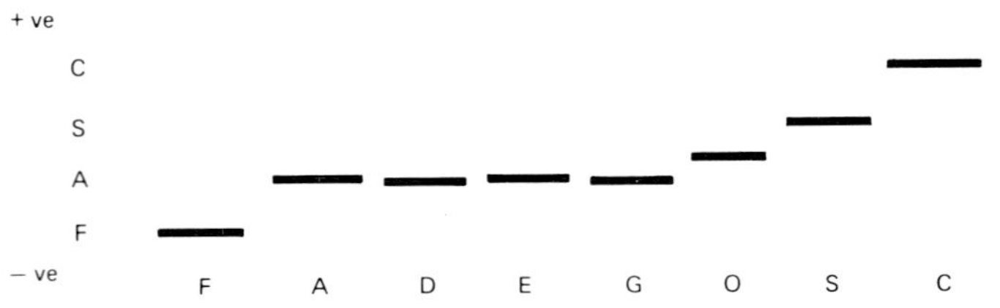

Figure 11.13 Relative mobilities of haemoglobin variants in citrate agar, pH 6.2

Globin-chain electrophoresis [105,106]

Clinically significant problems possibly remaining after electrophoresis on cellulose acetate, solubility testing and citrate agar electrophoresis are the differentiation of Hb G Philadelphia from Hb D, the distinction between the hybrid Hb S/SG and Hb SC and, in addition, the differentiation of Hb SO, SE and SC.

Globin-chain separation can be performed on cellulose acetate at acidic and/or alkaline pH in buffers containing 2-mercaptoethanol which cleaves haem from globin, and urea which severs the α from the non-α chain. Only small amounts of haemolysate are required and separation is achieved in 1–1.5 hours. Electrophoresis at both acid and alkaline pH reveals most information but most problems can be resolved at acid pH. Discontinuous buffer systems can be used but satisfactory results can be obtained using a single buffer.

Reagents

1. Haemolysing reagent: 1 g tetrasodium EDTA and 0.2 g KCN in 1 litre of deionized water.
2. Citric acid solution: 300 g/l.
3. Stain: 5 g Ponceau S in 1 litre trichloroacetic acid (50 g/l).
4. Differentiator: 30 ml glacial acetic acid to 970 ml water.
5. Tris-EDTA-boric acid-citrate buffer, pH 6.3: 10.2 g Tris (hydroxymethyl) methylamine, 0.6 g EDTA, 3.2 g boric acid in 1 litre deionized water. Dilute 1 in 3 with water. Dissolve 36 g urea in about 65 ml buffer and adjust to pH 6.3 by adding citric acid solution; make up to 100 ml.

Preparation of samples

Add 3 volumes of haemolysing reagent to 1 volume packed red cells. To 20 μl haemolysate add 20 μl urea buffer and 10–20 μl of 2-mercaptoethanol. Stand for 30 minutes before application but not longer than 4 hours.

Preparation of cellulose acetate

Soak membranes overnight in the urea-mercaptoethanol buffer (7 mM mercaptoethanol), drain and blot. If Mylar-backed gels (Helena Laboratories) are used, prolonged soaking in the presence of mercaptoethanol may soften the Mylar backing; soak in urea buffer alone overnight and for 1 hour in urea + mercaptoethanol buffer, drain and blot.

Electrophoresis
Fill the electrophoresis reservoirs with the urea buffer after adding 0.5 ml 2-mercaptoethanol. Apply 2 μl of samples about 1 cm from anodal end if using gels and about 3 cm if using acetate sheets. Assemble the wicks, sheets or gels and in the case of gels cover with a glass plate. Apply 200 V for 1–1.5 hours. Haem-containing bands will rapidly move to the anode and into the buffer. After completing the separation remove the plate or sheet, stain for a few minutes and differentiate with dilute acetic acid.

Control samples containing Hbs A, S and C must be run alongside the test samples or an AFSC mixture.

Results
The relative mobilities of the normal globin chains and certain abnormal variants and combinations are shown in *Figure 11.14*. Fuller illustration of other globin chain mobilities are available[106,107].

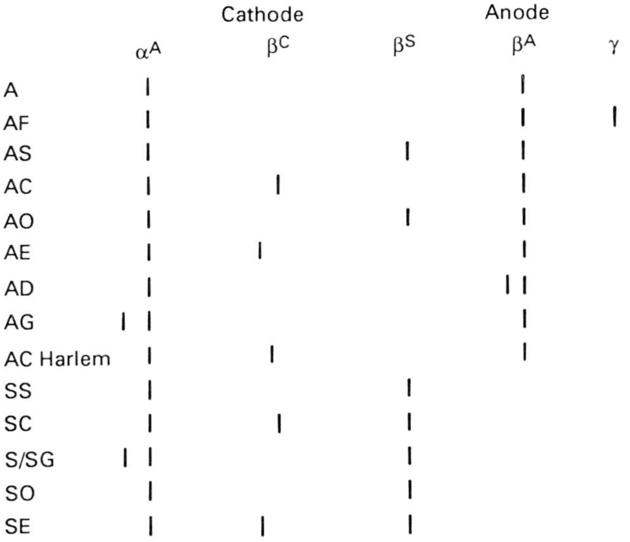

Figure 11.14 Relative mobilities of various globin chains by cellulose acetate electrophoresis in acid urea-mercaptoethanol buffer pH 6.3

Demonstration of unstable haemoglobin

The most reliable approach to demonstrating this group of variants is the use of stability or precipitation tests. Fresh blood samples or whole-blood samples stored at 4°C should be used; haemolysates are prepared simply by the addition of water followed by centrifugation to remove red-cell stroma but this is not essential. Extraction with organic solvent must not be used.

Isopropanol precipitation test[108]

Principle
Haemolysate is mixed with an isopropanol–Tris buffer, pH 7.4, and incubated at 37°C for 30 minutes. The test is sensitive and false-positive results occur, possibly

due to the presence of Hi. The presence of Hb F is particularly associated with precipitation probably because Hb F is more readily converted to Hi than Hb A. The addition of potassium cyanide to the haemolysate reduces the number of false positives. Storage of whole-blood samples at 4°C prior to testing also appears to reduce the number of false positives [109].

Reagent
Isopropanol–Tris buffer: 12.1 g Tris (hydroxymethyl) methylamine dissolved in 600 ml distilled water and adjusted to pH 7.4 with 1 mol/l HCl. To 83 ml of buffer is added 17 ml isopropanol.

Method
2 ml of reagent is pipetted into each of two tubes and warmed to 37°C. 0.2 ml of test haemolysate (10 g/dl containing 0.02 ml of 20 g/l KCN) is added to one tube and 0.2 ml of a control lysate to the other. Stopper, mix and leave at 37°C for 30 minutes.

Interpretation
A positive result is the appearance of a flocculent precipitate. The control tube should remain clear. The test is simple and rapid but false-positive results occur and all positive results should be confirmed with the more specific heat stability test.

Zinc acetate precipitation test [110]

Principle
The addition of haemolysate to a solution of buffered zinc acetate in the proportion of 3.5 mol zinc : 1 mol haemoglobin results in precipitation of the haemoglobin if it is an unstable variant.

Reagents
1. Haemolysate: 10 g/dl.
2. 0.003 M zinc acetate.
3. Tris(trimethamine) buffer: 0.1 M pH 7.4.

Method
Mix 0.35 ml zinc acetate solution and 1.45 ml Tris buffer. Add 0.2 ml haemolysate, mix and incubate for 30 minutes at 37°C.

Interpretation
With unstable haemoglobin immediate flocculation is seen which settles as a precipitate by the end of the incubation period. No precipitation is seen when up to 20% Hb F is present or with 3% methaemoglobin. It may therefore be the preferred test for aged haemolysates.

Note
Zinc acetate precipitation is useful for concentrating dilute solutions of haemoglobin. Stable haemoglobin solutions will precipitate when the ratio of zinc to haemoglobin is 10:1. The precipitated haemoglobin can be redissolved in EDTA solution [110].

Heat stability test

Principle
Normal haemoglobin is stable when heated at 50°C at pH 7.4. Unstable haemoglobin is precipitated under the same conditions.

Reagent
Tris–HCl buffer: Dissolve 6.05 g Tris (hydroxymethyl) methylamine in about 600 ml distilled water. Adjust the pH to 7.4 with 1 mol/l HCl (about 36 ml) and make up to 1 litre.

Method
To 1 ml of buffer add 0.8 ml distilled water and 0.2 ml haemolysate (10 g/dl). Haemolysate containing KCN is unsatisfactory. A control lysate is treated in the same way. Mix and incubate at 50°C. If unstable haemoglobin is present a copious flocculent precipitate will be formed within 60 minutes with further formation up to 180 minutes. No, or minimal precipitation is formed with the control haemolysate. Hb F is stable. The proportion of unstable haemoglobin may be measured by comparing the amount of haemoglobin in the supernatant with that present before heating.

Interpretation
The test is apparently sensitive and specific for unstable haemoglobin; other haemolytic anaemias associated with Heinz-body formation due to oxidative stress give negative results. The need for a water bath at 50°C is a minor disadvantage. The precipitated haemoglobin may be used for further characterization of the variant.

Electrophoresis in the demonstration of unstable haemoglobins

The majority of unstable variants migrate as Hb A. Unstable variants always occur as a minor component due to the selective loss of the abnormal haemoglobin from the red cells in the form of Heinz bodies or, in the case of Hb H, by the intracellular degradation of free β chains. Although only a minority of unstable variants are cathodic to Hb A, haem-depleted bands are apparently always present and may be demonstrated by protein staining of the electrophoretic strip or gel [111].

Other tests for unstable haemoglobins

In vitro Heinz-body formation is induced more readily than in normal blood after incubation or on the addition of phenylhydrazine but the finding is not specific.

Haemoglobin A_2 is often increased in unstable β-chain abnormalities due to loss of unstable haemoglobin from the cells.

Oxygen affinity studies can indicate unstable haemoglobins, as high or low affinities occur, often with altered haem–haem interaction.

Demonstration of haemoglobin S

The presence of Hb S can be shown by electrophoresis (*see* page 367) or by its insolubility in the reduced state either by the microscopic demonstration of sickling or by the demonstration of reduced solubility by precipitation in concentrated buffer containing a reducing agent.

Sickling test

One drop of whole blood is mixed on a slide with three drops of freshly prepared 20 g/l sodium dithionite, sealed under a cover-slip and incubated at 37°C. Typical sickle cells may be seen after 20 minutes particularly at the margin of the preparation. The sickle-cell appearance is preceded by the presence of 'holly-leaf' forms which may persist if the proportion of Hb S is less than 30% which can occur when the sickle-cell trait (Hb AS) coexists with iron deficiency or α_1-thalassaemia trait. In addition to Hb S, other variants cause sickling – Hb C Harlem and Hb C Ziguinchor – and have low solubility, but are rare in comparison with Hb S. Though deceptively simple, false results may be recorded.

False-positive reports can be due to confusion with abnormally shaped such as acanthocytes and crenated cells. Drying of the preparation with intracellular crystallization may also be mistaken for sickling.

False-negative results can be due to the reducing agent not being freshly prepared or when the number of cells containing Hb S is low, e.g. after transfusion, in cord blood, or in infant's blood, when the proportion of Hb S in individual cells is low, e.g. in iron deficiency or α_1-thalassaemia trait, or in the presence of Hb F in every cell which will inhibit sickling. Plasma is necessary for the sickling phenomenon and washed cells should not be used. Although of academic and educational interest, sickling as a screening test has been virtually replaced by solubility testing partly for convenience and partly because of the possibility of false results.

Solubility tests for Hb S

The tests are based on that of Itano[112] using the principle that deoxy-Hb S (and Hb C Harlem) is less soluble in concentrated phosphate buffers than all other haemoglobins. Haemolysate or whole blood can be used, each having advantages. The use of whole blood is quicker but may introduce errors which are eliminated by the use of washed red cells or haemolysates of standard haemoglobin concentration.

Method using whole blood[113]

Buffer (2.24 mol/l, pH 6.7)
Dipotassium hydrogen phosphate (K_2HPO_4) 220.3 g; potassium dihydrogen phosphate (KH_2PO_4) 132.45 g; saponin (BDH) 5 g; water 1 litre.

Method
To 1 ml of buffer *at room temperature* is added 10 mg of sodium dithionite in a 75 × 10 mm tube. 0.02 ml whole blood is added, mixed and allowed to stand for 3 minutes. Control negative and positive blood samples should be set up with each test.

Reading of results
The presence of Hb S may be demonstrated in three ways:

1. *Turbidity* Blood not containing Hb S will appear as a purplish solution that is transparent but not crystal clear. A positive result is seen as a clearly turbid

solution through which it is difficult to distinguish a black and white lined background.

2. *After centrifugation* Negative results are seen as a clear purple solution with a thin 'scum' of precipitated protein and red-cell stroma. A positive result is seen as a clear or slightly pink fluid with a thick brown surface layer.
3. *Microscopically* Precipitated plasma proteins appear as amorphous material, red cells that contained Hb A appear as ghosts, cells containing Hb S appear intact. Contrary to the generally held view, saponin does not allow Hb S to escape from the cell to be precipitated from solution but allows the dithionite buffer to enter the cell with resulting intracellular Hb S precipitation[114]. Microscopy can therefore be used to confirm visual reading and is particularly useful in neonatal samples with small numbers of cells containing Hb S.

Notes

When assessed solely by turbidity *false-positive* results may be due to cell debris, increased amounts of plasma protein in anaemic bloods, paraproteinaemias or due to Heinz bodies in unstable haemoglobin disorders. *False-negative* results can be due to lack of turbidity when haemoglobin concentration is less than 7 g/dl (which should be corrected by removing excess plasma rather than increasing the volume of blood added), a low proportion of Hb S in cord blood or by inactive reagents; false-negative results may also be found after transfusion and in samples from infants. Deterioration of the dithionite, unsuitable saponin, not using truly anhydrous salts for preparing the buffer and not allowing the buffer to come to room temperature are examples of technical failures. Experience is necessary to eliminate observer error.

The use of washed red cells eliminates the errors due to plasma proteins and insufficient red cells. Using haemolysates of washed cells eliminates error due to Heinz bodies or to the presence of Hb H. An error-free method using haemolysate which also allows quantitation of Hb S has been described[115]. Errors due to interfering plasma components and to anaemia can be eliminated by adding 10 μl of sedimented red cells instead of 20 μl of whole blood.

Modifications of 'standard' solubility tests include a micromethod using microtitre plates to reduce costs when commercial reagents are used[116] and an automated method using autoanalyser equipment for handling large numbers of samples[117]. The differentiation of heterozygous and homozygous Hb S samples can be achieved by modified solubility testing followed by centrifugation[118].

Demonstration of the red-cell defect in paroxysmal nocturnal haemoglobinuria

The diagnosis of PNH depends upon the demonstration of the undue susceptibility of the red cells to lysis by complement. A variety of *in vitro* tests have been described: the acidified serum test (Ham's test), sucrose lysis test, the addition of thrombin in the presence of inulin, lysis by high-titre cold antibodies, by the addition of cobra venom or simply by increased lysis when incubating at 37°C. Of these only the acidified serum test and the sucrose lysis test will be considered on the basis of specificity, sensitivity and ease of performance.

Acidified serum test

Principle

The test red cells are suspended in normal serum acidified to between pH 6.5 and 7.0, incubated at 37°C and examined for haemolysis. Lysis is induced by activation of the alternative pathway of complement activation.

Samples

Red cells can be used from clotted or defibrinated blood or from blood collected into any anticoagulant including cells stored for up to 3 weeks in ACD if kept sterile.

Serum should be free from haemolysis to facilitate reading of the tests. This is no problem with normal serum but serum from a case of PNH may show haemolysis. Normal sera differ greatly in their lysis of PNH cells and it is important to select sera known to be strongly lytic. As ABO-compatible serum is required, a group AB member of staff whose serum shows satisfactory lysis would be ideal. Alternatively persons of each ABO group should be tested beforehand. If PNH red cells are not available for selection of sera, 'PNH-like' red cells prepared by treatment with 2-aminoethylisothiouronium bromide (AET) can be used (*see* page 378). Sera should be fresh and used within a few hours or may be stored at −70°C; deterioration occurs within a few days at −20°C.

Method

Although essentially a simple test the significance of the results depends upon adequate controls. The test is set up as shown in *Table 11.14*.

Table 11.14 Reagents and amounts used in acidified serum test

Reagents	*Test* (ml)			*Controls* (ml)		
	1	*2*	*3*	*4*	*5*	*6*
Fresh normal serum	0.5	0.5	0	0.5	0.5	0
Inactivated normal serum	0	0	0.5	0	0	0.5
0.2 mol/l HCl	0	0.05	0.05	0	0.05	0.05
50% patients cells	0.05	0.05	0.05	0	0	0
50% normal cells	0	0	0	0.05	0.05	0.05
Results (lysis):						
Typical PNH	trace	+++	−	−	−	−
Other cell defect, e.g. spherocytosis	−	+	+	−	−	−
Lysin in 'normal' serum	+++	+++	−	+++	+++	−

Notes

1. Normal serum is inactivated by heating at 56°C for 30 minutes.
2. Red cells are washed twice with isotonic saline.
3. Cells should be added directly into the serum and not allowed to run down the side of the tube.
4. The cell–serum mixtures are incubated at 37°C for 1 hour and then centrifuged. The cells should be gently re-suspended during the incubation period.

5. Lysis may be quantitated by measuring the haemoglobin in the supernatants against '100% lysis' prepared by adding 0.05 ml of cells to 0.55 ml of water followed by suitable dilution of supernatants and '100% lysis' in Drabkin's solution and reading in a photometer at 540 nm using the original serum as a blank.
6. The addition of thrombin to the test to enhance lysis has been recommended but in practice is not of significant benefit in diagnosis.
7. A further modification which appears to eliminate the variability of normal sera is the addition of magnesium ions in the form of magnesium chloride at a final concentration of 0.3 mmol/l Mg^{2+} [119].

Interpretation

PNH cannot be diagnosed unless a properly controlled positive acidified serum test is demonstrated. The test may be considered specific if the only other known cause of a positive test – i.e. congenital dyserythropoietic anaemia type II (hereditary erythroblast multinuclearity with a positive acid serum test (HEMPAS)) – is excluded. Unlike PNH, however, HEMPAS red cells will not be lysed by their own serum and will only be lysed by about 30% of normal sera (*see* page 405). Strictly, the patient's serum should be included in the acidified serum test as a further control but occasionally the serum from cases of PNH may produce a negative result possibly due to complement depletion. This step would also make the test unnecessarily complex, particularly as HEMPAS is a rare disorder. The possibility of HEMPAS should, however, be excluded whenever a positive test is obtained. A further difference between the two disorders is that the sucrose lysis test (*see* below) is negative in HEMPAS.

Lysis of PNH cells is never complete and may be as little as 5% or even less. A possible cause of a false-negative test is the presence of iron deficiency [120], the test becoming positive when the deficiency is corrected.

The sucrose haemolysis and 'sugar-water' tests

Principle

Erythrocytes from patients with PNH haemolyse when incubated in isotonic solutions of low ionic strength provided a small amount of serum (complement) is present in the reaction mixture. Lysis is induced by activation of the classical pathway of complement lysis.

The 'sugar-water' test [121]

Sugar-water 10 ml granulated commercial sugar is lightly packed by tapping in a graduated tube and dissolved in a final volume of 100 ml. It is prepared *fresh* as required.

Sample Citrated or oxalated whole blood. Do not use defibrinated, EDTA, heparinized blood or blood without anticoagulant.

Method Add 0.1 ml whole blood to 0.9 ml sugar solution. Mix immediately and leave for 30 minutes at room temperature. Centrifuge and inspect the supernatant.

Interpretation If no haemolysis is present the patient probably does not have PNH, provided that multiple transfusions have not greatly reduced the proportion of patient's cells. If there is haemolysis it is essential to perform the sucrose haemolysis test.

The sucrose haemolysis test[122,123]

Sucrose solution Iso-osmotic sucrose solution, 92.4 g/l of reagent grade sucrose in water. The solution may be stored at 4°C for up to 3 weeks. Phosphate buffer pH 6.1 (910 ml 10.05 mol/l NaH_2PO_4, 90 ml 0.05 mol/l Na_2HPO_4) has been used instead of distilled water.

Sample 50% saline suspension of washed patient's red cells.

Method Two tubes are set up containing 0.05 ml of fresh normal group AB or ABO-compatible serum diluted in 0.85 ml of sucrose solution and 0.85 ml of isotonic NaCl, respectively. To each tube is added 0.1 ml of washed patient's red cells. Mix promptly and leave at room temperature for 30 minutes. Centrifuge and inspect the supernatant. If haemolysis is present determine the % haemolysis using the serum–saline supernatant as a blank and 0.1 ml of cells in 0.9 ml water which represents 100% lysis.

Interpretation Less than 5% haemolysis is probably inconsequential; 5–10% haemolysis is border-line and greater than 10% appears to be diagnostic of PNH. Weak positive results have been described in myeloblastic leukaemia, myelosclerosis and other dyserythropoietic anaemias. The test is therefore less specific for PNH than the acidified serum test but appears to be more sensitive and is not apparently influenced by concurrent iron deficiency. The acidified-serum and sucrose lysis tests have been compared with particular respect to the choice of serum and the use of several normal random sera for each test has been recommended[124]. The degree of haemolysis usually parallels the acidified serum test. The sucrose lysis test is characteristically *negative* in HEMPAS.

Preparation of PNH-like cells by treatment with 2-aminoethylisothiouronium bromide (AET)

Normal red cells treated with AET are virtually identical with true PNH cells by *in vitro* testing. They can be used as a positive control and for screening normal sera for use in the acidified serum test.

Method[125] Blood collected into ACD is washed twice with isotonic NaCl and one volume of cells is added to four volumes of AET (80 g/l adjusted to pH 8.0 with 5 mol/l NaOH) in a 75 × 12 mm glass tube and stoppered, mixed gently and placed at 37°C for exactly 19 minutes and then washed repeatedly until the supernatant is clear. The first centrifugation should be for a short time at low speed as the cells tend to stick together and have to be re-suspended by shaking. After washing, the cells are ready for use.

Tests for disorders of the pentose phosphate pathway

Deficiency of G6PD is the most common disorder of the pentose phosphate pathway. The high incidence of G6PD deficiency and its association with drug-induced haemolytic anaemia, neonatal jaundice, favism and the less common non-spherocytic haemolytic anaemias have resulted in a variety of screening methods to detect a deficiency of the enzyme. These include the methaemoglobin reduction test of Brewer, the Brilliant Cresyl Blue decolorization test of Motulsky and other dye reduction procedures, the ascorbate–cyanide method of Jacob and Jandl and the fluorescent spot technique of Beutler.

Most of the methods are efficient in detecting male hemizygotes and female homozygotes but for the recognition of female heterozygotes are less reliable and indeed assay techniques may fail to detect heterozygotes because of individual gene expression and genetically determined control of normal enzyme levels. A further limitation of screening tests can be the difficulty in diagnosis following a haemolytic episode in a person with a mild form of deficiency. National quality assessment surveys have also shown that certain methods give misleading results when performed by different laboratories. As neither screening tests nor assays can reliably detect heterozygotes, methods which demonstrate G6PD activity at a cellular level are valuable, particularly for family studies.

A screening test should be relatively simple, rapid and reliable within the limitations of gene expression mentioned above. The ICSH recommend the fluorescent spot test of Beutler and Mitchell [126].

Fluorescent spot test for G6PD deficiency

Principle

In the presence of G6PD, NADP will be reduced to NADPH which fluoresces under long-wave ultraviolet light.

Blood samples

Blood anticoagulated with EDTA, heparin, ACD or CPD is suitable. Samples may be stored *as whole blood* for 21 days at 4°C or 5 days at 25°C. Blood collected and dried on blotting paper may be used.

Reagents

1. Glucose-6-phosphate, sodium salt 10 mmol/l: 305 mg in 100 ml water.
2. β-NADP, 7.5 mmol/l: 55.7 mg in 10 ml water.
3. Saponin (Sigma): 1 g in 100 ml water.
4. Tris–HCl buffer, 750 mmol/l, pH 7.8: 90.8 g Tris (hydroxymethyl) aminomethane in 250 ml water. Add 33 ml 1 mol/l HCl and water to 1 litre.
5. Oxidized glutathione, 8 mmol/l: 49 mg in 10 ml water.
6. Working reagent: mix G6P 200 μl, NADP 100 μl, saponin 200 μl, Tris buffer 300 μl, glutathione 100 μl, water 100 μl. The reagent is stable for 2 years at −20°C and for at least 2 months at 4°C.

Method

10 μl whole blood are added to 100 μl reagent (alternatively a punched disc of blotting paper containing approximately 10 μl blood may be used). The blood–reagent mixture is allowed to stand at room temperature for between 5 and 10 minutes (if the ambient temperature is very high, 5 minutes is suitable). The mixture is spotted on Whatman No 1 filter paper, *allowed to dry thoroughly,* and examined visually under long-wave ultraviolet light.

Interpretation

Normal samples fluoresce brightly while deficient samples show little or no fluorescence. Intermediate degrees of fluorescence may be seen in blood from heterozygotes or from patients with mild G6PD variants who have recently undergone haemolysis.

Controls

As samples are stable for at least 4 weeks at 4°C, blood from a known deficient subject collected into ACD is the most suitable abnormal control. Normal and deficient controls should be set up with each test or batch of tests.

Note

The higher G6PD activity in reticulocytes and in the younger red-cell population of cord blood may be disregarded if the sample is spun in capillary tubes in a microhaematocrit centrifuge and a bottom portion containing approximately 5 μl of blood is broken off and the contents released into the reagent.

Other screening tests

The fluorescent spot test is for practical purposes specific for G6PD as it depends on the generation of NADPH. The earlier Brilliant Cresyl Blue decolorization test [127] is also dependent on NADPH formation but national quality assessment surveys show that incorrect results are more frequent than with the fluorescent spot test and are possibly due to variation in the batches of dye used.

The methaemoglobin reduction test [128] reflects the ability of intact red cells to reduce Hi, formed by the addition of sodium nitrite, by the action of NADPH-dependent methaemoglobin reductase and is therefore less specific than either the fluorescent or dye decolorization techniques. It has, however, been demonstrated to be superior to the Brilliant Cresyl Blue test in detecting heterozygotes for G6PD deficiency.

The ascorbate–cyanide test [129] is also dependent on enzymes and intermediates other than G6PD and in particular on the amount of GSH. As with the methaemoglobin reduction test it is probably superior to the more specific tests in detecting G6PD-deficient heterozygotes. An additional advantage as a screen for the activity of the pentose phosphate pathway is that low levels of GSH due to deficiency of glutathione synthetase or γ-glutamyl-cysteine synthetase can also be demonstrated. The ability of the test to detect heterozygotes for G6PD deficiency is improved by the demonstration, after completion of the standard test, of Heinz bodies in the G6PD-deficient cell population[130] irrespective of the degree of X-chromosome inactivation. The ascorbate–cyanide test is described for the reasons stated above.

Ascorbate–cyanide screening test [129]

Principle

Sodium cyanide added to blood inhibits catalase and allows hydrogen peroxide to be generated from the coupled oxidation of HbO_2 and the added ascorbate. The hydrogen peroxide generated will convert HbO_2 to Hi unless it is reduced by glutathione peroxidase, a reaction that requires GSH as the proton donor.

Reagents

1. Ascorbate: 10 mg sodium ascorbate and 5 mg glucose are dispensed into each of a number of small tubes. The tubes are stoppered and stored at −20°C.
2. Sodium cyanide: 500 mg NaCN are dissolved in 50 ml water and 20 ml of iso-osmotic phosphate buffer pH 7.4 added. The solution is neutralized with 2 mol/l HCl and the volume made up to 100 ml with water. The solution is stable indefinitely at 20°C.

Method

Blood collected into EDTA is preferred, though heparin is suitable (but not oxalate). The sample is aerated to a bright red colour and 2 ml added to a tube containing ascorbate and glucose and 0.1 ml cyanide solution added. The mixture is incubated, without a stopper, at 37°C preferably with agitation and is thoroughly mixed after 2 hours and again after 3–4 hours, its colour being noted on each occasion. Control samples of normal and G6PD-deficient blood must be tested in parallel. Normal blood darkens slowly over several hours. A positive reaction is seen by the blood becoming brown within 1–2 hours. Intermediate reactions may be seen between 2 and 3 hours. The change in colour is not very great and experience is required to detect the end-point which may best be appreciated by gently shaking the tubes and observing the colour of the film of blood on the side of the tube.

Supplementary test [130]

One drop of the cell suspension is added to two drops of methyl violet (5 g/l) and after 10 minutes a drop is transferred to a slide and examined under a cover-slip. Normal blood will not show any inclusions. Homozygotes and hemizygotes for G6PD deficiency will show inclusions in virtually all cells. Positive results due to defects other than G6PD will also show inclusions in virtually all cells. G6PD-deficient heterozygotes will show a variable proportion of cells with inclusions. Microscopic examination will be advantageous following transfusion or after a haemolytic episode when screening tests or assays are difficult to interpret.

Notes

1. A positive result with a dual cell population is characteristic of a G6PD-deficient heterozygote or a transfused homozygote or hemizygote.

2. A positive result with all cells containing inclusions may be homozygous or hemizygous for G6PD deficiency *or* due to an alternative cause. Estimation of GSH is indicated.
3. The demonstration of G6PD deficiency in individual cells may be the only way of identifying heterozygotes with certainty.

The method described above depends on the formation of Heinz bodies in deficient cells. An alternative approach is to induce methaemoglobin (Hi) formation by exposure to sodium nitrite. The reconversion of Hi to HbO_2 depends on G6PD activity which is demonstrated by the formation of insoluble formazan from soluble tetrazolium[131–133] or by a hydrogen peroxide elution technique in which Hi is eluted from the red cells but HbO_2 is not[134]. In heterozygotes a mosaicism is seen of stained or non-eluted cells with G6PD activity and non-staining or eluted ghosts lacking G6PD activity. Extremes of lyonization may cause difficulty in interpretation.

Screening test for pyruvate kinase deficiency

Although PK variants are extremely heterogeneous in their characteristics the majority will be demonstrated by failure of conversion of NADH to NAD at conventional substrate concentration, temperature and pH and can be detected by a fluorescent screening test[135].

Principle

In the presence of PK a phosphate group is transferred from phosphoenolpyruvate to ADP to form pyruvate and ATP. LDH catalyses the reduction of pyruvate to lactate with the oxidation of NADH to NAD with loss of fluorescence.

Reagents (also available in kit form from Sigma)

1. Phosphoenolpyruvate (PEP) (tricyclohexylammonium salt): 150 mmol/l 249 mg in 5 ml water. Adjust to pH 7–8 with 0.2 mol/l NaOH using pH paper. Store at −20°C.
2. ADP, 30 mmol/l: 150 mg ADP disodium salt in 5 ml water. Adjust to pH 7–8 with 0.2 mol/l NaOH using pH paper. Store at −20°C.
3. NADH, 15 mmol/l: add 0.9 ml water to a 10 mg pre-weighed vial of NADH-disodium salt (Sigma). Adjust to pH 7–8 with 0.2 mol/l NaOH using pH paper. Prepare fresh for each test or batch.
4. $MgSO_4$, 80 mmol/l: 98 mg $MgSO_4.7H_2O$, in 5 ml water.
5. Potassium phosphate buffer, pH 7.4: 250 mmol/l.

Blood sample

Blood collected into EDTA, heparin or ACD is centrifuged and the plasma and buffy coat carefully aspirated to remove the majority of leucocytes. A 20% suspension is prepared by adding four volumes of isotonic NaCl.

Procedure

20 µl cell suspension is added to 200 µl reagent and incubated at 37°C. After 20 minutes a drop of the reaction mixture is spotted on Whatman No 1 filter paper, *allowed to dry completely* and examined under long-wave ultraviolet light. Ideally normal and deficient blood should be similarly tested as controls. As a minimum a normal blood should be included.

Interpretation

Normal samples will show little or no fluorescence whereas deficient samples will fluoresce brightly.

Assay procedures for red-cell enzymes

Because of the great variety of techniques and the varying conditions of red-cell enzyme assay the ICSH have recommended methods of analysis[79] while at the same time acknowledging that alternative methods can be reliable and that modification may be desirable.

The use of a single haemolysate for multiple assays, a common buffer system and common substrate and co-factor solutions in the performance of all the assays was sought whenever possible with correction factors for temperatures other than 37°C.

The descriptions of the performance of assays covers a large number of enzymes but is unfortunately somewhat terse and, for the non-expert, difficult to follow. A final volume of 1 ml is recommended using 0.1 ml volumes of reagents unless otherwise specified, the final volume being made up to 1 ml with water. The molarities given are final concentrations and therefore reagents are prepared at 10 times the concentration stated. The scope of this book allows consideration only of those enzymes most commonly deficient, i.e. G6PD and PK.

Collection and storage of samples

EDTA, ACD and heparin are each generally satisfactory though ACD is preferred if prolonged storage (over 20 days) is necessary. Almost always, red-cell enzymes and other constituents are more stable in whole blood than in haemolysates. All enzymes are stable for 24 hours at room temperature or 6 days at 4°C. With the exception of phosphofructokinase, triose phosphate isomerase, adenosine deaminase and glyceraldehyde-phosphate-dehydrogenase, samples are stable for over 20 days in ACD at 4°C. Samples in transit should not be frozen as this will disrupt leucocytes and platelets as well as cause haemolysis and invalidate some assay results.

Deficiencies of some red-cell enzymes, e.g. G6PD, are reflected in the leucocytes and therefore removal of leucocytes is not strictly necessary. Most other red-cell enzyme activities are lower than those of leucocytes and platelets. When this difference is large and when leucocytes are unaffected by a red-cell deficiency, e.g. PK, it is essential that red-cell preparations are virtually free of leucocytes and platelets. The technique of centrifuging whole blood and removing the buffy layer is not satisfactory and may result in loss of the upper layer of reticulocytes. Filtration through a mixture of microcrystalline cellulose and α-cellulose is simple and rapid and the column can be prepared and stored[136].

Separation of red cells from whole-blood samples

Equal weights of microcrystalline cellulose (Sigmacell 50) and α-cellulose (both obtained from Sigma) are mixed with 0.154 mol/l NaCl. The plunger of a 5 ml plastic syringe is removed and the barrel fixed in a vertical position. A small circle of filter paper is placed in the bottom of the syringe and cellulose slurry poured to the 2 ml mark. The bed is washed with 5 ml of 0.154 mol/l NaCl and 1 ml of anticoagulated whole blood is allowed to flow into the column and the effluent collected in a centrifuge tube. The remaining red cells are washed through the column with 2–5 ml of 0.154 mol/l NaCl. The cell suspension is washed twice with ice-cold 0.154 mol/l NaCl and re-suspended as an approximately 50% cell suspension.

Haemolysate is prepared by adding 0.2 ml cell suspension to 1.8 ml 'stabilizing solution' containing 2.7 mmol/l EDTA (pH 7.0) and 0.7 mmol/l 2-mercaptoethanol (10 ml of 0.27 mol/l EDTA, 0.5 ml 2-mercaptoethanol to 1 litre water). The haemolysate is frozen rapidly in a dry-ice acetone bath or in methanol at −20°C and thawed in a beaker of water at room temperature and is then ready for assay as '1 in 20' haemolysate. It should not be centrifuged as loss of stromal-bound enzymes may occur. Any further dilution of the haemolysate is made with stabilizing solution which is itself stable for at least 10 days at 4°C. Most enzymes in the haemolysate are stable for at least 8 hours at 0°C although G6PD will lose about 25% activity in 6 hours and should therefore be assayed without delay. The haemoglobin content is determined as HiCN by diluting 1 in 10 and by comparison with a standard HiCN solution. The Hb concentration is expressed as g/l.

Expression of enzyme activity

Activity may be expressed as enzyme units (EU)/ml red cells, as EU/10^{10} red cells or EU/g Hb. Expression as EU/ml red cells demands determination of the PCV, with its inherent errors, of the 50% cell suspension, plus the errors of the subsequent dilution of the haemolysate. Haemoglobin measurement of actual haemolysate used in the assay is simple and readily available though it is the least logical. Enumeration of red cells in the washed suspension can be accurately performed with electronic counters. Activity per g Hb and per 10^{10} red cells will obviously be similar when red cells are of normal volume and haemoglobin content. When volume and haemoglobin content are discrepant, correction factors may be applied using MCV, MCH and MCHC values obtained from routine testing of the patient's blood[137].

Assay of glucose-6-phosphate dehydrogenase

Principle

G6PD catalyses the oxidation of glucose-6-phosphate to 6-phosphogluconolactone which quickly hydrolyses to 6-phosphogluconate (6-PGA):

$$\text{glucose-6-P} + \text{NADP} + \xrightarrow{\text{G6PD}} \text{6-PGA} + \text{NADPH} + \text{H}^+$$

The activity of G6PD is determined from the rate of reduction of NADP brought about by this reaction. NADPH is determined by measuring the rate of change in optical density at 340 nm. Ideally the reaction should be followed at 37°C but tests may be carried out at 25°C and appropriate correction factors applied (*see* page 386). The conversion of 6-PGA to ribulose-5-P by 6-phosphogluconate dehydrogenase (6-PGD) results in further reduction of $NADP^+$ and therefore true G6PD activity can be determined by adding 6-PGA together with G6P to the assay system and subtracting from the total rate of NADP reduction the rate of reduction in a system to which 6-PGA alone has been added.

Reagents

1. 1 mol/l Tris-HCl, 5 mmol/l EDTA buffer, pH 8.0: dissolve 30.25 g Tris and 0.42 g disodium EDTA in about 200 ml water. Adjust to pH 8.0 with 5 mol/l HCl at 25°C. Dilute to 250 ml with water.
2. Magnesium chloride, 0.1 mol/l: dissolve 5.08 g $MgCl_2 . 6H_2O$ in 250 ml water.
3. NADP, 2 mmol/l: add 6.5 ml water to a 10 mg pre-weighed vial of NADP (Sigma).
4. Glucose-6-phosphate disodium salt hydrate, 6 mmol/l: weigh 20.6 mg glucose-6-phosphate (disodium salt) and add 10 ml water.
5. 6-Phosphogluconate (trisodium salt), 6 mmol/l: 22.7 mg in 10 ml water.

All reagents are stable at −20°C for several months or at 4°C if no mould forms.

Method

Four cuvettes are prepared as shown in *Table 11.15*.

Follow the change in absorbance at 340 nm at 1 minute intervals for 10 minutes with full-scale absorbance set at 1.0. Select a straight part of the curve and calculate ΔA (increase in absorbance per minute).

Table 11.15 Preparation of cuvettes for glucose-6-phosphate (G6PD) dehydrogenase assay

Reagent	*Cuvette*			
	6-PGD assay		*6-PGD + G6PD assay*	
	1 (*Blank*, μl)	*2* (*Test*, μl)	*3* (*Blank*, μl)	*4* (*Test*, μl)
Tris-HCl-EDTA	300	300	300	300
$MgCl_2$	300	300	300	300
NADP	300	300	300	300
Haemolysate '1 in 20'	60	60	60	60
Water	2.04 ml	1.74 ml	2.04 ml	1.44 ml
[Incubate at 37°C or 25°C for 10 minutes]				
G6P	–	–	–	300
6-PGA	–	300	–	300

G6P = Glucose-6-phosphate; 6-PGA = 6-phosphogluconate; 6PGD = 6-phosphogluconate dehydrogenase.

Notes

1. The volumes may be scaled down if suitable cuvettes are available. (The ICSH recommended methods are based on a final volume of 1 ml.)
2. Assays at low concentrations of substrate are made by adding one-tenth the amount of substrate with appropriate increase in the volume of water.

Calculation

The international unit of enzyme activity is defined as the decrease in substrate or formation of product (or co-enzyme change) and is expressed in $\mu mol.min^{-1}.l^{-1}$.

Molar absorbance of NADPH = 6.22×10^3.

$$\text{Therefore if } \Delta A = 1 \text{, this represents } \frac{1}{6.22 \times 10^3}\ mol.min^{-1}.l^{-1}$$

$$\text{or } \frac{1000}{6.22}\ mol.min^{-1}.l^{-1}.$$

$$\text{Therefore enzyme activity} = \frac{\Delta A \times 1000}{6.22} \times \frac{3000}{60}\ \mu mol.min^{-1}.l^{-1}$$

where 3000 = cuvette volume and 60 = µl haemolysate added.

$$\text{Or enzyme activity/g Hb} = \frac{\Delta A \times 8040}{\text{Hb (g/l)}}$$

G6PD activity is obtained by subtracting 6PGD activity alone from the activity measured when both substrates are added.

Normal ranges [79]

Corrected for 6PGD activity EU/g Hb = 8.34 ± 1.59 at 37°C. For reactions at 25°C multiply by 0.559.

Not corrected for 6PGD activity (cuvettes 1 and 2 only) EU/g Hb = 12.1 ± 2.09 at 37°C. For reactions at 25°C multiply by 0.504. Normal ranges for a low-substrate system have been determined [79].

Assay of pyruvate kinase

Principle

Phosphoenolpyruvate (PEP) is converted to pyruvate by PK in the presence of ADP. Pyruvate is converted to lactate by lactate dehydrogenase (LDH) in the presence of NADH. The conversion of NADH to NAD^+ is followed by change of absorbance at 340 nm. Though the majority of cases have low residual PK activity the marked heterogeneity of PK deficiency may be associated with normal or even increased PK activity. The additional 'low-assay' system described is to demonstrate those that are inefficient at low concentrations of PEP in the presence of the allosteric effector fructose-1-6-diphosphate.

Blood samples

The haemolysate must be free of leucocytes and platelets as described previously (*see* page 384). Haemolysate should be dialysed 1:1000 against stabilizing solution for 6 hours.

Reagents

1. Tris-EDTA-HCl and $MgCl_2$: as for G6PD assay.
2. Potassium chloride, 1 mol/l: 7.45 g KCl in 100 ml water.
3. NADH, 2 mmol/l: add 3.25 ml water to 5 mg pre-weighed vial of NADH (Sigma). Prepare fresh for each assay and store at 0°C before use.
4. ADP, 15 mmol/l: 72 mg ADP-sodium salt . $1H_2O$ (Sigma) in 10 ml water. Store at −20°C.
5. Lactic dehydrogenase (LDH): 90 units in 1.5 ml water.
6. Phosphoenolpyruvate, 50 mmol/l: 135 mg PEP-trisodium salt (anhydrous) in 10 ml water. Store at −20°C.

Method 1

Two cuvettes are set up as shown in *Table 11.16*.

Table 11.16 Preparation of cuvettes for pyruvate kinase assay

Reagent	*Cuvette 1 (blank)* (μl)	*Cuvette 2 (test)* (μl)
Tris-EDTA-HCl	300	300
$MgCl_2$	300	300
KCl	300	300
NADH	300	300
ADP	–	300
LDH	300	300
Haemolysate '1 in 20'	60	60
Water	1.14 ml	0.84 ml

Incubate the cuvettes for 10 minutes at 37° or 25°C. Start the reaction by adding 300 μl PEP to each cuvette. Follow decrease in absorbance at 340 nm at 1 minute intervals for 10 minutes with the absorbance range set at 1.0. Select a straight part of the curve and calculate ΔA (the decrease in absorbance per minute).

Calculation As for G6PD assay.

Method 2 – Low-substrate system

Additional reagents:
1. ADP, 6 mmol/l: to 6 ml 15 mmol/l ADP add 9 ml water.
2. Fructose-1,6-diphosphate, 5 μmol/l: a stock 1 mmol/l solution is prepared by dissolving 3.4 mg FDP in 10 ml water. Dilute 1 in 200 for use.
3. PEP, 2.5 mmol/l: to 1 ml 50 mmol/l PEP add 19 ml water.

Table 11.17 Preparation of cuvettes for pyruvate kinase assay with low-substrate system

Reagent	*Cuvette 1* (μl)	*Cuvette 2* (μl)
Tris-EDTA-HCl	300	300
$MgCl_2$	300	300
KCl	300	300
NADH	300	300
ADP	–	300
LDH	300	300
Haemolysate '1 in 20'	60	60
FDP	300	300
Water	0.84 ml	0.54 ml

FDP = Fructose di-phosphate.

Method (*Table 11.17*)
Incubate for 10 minutes at 37°C or 25°C.
Start by addition of 300 μl PEP and proceed as for standard assay.

Normal range [79]

EU/g Hb = 15.0 ± 1.99 at 37°C. For reactions at 25°C multiply by 0.432.

Low-substrate with FDP 43.5 ± 2.46% of above value at 37°C. Multiply by 1.063 for reactions at 25°C.

Notes

1. Although the majority of PK variants will show low activity in the systems described a normal value does not exclude an abnormal PK variant. Additional studies which are normally outside the scope of most haematology laboratories can be employed including determination of alternative pH optimum, electrophoresis, heat stability, etc. The ICSH have published recommended methods for the characterization of PK variants [138].
2. As normal assay values may be found with some PK variants the assay of 2,3-DPG can be helpful in deciding whether to pursue the possibility of a PK variant. Characteristically 2,3-DPG levels in PK deficiency are 2–3 times the normal value.
3. In the preparation of reagents, full allowance must be made for variation in molecular weight due to state of hydration, type of salt and assay of purity.

Pyrimidine-5′-nucleotidase activity

Pyrimidine-5′-nucleotidase (P5N) is probably the third most common cause of hereditary non-spherocytic haemolytic anaemia, is important in the pathogenesis of the anaemia of lead poisoning and is of interest in certain other dyserythropoietic anaemias.

The ICSH have recommended two methods for the assay of P5N [139]. A radiometric method [140] is considered to be the better but uses ^{14}C-labelled cytidine. An alternative colorimetric method is also described but has possible problems of specificity. However, an ultraviolet absorption screening test for P5N activity has been recommended[141].

Principle

The nucleotides of normal red cells consist largely of purine derivatives (adenine and small amounts of guanine). The levels of the pyrimidine nucleotides (cytidine and uridine) are extremely low. Acidic solutions of cytidine have an absorption maximum of 280 nm while adenine, guanine and uridine nucleotides have an absorption maximum at about 260 nm. The position of the absorption maxima at 260 nm is shifted to 270 nm in P5N-deficient cells due to the accumulation of cytidine nucleotides. The reduced absorbance ratio of 260 nm to 280 nm implies P5N deficiency with the exception of CDP-choline accumulation which can occur despite normal P5N deficiency.

Sample preparation

Blood freshly collected in EDTA is centrifuged at 3000 *g* for 5 minutes, the plasma removed, and the cells washed three times with ice-cold 9 g/l NaCl solution. One ml of a 50% suspension of the washed red cells is added to 4 ml of ice-cold 4% perchloric acid (PCA) solution. The specimens are shaken vigorously for approximately 30 s. The clear supernatant obtained after centrifugation at 3000 *g* for 15 minutes is transferred to a small test tube. A blank extract is prepared by adding 1 ml of 9 g/l NaCl to 4 ml of the 4% PCA solution.

Procedure

500 µl of water and 300 µl of 1 mol/l glycine buffer, pH 3.0 are added to each of two cuvettes, one for the sample and one for the blank. The sample cuvette is read against the blank cuvette at 260 and 280 nm, giving readings of 260_B and 280_B. Next, 200 µl of the blank PCA extract are added to the blank cuvette while the PCA extract from the red cells is added to the sample cuvette. The reading of the blank cuvette is adjusted to 0 at 260 nm, and the sample cuvette is read, giving the value 260_S. The procedure is then repeated at 280 nm, giving the reading 280_S.

The A_{260}/A_{280} absorbance ratio (R) is calculated by the formula:

$$R = \frac{260_S - 260_B}{280_S - 280_B}$$

Interpretation

The ratio (R) of freshly collected blood from ten normal individuals was found to be 3.22 ± 0.10 (mean ±SD). In P5N deficiency, the value was 1.22 ± 0.14 (n = 10). After storage at 4°C for 5 days, the mean value of the normal samples had fallen to 2.44, SD 0.16 (n = 10). These values vary slightly between instruments. It may therefore be necessary for an individual laboratory to establish its own reference values.

Assay of intermediate compounds

Certain enzymes are either difficult to assay or may not show decreased activity in conventional assay systems. Furthermore, when the 'common' enzyme deficiencies have been excluded, it is useful to have an indication of which glycolytic pathway may be affected or the possible location of a defect in a particular pathway. The assay of intermediate compounds is a possible approach.

The ICSH have published recommended methods[139] for the assay of 2.3-diphosphoglycerate (2.3-DPG), adenosine-5′-triphosphate (ATP) and reduced glutathione (GSH). However, as with previously recommended methods for enzyme assay[79], the methods are not easy to understand and reproduce and the preparation of certain reagents is not sufficiently detailed or not described. This section is therefore confined to consideration of the rationale and principles involved.

2.3-DPG is an intermediate of the Embden–Myerhof pathway. An accumulation of 2.3-DPG is characteristically seen in most cases of pyruvate kinase (PK) deficiency. Conversely, when an enzyme defect is 'proximal' to 2.3-DPG, a lowered level of the compound may be demonstrated. In the recommended method 2.3-DPG is dephosphorylated by monophosphoglyceromutase (MPGM) in the presence of phosphoglycolate with the formation of 3-phosphoglycerate (3-PG). The 3-PG is then estimated through the 'backward' phosphoglycerate kinase (PGK) and glyceraldehyde 3-phosphate dehydrogenase (GAPD) reactions.

ATP is also decreased in PK deficiency. ATP content is measured using hexokinase and G6PD reactions. Hexokinase phosphorylates glucose with ATP in the presence of Mg^{2+} to glucose-6-phosphate; G6PD catalyses the dehydrogenation of G6P with NADP to give 6-phosphogluconolactone and NADPH. The resulting change in absorption from the reduction of NADP to NADPH is measured at 340 nm.

Reduced glutathione (GSH) is of particular value. The haemolysis associated with G6PD deficiency is due to reduction in the level of GSH or reduced GSH stability. Two enzymes, γ-glutamylcysteine synthetase and glutathione synthetase are involved in glutathione synthesis and GSH is markedly reduced if either of these enzymes is deficient. GSH levels are markedly increased in P5N deficiency. Assay of GSH is straightforward and is described.

Assay of reduced glutathione (GSH) [139]

Principle

GSH readily reduces 5,5′-dithiobis (2-nitrobenzoic acid) (DTNB) to form a deeply coloured yellow anion, absorbance being measured at 412 nm.

Sample preparation and assay

The PCV of EDTA-whole blood is measured. 0.2 ml is added to 1.8 ml of water and 3 ml metaphosphoric acid is added (1.67 g glacial metaphosphoric acid, 0.2 g disodium EDTA, 30 g NaCl, water to 100 ml). Stand for 5–10 minutes and filter through a Whatman No. 42 filter paper. To 4 ml 0.3 mol/l $Na_2HPO_4 . 2H_2O$ (53.4 g/l) add 1 ml of filtrate. A blank filtrate is prepared by adding 2 ml water to 3 ml metaphosphoric acid solution. The absorbance at 412 nm is measured within 5 minutes after the addition of 0.5 ml DTNB reagent (20 mg DTNB in 100 ml 10 g/l trisodium citrate solution) to the blank (A_B) and the sample filtrate (A_S).

Calculation
The blood is diluted by the following factor (F):

$$F = \frac{4.8 + (0.8 \times 0.2)}{0.2} \times \frac{5.5}{1.0} = 136.4$$

The GSH concentration (C) in red cells in mg/100 ml red cells is calculated as:

$$C = \frac{A_S - A_B}{13\,600} \times 136.4 \times 307 \times 100 \times \frac{1}{\text{PCV}}$$

where 13 600 is the molar extinction coefficient of the yellow anion produced when GSH interacts with DTNB; 136.4 is the dilution factor; 307 is the molecular weight of GSH; and PCV is expressed as l/l.

Reference values
The red cells contain 68.5 ± 10.8 mg GSH per dl (n = 10, mean ±SD).

References

1. Banga, J. P., Pinder, J. C., Gratzer, W. B., Linch, D. C. and Huehns, E. R. (1979) An erythrocyte membrane abnormality in march haemoglobinuria. *Lancet,* **ii**, 1048–9
2. Chilcote, E., Le Beau, M. M., Dampier, C. *et al.* (1989) Association of red-cell spherocytosis with deletion of the short arm of chromosome 8. *Blood,* **69**, 156–9
3. Agre, P., Orringer, E. P. and Bennett, V. (1982) Deficient red-cell spectrin in severe, recessively inherited, spherocytosis. *N. Engl. J. Med.,* **306**, 1155–62
4. Becker, P. S. and Lux, S. E. (1985) Hereditary spherocytosis and related disorders. *Clin. Haematol.,* **14**, 15–43
5. Lefrere, J. J., Courouce, A. M., Girot, R., Bertrand, Y. and Soulier, J. P. (1986) Six cases of hereditary spherocytosis revealed by human parvovirus infection. *Br. J. Haematol.,* **62**, 653–8
6. Palek, J. and Lux, S. E. (1983) Red cell membrane skeletal defects in hereditary and acquired hemolytic anaemia. *Sem. Haematol.,* **20**, 189–224
7. Palek, J. (1985) Hereditary elliptocytosis and related disorders. *Clin. Haematol.,* **14**, 45–87
8. Coetzer, T., Lawler, J., Prchal, J. T. and Palek, J. (1987) Molecular determinants of clinical expression of hereditary elliptocytosis and pyropoikilocytosis. *Blood,* **70**, 766–72
9. Lambert, S. and Zail, S. (1987) A new variant of the subunit of spectrin in hereditary elliptocytosis. *Blood,* **69**, 473–8
10. Morle, L., Alloisio, M. T., Ducluzeau, B. *et al.* (1988) Spectrin Tunis ($\alpha^{I/78}$): a new variant that causes asymptomatic hereditary elliptocytosis in the heterozygous state. *Blood,* **71**, 508–11
11. McGuire, M., Smith, B. L. and Agre, P. (1988) Distinct variants of erythrocyte protein 4.1 inherited in linkage with elliptocytosis and Rh type in three white families. *Blood,* **72**, 287–93
12. Iarocci, T. A., Wagner, G. M., Mohandas, N., Lane, P. A. and Mentzner, W. C. (1988) Hereditary poikilocytic anemia associated with the co-inheritance of two alpha spectrin abnormalities. *Blood,* **71**, 1390–6
13. Zarkowsky, H. S. (1979) Heat-induced erythrocyte fragmentation in neonatal elliptocytosis. *Br. J. Haematol.,* **41**, 515–18
14. Douglass, C. C. and Twomey, J. J. (1970) Transient stomatocytosis with haemolysis: a previously unrecognised complication of alcoholism. *Ann. Intern. Med.,* **72**, 159–64
15. Lande, W. M. and Mentzner, W. C. (1985) Haemolytic anaemia associated with increased cation permeability. *Clin. Haematol.,* **14**, 89–103
16. Eber, S. W., Lande, W. M., Iarocci, T. A. *et al.* (1989) Hereditary stomatocytosis: consistent association with an integral membrane protein deficiency. *Br. J. Haematol.,* **72**, 452–5
17. Lock, S. P., Smith, R. S. and Hardisty, R. M. (1961) Stomatocytosis: a hereditary red-cell anomaly associated with haemolytic anaemia. *Br. J. Haematol.,* **7**, 303–14

18. Wiley, J. S., Ellory, J. C., Shuman, M. A., Shaller, C. C. and Cooper, R. A. (1975) Characteristics of the membrane defect in the hereditary stomatocytosis syndrome. *Blood,* **46**, 337–56
19. Sturgeon, P. (1970) Haematological observations on the anemia associated with blood type Rh null. *Blood,* **36**, 310–20
20. Glader, B. E., Fortier, N. L. and Snyder, L. M. (1976) Hereditary hemolytic anaemia associated with RBC K-loss and dehydration: A family study. *Clin. Res.,* **24**, 309 (abstract)
21. Beutler, E. (1978) Why has the autohaemolysis test not gone the way of the cephalin flocculation test? *Blood,* **51**, 109–10
22. Kasper, M. L., Miller, W. J. and Jacob, H. S. (1986) G6PD-deficiency infectious haemolysis: a complement dependent innocent bystander phenomenon. *Br. J. Haematol.,* **63**, 85–91
23. Beutler, E. (1979) Red-cell enzyme defects as non-disease and diseases. *Blood,* **54**, 1–7
24. Luzatto, L. (1975) Inherited haemolytic states: glucose-6-phosphate dehydrogenase deficiency. *Clin. Haematol.,* **4**, 83–108
25. Gordon-Smith, E. C. (1980) Drug induced oxidative haemolysis. *Clin. Haematol.,* **9**, 557–86
26. Beutler, E. (1978) *Hemolytic Anemia in Disorders of Red-cell Metabolism.* New York: Plenum
27. Konrad, P. N., Richards, F., Valentine, W. N. and Paglia, D. E. (1972) γ-glutamyl-cysteine synthetase deficiency. *N. Engl. J. Med.,* **286**, 557–61
28. Beutler, E., Moroose, R., Kramer, L., Gelbart, T. and Forman, L. (1990) Gamma-glutamylcysteine synthetase deficiency and hemolytic anemia. *Blood,* **75**, 271–3
29. Boivin, P., Galand, C., André, R. and Deray, J. (1966) Anémies hémolytiques congénitals avec déficit isolé en glutathion reduit par déficit en glutathion synthetase. *Nouv. Rev. Fr. Hematol.,* **6**, 859–65
30. Valentine, W. N. and Paglia, D. E. (1979) Non-recessively transmitted non-spherocytic hereditary haemolytic anaemia associated with increased red-cell glutathione. *Br. J. Haematol.,* **42**, 231–7
31. Valentine, W. N., Fink, K., Paglia, D. E., Harris, S. R. and Adams, W. S. (1975) Hereditary hemolytic anemia with human erythrocyte pyrimidine-5-nucleotidase deficiency. *J. Clin. Invest.,* **54**, 866–79
32. Torrance, J. D. and Whittaker, D. (1979) Distribution of erythrocyte nucleotides in pyrimidine 5′ nucleotidase deficiency. *Br. J. Haematol.,* **43**, 423–8
33. Valentine, W. N. (1979) Hemolytic anaemias and inborn errors of metabolism. *Blood,* **54**, 549–59
34. Eaton, W. A. and Hofrichter, J. (1987) Hemoglobin S gelation and sickle cell disease. *Blood,* **70**, 1245–66
35. Liu, S-C., Zhai, S. and Palek, J. (1988) Detection of hemin release during hemoglobin S denaturation. *Blood,* **71**, 1755–8
36. Horn, M. E. C., Dick, M. C., Frost, B. *et al.* (1986) Neonatal screening for sickle cell diseases in Camberwell: results and recommendations of a two year pilot study. *Br. Med. J.,* **292**, 737–40
37. British Society for Haematology (1988) Guidelines for haemoglobinopathy screening. *Clin. Lab. Haematol.,* **10**, 87–94
38. Beutler, E. (1986) Hemoglobinopathies associated with unstable hemoglobin. In *Haematology,* 3rd edn (eds W. J. Williams, E. Beutler, A. J. Erslev and M. A. Lichtman), pp. 609–17. Singapore: McGraw-Hill
39. Grimes, A. J. and Meisler, A. (1962) Possible cause of Heinz bodies in congenital Heinz body anaemia. *Nature (Lond.),* **194**, 190–1
40. Winterbourn, C. C. and Carrell, R. W. (1974) Studies of hemoglobin denaturation and Heinz body formation in the unstable hemoglobins. *J. Clin. Invest.,* **54**, 678–89
41. Stern, M. and Rosse, W. F. (1979) Two populations of granulocytes in paroxysmal nocturnal haemoglobinuria. *Blood,* **53**, 928–34
42. Aster, R. H. and Enright, S. E. (1969) A platelet and granulocyte membrane defect in paroxysmal nocturnal hemoglobinuria: usefulness for detection of platelet antibodies. *J. Clin. Invest.,* **48**, 1199–210
43. Dessypris, E. N., Clark, D. A., McKee Jr, L. C. and Krantz, S. B. (1983) Increased sensitivity to complement of erythroid and myeloid pregenitors in paroxysmal nocturnal hemoglobinuria. *N. Engl. J. Med.,* **309**, 690–3

44. Rosse, W. F. (1973) Variations in the red-cells in paroxysmal nocturnal haemoglobinuria. *Br. J. Haematol.*, **24**, 327–42
45. Chua, C., Hoffmann, E. M., Adams, J. P. and Rosse, W. F. (1980) Inhibitors of complement derived from the erythrocyte membrane in paroxysmal nocturnal haemoglobinuria. *Blood,* **55**, 772–6
46. Ninomiya, H., Abe, T., Shichishimat, T., Terasawa, T. and Fujita, T. (1988) Decay-accelerating factor (DAF) on the blood-cell membranes in patients with paroxysmal nocturnal haemoglobinuria (PNH): measurement by enzyme-linked immunoadsorbent assay (ELISA). *Br. J. Haematol.*, **69**, 81–7
47. Sirchia, G. and Lewis, S. M. (1975) Paroxysmal nocturnal haemoglobinuria. *Clin. Haematol.*, **4**, 199–229
48. Rosse, W. F. (1989) Paroxysmal nocturnal haemoglobinuria: the biochemical defects and the clinical syndrome. *Blood Rev.*, **3**, 192–200
49. Petz, L. D. and Branch, D. R. (1985) Drug-induced immune hemolytic anemia. In *Methods in Haematology No. 12, Immune Haemolytic Anemias* (ed. H. Chaplin), pp. 47–94. New York: Churchill Livingstone
50. Petz, L. D. (1985) Drug-induced immune hemolysis. *N. Engl. J. Med.*, **313**, 510–12
51. Worrledge, S. M. and Blajchman, M. A. (1972) The autoimmune haemolytic anaemias. *Br. J. Haematol.*, **23** (Suppl.), 61–9
52. Petz, L. D. and Garratty, G. (1980) *Acquired Immune Hemolytic Anaemias.* New York: Churchill Livingstone
53. Wolach, B., Heddle, N., Barr, R. H., Zipursky, A., Mohan Pai, K. R. and Blajchman, M. A. (1981) Transient Donath–Landsteiner haemolytic anaemia. *Br. J. Haematol.*, **48**, 425–34
54. Issitt, P. D. (1985) Serological diagnosis and characteristics of the causative auto-antibodies. In *Methods in Haematology No. 12, Immune Haemolytic Anemias* (ed. H. Chaplin), pp. 1–45. New York: Churchill Livingstone
55. Garratty, G., Petz, L. D. and Hoops, J. K. (1977) The correlation of cold agglutinin titrations in saline and albumin with haemolytic anaemia. *Br. J. Haematol.*, **35**, 587–95
56. Rosse, W. F. and Adams, J. P. (1980) The variability of haemolysis in the cold agglutinin syndrome. *Blood,* **56**, 409–16
57. Issitt, P. D. and Pavone, B. G. (1978) Critical re-examination of the specificity of auto-anti-Rh antibodies in patients with a positive direct antiglobulin test. *Br. J. Haematol.,* **38**, 63–74
58. Cooper, R. A. (1970) Lipids of human red-cell membrane: normal composition and variability in disease. *Sem. Haematol.*, **7**, 296–322
59. Goebel, K., Goebel, F. D., Schubotz, R. and Schneider, J. (1977) Red-cell metabolic membrane features in haemolytic anaemia of alcoholic liver disease (Zieve's syndrome). *Br. J. Haematol.,* **35**, 573–85
60. Reinhart, W. H., Gossi, U., Butikofer, P. *et al.* (1989) Haemolytic anaemia in analpha-lipoproteinaemia (Tangier disease): morphological, biochemical and biophysical properties of the red blood cells. *Br. J. Haematol.*, **72**, 272–7
61. Fehr, J. and Knob, M. (1979) Comparison of red-cell creatine level and reticulocyte count in appraising the severity of haemolytic processes. *Blood,* **53**, 966–76
62. Panzer, S., Kronik, G., Lechner, K. *et al.* (1982) Glycosylated hemoglobins (GHb): an index of red-cell survival. *Blood,* **59**, 1348–50
63. Drysdale, H. C., Emerson, P. M. and Holmes, A. (1979) An improved method for the measuremment of red-cell survival using non-radioactive chromium. *J. Clin. Pathol.*, **32**, 655–9
64. Ricketts, C., Cavill, I. and Napier, J. A. F. (1977) The measurement of red-cell life-span using ^{59}Fe. *Br. J. Haematol.,* **37**, 403–8
65. Hutcheon, A. W., Horton, P. W., Orr, J. S. and Dagg, J. H. (1977) The assessment of red-cell survival in normal subjects and in patients with haemolytic disorders and ineffective erythropoiesis using the radioiron occupancy principle. *Br. J. Haematol.,* **37**, 195–205
66. Sears, D. A. and Weed, R. I. (1969) Diisopropylfluorophosphate is not a specific label for the red-cell membrane. *Blood,* **34**, 376–9
67. International Committee for Standardisation in Haematology (1980) Recommended method for red-cell survival studies. *Br. J. Haematol.*, **45**, 659–66

68. International Committee for Standardisation in Haematology (1975) Recommended methods for surface counting to determine sites of red-cell destruction. *Br. J. Haematol.*, **30**, 249–54
69. Bowring, C. S. (1981) *Radionuclide Tracer Techniques in Haematology*. London: Butterworths
70. Hodgson, R. and Sewell, P. (1965) Determination of serum haptoglobin concentration; a simple, rapid, gel-filtration method. *J. Med. Lab. Technol.*, **22**, 130–4
71. Owen, J. A., Better, F. C. and Hoban, J. (1960) A simple method for the determination of serum haptoglobin. *J. Clin. Pathol.*, **13**, 163–4
72. Hall, R. (1964) A simple and rapid method for estimation of haptoglobins in serum. *J. Med. Lab. Technol.*, **21**, 64–65
73. Griffiths, K. D. (1986) Tetramethylbenzidine – a sensitive stain for haemoglobin electrophoresis. *Clin. Lab. Haematol.*, **8**, 337–40
74. Chong, G. C. and Owen, J. A. (1967) Determination of methaemalbumin in plasma. *J. Clin. Pathol.*, **20**, 211–12
75. Dacie, J. V. and Lewis, S. M. (1984) *Practical Haematology*, 6th edn, p. 144. London: Churchill Livingstone
76. Dacie, J. V. and Lewis, S. M. (1984) *Practical Haematology*, 6th edn, pp. 139–40. London: Churchill Livingstone
77. Johnson, K. R., Ingle, A. R. and Payne, R. B. (1971) A method for measuring haemoglobin at low concentration in the presence of plasma inhibitors. *Clin. Chim. Acta*, **32**, 279–83
78. Van Assendelft, O. W. (1970) *Spectrophotometry of Haemoglobin Derivatives*. Assen: Royal Van Gorcum
79. International Committee for Standardisation in Haematology (1977) Recommended methods for red-cell enzyme analysis. *Br. J. Haematol.*, **35**, 331–40
80. Board, P. G. and Pidcock, M. E. (1981) Methaemoglobinaemia resulting from heterozygosity for two NADH-methaemoglobin reductase variants: characterisation as NADH-ferricyanide reductase. *Br. J. Haematol.*, **47**, 361–70
81. Hirano, M., Matsuki, T., Tanishima, K. *et al.* (1981) Congenital methaemoglobinaemia due to NADH methaemoglobin reductase deficiency: successful treatment with oral riboflavin. *Br. J. Haematol.*, **47**, 353–9
82. Lehmann, H. and Huntsman, R. G. (1974) *Man's Haemoglobins*, 2nd edn, pp. 213–15. Oxford: North Holland
83. Dacie, J. V. and Lewis, S. M. (1984) *Practical Haematology*, 6th edn, pp. 148–9. London: Churchill Livingstone
84. Park, C. M. and Nagel, R. L. (1984) Sulfhemoglobinemia. Clinical and molecular aspects. *N. Engl. J. Med.*, **310**, 1579–84
85. Petz, L. D. and Garratty, G. (1980) In *Acquired Immune Haemolytic Anaemias*. London: Churchill Livingstone
86. Freedman, J. (1979) False positive antiglobulin tests in healthy subjects and in hospital patients. *J. Clin. Pathol.*, **32**, 1014–18
87. Worrledge, S. M. (1978) The interpretation of a positive direct antiglobulin test. *Br. J. Haematol.*, **39**, 157–62
88. Huh, Y. O., Liu, F. J., Rogge, K. *et al.* (1988) Positive direct antiglobulin test and high serum immunoglobulin G values. *Am. J. Clin. Pathol.*, **89**, 197–200
89. Jamin, D., Schulman, I., Lam, H. T. *et al.* (1988) Production of a positive direct antiglobulin test due to Suramin. *Arch. Pathol. Lab. Med.*, **112**, 898–900
90. Rubin, H. (1963) Antibody elution from red blood cells. *J. Clin. Pathol.*, **16**, 70–3
91. Branch, D. R., Siok, S. Y., Hian, A. L. and Petz, L. D. (1982) A new elution procedure using chloroform, a non-flammable organic solvent. *Vox Sang.*, **42**, 46–53
92. Jenkins, D. E., Jr and Moore, W. H. (1977) A rapid method for the preparation of high potency auto and alloantibody eluates. *Transfusion*, **17**, 110–14
93. Bueno, R., Garratty, G. and Postoway, N. (1981) Elution of antibody from red-cells using xylene – a superior method. *Transfusion*, **21**, 157–62
94. Garratty, G., Petz, L. D. and Hoops, J. K. (1977) The correlation of cold agglutinin titrations in saline and albumin with haemolytic anaemia. *Br. J. Haematol.*, **35**, 587–95

95. Zanella, A., Izzo, C., Rebulla, P., Zanuso, F., Perroni, L. and Sirchia, G. (1980) Acidified glycerol lysis test: a screening test for spherocytosis. *Br. J. Haematol.,* **45**, 481–6
96. Rutherford, C. J., Postlewaight, B. F. and Hallowes, M. (1986) An evaluation of the acidified glycerol lysis test. *Br. J. Haematol.,* **63**, 119–21
97. Hoffmann, J. J. M. L., Swaak-Lammers, N., Bucx, M. J. L. and Breed, W. P. M. (1987) Evaluation of the acidified glycerol lysis test. *Br. J. Haematol.,* **65**, 252
98. Vettore, L., Zanella, A., Molaro, G. *et al.* (1984) A new test for the laboratory diagnosis of spherocytosis. *Acta Haematol.,* **72**, 258–63
99. British Society for Haematology (1988) Guidelines for haemoglobinopathy screening. *Clin. Lab. Haematol.,* **10**, 87–94
100. International Committee for Standardisation in Haematology (1988) Recommendations for neonatal screening for haemoglobinopathies. *Clin. Lab. Haematol.,* **10**, 335–45
101. Scott, R. B. (1970) Rapid technique for preparation of haemoglobin solutions for electrophoresis. *Am. J. Clin. Pathol.,* **54**, 78–81
102. International Committee for Standardisation in Haematology (1977) Recommendations for abnormal haemoglobin standard. *Br. J. Haematol.,* **35**, 161–4
103. Schneider, R. G., Hosty, T. S., Tomlin, G. and Atkins, R. (1974) Identification of hemoglobin and hemoglobinopathies by electrophoresis on cellulose acetate plates impregnated with citrate agar. *Clin. Chem.,* **20**, 74–7
104. Milner, P. F. and Gooden, H. M. (1975) Rapid citrate–agar electrophoresis in routine screening for haemoglobinopathies using a simple haemolysate. *Am. J. Clin. Pathol.,* **64**, 58–64
105. Ueda, S. and Schneider, R. G. (1969) Rapid identification of polypeptide chains of haemoglobin by cellulose acetate electrophoresis of haemolysate. *Blood,* **34**, 230–5
106. Schneider, R. G. (1974) Differentiation of electrophoretically similar haemoglobin such as S, D, G and P; or A_2, C, E or O by electrophoresis of the globin chains. *Clin. Chem.,* **20**, 1111–15
107. International Committee for Standardisation in Haematology (1978) Recommendations of a system for identifying abnormal haemoglobins. *Blood,* **52**, 1065–7
108. Carrell, R. W. and Kay, R. (1972) A simple method for the detection of unstable haemoglobins. *Br. J. Haematol.,* **23**, 615–19
109. Brosious, E. M., Morrison, B. Y. and Schmidt, R. M. (1976) Effects of haemoglobin F levels, KCN and storage on the isopropanol precipitation test for unstable haemoglobins. *Am. J. Clin. Pathol.,* **66**, 878–82
110. Carrell, R. W. and Lehmann, H. (1981) Zinc acetate as a precipitant of unstable haemoglobins. *J. Clin. Pathol.,* **34**, 796–9
111. White, J. M. (1974) The unstable haemoglobin disorders. *Clin. Haematol.,* **3**, 333–56
112. Itano, H. A. (1953) Solubility of naturally occurring mixtures of human hemoglobins. *Arch. Biochem. Biophys.,* **47**, 148–59
113. Cook, A. and Raper, A. B. (1971) The solubility test for Hb S: a cheap and rapid method. *Med. Lab. Technol.,* **28**, 373–6
114. Barnard, D. L. and Webber, R. C. (1979) The basis of the rapid solubility test for Haemoglobin S. (Abstract.) *Br. J. Haematol.,* **41**, 610
115. Efremov, G. D. and Huisman, T. H. J. (1974) The laboratory diagnosis of the haemoglobinopathies. *Clin. Haematol.,* **3**, 550–1
116. Powell, J. B. and Beach, D. J. (1971) A modification of the 'Sickledex' test for Haemoglobin S. *Clin. Chem.,* **17**, 1055–6
117. Canning, D. M., Crane, R. S., Huntsman, R. G. and Yawson, G. I. (1972) An automated screening technique for the detection of sickle-cell haemoglobin. *J. Clin. Pathol.,* **25**, 330–4
118. Huntsman, R. G., Barclay, G. P. T., Canning, D. M. and Yawson, G. I. (1970) A rapid whole blood solubility test to differentiate the sickle cell trait from sickle cell anaemia. *J. Clin. Pathol.,* **23**, 781–3
119. May, J. E., Rosse, W. and Frank, M. M. (1973) Paroxysmal nocturnal haemoglobinuria. Alternate complement pathway-mediated lysis induced by magnesium. *N. Engl. J. Med.,* **289**, 705–9
120. Kann, H. E., Mengel, C. E. and Wall, R. L. (1967) Paroxysmal nocturnal haemoglobinuria 'obscured' by the presence of iron deficiency. *Ann. Intern. Med.,* **67**, 593–6

121. Hartmann, R. C. and Jenkins, D. E., Jr. (1966) The 'sugar-water' test for paroxysmal nocturnal haemoglobinuria. *N. Engl. J. Med.*, **275**, 155–7
122. Hartmann, R. C., Jenkins, D. E., Jr. and Arnold, A. B. (1970) Diagnostic specificity of the sucrose haemolysis test for paroxysmal nocturnal haemoglobinuria. *Blood*, **35**, 462–75
123. Dacie, J. V. and Lewis, S. M. (eds) (1975) *Practical Haematology*, 5th edn, pp. 309–10. London: Churchill Livingstone
124. Sirchia, G., Marubini, E., Mercuriali, F. and Ferrone, S. (1973) Study of two *in vitro* diagnostic tests for paroxysmal nocturnal haemoglobinuria. *Br. J. Haematol.*, **24**, 751–9
125. Sirchia, G., Ferrone, S. and Mercuriali, F. (1965) The reaction of two sulfhydryl compounds on normal human red-cells. Relationship to red-cells of paroxysmal nocturnal haemoglobinuria. *Blood*, **25**, 502–10
126. International Committee for Standardisation in Haematology (1979) Recommended screening test for glucose-6-phosphate dehydrogenase (G-6-PD) deficiency. *Br. J. Haematol.*, **43**, 469–77
127. Motulsky, A. G., Kraut, J. M., Thieme, W. T. and Musto, D. F. (1959) Biochemical genetics of glucose-6-phosphate dehydrogenase deficiency. *Clin. Res.*, **7**, 89–90
128. Brewer, G. J., Tarlow, A. R. and Alving, A. S. (1960) Methemoglobin reduction test. A new, simple *in vitro* test for identifying primaquine sensitivity. *Bull. World Hlth. Org.*, **22**, 633–40
129. Jacob, H. S. and Jandl, J. H. (1966) A simple visual screening test for glucose-6-phosphate dehydrogenase deficiency employing ascorbate and cyanide. *N. Engl. J. Med.*, **274**, 1162–7
130. Deacon-Smith, R. (1982) The ascorbate-cyanide test and the detection of females heterozygous for glucose-6-phosphate dehydrogenase deficiency. *Med. Lab. Sci.*, **39**, 139–43
131. Fairbanks, V. F. and Lampe, L. T. (1969) A tetrazolium-linked cytochemical method for estimation of glucose-6-phosphate dehydrogenase activity in individual erythrocytes: application in the study of heterozygotes for glucose-6-phosphate deficiency. *Blood*, **31**, 589–603
132. Van Noorden, C. J. F. and Vogels, I. M. C. (1985) A sensitive cytochemical staining method for glucose-6-phosphate dehydrogenase activity in individual erythrocytes. *Br. J. Haematol.*, **60**, 57–63
133. Vogels, I. M. C., Van Noorden, C. J. F., Wolf, B. H. M. *et al.* (1986) Cytochemical determination of heterozygous glucose-6-phosphate dehydrogenase deficiency in erythrocytes. *Br. J. Haematol.*, **63**, 402–5
134. Gall, J. C. Jr, Brewer, G. J. and Dern, R. J. (1965) Studies of glucose-6-phosphate dehydrogenase activity of individual erythrocytes: the methemoglobin elution test for identification of females heterozygous for G6PD deficiency. *Am. J. Hum. Genet.*, **17**, 359–68
135. Beutler, E. (1966) A series of new screening procedures for pyruvate kinase deficiency, glucose-6-phosphate dehydrogenase deficiency and glutathione reductase deficiency. *Blood*, **28**, 553–62
136. Beutler, E., West, C. and Blume, K. G. (1976) The removal of leukocytes and platelets from whole blood. *J. Lab. Clin. Med.*, **88**, 328–33
137. Beutler, E. (1984) *Red Cell Metabolism. A Manual of Biochemical Methods*, 3rd edn. Orlando: Grune and Stratton
138. International Committee for Standardisation in Haematology (1979) Recommended methods for the characterisation of red-cell pyruvate kinase variants. *Br. J. Haematol.*, **43**, 275–86
139. International Committee for Standardisation in Haematology (1989) Recommended methods for an additional red cell enzyme (pyrimidine-5′-nucleotidase) assay and the determination of red cell adenosine-5′-triphosphate, 2.3-diphosphoglycerate and reduced glutathione. *Clin. Lab. Haematol.*, **11**, 131–8
140. Torrance, J., West, C. and Beutler, E. (1977) A simple, rapid radiometric assay for pyrimidine-5′-nucleotidase. *J. Lab. Clin. Med.*, **90**, 563–8
141. International Committee for Standardisation in Haematology (1989) Recommended screening test for pyrimidine-5′-nucleotidase deficiency. *Clin. Lab. Haematol.*, **11**, 55–6

Chapter 12

Anaemias. IV. Refractory anaemias

'Refractory anaemia' was a term used to describe anaemias of unknown aetiology and characterized by failure to respond favourably to substances which cure the great majority of anaemias[1]. The types of anaemia fulfilling this definition have narrowed dramatically with better understanding and improved diagnosis but there remains a heterogeneous group of anaemias which are well characterized by haematological criteria. This group includes anaemias due to bone-marrow failure or primary dyserythropoiesis. It also serves as a convenient depository for those anaemias which do not fall conveniently into simple classifications!

Aplastic anaemia

Definition

Aplastic anaemia has been defined as 'a syndrome of peripheral blood pancytopenia, without dominant peripheral blood destruction, associated with hypocellularity of haemopoietic tissue in both intramedullary and extramedullary sites and without bone-marrow fibrosis or invasion by malignant cells'[2]. This definition is clearly worded to exclude cytopenias due to immune destruction of circulating cells, the proliferative red cell or leucocyte disorders, myelofibrosis, non-haemopoietic malignancy and hypersplenism.

The definition implies a failure of haemopoiesis due to a quantitive or qualitative disorder of stem-cell proliferation, failure of humoral stimulation or inhibition of cell growth and multiplication.

Causes of aplastic anaemia

Ionizing radiation, chemicals, drugs, cytotoxic viruses and immune mechanisms are established causes of bone-marrow failure. Damage due to irradiation, cytotoxic drugs and chemicals may be reversible if the exposure is limited. Many examples of drug-induced aplasia appear to be idiosyncratic, not related to dose and often irreversible. Aplastic anaemia is associated with virus infections (notably non-A, non-B hepatitis), drugs or chemicals (chloramphenicol, phenylbutazone, gold and industrial solvents are most frequently implicated) but it is nevertheless an infrequent complication. The remaining 70% of cases are apparently 'idiopathic' and immune mechanisms are possibly involved. The immune mechanisms for which there is evidence are antibody inhibition, T cell suppression, inhibition of cell growth by monocyte-macrophages and the overproduction of lymphokines. It is suggested that a single immunological cause is unlikely; rather the entire immune system is activated[3]. A congenital or familial form of aplastic anaemia in children, and associated with anatomical malformations, is known as Fanconi's anaemia.

An interesting horticultural analogy has been applied to aplastic anaemia[4]. For successful plant growth there are three major requirements – soil, seed and nutrients – and if one or more is inadequate, stunted or no growth is the result. For 'soil' may be substituted bone-marrow structure and microenvironment, the 'seed' is the pluripotent stem cell or committed progenitor cell and for 'nutrients' substitute haematinic or humoral factors.

Laboratory features

Blood changes

Pancytopenia, a reduction in the numbers of circulating red cells, platelets and leucocytes, is the classic presentation which when severe results in the symptoms of anaemia, haemorrhagic phenomena and susceptibility to infection.

The red-cell changes are macroanisocytosis often with dyserythropoietic features. The reticulocyte count is typically low and is particularly obvious when expressed in absolute numbers or as a corrected reticulocyte count. A low reticulocyte count may precede the appearance of anaemia.

The thrombocytopenia is often severe and in contrast to immune thrombocytopenia the platelets are small with few, if any, large forms.

The leucopenia is mainly due to a neutropenia usually below 1.5×10^9/l and in severe aplasia less than 0.5×10^9/l. Morphology may be normal though toxic granulation may be associated with infection and coarse, reddish granulation has also been reported. Other leucocyte lines may also be reduced and of particular interest is the absolute lymphocyte count which is less than 1.0×10^9/l in 10–45% of cases; morphology is usually normal.

The lymphopenia is due to B-cell depletion and may therefore be expected to be associated with reduced immunoglobulin levels.

Severe monocytopenia (less than 0.02×10^9/l) may be present and has been reported as being associated with a poor prognosis due to infection.

The differential laboratory diagnosis at this stage is mainly between aplasia, aleukaemic leukaemia and possibly bone-marrow failure associated with megaloblastic change. Accurate cell counting is important as prognosis and consequently the approach to treatment can be related to the severity of the pancytopenia[5].

Bone-marrow appearances

The diagnosis of aplastic anaemia by exclusion of other causes of pancytopenia depends on the examination of bone-marrow samples. Although typically the bone-marrow aspirate or trephine biopsy is hypocellular, considerable variation in cellularity may be found at different biopsy sites and more than one biopsy may be necessary to establish the true picture[6].

Films of aspirated marrow are typically hypocellular with an absence of marrow fragments at the tail of the film or fragments of fatty tissue with only small amounts of haemopoietic tissue. Occasionally fragments of normal cellularity or even hypercellular particles may be aspirated. Differential counts of the various cell lines are of value and in particular the proportion of lymphocytes; a high proportion (about 70%) of lymphocytes appears to carry a poor prognosis[6]. It has been suggested that high lymphocyte counts may be associated with an autoimmune process. The dyserythropoietic aspects of erythroblast morphology in aplastic anaemia have been emphasized[7]. Iron staining usually demonstrates iron-loaded macrophages which after multiple transfusions can be a striking feature.

The evaluation of trephine biopsies is not without problems and an adequate biopsy of at least 1 cm is necessary due to variation in cellularity in closely adjacent sites. Hypercellular foci consisting of granulopoietic or erythropoietic tissue or both may be present in otherwise predominantly hypocellular marrow.

Erythrokinetics

Studies with radio-iron show a delayed plasma iron clearance, reduced iron turnover and iron utilization, often with ineffective erythropoiesis. Surface counting patterns show a slowly falling heart count and little or no uptake over the sacrum or spleen, with most of the injected activity being accumulated in the liver (*Figure 12.1*). It is emphasized that this pattern only reflects the reduced erythroid activity of the marrow and absence of extramedullary erythropoiesis in the spleen; other disorders associated with reduced erythropoiesis in the bone marrow could give a similar pattern. Red-cell survival studies usually show a shortened red-cell life span as might be expected in the presence of significant dyserythropoiesis.

Cell culture

The techniques of *in vitro* cell culture have been applied to aplastic anaemia and have supported the concept of defective proliferative potential of pluripotent stem cells by showing a reduction or absence of progenitor cells capable of forming colonies of the granulocyte–macrophage series (CFU–GM) and erythroid series (CFU–E and BFU–E). There is no response to specific growth factors such as GM–CSF, IL-3 and Epo. In contrast, the serum of patients with severe aplastic anaemia has increased levels of humoral growth factors. Decreased levels of IL-1 probably reflect monocyte depletion[8]. Cell culture has also been used to attempt to identify or differentiate those cases of aplasia due to autoantibodies or suppressor T lymphocytes. The technique has also been applied to the assessment of bone-marrow transplantation in aplastic anaemia[8].

Additional studies

Test for PNH (*see* page 375)

The association of bone-marrow hypoplasia with PNH is well established. Red cells from cases with aplastic or hypoplastic anaemia should routinely be tested for the PNH defect as aplasia may precede the manifestations of PNH. After treatment with anti-lymphocyte globulin (ALG) the development of PNH is a frequent complication[9].

Neutrophil alkaline phosphatase (NAP)

In aplastic anaemia NAP activity is raised, sometimes markedly, while in PNH NAP activity is typically low and may provide additional evidence of the future development of PNH.

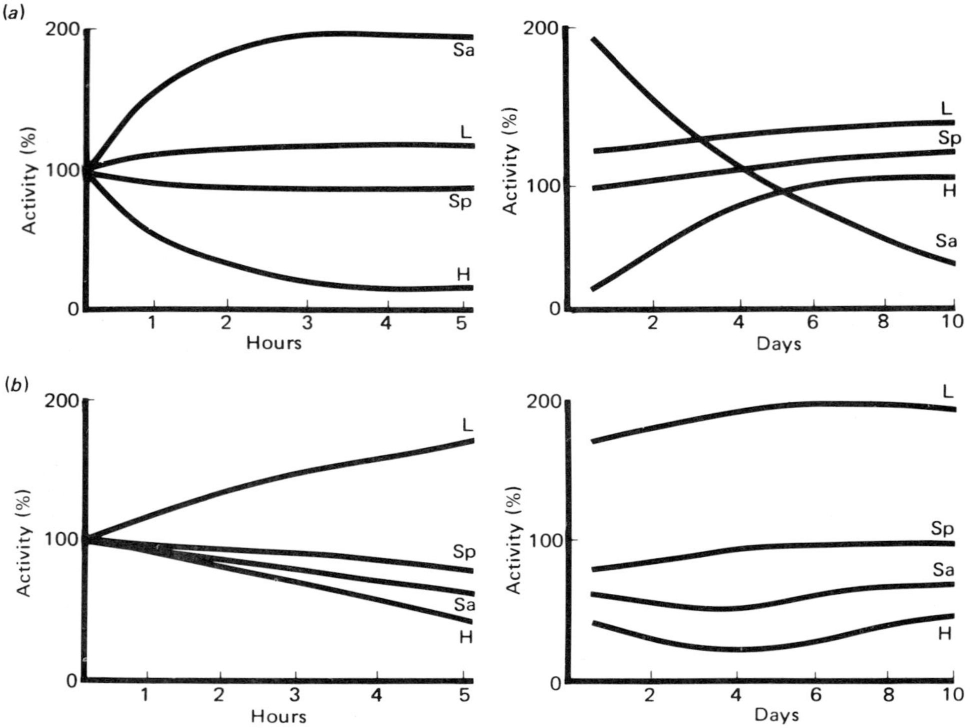

Figure 12.1 Surface counting patterns after intravenous injection of ^{59}Fe-labelled transferrin. H = Heart; L = liver; Sa = sacrum; Sp = spleen. (*a*) Normal subject; there is a rapid fall of activity over the heart as the ^{59}Fe is cleared from the plasma though activity does not fall to very low levels due to ^{59}Fe being taken up by the sternum and ribs. Sacral activity begins to decline after 1–2 days as red cells are released into the circulation, a process that reaches a plateau after 10–12 days. (*b*) The pattern in aplastic anaemia; the injected iron accumulates in the liver with little or no increase in sacral activity. Heart counts fall slowly. There is little increase in heart activity in the following days which indicates failure of the red-cell production

Hb F levels

Hb F values up to 20% have been found, particularly in children, and were thought to be of prognostic significance. It may be more informative to report Hb F levels as concentration, i.e. in g/dl. As small increases may be significant, particularly in adults, sensitive techniques should be used and an immunological approach is suggested. As the origin of the Hb F is probably clonal[10] the presence of F-containing cells may be demonstrated, but not quantitated, by the Kleihauer technique or by immunofluorescence using a labelled anti-Hb F serum.

Cytogenic studies

Non-specific abnormalities such as chromosome breaks, gaps, constrictions, translocations and exchanges, may be found in preparations from bone marrow and may have prognostic significance in respect of leukaemic transformation.

Pure red-cell aplasia

This variant of aplastic anaemia may be hereditary or acquired. The hereditary form, or Blackfan–Diamond syndrome, presents at birth or in the first weeks of life as an autosomal dominant defect and some cases have other congenital abnormalities which may cause confusion with the Fanconi type of aplasia. The anaemia is often severe with macrocytosis and a low reticulocyte count. Granulocytes and platelets are typically normal though low-normal values may be seen. The bone marrow shows few erythroblasts. Cell culture has shown normal numbers of progenitor cells which respond *in vitro* to erythropoietin. Response to immunosuppressive therapy suggests a possible immunological basis.

Acquired pure red-cell aplasia in the adult may be caused by mechanisms similar to those causing aplastic anaemia, i.e. drugs, chemicals and infections. Additionally, however, an immune basis can be inferred in about 50% of cases by association with thymoma, by response to immunosuppressive therapy or by the demonstration of an antibody against erythropoietin or even against the progenitor BFU–E cells. Other manifestations of an autoimmune process such as antinuclear antibodies, auto-immune haemolytic anaemia, platelet or leucocyte antibodies and hypo-gammaglobulinaemia may be demonstrated[11].

Pure white-cell aplasia

Agranulocytosis in the blood is a relatively frequent occurrence, is usually associated with drugs, and is usually reversible on cessation of drug exposure. Selective aplasia of the granulocyte series is uncommon and there is evidence that antibody-mediated inhibition of CFU–GM formation is the mechanism involved[12,13]

Dyserythropoietic anaemias

A qualitative or dysplastic disorder of haemopoiesis is referred to as dyshaemopoiesis and when mainly confined to the erythroid series may be termed dyserythropoiesis and the resulting anaemia a dyserythropoietic anaemia[14]. The cause of the anaemia in dyserythropoiesis is ineffective erythropoiesis (*see* page 222) which occurs when an apparently active erythropoietic series fails to deliver adequate numbers of red cells to the circulation; that proportion of total erythropoiesis which does not appear in the circulation being the ineffective fraction. Anaemias in which dyserythropoiesis is the major mechanism are:

1. Hereditary – thalassaemia.
2. Congenital (some inherited) – types I, II, III; variants or mixed types.
3. Acquired – megaloblastosis, severe iron deficiency, primary sideroblastic anaemia, erythroleukaemia, myelodysplasia.

Ineffective erythropoiesis is also found in a variety of anaemias not primarily due to a qualitative defect, e.g. aplastic anaemia, myelofibrosis and some leukaemias. Megaloblastic anaemia (*see* Chapter 10), the thalassaemia syndromes and severe iron deficiency (*see* Chapter 9) have already been considered in detail, but to provide a balanced account some aspects are included again.

Laboratory recognition of dyserythropoiesis

Morphological features

Blood changes

With the specific exceptions of the thalassaemias and iron deficiency, dyserythropoiesis is usually associated with macroanisocytosis and poikilocytosis often with oval cells and 'tear-drops'. Dimorphism may be a feature of primary acquired sideroblastic anaemia but not necessarily so. Basophilic stippling is often present (*see Figure 12.2*).

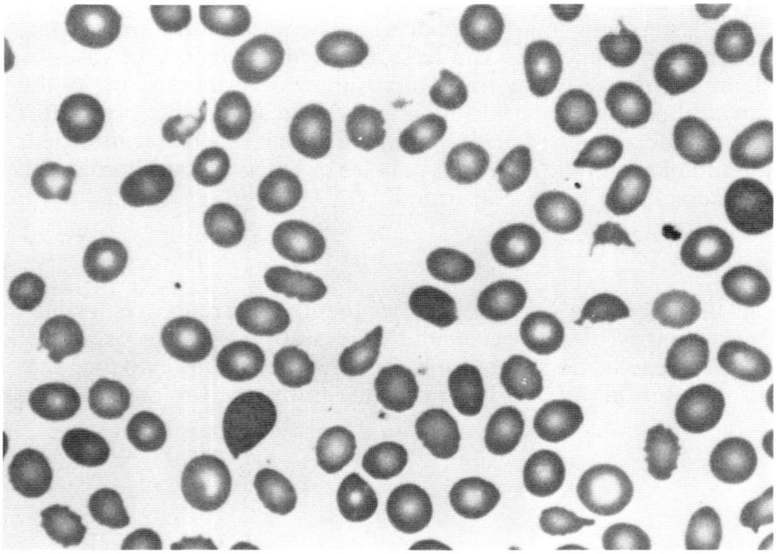

Figure 12.2 Blood film. Dyserythropoiesis. Macroanisocytosis, oval and tear-drop poikilocytosis, basophilic stippling. ×550

Bone marrow

Typically and by definition, the erythroid series is active though there may be maturation arrest at the early or intermediate stages of development. The classic example of abnormal erythroblast morphology is megaloblastic change though not necessarily due to disturbance of the folate/B_{12} metabolic pathways. Giant or multinucleated 'megaloblasts' are characteristic of congenital dyserythropoietic anaemia (CDA) type III. Cytoplasmic 'bridging' though found occasionally in normal marrow may be an obvious feature and is clearly different from the nuclear bridges that characterize CDA type I. Nuclear lobulation and fragmentation may be seen. Multinucleated erythroblasts are not specific to any particular type of dyserythropoiesis but binucleated cells are characteristic of CDA type II (HEMPAS).

Vacuolation of the erythroblast cytoplasm is sometimes a feature of erythroleukaemia. Foamy vacuolation is found in primary sideroblastic anaemia and precipitated globin chains are a feature of homozygous β-thalassaemia. Many abnormalities of the erythroblast nucleus and cytoplasm can be seen in stained films by light microscopy; by transmission electron microscopy further abnormalities such as nuclear clefting, enlargement of nuclear pores and cytoplasmic peripheral cisternae may be demonstrated.

Cytochemical abnormalities

Cytochemical techniques are of value in recognizing dyserythropoiesis, the most useful being iron staining to demonstrate the increased number and size and abnormal distribution of intracellular iron granules seen in many dyserythropoietic states. The PAS reaction often shows diffuse positivity in disorders such as thalassaemia and severe iron deficiency and a more characteristic block-positivity due to glycogen in erythroleukaemia, the distribution often coinciding with the vacuolation seen in the stained film. Non-specific esterase activity can be demonstrated in megaloblasts and in the erythroblasts in erythroleukaemia.

Biochemical changes

Intramedullary destruction of erythroblasts containing haemoglobin and consequent haemoglobin catabolism results in biochemical evidence of haemolysis similar to that resulting from the destruction of circulating erythrocytes. Unconjugated bilirubin level is increased and has been termed 'shunt' bilirubin. Some examples of CDA were initially diagnosed as disorders of bilirubin conjugation such as Gilbert's disease or Dubin–Johnson syndrome. Increased excretion of stercobilinogen and urobilinogen is found. Liberation of cytoplasmic enzymes from effete erythroblasts results in elevated levels of LDH, and of aldolase. The erythroblastic origin of the elevated serum LDH may be demonstrated electrophoretically by an increase in the anodal isoenzymes 1 and 2. Plasma aldolase is reported as being a more specific indication of erythroblast destruction. Serum iron and ferritin is often increased even in the absence of multiple blood transfusions.

Abnormal globin-chain synthesis

A variety of defects in globin-chain synthesis may be found. Synthesis of γ chains may persist in congenital dyserythropoiesis or may re-emerge in acquired types resulting in either case in elevated Hb F levels or at least the presence of red cells containing Hb F which can be demonstrated by the Kleihauer technique. Increased levels of Hb A_2 may be found. Imbalanced chain synthesis can result in the presence of Hb H most probably due to α-chain suppression but cases have been described with increased α- or β-chain synthesis.

Ferrokinetics using radio-iron

Tracer techniques using ^{59}Fe show an increased rate of plasma-iron clearance, plasma-iron turnover and erythron-iron turnover each reflecting the increased total erythropoiesis typically present in dyserythropoietic states. Of greater significance is the quantitation of the degree of ineffective erythropoiesis, the accurate measurement of which is a matter of debate and dispute due to the problem of quantitating the re-circulation of radio-iron into the iron pool from effete erythroblasts that have taken up the tracer or from destruction of labelled erythrocytes that have entered the circulation. Surface counting over the sacrum, liver, spleen and heart shows retention of sacral activity but at best must be regarded as qualitative evidence of ineffective erythropoiesis (*Figure 12.3*). Ferrokinetic techniques are described on page 408.

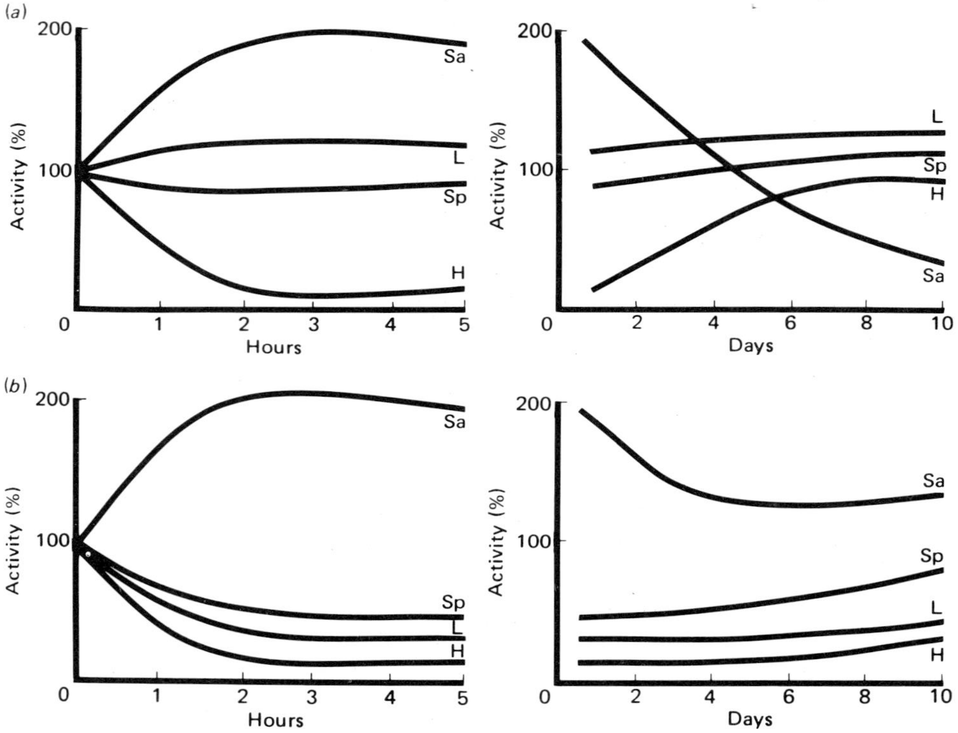

Figure 12.3 (*a*) Surface counting patterns in normal subjects after intravenous injection of ^{59}Fe-labelled transferrin. (*b*) Surface counting patterns in a patient with ineffective erythropoiesis. Iron is rapidly localized in the sacrum and the activity begins to fall after a few days with a slight rise in heart count. The level of sacral activity remains well above initial levels and represents destruction or retention of erythroblasts within the marrow. The slight rise in spleen activity represents destruction of labelled red cells. H = Heart; L = liver; Sa = sacrum; Sp = spleen

Kinetics of erythroblasts in interphase

The *in vitro* incorporation of tritiated thymidine (^{3}HTdr) to identify those erythroblasts synthesizing DNA (S phase), combined with quantitative microdensitometry of Feulgen-stained preparations to identify those cells in the post-mitotic/pre-synthesis phase (G_1) and those in the post-synthesis/pre-mitotic phase (G_2) has been used extensively in the study of dyserythropoietic anaemias. Despite differing aetiologies a general pattern has emerged: (1) an increase in the proportion of cells in G_2; (2) the presence of cells with DNA content between 2n (G_1) and 4n (G_2) which are not synthesizing DNA as judged by their failure to incorporate Tdr (U cells); and (3) the presence of cells with hypertetraploid DNA content (>4n).

Serological studies

Serological evidence of dyserythropoiesis is provided by reactions of the red cells with anti-I and anti-i and by the acidified serum test. Increased agglutination and/or lysis by anti-I and anti-i can be demonstrated in many dyserythropoietic states. A possible explanation of the increased reaction with anti-i is a shortened marrow transit time. In CDA types I and II, agglutination and lysis may approach the strength of reaction found with normal cord blood. The reactions with anti-I are less consistent and may reflect the use of different antisera.

The acidified-serum test is of particular importance in the recognition of CDA type II (HEMPAS). About 30% of normal sera will produce lysis of HEMPAS red cells in the acidified-serum test but, in contrast to PNH, lysis will not occur using the patient's own serum. The *antibody* responsible is termed anti-HEMPAS, is IgM, and is present in the serum of most normal adults; the majority of normal sera will agglutinate HEMPAS red cells at room temperature. The HEMPAS antigen is apparently hidden in normal cell membranes but is exposed in HEMPAS red cells.

Cytogenetics

Chromosome abnormalities involving the C group have been described in association with dyserythropoiesis and include trisomy 8, monosomy 7 and deletion of the long arm of chromosome 5 (5(q−)).

For a fuller account of many of the features described in the preceding sections, *see* Lewis and Verwilghen [15].

Congenital dyserythropoietic anaemia

The classification of CDA into types I, II and III on the basis of erythroblast morphology has been generally accepted and is supported by the application of the acidified-serum test.

CDA type I [16]

Probably the second most common form of CDA, the inheritance is autosomal recessive with the heterozygotes showing no haematological abnormality. Anaemia is mild to moderate with macrocytosis, anisocytosis, poikilocytosis and basophilic stippling. Cabot rings are said to be a feature but their presence probably depends on the method of Romanowsky staining. The bone marrow by definition shows erythroblast hyperplasia with a variety of morphological changes which in themselves are not specific for CDA type I but when present as outstanding features are considered diagnostic. Megaloblastoid changes are present together with appearances suggesting disturbance of karyokinesis – large cells with two nuclear segments of irregular mass suggesting incomplete nuclear division, binucleate cells with nuclei of differing size, structure and staining and the *presence of internuclear chromatin bridges*. Ring sideroblasts are not a feature. Haemoglobin studies and serological reactions are normal. Abnormality of nuclear histones has been suggested as the fundamental defect.

Studies in two cases of CDA I [17] demonstrated the ultrastructural appearance of multiple rounded electron-lucent areas within abnormally dense heterochromatin – the 'Swiss cheese' appearance. Intracytoplasmic inclusions indistinguishable from precipitated chains were demonstrated together with increased $\alpha:\beta$ chain synthesis ratios, arrest in DNA synthesis but no impairment of the methylation of deoxyuridylate. Abnormality of nucleoprotein synthesis was considered the likely defect.

CDA type II (HEMPAS) [18,19]

This form of CDA appears to be the most common and is inherited as an autosomal recessive with the heterozygotes being haematologically normal apart from showing an increased binding of anti-i to their red cells [19]. Affected subjects show a variable degree of anaemia, from near normal to moderately anaemic with variable jaundice. Anisocytosis with irregular poikilocytosis, some hypochromic cells, tear-drop poikilocytes and stippling are features of the blood film.

The bone marrow shows erythroblast hyperplasia and the morphology of the proerythroblasts and basophilic erythroblasts is normal. Between 10 and 35% of intermediate and late erythroblasts have two morphologically normal nuclei not connected by chromatin bridges. Less than 10% of erythroblasts show multinuclearity. Ring sideroblasts are not seen. Transmission electron microscopy discloses cytoplasmic cisternae which give the appearance of a double cytoplasmic membrane. Gaucher-like cells containing needle-shaped, birefringent crystalline inclusions may be seen. A defect in cytokinesis has been suggested as the cause of the bi-nuclearity. Abnormalities of membrane proteins have been described [20–22] and have centred on decreased glycosylation of band 3 and possibly band 4.5 and glycophorin A. In addition to the abnormal glycosylation, accumulation of glycolipids has been demonstrated [23], both possibly resulting from prolongation of the G_1 and M stages of the cell cycle.

The serological findings of increased agglutination and lysis and the reactions in the acidified-serum test using a selection of normal sera has been referred to previously. In contrast to PNH the cells in HEMPAS react as a single population. Altered $\alpha:\beta$ globin-chain ratios have been reported.

CDA type III [24,25]

This is the rarest form of CDA in the I, II, III classification and is inherited as an autosomal dominant. The blood film shows gross anisocytosis, macrocytosis, poikilocytosis and stippling. The bone marrow is also grossly abnormal with giant erythroblasts or megaloblasts having up to 12 nuclei. Lobulation, budding and karyorrhexis are common. Ring sideroblasts are not seen and the PAS reaction is reported as being negative. Granulocytes and platelets are normal. The acidified-serum test is negative but strong agglutination and lysis is obtained with anti-i.

Studies of one case of CDA III [26] indicated that the abnormality of erythropoiesis resulted from disturbances during mitosis and the G_2 phase. As in CDA I and II, there is unbalanced globin-chain synthesis with precipitated chains in the erythroblasts [27].

Variants of CDA

Perhaps inevitably, since the original classification of the CDAs there have been reports of CDAs that do not fit into the I, II, III categories. Variants may be separated on the basis of their reaction in the acidified-serum test[28] but with variation in the pattern of inheritance and morphology. Further variants include the presence of cytoplasmic vacuolation[29], associated granulocyte and platelet membrane abnormalities[30], a defect in the membrane transport of 5-methyltetrahydrofolate associated with type III morphology[31] and a family with 'mixed' morphological features and autosomal dominant inheritance[32]. A family with CDA and ringed sideroblasts has been described[33].

Primary acquired sideroblastic anaemia (PASA)

Acquired clonal proliferative disorders with a greater or lesser tendency to transform into acute leukaemia are now usually referred to as 'myelodysplastic syndromes' or MDS (Chapter 13). This is true of PASA but the usual presentation is of a refractory dyserythropoietic anaemia and is therefore included in this chapter.

This form of sideroblastic anaemia is most often found in the elderly and probably has a higher incidence than either myeloma or chronic granulocytic leukaemia. The tendency in some texts to accept a common aetiology for all types of sideroblastic anaemia is not justified from clinical, morphological, erythrokinetic or biochemical studies.

The anaemia may be mild or severe, stable or progressive with some patients having a transfusion requirement and others not. Unlike the microcytic, hypochromic and dimorphic picture of the hereditary form, PASA is usually macrocytic with anisocytosis and poikilocytosis (*Figure 12.4*) and although a microcytic population is often present it is not a constant feature. Basophilic stippling is often present and normoblasts may be seen, often poorly haemoglobinized with patchy vacuolation. Leucocytes and platelets are usually

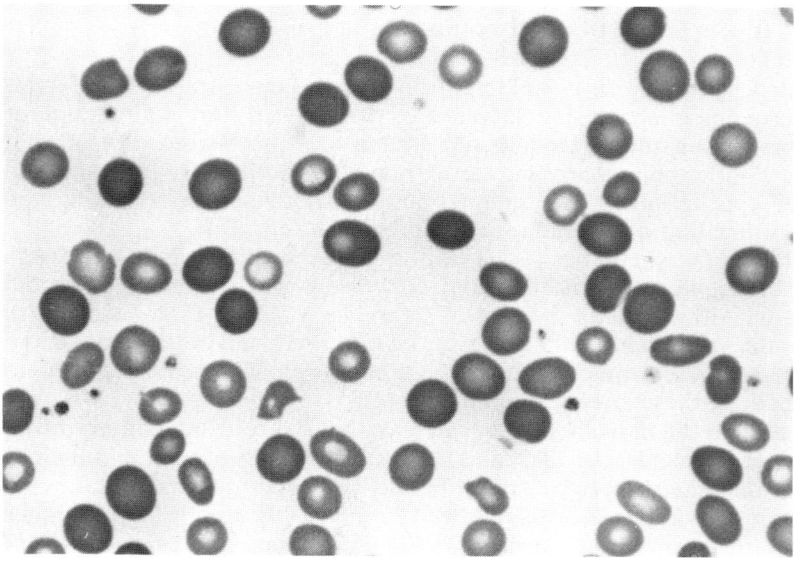

Figure 12.4 Blood film. Primary sideroblastic anaemia. Marked anisocytosis, overall macrocytosis with a hypochromic red-cell population. ×550

normal though some significance has been attached to the presence of a thrombocytosis[34]. The corrected reticulocyte count is not increased. The overall impression of the blood film is of anaemia due to dyserythropoiesis rather than from a failure of haemoglobin synthesis.

The bone marrow characteristically shows erythroid hyperplasia with a proportion of the more mature normoblasts showing poor haemoglobinization. Megaloblastic features are not uncommon and are due to secondary folate deficiency due to an increased folate requirement as is found in other chronic anaemias with increased erythroid activity. Iron staining shows the presence of ring sideroblasts which are typically found in all stages of erythroblast development in contrast to the hereditary and secondary sideroblastic anaemias in which the rings are usually confined to the late normoblasts[35]. From an investigative standpoint it may be reasonably stated that if ring sideroblasts are found in all erythroblast stages then family studies to establish the hereditary type are not justified. The PAS reaction in PASA may show diffuse positivity. Although PASA is a chronic anaemia, refractory or only partially responsive to haematinics, about 10% of cases terminate as acute leukaemia usually of myelomonocytic type though myeloblastic or even more rarely megakaryoblastic transformation can occur. In some cases of PASA minor changes in the leucocytes such as agranular and pseudo-Pelger neutrophils may precede leukaemic transformation.

The cause of the mitochondrial iron-loading is uncertain. Failure of haem synthesis has been the general view but severe haem synthetase deficiency is not associated with sideroblasts and, as iron uptake by erythroblasts in PASA is essentially normal, the defect may be an abnormality of mitochondrial iron metabolism. This could result in free radical formation and consequent lipid and protein damage. Mitochondrial enzyme defects would then be secondary to the iron-loading rather than the cause[36].

Ferrokinetics in the study of erythropoiesis

Radio-iron added to plasma *in vitro* binds firmly to the unsaturated transferrin. Following intravenous injection the clearance of the labelled iron is a function of the macrophages of the reticuloendothelial system and the degree of erythroid activity, whether in the bone marrow or in extramedullary sites. By following the radioactivity of appropriate blood samples and by body-surface counting the movement and utilization of the radio-iron can be followed.

In iron depletion or when there is erythroid hyperplasia the rate of plasma clearance will be greater than normal and conversely when there is erythroid hypoplasia or tissue-iron loading the rate of clearance is slower than normal. An increased rate of iron clearance will, however, be observed with both effective and ineffective erythropoiesis and iron utilization measurements are necessary to differentiate between these states.

It is recognized that the movement between plasma, erythroid and non-erythroid compartments is complex (*Figure 12.5*) and that measurements of total plasma iron turnover do not distinguish betwen erythroid and non-erythroid iron uptake and that the iron utilized by red cells is also derived from both sources. The techniques and calculations for plasma iron clearance (PIC) and plasma iron turnover (PIT) together with red-cell iron utilization are described and can contribute useful information. More precise data may be obtained by extended measurements of the

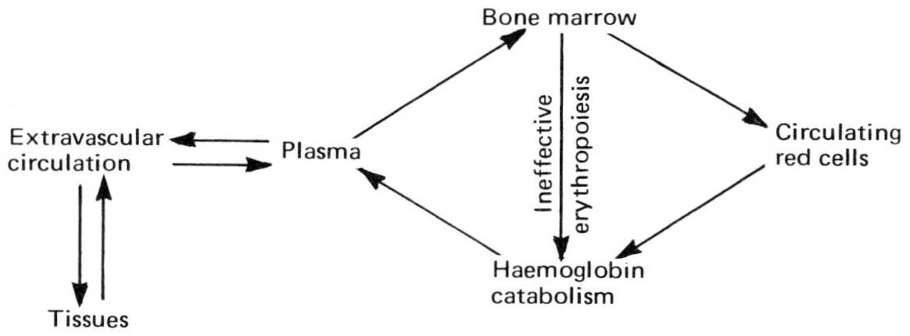

Figure 12.5 A model of iron kinetics

plasma clearance curve and in particular the ineffective iron turnover (IIT) as an indication of ineffective erythropoiesis[37]. The calculations may be extended to measure mean red-cell life span if a 'steady state' exists. Such studies require considerable computer capability and do not appear to have been widely applied. The clinical value of extended studies has not been clearly demonstrated and the fundamental principles can be reasonably considered to be disputed[38,39].

Method

Labelling of plasma with radio-iron

Choice of isotope

The most widely used and readily available radioisotope of iron is ^{59}Fe. Its half-life (T_{50}) of 45 days makes it suitable for extended erythrokinetic studies and it emits high-energy γ rays which are easily detected by surface counting. Because of its short half-life ^{52}Fe can only be used in the early stages of a ferrokinetic study but it is most useful for imaging functional erythropoietic tissues. ^{55}Fe has a half-life of 3 years and emits low-energy photons and is thus not widely used. ^{59}Fe is available as ferric citrate or ferric sulphate in sterile isotonic NaCl with specific activity up to 30 μCi/μg (1.11 MBq); activities over 10 μCi/μg (0.37 MBq) should be used.

Technique

The usual dose is 0.05 μCi/kg (0.0018 MBq), a level of activity that permits body surface counting. An appropriate amount of activity is added drop-wise with continual swirling and aseptic precautions to 5–10 ml heparinized plasma. The unsaturated iron binding capacity of the patient's serum should have been previously determined and should exceed 18 μmol/l (100 μg/dl). If below this level, ABO-compatible plasma (HBsAg, HIV negative) should be obtained from a normal donor. The plasma and radio-iron are incubated at 37°C for 30 minutes. Unbound ^{59}Fe may be removed by passage through an anion exchange resin[40].

If the red-cell utilization is to be calculated it is necessary to know the red-cell volume of the patient. This may be calculated from the plasma volume as described later, or in certain circumstances determined separately using ^{51}Cr or ^{99m}Tc labelling of red cells.

The preparation of standards is necessary to determine the total radioactivity injected. Weighing of the syringe is more accurate than estimates of volumes delivered from the syringe. Weigh the syringe containing the labelled plasma to the nearest mg. Transfer approximately 1 ml plasma to a volumetric flask and re-weigh the syringe and needle. Make up the volume of plasma to 100 ml with 1% diNaEDTA and deliver duplicate 2 ml volumes into counting tubes. Before injecting the labelled plasma collect blood for measurements of plasma iron, iron-binding capacity and PCV. Use 2 ml plasma and 4 ml blood for background determination. After injection re-weigh the syringe and needle to determine the exact weight of labelled plasma injected.

Blood sampling and radioactivity measurements

Collect 5 ml blood samples from the opposite limb at 5, 10 and 15 minutes after injection and further samples at approximately 30, 60, 90 and 120 minutes. These times are not critical but the exact time of sampling should be noted and ideally should be collected within the anticipated half-time of clearance. Separate the plasmas and accurately measure 2 ml into separate counting vials. Measure the ^{59}Fe activity in a well-scintillation counter together with the activity of the background plasma and the 2 ml diluted standard. Sufficient counts should be obtained to give a counting error of less than 3%. For red-cell incorporation studies duplicate 5 ml blood samples are obtained on day 14. The PCV is determined and 4 ml measured into a counting vial with saponin to achieve lysis and prevent cell sedimentation. If there is significant shortening of red-cell survival, iron utilization may be underestimated by taking a single sample at day 14 due to loss of labelled cells from the circulation. The curve of red-cell incorporation may be constructed by taking samples at 2-day intervals during the first 14 days. Each 4 ml whole-blood sample is counted alongside the 4 ml background sample and the 4 ml standard.

Calculations

Parameters of plasma transport

The injected dose of ^{59}Fe is calculated from the 2 ml standard by:

$$\text{Injected } ^{59}\text{Fe (cpm)} = \frac{\text{standard } ^{59}\text{Fe (cpm/ml)} \times \text{weight of dose} \times 100}{\text{weight of standard}}$$

All counts are corrected by deduction of background. As plasma iron clearance is exponential, plot the activity of the plasma samples on semi-logarithmic paper against time in minutes. Activity at T_0 is obtained by extrapolation of the initial points of the curve to the *y* axis (ordinate).

PIC is determined from the graph by the time taken for the activity at T_0 to fall by one half and is expressed in minutes. A least-squares fitting procedure may be used to obtain the best fit for the observed values. The normal range is quoted as 60–140 minutes[41] or 64–101 with a mean of 86 minutes[42].

Plasma volume is calculated from:

$$\text{Plasma volume (ml)} = \frac{\text{injected } ^{59}\text{Fe}}{T_0 \text{ plasma } ^{59}\text{Fe (cpm/ml)}}$$

Red-cell mass is calculated from plasma volume and PCV assuming a whole-body:venous PCV ratio of 0.9 by:

$$\text{Red-cell mass (ml)} = \frac{\text{plasma volume (ml)} \times 0.9 \times \text{PCV (l/l)}}{1000 - (0.9 \times \text{PCV})}$$

Plasma iron turnover (PIT) or the amount of iron flowing through the plasma each day is calculated on the basis of a single exponential clearance by multiplying the fractional clearance by the plasma iron concentration where fractional clearance is calculated by dividing the natural log of 2 (0.693) by the PIC in minutes and converting from minutes to days:

$$\text{PIT } (\mu\text{mol/l plasma}) = \frac{0.693 \times 24 \times 60 \times \text{plasma iron } (\mu\text{mol/l})}{\text{PIC } (\text{T}_{50} \text{ min})}$$

$$= \frac{\text{plasma iron } (\mu\text{mol/l}) \times 1000}{\text{PIC } (\text{T}_{50} \text{ min})}$$

As plasma iron turnover is proportional to body weight the PIT can be expressed to obtain a value independent of body weight:

$$\text{PIT } ((\mu\text{mol/l blood})^{-1}.\text{day}^{-1}) = \frac{\text{plasma iron } (\mu\text{mol/l}) \times 1000 \times 0.9 \times \text{PCV (l/l)}}{\text{PIC } (\text{T}_{50} \text{ min})}$$

Normal range = 72–144 μmol.(l whole blood)$^{-1}$.day^{-1}[40] or 104–152 μmol.(l whole blood)$^{-1}$.day^{-1}, mean 125 μmol.(l whole blood)$^{-1}$.day^{-1}[42]. Further corrections can be made if blood volume per unit body weight is abnormal[43].

Red-cell iron utilization (% RCIU)
Recalculate the injected dose of ^{59}Fe using the 4 ml standard. The red-cell utilization of any whole-blood sample is calculated by converting the ^{59}Fe for each 4 ml blood sample to cpm/ml packed cells by:

$$\text{Red-cell } ^{59}\text{Fe (cpm/ml red cells)} = \frac{\text{blood activity (cpm)}}{\text{PCV (l/l)} \times 4}$$

$$\text{RCIU } (\%) = \frac{\text{red-cell activity} \times \text{red-cell mass} \times 100}{\text{injected } ^{59}\text{Fe activity}}$$

If additional samples have been collected the values for each blood sample are calculated as above and plotted on arithmetic paper against time in days. RCIU is taken as the maximum value obtained during the period of study. Normal range = 70–80% [41] or 74–86% [42]. In aplasia the value may be as low as 10–15% and in ineffective erythropoiesis in the order of 30–50% [40].

The additional parameter of *marrow transit time* (MTT) may be calculated as the time taken for half the maximum red-cell incorporation by expressing each point on the red-cell incorporation curve as a fraction of maximum utilization and plotting the reciprocal of these values on semi-log paper against time in hours[43]. The normal value is 80 hours.

For additional details of ferrokinetic measurements and discussion of their significance the reader is referred to Cook and Finch[43] and Bowring[44].

Surface counting following injection of plasma labelled with ^{59}Fe

It is usual and useful to combine surface scintillation counting of ^{59}Fe activity with the blood and plasma studies already described. The organs or sites studied are bone marrow (represented by the sacrum), liver, spleen and heart (representing activity in the plasma). Use is made of suitably shielded and collimated scintillation crystals. The positioning of the counters depends largely on the type of equipment available, which may range from hand-held counters with crystals about 2 cm in diameter to those of 5 cm or more requiring staging or gantries for support. Various anatomical features have been used to ensure optimum detection of organ activity, the basic principles being accurate and reproducible positioning of the external counter over the organ while avoiding as far as possible the activity from other major blood-filled structures. For hand-held counters the following positions are recommended:

Heart:	Vertically over the third interspace at left sternal border.
Liver:	Half-way between mid-clavicular and anterior axillary lines on the right side of the body, 3–4 cm above the costal margin.
Spleen:	The site of maximum activity should be selected on the first occasion by means of a preliminary count for a few seconds over each of several adjacent sites; this position is then marked as the point for subsequent counting.
Sacrum:	Vertically over the sacrum slightly below the posterior superior iliac spine.

The points selected should be marked with indelible ink to ensure correct positioning on each occasion. When there is gross enlargement of the liver or spleen these positions may be modified to avoid the rib-cage altogether. Alternative positioning for larger single or dual detectors has been recommended by the ICSH[45].

The actual counting procedure will depend upon whether one or multiple detectors are employed, but as many separate counts as possible are made at the beginning of the study to allow extrapolation of activity to 0 time. Establishing the initial level of activity is essential and this is made more difficult if plasma clearance is abnormally rapid and only one counter is available. Background counts are determined at each site before injection of the radio-iron. The critical times for counting are:

1. Immediately after injection.
2. At the time of minimal blood activity.
3. At maximal red-cell utilization.

During the first day the times of counting can be similar to those of blood sampling, then daily for 5 days and then alternate days up to 15 days. The extrapolated 0 time values are adjusted to 100% and subsequent counts related to this value. Observed activity each day is corrected for decay from 0 time.

Representative patterns of activity are shown in *Figure 12.3*. The findings in uncomplicated haemolytic anaemia are not illustrated but would show rapid sacral uptake with an earlier plateau and more rapid release into the circulation. The activity graphs may then vary considerably depending upon the rate of haemolysis and whether there is sequestration in the spleen.

Leucoerythroblastic reactions and leucoerythroblastic anaemia

The term leucoerythroblastic anaemia (LEA) was first used in 1905[46] to describe an anaemia associated with immature granulocytes and erythroblasts in the blood of a patient with carcinomatosis. The concept became established some 30 years later by reports of LEA in patients with other bone-marrow replacements[47,48].

In the intervening years LEA had been described in myelofibrosis, lipid storage disorders, osteopetrosis and leukaemia. Textbooks have adhered to the concept that leucoerythroblastic reactions are mainly associated with bone-marrow replacement[49,50]. This view has persisted despite several publications to the contrary and the introduction of the term 'leucoerythroblastosis' in recognition of the fact that anaemia may be slight or even absent[51]. The causes of leucoerythroblastic reactions can be grouped as follows:

1. Malignant infiltration of bone marrow, e.g. carcinomatosis, myelomatosis, lymphoma and acute leukaemia.
2. Non-malignant infiltration of bone marrow, e.g. myelofibrosis, osteopetrosis, and lipid-storage disorders.
3. Associated with anaemia due to:
   (a) haemorrhage;
   (b) haemolysis;
   (c) megaloblastosis.
4. Systemic infection.
5. Cardiopulmonary disease, e.g. acute myocardial infarction, cor pulmonale, ventricular failure, congestive cardiac failure and respiratory failure.
6. Miscellaneous, e.g. renal transplants, polycythaemia vera, post-splenectomy, neonates and associated with response to haematinic therapy.

In general hospital practice probably the commonest cause of leucoerythroblastic reactions are those due to cardiopulmonary disease and not those due to bone-marrow infiltration by non-haemopoietic elements; this can therefore pose problems in interpretation.

Laboratory aspects of leucoerythroblastic reactions

What constitutes a leucoerythroblastic reaction has not been adequately defined in either qualitative or quantitative terms. The observation of a single normoblast during a routine 100-cell differential satisfies the 'erythroblastic' aspect but what constitutes an immature granulocyte in the context of the 'leuco-' element is open to different interpretations. The presence of less than 1% metamyelocytes and myelocytes has been accepted[52]. Other series record the presence of immature granulocytes without stating their frequency[53]. Metamyelocytes are common in a wide variety of disorders and consequently their presence is of limited significance, whereas the more immature myelocytes and promyelocytes assume a greater significance. *Table 12.1* shows the occurrence of the three stages of immature

Table 12.1 Occurrence of immature granulocytes in two groups of patients with leucoerythroblastic reactions. For interpretation, see text

Granulocyte	*Cardiopulmonary disease (24 patients) (%)*	*Malignant bone-marrow infiltration (14 patients) (%)*
Metamyelocytes	100	85*
Myelocytes	30	85
Promyelocytes	5	65

*Not all patients had metamyelocytes despite having myelocytes, promyelocytes or both.

granulocytes in a group of patients with marrow infiltration and a group with cardiopulmonary disorders; myelocytes and promyelocytes are most frequently seen in the patients with bone-marrow infiltration.

It has been suggested[54] that in leucoerythroblastic anaemia associated with bone-marrow infiltration the number of erythroblasts in the blood is out of proportion to the degree of erythropoietic activity as reflected by the reticulocyte count. *Figure 12.6* shows the normoblast:reticulocyte ratio in the two groups of patients in *Table 12.1*. Normoblast numbers were derived from the total and differential nucleated cell count and expressed in absolute numbers per μl; the reticulocytes in thousands per μl derived from a standard reticulocyte count and the total red-cell count. The normoblast:reticulocyte ratio is clearly greater in the malignant group though there is considerable overlap with the cardiopulmonary

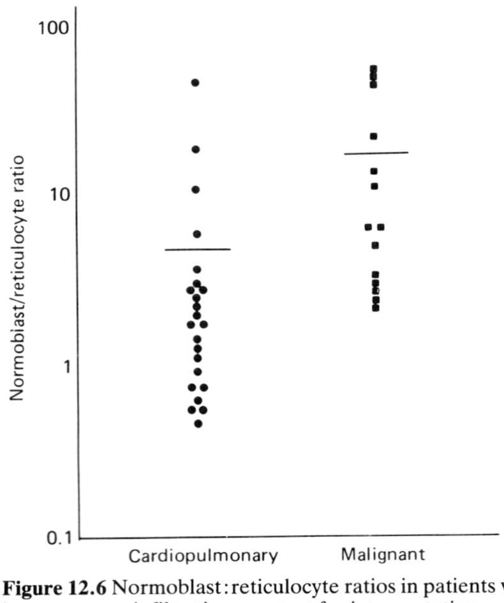

Figure 12.6 Normoblast:reticulocyte ratios in patients with cardiopulmonary disease and malignant bone-marrow infiltration; see text for interpretation

patients. The normoblast:reticulocyte ratio in response to haemorrhage or haemolysis is usually low.

Mechanisms of leucoerythroblastosis

Immature granulocytes and erythroblasts are not normally released from the bone marrow. The mechanisms controlling release are complex but certainly depend on the microanatomy of the bone marrow and the marrow–blood barrier (MBB) (*see* page 3). If the microstructure of the marrow is disordered either due to hyperplasia or the presence of 'foreign' cells or structures, the function of the MBB is disturbed thus allowing the release of immature cells.

Leucoerythroblastic reactions are common in myelofibrosis and in this disorder not only is there disturbed bone-marrow architecture but also extramedullary haemopoiesis, particularly in the spleen. It is likely that haemopoiesis in extramedullary sites is not subject to the same controls as the bone marrow and therefore leucoerythroblastic reactions are a feature of extramedullary haemopoiesis.

The occurrence of leucoerythroblastic reactions in cardiopulmonary disease has been shown to correlate with pO_2 levels of arterial blood and may therefore be due to acute hypoxic states.

References

1. Bomford, R. R. and Rhoads, C. P. (1941) Refractory anaemia. *Quart. J. Med.*, **10**, 175–281
2. Geary, C. G. and Testa, N. G. (1979) Pathophysiology of marrow hypoplasia. In *Aplastic Anaemia* (ed. C. G. Geary), p. 2. London: Baillière Tindall
3. Nissen-Druey, C. (1989) Pathophysiology of aplastic anaemia. *Clin. Haematol.*, **2**, 37–49
4. Lancet (1977) Aplastic anaemia, seed or soil? *Lancet*, **ii**, 748–50
5. Camitta, B. M., Storb, R. and Thomas, E. D. (1982) Aplastic anaemia (first of two parts): pathogenesis, diagnosis, treatment and prognosis. *N. Engl. J. Med.*, **306**, 645–52
6. Frisch, B. and Lewis, S. M. (1974) The bone marrow in aplastic anaemia: diagnostic and prognostic features. *J. Clin. Pathol.*, **27**, 231–41
7. Lewis, S. M. (1979) Dyserythropoiesis in aplastic anaemia. In *Aplastic Anaemia* (ed. C. G. Geary) pp. 82–107. London: Baillière Tindall
8. Gascon, P. and Scala, G. (1988) Decreased interleukin 1 production in aplastic anaemia. *Am. J. Med.*, **85**, 668–74
9. Tichelli, A., Gratwohl, A., Wursh, A., Nissen, C. and Speck, B. (1988) Late haematological complications in severe aplastic anaemia. *Br. J. Haematol.*, **69**, 413–18
10. Weatherall, D. J. (1977) Foetal haemoglobin production or foetal erythropoiesis in dyserythropoietic anaemias. In *Dyserythropoiesis* (eds S. M. Lewis and R. L. Verwilghen), pp. 427–9. London: Academic Press
11. Geary, C. G. (1979) Red-cell aplasia. In *Aplastic Anaemia* (ed. C. G. Geary), pp. 195–229. London: Baillière Tindall
12. Fitchen, J. H. and Cline, M. J. (1980) Serum inhibitors of myelopoiesis. *Br. J. Haematol.*, **44**, 7–16
13. Levitt, L. J., Ries, C. A. and Greenberg, P. L. (1983) Pure white cell aplasia: antibody mediated inhibition of granulopoiesis. *N. Engl. J. Med.*, **308**, 1141–6
14. Lewis, S. M. and Verwilghen, R. L. (1972) Dyserythropoiesis and dyserythropoietic anaemia. *Br. J. Haematol.*, **23**, 1–4
15. Lewis, S. M. and Verwilghen, R. L. (eds) (1977) *Dyserythropoiesis*. London: Academic Press
16. Heimpel, H. (1977) Congenital dyserythropoietic anaemia, Type I. In *Dyserythropoiesis* (eds S. M. Lewis and R. L. Verwilghen), pp. 55–70. London: Academic Press
17. Wickramasinghe, S. N. and Pippard, M. J. (1986) Studies of erythroblast function in congenital dyserythropoietic anaemia type I: evidence of impaired DNA, RNA, and protein synthesis and unbalanced globin chain synthesis in ultrastructurally abnormal cells. *J. Clin. Pathol.*, **39**, 881–90
18. Verwilghen, R. L., Lewis, S. M., Dacie, J. V., Crookston, J. H. and Crookston, M. C. (1973) HEMPAS. Congenital dyserythropoietic anaemia (Type II). *Q. J. Med. (New Ser.)*, **42**, 257–78
19. Punt, K., Borst-Eilers, E. and Nijessen, J. G. (1977) Congenital dyserythropoietic anaemia, Type II (HEMPAS). In *Dyserythropoiesis* (eds S. M. Lewis and R. L. Verwilghen), pp. 71–81. London: Academic Press
20. Baines, A. J., Banga, J. P. S., Gratzer, W. B., Linch, D. C. and Huehns, E. R. (1982) Red cell membrane protein anomalies in congenital dyserythropoietic anaemia type II (HEMPAS). *Br. J. Haematol.*, **50**, 563–74
21. Mawby, W. J., Tanner, M. J. A., Anstee, D. J. and Clamp, J. R. (1987) Incomplete glycosylation of erythrocyte membrane protein in congenital dyserythropoietic anaemia type II (CDA II). *Br. J. Haematol.*, **55**, 357–68

22. Pothier, B., Morle, L., Alloisio, N. *et al.* (1987) Aberrant pattern of red cell membrane and cytosolic proteins in a case of congenital dyserythropoietic anaemia. *Br. J. Haematol.*, **66**, 393–400
23. Zdebska, E., Anselstetter, V., Pacuska, T. *et al.* (1987) Glycolipids and glycopeptides of red cell membranes in congenital dyserythropoietic anaemia type II (CDA II). *Br. J. Haematol.*, **66**, 385–91
24. Wolff, J. A. and von Hofe, F. H. (1951) Familial erythroid multinuclearity. *Blood*, **6**, 1274–83
25. Goudsmit, R. (1977) Congenital dyserythropoietic anaemia, Type III. In *Dyserythropoiesis* (eds S. M. Lewis and R. L. Verwilghen), pp. 83–92. London: Academic Press
26. Wickramasinghe, S. N., Parry, T., Williams, C., Bond, A. N., Hughes, M. and Crook, S. (1982) A new case of congenital dyserythropoietic anaemia type III: a study of the cell cycle distribution and ultrastructure of erythroblasts and of nucleic acid synthesis in marrow cells. *J. Clin. Pathol.*, **35**, 1103–9
27. Wickramasinghe, S. N. and Goudsmit, R. (1987) Precipitation of beta-globin chains within the erythropoietic cells of a patient with congenital dyserythropoietic anaemia type III. *Br. J. Haematol.*, **65**, 250–1
28. David, G. and van Dorpe, A. (1977) Aberrant congenital dyserythropoietic anaemias. In *Dyserythropoiesis* (eds S. M. Lewis and R. L. Verwilghen), pp. 93–100. London: Academic Press
29. Kenny, M. W., Ibbotson, R. M., Hand, M. J. and Tector, M. J. (1978) Congenital dyserythropoietic anaemia with unusual cytoplasmic inclusions. *J. Clin. Pathol.*, **31**, 1228–33
30. Lowenthal, R. M., Marsden, K. A., Dewar, C. L. and Thompson, G. R. (1980) Congenital dyserythropoietic anaemia (CDA) with severe gout, rare Kell phenotype and erythrocyte, granulocyte and platelet membrane reduplication, a new variant of CDA Type II. *Br. J. Haematol.*, **44**, 211–20
31. Howe, R. B., Branda, R. F., Douglas, S. D. and Brunning, R. D. (1979) Hereditary dyserythropoiesis with abnormal membrane folate transport. *Blood*, **54**, 1080–90
32. Sansone, G. (1978) A new type of congenital dyserythropoietic anaemia. *Br. J. Haematol.*, **39**, 537–43
33. Brien, W. F., Mant, M. J. and Etches, W. S. (1985) Variant congenital dyserythropoietic anaemia with ringed sideroblasts. *Clin. Lab. Haematol.*, **7**, 231–7
34. Streeter, R. R., Presant, C. A. and Reinhard, E. (1977) Prognostic significance of thrombocytosis in idiopathic sideroblastic anaemia. *Blood*, **50**, 427–32
35. Hall, R. and Losowsky, M. S. (1966) Distribution of erythroblast iron in sideroblastic anaemia. *Br. J. Haematol.*, **12**, 334–40
36. Jacobs, A. (1986) Primary acquired sideroblastic anaemia. *Br. J. Haematol.*, **64**, 415–18
37. Ricketts, C., Jacobs, A. and Cavill, I. (1975) Ferrokinetics and erythropoiesis in man: the measurement of effective erythropoiesis, ineffective erythropoiesis and red-cell lifespan using ^{59}Fe. *Br. J. Haematol.*, **31**, 65–75
38. Orr, J. S., Horton, P. W., Hutcheon, A. W. and Dagg, J. H. (1979) Erythropoiesis and iron kinetics. *Br. J. Haematol.*, **42**, 155–7
39. Cavill, I. and Ricketts, C. (1979) Erythropoiesis and iron kinetics. *Br. J. Haematol.*, **42**, 158
40. Cavill, I. (1971) The preparation of ^{59}Fe-labelled transferrin for ferrokinetic studies. *J. Clin. Pathol.*, **24**, 472–74
41. Dacie, J. V. and Lewis, S. M. (1975) *Practical Haematology*, 5th edn, pp. 445–50. London: Churchill Livingstone
42. Finch, C. A., Delbelbeiss, K., Cook, J. D. *et al.* (1970) Ferrokinetics in man. *Medicine*, **49**, 17–53
43. Cook, J. D. and Finch, C. A. (1980) Ferrokinetic measurements. In *Iron. Methods in Hematology* (ed. J. D. Cook) No **1**, pp. 134–47. London: Churchill Livingstone
44. Bowring, C. S. (1981) *Radionuclide Tracer Techniques in Haematology*. London: Butterworths
45. ICSH (1975) Recommended methods for surface counting to determine sites of red-cell destruction. *Br. J. Haematol.*, **30**, 249–54
46. Cabot, R. C. (1904) *A Guide to the Clinical Examination of the Blood*. New York: Wood
47. Vaughan, J. M. (1936) Leucoerythroblastic anaemia. *J. Pathol. Bacteriol.*, **42**, 541–64
48. Vaughan, J. M. and Harrison, C. V. (1939) *J. Pathol. Bacteriol.*, **48**, 339–52
49. Hoffbrand, A. V. and Lewis, S. M. (1981) *Postgraduate Haematology*, 2nd edn, p. 414. London: Heinemann

50. De Gruchy, C. G. (1970) *Clinical Haematology in Medical Practice*, 3rd edn, p. 457. Oxford: Blackwell
51. Wintrobe, M. M. (1951) *Clinical Haematology*, 3rd edn, p. 548. Philadelphia: Lea and Febiger
52. Retief, F. P. (1964) Leuco-erythroblastosis in the adult. *Lancet,* **i**, 639–42
53. Weick, J. K., Hagedon, A. B. and Linman, J. W. (1974) Leucoerythroblastosis. Diagnostic and prognostic significance. *Mayo Clin. Proc.,* **49**, 110–13
54. De Gruchy, C. G. (1970) *Clinical Haematology in Medical Practice*, 3rd edn, p. 458. Oxford: Blackwell

Chapter 13

Leukaemia and the proliferative disorders

The proliferative disorders arise in a single cell which assumes the capability for unregulated replication and expansion. The abnormality may originate in a pluripotent stem cell resulting in the proliferation of one or more cell lines as in myeloproliferative diseases. Alternatively, the change may occur at some stage in the pathway of a differentiated cell line which may be the mechanism in certain lymphoproliferative disorders. At whichever stage of cell development the result is the development of a clone of abnormal cells, sometimes having an identifiable monoclonal marker. The evidence for pluripotent stem-cell clonal origin of the myeloproliferative disorders is based on the presence of a chromosomal marker in all cell lines, the metamorphosis of a proliferation of one cell line to another, and that only one of the X-linked G6PD enzymes A or B is present in leukaemic cells of female heterozygotes. Clonal proliferations may result in cell lines incapable of differentiation beyond the blast-cell stage or retaining the ability to differentiate to mature cells.

Leukaemia is characterized by proliferation of blast cells or mature leucocytes with release of cells into the circulation, whereas expansion and differentiation of the red cells, platelets and marrow fibroblasts is termed 'non-leukaemic myeloproliferation'. In addition to hyperplasia, clonal abnormalities can give rise to dysplasia or 'myelodysplasia' which may progress to overt leukaemia. The terms 'acute' and 'chronic' strictly refer to the clinical course of untreated disease but coincide with the leukaemic cell type – acute leukaemias are associated with poorly differentiated cells of 'blast' type whereas in the chronic leukaemias the proliferating cells are well differentiated. Lymphatic tumours or lymphomas are not necessarily associated with bone-marrow replacement and are not characterized by a leukaemic blood picture.

A primary classification of the leukaemias and proliferative disorders is:

1. Leukaemia:
   (a) acute;
   (b) chronic.
2. Non-leukaemic myeloproliferation.
3. Myelodysplasia.
4. Lymphoma.
5. Myeloma and related disorders.

Aetiology

The intensive and continuing search for the cause or causes of irreversible cell proliferation has implicated environmental, infective, genetic and host factors.

Ionizing radiation

The association of ionizing radiation by occupational, diagnostic and therapeutic exposure was confirmed by the nuclear explosions at Hiroshima and Nagasaki [1]. All types of acute leukaemia together with chronic myeloid leukaemia and myelodysplasia have been described. The incidence of leukaemia appears to be related to age at exposure. Childhood leukaemia may be associated with inherited chromosomal changes induced in the sperm or ova of parents exposed to radiation [2].

Comparison of *de novo* and radiogenic leukaemias shows differences in the incidence of the different types of acute leukaemia.

Chemicals and drugs

It is clear that industrial exposure to benzene carries a 5–10 times higher risk of developing acute or chronic leukaemia, lymphoproliferative disorder, myeloma or aplastic anaemia [3, 4], probably by inducing chromosome damage. Alkylating drugs such as melphalan, busulphan, chlorambucil and cyclophosphamide, used for treating malignant disease, are associated with an increased incidence of leukaemia with a peak 3–5 years after the start of treatment. A myelodysplastic phase often precedes the development of overt leukaemia.

Viruses

RNA tumour viruses (retroviruses) can induce a variety of neoplasias in animals. Acute endogenous viruses carry specific sequences (oncogenes, onc-genes, v-*onc*) coding for a protein required for the initiation and maintenance of the transformed cell.

Chronic endogenous viruses induce the majority of naturally occurring leukaemias. These viruses do not carry onc-genes and probably induce leukaemia by promoting the expression of onc-genes in the host cell [5].

The evidence for viral aetiology of human lymphomas is the T lymphocyte leukaemia virus (HTLV I) which shows similarity to bovine leukaemia virus (BLV). Evidence of sub-groups has resulted in the designation of HTLV II which has been associated with hairy-cell leukaemia in humans. The widely encountered Epstein–Barr DNA virus (EBV) or the herpes group of viruses causes the self-limiting lymphocyte proliferation in infectious mononucleosis and has been incriminated in the occurrence of Burkitt's lymphoma.

Oncogenes

Oncogenes are tumour-associated DNA sequences. Cellular oncogenes (c-*onc*) are, in the main, partially homologous to viral oncogenes (v-*onc*) and are also referred to as proto-oncogenes. These genes are normal cell genes with a physiological role in the regulation of proliferation and differentiation and require activation to cause neoplasias. The retrovirus-associated oncogenes (v-*onc*) are almost all hybrids of the coding regions from cellular oncogenes linked to the coding region of essential viral genes[6]. In *normal* cells, cellular oncogenes are not related or linked to retroviral sequences.

Retroviral oncogenes can initiate and maintain malignant cell proliferation by the result of increased amount of gene product. This is referred to as the *single-step* hypothesis. Alternatively DNA and chronic leukaemia viruses do not transform to proliferate directly but appear to act by indirect mechanisms which require that an activated proto-oncogene may operate as an initiation gene requiring another gene (viral or cellular) in a *multi-step* process.

Proto- and viral oncogenes code for products associated with cell replication-growth factors, receptors, signal transducing proteins, etc., or can induce independence of the requirement for growth factors[7]. Chromosomal translocations in haemopoietic malignancies are associated with the movement of cellular oncogenes and relocation and possibly rearrangement with other genes resulting in altered gene expression.

Table 13.1 shows examples of the nomenclature, origin and association of some of the many oncogenes of haemotological significance.

Table 13.1 Examples of the nomenclature, origin or relationship and haematological association of certain oncogenes

Oncogene	*Origin*	*Association*
c-*abl*	Homologue of Ableson murine leukaemia virus	CML
c-*sis*	Homologue of simian sarcoma virus	CML
c-*myc*	Homologue of MC-29 avian acute leukaemia virus	AML-M3
c N-*ras*	Rodent Harvey sarcoma virus	AML, ALL
v-*myb*	Chicken leukaemia virus	Myeloblast
v-*fes*	Feline sarcoma virus	Pre-B lymphoblast
v-*src*	Mouse Rous sarcoma virus	Pre-B pre-T lymphoblast

Host factors

There is a higher frequency of leukaemia in disorders associated with congenital chromosomal abnormalities. Down's syndrome (mongolism, trisomy 21) is the clearest example which carries a 15 times higher risk than normal children and has a higher frequency of acute myeloid leukaemia than usual in this age group. The risk of acute leukaemia in Down's patients increases with age. Klinefelter's syndrome (XXY) and Patau's syndrome (D trisomy) also have an increased risk of leukaemia. Fanconi's anaemia (congenital pancytopenia, chromosome fragility), Bloom's syndrome (pancytopenia with anatomical abnormalities and chromosome fragility) and ataxia telangiectasia (immunodeficiency with chromosomal fragility) are other conditions with a higher risk of acute leukaemia. The latter condition is particularly relevant in indicating the role of impaired immunological surveillance in the aetiology of acute leukaemia. Other inherited immunodeficiencies, e.g. congenital X-linked agammaglobulinaemia, Wiskott–Aldrich syndrome, Di George's syndrome and severe combined immunodeficiency, have each been linked with increased risk of acute lymphoblastic leukaemia.

An increased risk has been shown in siblings of patients and one in five monozygotic twins may develop leukaemia within a year of diagnosis in the other twin. Although environmental factors could be involved a genetic basis is the more likely.

Epidemiology

With one notable exception the proliferative disorders are most frequent in adults. The exception is acute lymphoblastic leukaemia (ALL) of which over 80% of cases occur under the age of 15 years and have features different from ALL in adults. Conversely, over 85% of cases of AML occur in adults (those aged over 15 years). Many proliferative disorders have their highest frequency in the elderly. Sex differences are seen; for example, CLL is more frequent in males. Variations in the distribution of certain proliferative disorders throughout the world have been recorded but whether due to ethnic or geographical differences is not entirely clear. There are many reports of 'clusters' of the same disorder within quite small areas, which suggests transmissible or environmental agents.

Acute leukaemia

Laboratory presentation

Although acute leukaemia may be recognized as a chance finding during the routine investigation of an unrelated or relatively trivial clinical symptom, the majority are diagnosed by the investigation of a symptom or symptoms directly attributable to the leukaemic process, i.e. anaemia, haemorrhagic phenomena, fever or infection.

The anaemia is usually normochromic and normocytic or slightly macrocytic and with a low reticulocyte count. Thrombocytopenia is often severe and is responsible for the skin and mucous membrane haemorrhages, although in acute promyelocytic leukaemia (APML) (*see* below) disseminated intravascular coagulation is a feature. The leucocyte count is usually raised but not commonly over 50×10^9/l. Higher leucocyte counts are related to poor prognosis in ALL in children. The leucocyte count may be within the normal range or a leucopenia may be present. In the latter presentation further investigation must exclude aplastic anaemia by bone-marrow biopsy, but on occasions even the marrow biopsy appearances may be difficult to interpret. Blast cells are typically seen in the blood film but may be scanty particularly when the presentation is aleukaemic. Films made from the buffy layer of centrifuged blood may be useful. An alternative approach for concentrating the leucocytes is to allow the red cells of an anticoagulated blood sample to settle and obtain a cytocentrifuge preparation from the supernatant, leucocyte-containing plasma. The identification of proliferating blasts is important and is related to the clinical course, treatment and prognosis. The clinical features of acute leukaemia may suggest which cell line is involved but the classification of the acute leukaemias is essentially laboratory orientated and is based on blast-cell morphology in Romanowsky-stained blood and bone-marrow films, cytochemistry, immunological identification of cell markers, chromosome studies and, perhaps, transmission electron microscopy.

Morphological classification of acute leukaemias

Early classifications of the acute leukaemias were hampered by inconsistent morphological criteria and limited cytochemical techniques. The general acceptance of the FAB (French–American–British cooperative group) morphological classification [8] has improved concordance between observers. The classification separates the acute lymphoblastic leukaemias (ALL) from the remaining acute non-lymphocytic (ANLL) or acute myeloid leukaemias (AML) by morphological and cytochemical criteria and further characterizes categories within each major group. ALL was divided into L1–3 and AML into M1–6. Blood films alone are not considered adequate and bone-marrow preparations are specified.

The original criteria of the L1 and L2 subgroups have been modified [9], a variant of M3 (M3v) has been recognized [10, 11] and a further category added, i.e. megakaryoblastic (M7) [12]. The criteria for M7 represented a significant departure for the FAB group in that ultrastructural cytochemistry and/or immunological techniques are required.

The concept of pre-leukaemic or myelodysplastic states was clarified since the original FAB classification and resulted in proposals for classifying the myelodysplastic syndromes (MDS) [13] and included distinction between Type I and Type II myeloblasts.

Revised criteria for the classification of AML [14] included the use of Type I and II blasts, rigid quantitation of the proportions of blasts and erythroblasts, the recognition of an additional variant of the myelomonocytic (M4) type associated with eosinophils (M4 eos), specification that 500 cells must be counted, consideration of cytogenetic data and the optional use of serum lysozyme estimations.

The departure from light microscopy and simple cytochemistry and the proposed revised criteria for AML have been questioned [15, 16] as being not readily available, inconsistent or too rigid. Certainly the classification of AML is now complex, and whether the result is improved concordance remains to be seen.

Criteria of the FAB classification

This section is reproduced largely from the original and amended proposals.

Acute lymphoblastic leukaemias

The criterion for inclusion in the lymphoblastic group is less than 3% peroxidase or Sudan Black-positive blasts which allows for a small residual population of normal myeloid blasts. A poorly differentiated monocytic leukaemia (M5a) with no peroxidase activity may be confused with L2 but may be recognized by sodium fluoride-sensitive non-specific esterase activity.

The original morphological criteria of cell size, appearance of nuclear chromatin, nuclear shape, presence and number of nucleoli and the amount, basophilia and vacuolation of the cytoplasm, defined three types (L1, L2 and L3) (*Table 13.2*). Subsequent experience of the FAB and other groups indicated that although there was little difficulty in the identification of L3 the degree of agreement of L1 and L2 was less satisfactory due to some criteria being too rigid or too lax and to difficulty in defining others. Revised criteria with a scoring system were recommended for L1 and L2 [9] using only bone-marrow films and based on: (1) nuclear:cytoplasmic

Table 13.2 'Lymphoblastic' leukaemias – 1976 criteria

Cytological features	*L1*	*L2*	*L3*
Cell size	Small cells predominate	Large, heterogeneous in size	Large and homogeneous
Nuclear chromatin	Homogeneous in any one case	Variable – heterogeneous in any one case	Finely stippled and homogeneous
Nuclear shape	Regular, occasional clefting or indentation	Irregular; clefting and indentation common	Regular – oval to round
Nucleoli	Not visible or small and inconspicuous	One or more present, often large	Prominent; one or more vesicular
Amount of cytoplasm	Scanty	Variable; often moderately abundant	Moderately abundant
Basophilia of cytoplasm	Slight or moderate, rarely intense	Variable; deep in some	Very deep
Cytoplasmic vacuolation	Variable	Variable	Often prominent

(N/C) ratio; (2) the presence, prominence and frequency of nucleoli; (3) nuclear membrane outline (nuclear shape); and (4) cell size.

Revised classification criteria and scoring system

For N/C ratio and nucleoli, criteria for positive (+) and negative (−) scores are established, while for nuclear membrane regularity and cell size, only negative (−) or zero (0) scores are used. Intermediate or indeterminate criteria were not scored. The maximum positive score in any one case is two (+2) and the maximum negative score is four (−4). By definition, a total score of 0 to +2 establishes a diagnosis of L1, whereas a total score of −1 to −4 indicates a diagnosis of L2 (*Table 13.3*).

Details as to how to employ the classification and scoring systems and examples with each of the criteria are given below.

Table 13.3 Revised classification of L1 and L2 ALL

Criteria	*Score*
Nuclear:cytoplasmic ratio high in > 75% cells*	+1
Nuclear:cytoplasmic ratio low in > 25% cells	−1
Nucleoli absent or inconspicuous in > 75% cells	+1
Nucleoli present in > 25% cells	−1
Irregular nuclear membrane in < 25% cells	0
Irregular nuclear membrane in > 25% cells	−1
Large cells < 50% of total†	0
Large cells > 50% cells	−1
Totals possible	+2 to −4

* Cytoplasm occupies < 20% of cell surface.
† Large = more than 2× diameter of small lymphocyte.
FAB type L1 = 0, 1 or 2; L2 = −1, −2, −3, −4.

Nuclear:cytoplasmic (N/C) ratio In all cases the N/C ratio applies to the individual leukaemic cell regardless of its shape or size.

High N/C ratio – The cells have a narrow rim of cytoplasm or appear to have none at all, or scanty cytoplasm limited to a small portion of the perimeter of the cell. The cytoplasm occupies less than 20% of the surface area of the cell.

Low N/C ratio – The cytoplasm occupies 20% or more of the surface area of the cell.

Scoring system – (*Table 13.3*) (+) means that 75% or more of the cells have a high N/C ratio; (−) means that 25% or more of the cells have a low N/C ratio, and cells not conforming to either of the above categories are not scored.

Examples – (i) A case in which 75% of the cells have a high N/C ratio, 5% an intermediate ratio and 20% a low ratio would be scored as (+). (ii) A case in which 20% of the cells have a high N/C ratio, 55% an intermediate ratio and 25% a low ratio would be scored as (−). (iii) A case in which 50% of the cells have a high N/C ratio, 10% a low ratio and 40% an intermediate ratio would not be scored.

Nucleoli – *Small nucleoli* are ill defined, often incomplete and not sharply differentiated from the surrounding chromatin.

Prominent nucleoli are large, vesicular and often have perinucleolar chromatic condensation.

Scoring system – (+) means that 75% or more of the cells do not have a visible nucleolus or may have a single small nucleolus; (−) means that 25% or more of the cells have one or more prominent nucleoli. When the proportion of indeterminate cells precludes either (+) or (−) rating, this feature is not scored.

Examples – (i) A case in which 80% of the cells have no visible nucleolus or a single small nucleolus and 20% have one or more prominent nucleoli would be scored as (+). (ii) A case in which 70% of the cells have no visible nucleolus or a single small nucleolus and 30% have one or more prominent nucleoli would be scored as (−).

Nuclear membrane outline – *Regular* nuclei may be round or angular or may have narrow clefts, folds or indentations that do not distort the overall continuity of the outline.

Irregular nuclei may be reniform, or their outlines may be grossly distorted by irregularities, such as wide notches or pits which may be restricted to only part of the nuclear outline.

Scoring system – (−) means that 25% or more of the cells have an irregular nuclear membrane outline; no score is given when 75% or more of the cells have a regular nuclear membrane outline with a degree of irregularity insufficient for a (−) score.

Examples – (i) A case in which 60% of the cells have a regular nuclear membrane outline, 30% irregular and 10% an intermediate nuclear membrane outline would be scored as (−). (ii) A case in which 80% of the cells have a regular nuclear membrane outline, 10% irregular and 10% indeterminate would not be scored.

Cell size – Large cells have a diameter at least twice that of the small lymphocyte. Heterogeneity of cell size score is not considered significant unless 50% or more of the cells are large.

Scoring system – (−) means that 50% or more of the cells are *large*; all other cases are not scored.

Features of L3 (Burkitt type) The cells are large and characteristically homogeneous. They have a dense but finely stippled nuclear chromatin. The nucleus is oval to round and regular. One or more prominent vesicular nucleoli are present in the majority of cells. The cytoplasm is moderately abundant and completely surrounds the nucleus. Intense cytoplasmic basophilia is present in every cell. L3 is characteristically homogeneous in respect of every feature listed, both from case to case and in an individual case. A high mitotic index (about 5%) is characteristic. Prominent cytoplasmic vacuolation is often present in a majority of the cells; vacuolation may also be present in L1 and L2 but is usually less prominent.

General aspects

The revised criteria resulted in an increase in overall concordance within the FAB group from 63 to 84% [9]. By the use of reference drawings to illustrate cytoplasmic content of 15%, 20% and 25% in determining nuclear:cytoplasmic ratios, and by studying 100–200 blasts, 92% concordance was achieved within three observers [17]. This level of agreement has been confirmed [18].

Although there have been reports to the contrary, most series using the revised FAB classification have shown that lymphoblast morphology is an independent prognostic variable [9, 18]. FAB L2 is associated with poorer remission and higher relapse rates than L1. The prognosis for L3 is uniformly poor.

A significant difference in the incidence of the ALL morphological groups is found: 70–85% of childhood ALL is of L1 type, 15–25% is L2 and 1–3% L3. In adults (>15 years) the converse is found with about 65% being L2 type. There is no age difference in the incidence of L3. Immunological cell markers indicate that childhood ALL can be divided into four sub-groups: common (c)ALL (70%), T cell ALL (15%), B cell ALL and 'early B-precursor ALL', formerly 'non-T non-B' or 'null' ALL [19]. In adults the majority (aproximately 75%) of cases of ALL are of the 'early B-precursor' type.

Although the great majority of cALL have L1 morphology, there is no clear correlation between T-ALL and the L1 and L2 morphological categories.

Acute myeloid leukaemias

Seven main types (M1, M2, M3, M4, M5, M6 and M7) are defined according to (1) the direction of differentiation along one or more cell lines and (2) the degree of maturation of the cells. Thus M1, M2 and M3 show predominantly granulocytic differentiation and differ from one another in the extent and nature of granulocytic maturation; M4 shows both granulocytic and monocytic differentiation. M5 shows predominantly monocytic differentiation, M6 predominantly erythroblastic differentiation and M7 megakaryoblastic.

Two types of blasts have been defined [13]:

Type I These blasts vary from cells indistinguishable from myeloblasts to cells of various size which may be unclassifiable. Cytoplasmic granules are always absent. These cells usually have prominent nucleoli and an uncondensed chromatin pattern. The nuclear/cytoplasmic ratio of the smaller blasts tends to be higher (i.e. 0.8) than in the larger ones.

Type II These blasts have a few primary (azurophilic) granules. Otherwise they resemble type I blasts but the nuclear/cytoplasmic ratio tends to be lower and the nucleus remains in a central position.

When the following characteristics are present the cells are no longer considered to be type II blasts and are classified as promyelocytes: (i) eccentric nucleus; (ii) a developed Golgi apparatus (seen as a clear zone in the vicinity of the nucleus); (iii) more dense and/or clumped chromatin pattern; (iv) numerous granules; and (v) low N/C ratio. Deficiency of primary granules or their failure to take up the stain may result in a hypogranular or agranular promyelocyte which is recognized by the remaining four features.

Myeloblastic without maturation (M1)
The sum of blast cells types I and II must be 90% or more of the non-erythroid cells, with at least 3% of these blast cells being peroxidase or Sudan Black-positive. The remaining 10% of cells will be maturing granulocytic cells from promyelocytes onwards, or monocytes.

Myeloblastic with maturation (M2)
The sum of blast cells types I and II is from 30% to 89% of the non-erythroid cells; monocytes are less than 20% and the granulocytes, from promyelocytes to mature polymorphonuclear cells, are greater than 10%. Problems may arise in some cases that have early maturing cells with morphologic characteristics that do not conform to type I or type II blast cells, normal promyelocytes, or the hypergranular promyelocyte characteristic of M3. These cells have a fine nuclear chromatin, one or two nucleoli, and an abundant, often basophilic, cytoplasm with variable numbers of granules that sometimes coalesce. If these cells are less than 10% of the non-erythroid cells, the diagnosis remains M1. In some cases the proportion of these cells is greater than 10% and the diagnosis will become M2, even though few promyelocytes and later cells are present.

A variant of M2 is the presence of basophilic granules in the blast cells and in some of the maturing granulocytic cells in the blood and bone marrow. The variant has been designated M2 Baso.

Hypergranular promyelocytic leukaemia (M3)
Characteristic features of this disorder are: (1) the great majority of cells are abnormal promyelocytes, with a characteristic pattern of heavy granulation; (2) the nucleus varies greatly in size and shape and is often reniform or bilobed; (3) the cytoplasm of most of the cells is completely occupied by closely packed or even coalescent large granules staining bright pink, red or purple by Romanowsky dyes. In some cells the cytoplasm is filled with fine dust-like granules. Characteristic cells containing bundles of Auer rods ('faggots') randomly distributed in the cytoplasm are almost invariably present in the bone marrow and sometimes in the peripheral blood. The cytoplasm of the cells that contain faggots is often clear and pale staining but may also contain azurophilic granules.

The majority of cases of M3 fit this description, but an atypical form characterized by minimal rather than excessive granulation has been recognized. The most striking cytomorphological features of this 'M3 variant', M3v, relate to the nuclear configuration and to the relative scarcity of cells with heavy granulation and of cells containing multiple Auer rods ('faggot cells'). The nucleus of almost every cell in the peripheral blood is bilobed, multilobed or reniform, but the majority of cells are either devoid of granules or contain only a few azurophilic granules. However, at least a few cells with all the cytoplasmic features of typical M3 are present. If these are overlooked, the case is likely to be misdiagnosed as an atypical monocytic leukaemia. This atypical morphology is a feature of the peripheral blood cells. In the bone marrow the morphology is closer to that of typical M3. In contrast to typical M3, in which the leucocyte count is only rarely high and usually varies from slightly above the normal range to subnormal levels, M3v is commonly associated with markedly raised leucocyte counts (up to 200×10^9/l).

It is important that this less differentiated variant is recognized, as the measures that are generally considered essential in the management of typical M3 are equally essential in the variant form in reducing the risk of disseminated intravascular coagulation which is much higher in M3 than in the other forms of acute leukaemia. The chromosomal translocation, t(15;17), has been associated with cases of typical M3 [20], as well as in all the cases of the M3 variant studied [21]. It is important that all cases of this translocation in which the morphology is not that of typical M3 are assessed for the possibility of M3v.

Myelomonocytic (M4)

The diagnosis of M4 and its separation from M2 and M5 require assessment of both blood and bone-marrow films. In marrow, the blasts are >30% of the non-erythroid cells. The sum of myeloblasts, promyelocytes, myelocytes and later granulocytes is 30% or more but less than 80% of the non-erythroid cells. More than 20% of the non-erythroid cells are of the monocytic lineage at different stages of maturation; usually they are promonocytes and monocytes. When the monocytic cells exceed 80% the diagnosis is M5 (monocytic leukaemia). When the bone-marrow findings are as above and the blood monocyte count is 5×10^9/l or more, the diagnosis is M4. If the monocyte count is $<5 \times 10^9$/l a diagnosis of M4 can still be made if the bone-marrow findings are as described above and a significant monocyte component is confirmed by other tests such as serum lysozyme or combined esterase cytochemistry. The diagnosis of M4 is established if more than 20% of the bone-marrow precursors are monocytes as shown by cytochemical reactions or if the lysozyme concentration exceeds three times the reference value of the individual laboratory. If the bone marrow resembles that of M2, a diagnosis of M4 is still possible if the blood monocyte count exceeds 5×10^9/l or one or more of the above tests provides evidence for an increased monocytic component in the bone marrow.

In a small percentage of cases of M4, eosinophils are present in the bone marrow; they usually amount to 5% or more of non-erythroid cells. The eosinophils are abnormal and some have additional large basophilic (immature) granules and may have a single unsegmented nucleus. In contrast to normal eosinophils, these cells have positive reactions for chloracetate esterase and periodic acid–Schiff. Although rare, cells with these features can be identified in cases of M2, but overall the cases of M2 with eosinophils lack the abnormal granules seen in M4 with eosinophilia.

Monocytic (M5)

The diagnosis of M5 is based on the appearance of the bone marrow. One criterion suffices: 80% or more of the non-erythroid cells are monoblasts, promonocytes or monocytes. Two subtypes are recognized: poorly differentiated or monoblastic (M5a) and differentiated or monocytic (M5b).

For M5a 80% or more of the monocytic cells are monoblasts. The cells have delicate lacey chromatin, and one, occasionally up to three, large prominent vesicular nucleoli. The cytoplasm is voluminous, often shows one or more pseudopods, is basophilic and may contain rare azurophilic granules. The pseuopodia or buds may be more transluscent than the rest of the cytoplasm giving the appearance of a double membrane.

For M5b less than 80% of the monocytic cells are monoblasts, the remainder being promonocytes and monocytes but the proportion of monocytes in the blood is higher than in the marrow. The cells are similar to the monoblast but have a large nucleus with a cerebriform appearance; nucleoli may be present but the cytoplasm is less basophilic, has a greyish ground-glass appearance and fine azurophilic granules are scattered throughout.

In both types a few cells may contain Auer rods. The diagnosis must then be confirmed by the non-specific esterase reaction.

Erythroleukaemia (M6)

The erythropoietic component usually exceeds 50% of all the nucleated cells in the bone marrow, and the erythroblasts show, in varying degree, bizarre morphological features, especially multiple lobulation of the nucleus, with variation in size of the lobes, multiple nuclei, presence of one or more nuclear fragments, giant forms and megaloblastic features. Erythroblasts are often present in the blood.

The proportion of type I and II blasts must exceed 30% of the remaining non-erythroid cells. Auer rods may be seen. When 50% or more of all nucleated cells are erythroblasts and <30% of the non-erythroid cells are blasts, the diagnosis becomes myelodysplastic syndrome (MDS).

Megakaryoblastic (M7)

The blasts in megakaryoblastic leukaemia would be classified as lymphoblastic on the basis of negative peroxidase reaction or Sudan Black staining. The cells range from small and round with scanty cytoplasm and dense chromatin resembling L1 blasts to those that more closely resemble the blasts in L2, with or without granules, having 1–3 prominent and finely reticulated nuclear chromatin. There is heterogeneity in size with 20–30% of blasts being 2–3 times larger than normal lymphocytes. Cytoplasmic blebs and megakaryocytic fragments may be seen.

Megakaryoblastic leukaemia was described as acute myelofibrosis[22] and bone-marrow aspiration may be inadequate or even impossible. Blood films may therefore be used for diagnosis.

Additional cytochemical stains can be confusing. Non-specific esterase may suggest monocyte lineage; periodic acid–Schiff and acid phosphatase are frequently positive with a localized pattern. However, megakaryocytes are almost always negative for α-naphthyl butyrate esterase which distinguishes them from monocytes.

The platelet peroxidase reaction is almost always positive in M7, can be differentiated from myeloperoxidase by its inhibition by glutaraldehyde and formaldehyde and by its localization on the nuclear membrane and endoplasmic reticulum. Immunological demonstration of the platelet-specific membrane glycoproteins Ib and IIb/IIIa using monoclonal antibodies will establish the identity of megakaryoblasts and their numbers. A megakaryoblastic component of more than 30% is consistent with a diagnosis of M7[12].

General aspects
The quantitative criteria of the revised proposals for classification of AML are summarized in *Table 13.4.* A decision algorithm for the differential diagnosis of the acute myeloid leukaemias on the basis of the FAB classification is given in reference[14].

Table 13.4 Summary of the quantitative bone-marrow criteria proposed for the diagnosis of acute myeloid leukaemia subtypes* [14]

Bone-marrow cells	*M1* (%)	*M2* (%)	*M4* (%)	*M5* (%)	*M6* (%)
Blasts					
All nucleated cells	–	> 30	> 30	–	< 30 or > 30
Non-erythroid cells	90 (I + II)†	> 30	> 30	> 80‡	> 30
Erythroblasts, all nucleated cells	–	< 50	< 50	–	> 50
Granulocytic component§, non-erythroid cells	< 10	> 10	> 20‖	< 20	Variable
Monocytic component¶, non-erythroid cells	< 10	< 20	> 20	> 80‡	Variable

* Lysozyme estimations and cytochemical tests are required if the peripheral blood monocyte count is 5×10^9/l or more but the marrow suggests M2, and if the marrow suggests M4 but the peripheral blood monocyte count is less than 5×10^9/l (*see* text).
† Blasts type I and II, as previously described[13].
‡ Monoblasts in M5a; in M5b the predominant cells are promonocytes and monocytes.
§ Promyelocytes, myelocytes, metamyelocytes, and neutrophils.
‖ May include myeloblasts.
¶Promonocytes and monocytes.

In a study of 250 cases of AML classified according to the original FAB criteria[23], the distribution was M1 = 21%, M2 = 32%, M3 = 16%, M4 = 16%, M5 = 12% and M6 = 3%. The rate of remission was similar for M1, 2 and 3, about 60%, compared with 36–38% for M5 and M6.

One reason for the revision of the AML criteria is to obtain more accurate separation between MDS and AML because the need for chemotherapy and the type of therapeutic programmes are different for the two disorders.

Cytochemistry of acute leukaemias

The major problems in the morphological classification of acute leukaemia are:

1. The separation of the ALL types from the remainder and particularly from M1.
2. The identification of myeloblastic and monocytic cell lines.
3. The possibility of identifying cell lines within the L1 and L2 categories.

Cytochemical reactions are used to resolve these problems.

Myeloperoxidase and Sudan Black B

Myeloperoxidase is exclusive to the granulocytic and monocytic series and – though usually associated with the azurophil granules – positivity may be seen in the cytoplasm of cells devoid of granules, which possibly represents activity in the perinuclear space, endoplasmic reticulum, Golgi apparatus, or perhaps in granules not resolved by light microscopy. Though the specificity of Sudan Black B is uncertain it is clear that positive staining is closely equivalent to the myeloperoxidase reaction.

Myeloperoxidase, Sudan Black staining or both are therefore helpful in distinguishing ALL (L1, L2 and L3) from the myeloblastic and monocytic cell types (M1–M6) and in particular those examples of M1 that are devoid of azurophil granules. Additional features of the myeloperoxidase reaction in acute leukaemias are that Auer rods are strongly positive and that the neutrophils in AML (and other disorders) may show no activity. The positivity in the monocyte series is less than that of myeloblasts and is more finely granular and scattered, and in M5 the blasts may be totally negative. The reactions are negative in ALL.

Chloracetate esterase

The leucocyte isoenzymes of esterases 1, 2, 7 and 8 are known as the chloracetate esterases, and, with the substrate α-naphthyl AS-D chloracetate, activity is only found in the granulocyte series and in the abnormal erythroblasts of erythroleukaemia (M6). Activity develops during granulocyte maturation and appears at a later stage than myeloperoxidase activity. Chloracetate esterase activity may therefore be absent in undifferentiated myeloblasts which are peroxidase positive and is therefore of less value than peroxidase in differentiating M1 from L1 or L2. The main application of the demonstration of chloracetate esterase activity is in identifying M4 by differentiating the myeloblastic and monocytic cell lines.

Non-specific esterases

Non-specific esterases are represented by the isoenzymes 3, 4, 5 and 6. There is a choice of substrates each having different reaction characteristics. Naphthyl AS-acetate (NASA), naphthyl AS-D acetate (NASDA), α-naphthyl acetate (ANA) and α-naphthyl butyrate (ANB) have been used and fall into two groups. NASA and NASDA give positive results with granulocytes and monocytes; the reaction with monocytes (isoenzymes 4 and 5) is inhibited by the presence of sodium fluoride. ANA and ANB are virtually specific for the monocyte series and although also sensitive to sodium fluoride its addition is unnecessary as ANA and ANB do not show granulocyte activity (the specificity of ANB for monocytes is reportedly superior to ANA and was used for that purpose in the Technicon Hemalog D system). Non-specific esterase activity appears before either peroxidase or lysozyme activity. Although localized non-specific esterase activity is a feature of T lymphocytes there is no correlation between the *morphology* of L1, L2 and esterase activity. L3 cells are negative.

Combined or dual esterase reaction

The dual demonstration of chloracetate and non-specific esterases using contrasting coupling agents is useful in identifying the granulocytic and monocytic cells in M4 (acute myelomonocytic leukaemia).

Acid phosphatase

Seven isoenzymes of acid phosphatase are recognized – 0, 1, 2, 3, 3b, 4 and 5 – of which 1, 2, 3 and 4 are found in normal cell lines. Isoenzyme 3b is associated with both granulocyte and monocyte lineages. Fluoride inhibits all isoenzymes as does tartaric acid with the notable exception of isoenzyme 5 (*see* 'hairy cell' leukaemia, page 439). Acid phosphatase activity in AML is variable and diffuse, with some superimposed granularity, and is probably strongest in M5 but not sufficiently to allow subclassification. Auer rods are strongly positive.

In the peroxidase and esterase-negative acute leukaemias, L3 is consistently acid-phosphatase negative. Although a small proportion of cases show strong localized activity in blasts with T cell markers there is no correlation with L1/L2 morphology.

PAS reaction

The PAS reaction applied to haemic cells demonstrates glycogen. The reaction is of limited value in the classification of acute leukaemias with the exception of the strong granular or block positivity in the erythroblasts of M6 (erythroleukaemia). Positivity in the M1–M5 classes is variable and when present is diffuse or finely granular. The reaction has gained some support in the classification of ALL and certainly granular positivity in peroxidase/esterase negative blasts can support a morphological diagnosis of ALL. L3 are PAS-negative and there is no correlation between L1/L2 morphology and positive reactions. PAS-positive ALL is reported to have a better prognosis than PAS-negative cases and probably represent early B-precursor proliferations (non-B, non-T).

The cytochemical findings in acute leukaemia are summarized in *Table 13.5*.

Table 13.5 Summary of cytochemical findings in acute leukaemia

	Type of leukaemia								
Reaction	*L1–L2*	*L3*	*M1*	*M2*	*M3*	*M4*	*M5*	*M6*	*M7*
Peroxidase/Sudan Black	–	–	+	++	++	++	–/+	+ (in myeloid cells)	–
ANA esterase	–/+	–	–	–	–	–/+ (NaF sensitive)	++	–	+
Acid phosphatase	–/++	–	±	±	±	±	+	–	+
PAS	–/++	–	±	+ (diffuse)	+	+ (diffuse and/or granular)	+	++ (in erythroblasts)	+

ANA = α-naphthyl acetate; PAS = periodic acid–Schiff.

Other cytochemical reactions in acute leukaemias

Perls' Prussian Blue reaction for iron is useful for demonstrating the possible increased iron content and ring-sideroblast nature of the erythroblasts in M6, and in the classification of MDS.

Oil red O may be used to demonstrate lipid in the cytoplasmic vacuoles of L3.

5-nucleotidase has been reported to be a marker for megakaryoblasts[23] but activity and specificity has not been confirmed[24].

Neutrophil alkaline phosphatase is of no value in the diagnosis and classification of acute leukaemias.

Non-cytochemical enzyme markers in acute leukaemia

Lysozyme

This is associated with phagocytic cells and greatly elevated serum levels are found in monocytic leukaemias, with smaller increases in AML. Demonstration of cellular lysozyme by the lysis of *Micrococcus lysodeikticus* or by an immunological technique shows activity in segmented neutrophils and cells of the monocyte series. The enzyme appears later during maturation than non-specific esterase and acid phosphatase activity, and monoblasts may show no activity. The demonstration of lysozyme at a cellular level appears to offer little in the classification of acute leukaemias though serum levels can be used in the diagnosis of M5 and in monitoring progress of the disease.

Terminal deoxynucleotidyl transferase (terminal transferase, TdT) [25]

TdT is a DNA polymerase present in high concentration in lymphoid cells and may therefore be considered as a marker for ALL in the same way as myeloperoxidase is a marker for AML. The value of TdT has been established in the differentiation of acute leukaemias and in particular in undifferentiated leukaemia showing negative cytochemical reactions, in identifying the lymphoid nature of some 'blast-cell crises' in CGL (*see* page 450) and in mixed myeloid and lymphoid proliferations[26]. The preparation of antibodies to TdT and their use in immunological techniques allows identification of the presence of TdT at a single cell level with applications in the detection of CNS involvement and possibly the detection of early bone-marrow relapse.

Hexoseaminidase (Hex, N-acetyl-β-D-glucosaminidase)

This is a lysosomal hydrolase with differing isoenzyme patterns in leucocytes and a characteristic intermediate chromatographic peak (Hex I) which is almost exclusive to cALL.

Immunological classification of acute leukaemias

Developments in cellular immunology which commenced with the identification of the T, B and null subsets of normal lymphocytes, now extends to all haemopoietic cell lines. The development of the technology for the production of monoclonal antibodies (MoAb) has allowed the identification of cell markers at various stages of cell differentiation and has been particularly useful in the identification of subgroups of ALL.

The combination of the early techniques – demonstration of the receptor for sheep erythrocytes (E), the detection of cytoplasmic and surface membrane immunoglobulins, demonstration of TdT and the HLA-DR (Ia) antigen – together with the identification of cell antigens by MoAb, now allows a comprehensive approach to the identification and classification of acute leukaemias.

E-rosettes Receptors for sheep erythrocytes (E) were considered to be the 'gold standard' for T-cell lineage. The recognition of a pre-T cell differentiation antigen, a 40 000 d glycoprotein (gp40) recognized by a MoAb has made the rosetting technique unnecessary.

Cytoplasmic immunoglobulin (cIg) Demonstrated by immunofluorescence (IF) categorizes the pre-B ALL category of ALL.

Surface immunoglobulin by IF is a reliable marker of B-ALL.

HLA-DR (Ia)/class II determinant This antigen was originally identified in murine lymphocytes as glycoproteins of 28 000 and 33 000 d (p28,33). In humans the antigens are associated with the HLA-DR locus and are early markers of B-cell lineage and myeloid differentiation. The absence of the antigen is therefore a marker of T-cell lineage though 10% of cases of T-ALL express the antigen.

Terminal deoxynucleotidyl transferase (TdT) As described earlier, TdT is an early marker of T and B-cell ALL but is found in about 20% of AML[26].

Antibodies to cell markers

Initially antibodies were raised by immunizing rabbits with leukaemic cells, had 'in-house' designations, limited availability, and antibodies against the same or similar determinants had different names. The production of MoAbs[27] on a commercial scale inevitably led to different proprietary designations of antibodies with the same specificity. The confusing nomenclature has been addressed by a series of workshops which resulted in the use of the CD (clusters of differentiation) nomenclature which grouped together MoAbs on the basis of reactivity with

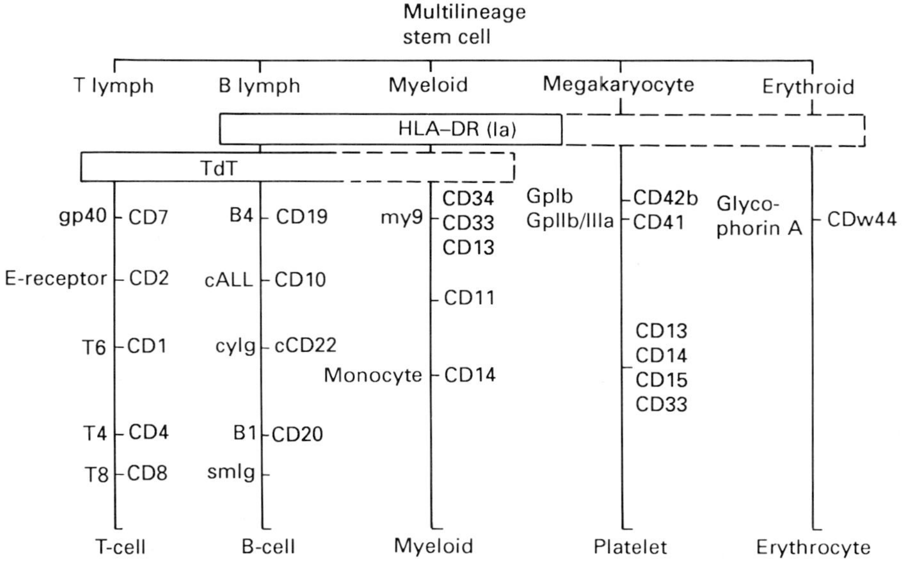

Figure 13.1 Haemopoietic cell lines and the relationship of CD antigens to stages of differentiation

different target cells and biochemical characteristics. In 1989 the CD nomenclature encompassed over 400 MoAbs in 89 designated clusters[28].

Although the initial objective was to produce MoAbs which selectively identified leukaemic cells, in many instances the antigens have been associated with the stages of differentiation of normal cells. *Figure 13.1* illustrates the major cell lines and the relationship of CD antibodies to the stages of differentiation.

Various strategies have been recommended for the differentiation of the acute leukaemias. Certain determinants are lineage-restricted markers and an initial separation into AML and B and T-cell ALL is one approach (*Table 13.6*).

Table 13.6 Lineage-restricted markers of acute leukaemia[29]

	CD19	*CD7*	*CD33*	*CD13*	*DR*	*TdT*
B-lineage	+	−	−	−	+	+†
T-lineage	−	+	−	−	−*	+
AML	−	−*	+	+	+	−*

* Exceptions in small proportion of cases.
† Negative in most mature (SmIg+) B-ALL.

T and B-ALL can be further subdivided. B lineage is shown in *Table 13.7* and T-cell lineage in *Table 13.8*.

Table 13.7 Relationship of B-ALL and cell markers

	TdT	*DR*	*CD19*	*CD10 cALL*	*CD20*	*SmIg*
Pro-B-ALL (null)	+	+	+	−	−	−
Common-B-ALL	+	+	+	+	−	−
Pre-B-ALL	+	+	+	+	+/−	−
Early B-ALL	−	+	+	+/−	+	+
Mature B-ALL	−	+	+	−	+	+

Table 13.8 Marker patterns in T-ALL

	TdT	*DR*	*CD7*	*CD2*	*cCD3*
Early T-precursor ALL	+	−	+	−	−
T cell ALL	+	−	+	+	+

The correlation between FAB morphology and membrane markers in AML is less distinct showing considerable cross-reaction[30]. CD14 is associated with M4, M5a and M5b; CD15 with M2, M3 and M4 and CD33 with undifferentiated (M0) and M1 types. Glycophorin A MoAb is specific for the erythroblasts in M6 and CD41 for the membrane glycoproteins of megakaryoblasts (M7). Confusion between T-ALL and AML may occur due to TdT and CD7 expression in a small proportion of AML. *Table 13.9* summarizes the relationship between FAB morphology and membrane markers in AML.

Table 13.9 Correlation of membrane markers with FAB classification in AML

Antibodies	*M1*	*M2*	*M3*	*M4*	*M5*	*M6*	*M7*
HLA-DR	+	+	−	+	+	+/−	+/−
CD34	+	+/−	−	+/−	+/−	−	+/−
CD33	+	+	+	+	+	+/−	+/−
CD13	+/−	+	+	+	+	−	+/−
CD11	−	+	+/−	+	+	−	?
CD15	−	+	+/−	+	+	+/−	+/−
CD14	−	+/−	−	+	+	−	+/−
Glycophorin A	−	−	−	−	−	+	−
CD41	−	−	−	−	−	−	+

Strategies have been developed to allow lineage identification with minimum numbers of antibodies. A panel of four MoAbs against CD7, CD19, CD33 and DR has been recommended[31] for initial phenotypic differentiation which can be supplemented as necessary. TdT, CD19 and cCD22 will identify almost all cases of B-precursor ALL and TdT, CD7, CD2 and cCD3 will deal similarly with T-ALL[32].

Gene rearrangements

Analysis of T-cell receptor (TCR) genes shows rearrangement in T-cell neoplasms. TCR chain gene is rearranged in all except those arrested at a very early stage of differentiation. Mature T-cell neoplasms with chain rearrangement include Sezary syndrome, peripheral T-cell lymphoma, mycosis fungoides and adult T-cell leukaemia[33].

Nearly all B-cell proliferations show immunoglobulin gene rearrangements. The majority of non-T non-B ALL are B-cell neoplasms[34]. TCR and immunoglobulin gene rearrangements are clear evidence of clonality of T or B lineage lymphocytic proliferations.

Chromosomes in acute leukaemia

Numerical abnormalities involving the loss or gain of a chromosome have been associated with acute leukaemias for many years. Improved methods for culturing leukaemic cells and high quality banding techniques to allow detailed analysis of chromosome structure have shown that consistent chromosomal abnormalities can be demonstrated in about two-thirds of acute leukaemias. Characteristic, non-random, but less consistent abnormalities are also found.

The commonest and most specific defects are translocations, deletions, inversions and trisomy. A translocation or inversion could place an oncogene next to an activating DNA sequence, a deletion could eliminate an oncogene suppressor and trisomy would carry extra gene dosage.

The FAB and immunological classifications have allowed more reliable associations between karyotype and the morphological and/or immunological types.

Acute lymphoblastic leukaemias

Because of the general lack of concordance between the FAB subtypes and the better defined immunological categories, cytogenetic classification is usually correlated with immunological categories. Most of the cytogenetic abnormalities are characteristic of either B or T lineage but some are found in both types and also in non-lymphoid proliferations [19].

The standard Philadelphia (Ph) translocation t(9;22)(q34;q11) (*see* page 446), or occasionally its variant forms, are associated with early B-precursor, cALL or pre-B ALL; a Ph rarely appears in T-cell ALL. Deletion del(6q) at various bands, mainly 6q15 and 6q21, is associated with cALL but is occasionally found in L3 and sometimes in T-ALL. Near haploidy is associated mostly with cALL. Translocations or deletions involving 12p12 are primarily seen in cALL. Translocation t(1;19)(q23;p13) is associated with pre-B ALL with L1 morphology. Translocations t(8;14)(q24;q32), t(8;22)(q24;q11) and t(2;8)(p12 or 13,q24) are associated with Burkitt's type (L3) and with a B-cell phenotype. The oncogene c-*myc* moves from 8 to the Ig heavy chain site at 14q32, to 22q11 to express λ light chain and to 8q24 for κ light chain. The translocation t(2;8) has been found in the pre-B cell phenotype.

Translocations or deletions involving 9p at bands p21 and p22 occur in early T precursor but also in pre-B ALL. Translocation t(11;14)(p13;q13) is a relatively infrequent rearrangement found in CD2+ T-ALL.

Acute myeloid leukaemias

In contrast to ALL, cytogenetic defects correlate well with FAB morphology [29] and are summarized in *Table 13.10*.

Table 13.10 The MIC classification of AML: karyotypic and morphological associations

Karyotype	*Typical morphology*	*Less frequent associations*	*Nomenclature*
t (8;21) (q22;q22)	M2		M2/t (8;21)
t (15;17 (q22;q12)	M3, M3v		M3/t (15;17)
t/del (11) (q23)	M5a	M5b, M4	M5a/t (11q)
inv/del (16) (q22)	M4Eo		M4Eo/inv (16)
t (9;22) (q34:q11)	M1	M2	M1/t (9;22)
t (6;9) (p21–22;q34)	M2 or M4 with basophils		M2/t (6;9)
inv(3) (q21;q26)	M1 with thrombocytosis	M2, M4, M7	M1/inv(3)
t (8;16) (p11;p13)	M5b with phagocytosis		M5b/t (8;16)
t/del (12) (p11–13)	M2 with basophils		M2Baso/t (12p)
+4	M4	M2	M4/+4

Abnormalities not associated with FAB subtype include:

Trisomy 8 (+8) is the most common anomaly in AML either alone or in association with other changes; as a sole anomaly it is most frequent in M1, M4 and M5 in that order of frequency.

Monosomy 7(7−) and del 7q(7q−) second most common anomaly and as a sole anomaly is seen predominantly in M2 and M4. Both 7− and 7q− are particularly associated with patients who have received cytotoxic drug therapy.

Deletion of 5q (5q−) variable breakpoints in the long arm of 5 and again is associated with cytotoxic exposure.

Loss of Y chromosome usually occurs as a normal phenomenon in ageing males.

Trisomy 21, 9q−, i(17q), trisomy 22 are well documented but rare associations with AML.

Additional chromosome abnormalities developing during the course of the disease have been associated with relapse and carry a poor prognosis.

Chronic leukaemias

Chronic lymphocytic leukaemia and leukaemic lymphoproliferative disorders

The great majority of chronic lymphoproliferative disorders involve the B-lymphocyte series. As the function of this cell line is the formation and secretion of antibodies, the term 'immunoproliferative disorders' has been applied. A small proportion of chronic lymphocytic proliferations are of T-cell origin and have distinct clinical and cytological features. A classification of the chronic lymphoproliferative disorders is as follows:

1. B-cell proliferations:
   (a) Common chronic lymphocytic leukaemia (B-CLL).
   (b) Prolymphocytic leukaemia (B-PLL).
   (c) Hairy-cell leukaemia (HCL), leukaemic reticuloendotheliosis (LRE).
   (d) Waldenström's macroglobulinaemia (WM).
   (e) Heavy chain disease.
2. T-cell proliferations:
   (a) Chronic lymphocytic leukaemia (T-CLL).
   (b) Prolymphocytic leukaemia (T-PLL).
   (c) Sezary syndrome.

By conventional morphological criteria normal B lymphocytes appear to be mature cells but from an immunological standpoint they are at an early stage of lymphocyte differentiation, which when fully expressed is exemplified by the plasma cell which actively synthesizes and secretes immunoglobulin. Malignant clonal proliferation can occur at each stage of maturation. Conventional morphological criteria of maturation in the stained blood film do not relate well to immunological status. The different stages of malignant B-cell proliferation are reflected by the involvement of different tissues, e.g. in B-chronic lymphocytic leukaemia (B-CLL) the bone marrow and blood are initially involved and the lymph nodes become involved later, while in B-prolymphocytic leukaemia (B-PLL) splenomegaly is a feature rather than lymph-node enlargement, with the marrow becoming involved later.

B-cell proliferation

B-cell chronic lymphocytic leukaemia (B-CLL)

This is the most common form of leukaemia in the Western world but is uncommon in the Orient. It is a disease of the elderly – it is very rare below the age of 40 years –

and shows the greatest sex difference of any leukaemia (male:female ratio, 2:1). The onset is insidious, and infection, anaemia or lymph-node enlargement may be the presenting symptom, but about one-quarter of cases are detected by routine blood examination for unrelated symptoms.

Blood picture

Anaemia may be moderate, mild or absent. Red cells are usually normocytic and normochromic though there is an established association of CLL with autoimmune haemolytic anaemia in which spherocytosis might be expected. The total leucocyte count is usually greater than 15×10^9/l but usually below 200×10^9/l. There is an absolute lymphocytosis and lymphocytes may comprise over 98% of the very high leucocyte counts. The cells are small with scanty cytoplasm. 'Smudge-cells' are usually a feature and represent lymphocytes disrupted during the spreading of a 'wedge-film'. Mixing one drop of 20% albumin with one drop of blood before spreading the film may prevent 'smudging'. The disrupted forms are not seen in 'spun-films'. The presence of an absolute lymphocytosis in a patient aged over 40 years is very suggestive of a lymphoproliferative disorder. The platelet count reflects the degree of bone-marrow involvement. The degree of anaemia, thrombocytopenia and lymphocyte numbers are parameters used in the clinical staging of CLL together with organ involvement [35]. The proliferating B cells are monoclonal and patients are seen with a monoclonal paraprotein in the serum that has the same characteristics as that found on the lymphocyte membrane. Monoclonal light chains may be found in urine [36]. Serum immunoglobulins are typically reduced which is reflected by reduced plasma viscosity and associated with recurrent infections.

The development of CLL to a more malignant form is not uncommon and may take the form of transformation into a 'prolymphocytoid' cell type with progression of the disease, the appearance of a lymphoma unrelated to CLL, or a blast-cell crisis resembling acute leukaemia though the latter is a rare event.

Immunological markers

The lymphocytes reflect their monoclonality by weak SmIg restricted to a single light-chain type. Membrane antigens detected by CD19, CD20 and CD21 are specific for B cells. T lymphocytes persist in B-CLL and in untreated cases the absolute numbers are increased. The T suppressor and helper subsets are related to the clinical stages of the disease and to the deficiency in immunoglobulins [37]. Although the mouse red cell rosetting test for B lymphocytes is not an essential marker, it is of value in the differentiation between B-CLL and the prolymphocytic form (*see* below). In B-CLL about 50% of lymphocytes form rosettes and the number is increased by prior treatment of the lymphocytes with neuraminidase.

Cytogenetics

The most frequent abnormality is trisomy 12 seen in 50% of cases [38]. The translocation t(11;14) is also often found.

Cytochemistry

This is of little value in identifying B-CLL particularly if techniques for immunological markers are available. The PAS reaction in B-CLL shows fine granular positivity in 80–90% of cells. Acid phosphatase and non-specific esterase activity is absent (cf. T cells). β-glucuronidase activity is low.

B-prolymphocytic leukaemia (B-PLL)

B-PLL is clinically distinct from B-CLL in having massive splenomegaly and little or no lymph gland involvement. It is found mainly in men over 60 years of age.

Blood picture

The leucocyte count is usually over 100×10^9/l and the prolymphocytes are larger than those of CLL with more cytoplasm and a single, distinct, prominent nucleolus in a less condensed nuclear chromatin. Transmission electron microscopy shows ultrastructural changes distinct from B-CLL [38]. The defining criterion for PLL is >55% prolymphocytes [39] and CLL as <10% prolymphocytes. Cases with 11–55% prolymphocytes have intermediate clinical and haematological features. The spleen may be the source of the proliferating cells.

Immunological markers

SIg immunofluorescence is stronger than that of CLL while the proportion of Mo-rosettes is less and, in contrast to CLL, does not increase when the lymphocytes are pre-treated with neuraminidase. The monoclonal antibody FMC 7 reacts strongly with PLL cells but weakly with most examples of B-CLL. Those cases of B-CLL which are positive are in prolymphocytoid transformation.

Cytochemistry

Similar to B-CLL though the PAS reaction is reported to show coarser granulation.

Cytogenetics

In five cases of B-PLL, the translocation t(6;12)(q15;p13) was present in each. This has not been reported in other proliferative disorders and supports the view that B-PLL is a distinct clinical entity [40].

Hairy-cell leukaemia (HCL) or leukaemic reticuloendotheliosis (LRE) [41–43]

HCL usually presents with pancytopenia and splenomegaly, most often in males between 40 and 60 years of age.

Morphology

The proliferating cells are almost always present in the blood and are relatively large with a moderate amount of grey-blue cytoplasm and fine surface projections which, although evident in Romanowsky-stained films, are more conspicuous by phase-contrast microscopy in wet preparations. The nucleus is somewhat irregular with fine chromatin. Bone marrow is characteristically difficult to aspirate. Trephine biopsy shows a characteristic histological appearance. Other morphological features are the demonstration of cytoplasmic ribosome–lamellar inclusions by transmission electron microscopy, adherence to glass and weak phagocytic activity.

The nature of hairy cells (HCs)

The B lymphoid lineage of HCs, originally determined by the expression of SmIg of light-chain restricted type, has been confirmed by B cell-specific antibodies. Although examples of HCL with T-cell characteristics have been described [44, 45], they are extremely rare and may represent a marker of an evolving T-cell proliferation.

The normal counterpart of the hairy cell has not been identified with certainty but studies with a 'specific' anti-HC MoAb have suggested that it may be an infrequent cell type produced transiently on B-cell activation.

Cytochemistry

Acid phosphatase activity is stronger in HCL than in other lymphoid cell lines and is resistant to the addition of tartrate (tartrate-resistant acid phosphatase, TRAP). TRAP is a characteristic of isoenzyme 5 of acid phosphatase. TRAP has been identified in other cell lines (e.g. B-PLL) and is therefore not specific for HCL. Furthermore, TRAP activity may be weak or even absent in a small proportion of otherwise typical cases of HCL.

Esterase activity with α-naphthyl butyrate (ANBE) as substrate is seen as fine scattered granules with coarser granules in a crescentic distribution. The activity is sodium-fluoride resistant. This pattern of activity of ANBE has been suggested as a reliable marker of HCL. The combined patterns of acid phosphatase and esterase activity are unique to HCL.

β-glucuronidase activity is negative in HCL in contrast to its presence in certain other chronic lymphoproliferative disorders.

Neutrophil alkaline phosphate activity is usually elevated and may be helpful in identifying atypical cases.

The PAS reaction is usually strong with both diffuse and granular patterns.

Ultrastructural peroxidase activity in unfixed cells can be demonstrated by electron microscopy. The peroxidase activity is distinct from myeloperoxidase and is located in the endoplasmic reticulum and perinuclear space.

Membrane markers

In the great majority of cases of HCL the cells can be shown to have B-cell characteristics by their ability to synthesize and secrete immunoglobulin, to form mouse red-cell rosettes, and positive reactions with anti-DR, FMC7 and other B-lineage specific antibodies. Immunoreactivity for S-100 protein has also been described[46, 47].

Waldenströms macroglobulinaemia (WM)

This uncommon B-lymphocyte proliferation is associated with the synthesis and secretion of monoclonal immunoglobulin which in most cases is IgM and which is mainly responsible for the clinical features of the disease. The blood-film appearances are dominated by massive rouleaux formation extending to the tail of the film and bluish 'background-staining' of the paraprotein.

The bone marrow, lymph nodes and spleen are infiltrated with the proliferating cells which typically have features between those of lymphocytes and plasma cells and the term 'plasmacytoid lymphocytes' has been applied. The cells are somewhat pleomorphic having a round nucleus with a tendency to irregular chromatin condensation without a nucleolus and with a moderate amount of rather opaque blue cytoplasm. Cytochemistry is not well documented but PAS-positive inclusions are seen. Cell markers are typical of B-lymphocyte type with the additional feature of cytoplasmic immunoglobulin (CIg). A small proportion of cells produces mouse red-cell rosettes. The concentration of monoclonal IgM (IgM paraprotein) in the serum is usually greater than 25 g/l and free light chains may be found in the urine. The haemorrhagic phenomena associated with WM are in part attributable to the macroglobulin interfering with normal protein interactions in the haemostatic process and in particular with the polymerization of fibrin monomer and blocking of platelet receptors.

The differential diagnosis is from other lymphoproliferative disorders associated with a paraprotein – heavy-chain disease and myeloma (*see* below).

Heavy-chain disease

This rare group of disorders is characterized by B-cell proliferation and the secretion of a protein consisting only of the heavy chain (or part of a heavy chain) of an immunoglobulin. The commonest type of heavy chain synthesized is the α chain of IgA followed in frequency by the γ chain, μ chain and δ chain. The differential diagnosis from WM is by the recognition of the absence of light chains from the paraprotein.

Myelomatosis

Neoplasms of the B-lymphocyte series resulting in *chronic leukaemia* have been considered in the previous section and it has been emphasized that the proliferations mainly involve B lymphocytes at relatively early stages of immunological development. Only the 'plasmacytoid' lymphocytes of WM and heavy-chain disease are consistently associated with the intracellular formation and secretion of monoclonal immunoglobulin (M-protein or paraprotein; M-protein refers to monoclonal immunoglobulin and *not* IgM, macroglobulin or myeloma protein).

The plasma cell represents the end-point of B-lymphocyte differentiation. Myelomatosis or multiple myeloma is a neoplastic monoclonal proliferation of plasma cells, with characteristic clinical, haematological and immunological features and is rarely frankly leukaemic. The homogeneity of the M-protein is evidence that the malignancy arises from a single B lymphocyte by one or more stimuli. Some M-proteins have been shown to have specificity for antigens to which patients have been previously exposed but the great majority of cases show no demonstrable specificity.

Clinical features

The disease is most common in the elderly and is only rarely diagnosed below the age of 40. The commonest symptom is bone pain, with anaemia and uraemia the major signs when bone pain is minimal or absent. Infection is also a frequent presenting symptom. Some cases are recognized by the chance detection of a paraprotein by routine protein electrophoresis. In symptomatic patients a diagnosis of myelomatosis can be established entirely on the results of laboratory tests. The clinical effects of myelomatosis are due to: (1) the effect of the proliferating cells on bone and bone marrow; and (2) the production of large quantities of immunoglobulin and free light chains (Bence–Jones protein).

Blood changes

Anaemia is usual and is typically normocytic and normochromic. The total leucocyte count may be normal, low or raised. The platelet count is normal or low.

The gross blood-film changes are attributed to the paraprotein. The macroscopic appearance of the stained film is an overall bluish-staining appearance which microscopically can be seen to be due to the bluish 'background staining' of the paraprotein. Gross rouleaux formation extending to the tail of the film also reflects the high immunoglobulin level which is also responsible for the very high ESR and PV. When only light chains are synthesized (light-chain disease, Bence–Jones myeloma) the ESR and PV changes are not seen and rouleaux formation and background staining are not prominent features. The differential leucocyte count may show a small number of plasma cells and when bone-marrow involvement is extensive a leucoerythroblastic picture (*see* Chapter 12) is to be expected. A marked leucocytosis due to circulating plasma cells is more suggestive of plasma-cell leukaemia (*see* page 444).

Bone-marrow appearance

Material is usually readily aspirated and may have a gelatinous consistency. The marrow is infiltrated with plasma cells which usually comprise over 30% of the nucleated cells though levels between 10 and 30% may be found. The morphology of the neoplastic cells is variable [48]. In some cases the cells are mainly typical plasma cells together with a small proportion having more copious cytoplasm and with binucleate or multinucleate forms. Other cases may show a predominantly abnormal morphology with larger, paler cells, often with the nucleus showing a single large nucleolus. These features should be regarded as malignant de-differentiation rather than 'plasmablast' or 'proplasmacyte' stages. In a large series of patients with myeloma, five morphological cell types were distinguished with the major group further divided into three subgroups [49].

Cytoplasmic inclusions and abnormalities are not uncommon in malignant plasma cells. Russell bodies are large hyaline inclusions which stain pink by Romanowsky dyes. Morular or 'Mott' cells show numerous grey-blue inclusions which probably represent accumulation of immunoglobulin. The only correlation with immunoglobulin class is the reported occurrence in IgA myeloma of plasma cells with red cytoplasm or 'flaming cells', but the appearance is not specific [50]. Normal plasma cells do not show phagocytic properties but in myeloma, phagocytosis of iron, red cells and nucleated cells have been described. Azurophilic cytoplasmic inclusions resembling Auer rods are sometimes seen. Crystalline inclusions are occasionally found.

Cytochemistry

The characteristic cytochemical property of myeloma cells is the presence of RNA which reflects the active protein synthesis and is demonstrated by pyroninophilia in the methyl green–pyronin technique (Unna–Pappenheim). The PAS reaction is negative, or weakly and diffusely positive; Russell bodies are weakly PAS positive and diastase resistant and therefore probably represent mucoprotein. Non-specific esterase activity is present but no differences are observed between cells secreting different types of immunoglobulin. Acid phosphatase activity is strong and using a scoring technique, a significant difference has been recorded between κ and λ light-chain subtypes [51].

Cytogenetics

Almost 50% of cases have an abnormal karyotype[51]. Trisomy 3, 5, 9 and 15 and monosomy 3 and 16 are common clonal abnormalities. Structural changes of 1 and 14 have been frequently reported. Translocations involving 14q+ are associated with other B-cell malignancies including t(8;14)(q24;q32). The association of t(8;14) abnormalities with IgA protein suggests a relationship between specific karyotype and type of myeloma protein, as is the location of the heavy chain on chromosome 6.

Immunoglobulins in myelomatosis

The characteristic features are:

1. A progressive increase of the M-protein in plasma.
2. Presence in the urine of monoclonal light chains (κ or λ) in addition to the M-protein in the plasma.
3. Reduced levels of normal plasma immunoglobulins.

The level of the plasma M-protein is related to the immunoglobulin type: IgG level is usually greater than 35 g/l, IgA level greater than 20 g/l. Levels of *normal* immunoglobulin are in the order of: IgM less than 0.5 g/l, IgA less than 1 g/l and IgG less than 6 g/l. The low levels of normal immunoglobulin predispose to recurrent infection. The incidence of the various monoclonal immunoglobulins broadly follows the normal concentrations of plasma immunoglobulins, i.e. IgG>IgA>IgM>IgD>IgE, with κ light chains being more frequent than λ (in approximate ratio 3:2). However in some larger series, examples of IgM myeloma are not recorded and proliferations secreting only Bence–Jones protein are found in 10–20% of cases. Occasionally cases are found with two paraproteins which represent the proliferation of two cell-clones. If the urine is concentrated before testing, Bence–Jones protein can be demonstrated in about 70% of those cases producing complete immunoglobulins. Recognition of the monoclonal nature of the paraproteins is usually by immunoelectrophoresis using specific antisera and the concentration is determined by radial immunodiffusion or quantitative immunoelectrophoresis. Monoclonal paraproteins can be demonstrated at a cellular level by immunological techniques using labelled specific antisera.

The production of Bence–Jones protein and its effect on renal function is a serious complication of myelomatosis. The light chains are present as monomers (molecular weight 22 000) or dimers (molecular weight 44 000) and are therefore capable of glomerular filtration and subsequent precipitation in the renal tubules. Daily urinary excretion is typically between 1 and 15 g but may occasionally reach 50 g. The average concentration of Bence–Jones protein in IgG and IgA myeloma with λ chains (IgGL and IgAL) is considerably higher than in those cases with κ chains (IgGK and IgAK).

Immunoglobulin levels have been shown to relate to the total tumour-cell mass. In IgG myeloma the concentration of paraprotein has been shown to double, on average, every 10 months and IgA levels to double every 6 months. These levels represent protein production from about 1 kg or 4.6×10^{11} plasma cells. It has been calculated that if the growth rate and paraprotein production of the malignant cells is constant, the time interval between initial detection of paraproteinaemia or Bence–Jones proteinuria and the onset of clinical myelomatosis is in the order of 33 years for IgG myeloma, 21 years for IgA and 11 years for Bence–Jones disease. It is likely that the growth rate of the tumour cell mass slows and that the above estimates are too long; nevertheless the developmental period clearly extends over many years.

The sequential measurement of plasma paraprotein levels is an important investigation in distinguishing myelomatosis from *benign monoclonal gammopathy* in an otherwise healthy subject, or the occasional occurrence of a monoclonal gammopathy in non-lymphoplasmacytic disorders. Benign monoclonal gammopathy is more common than myeloma and about 3% of persons over the age of 70 have a plasma M-component which unlike myelomatosis: (1) remains at a constant concentration even for many years; (2) is less than 25 g/l (3) is associated with normal levels of the other immunoglobulins; and (4) is not usually associated with Bence–Jones proteinuria. Using the technique of immuno-isoelectric focusing [53], 11% of individuals over the age of 45 years had evidence of a paraprotein compared with 2% by zonal and immunoelectrophoresis. Marrow infiltration with plasma cells is not present and the typical radiological bone changes are not found.

In addition to the renal changes due to Bence–Jones protein, the plasma paraproteins may result in symptoms due to hyperviscosity or cryoprecipitation. Haemostatic function is impaired due to interference by the paraprotein with platelet aggregation and adhesion and with fibrin polymerization. The phagocytic function of neutrophils is also compromised and possibly contributes to the frequency of infection in myelomatosis.

Plasma-cell leukaemia

It has been stated that the number of plasma cells in the blood in myeloma is usually small and frankly leukaemic pictures are most unusual. Plasma-cell leukaemia is an exceedingly rare disorder which presents as an acute leukaemia with bone-marrow failure and splenomegaly. The malignant plasma cells are typically poorly differentiated [54]. Paraprotein production follows the same pattern as myeloma with the gross blood-film changes, except when Bence–Jones protein only is secreted. Bone changes are not usual. The condition does not respond well to the therapeutic regimens used in myeloma.

T-cell proliferations

In mature cell CLL only 1–2% of cases are of T-cell type although 20% of prolymphocytic leukaemias show features characteristic of T-cell lineage [55]. Rare examples of T-HCL have been described [43].

T-cell chronic lymphocytic leukaemia (T-CLL)

Lymphadenopathy is not a feature and splenomegaly is less marked. The total lymphocyte count is rarely $>25 \times 10^9$/l. Neutropenia is common. The lymphocytes have abundant cytoplasm with azurophilic granules in contrast to the scanty cytoplasm of B-CLL, and show acid phosphatase activity. The disease has a very chronic clinical course which has questioned the neoplastic nature of T-CLL and the term ‘T-lymphocytosis’ has been used to describe the disorder. However, the homogeneity of the T cells judged by membrane phenotype suggests a clonal origin. The complex interrelationships of the chronic lymphoproliferative disorder and lymphomas has been comprehensively reviewed [56].

T-cell prolymphocytic leukaemia (T-PLL)

There are significant differences between the clinical and haematological presentation of B-PLL and T-PLL. Lymphadenopathy and skin lesions are a feature and splenomegaly is less common in the T-cell type. Leucocyte counts over 100×10^9/l are slightly more common. The nuclear outline of the cells is irregular in contrast to the round appearance in B-PLL.

Cytochemical studies show that α-naphthyl esterase, acid phosphatase and β-glucuronidase activities can be demonstrated in T-PLL compared with the negative findings in B-PLL. Membrane markers clearly show the T-cell lineage. Serum immunoglobulin levels are normal.

Cytogenetic studies in T-PLL[57] show the most frequent abnormality to be associated with 14q on which is located the T-cell receptor (TCR) κ-chain gene at q11 and the immunoglobulin heavy-chain gene at q32. The most frequent abnormalities are an inversion, inv(14)(q11;q32) and translocations involving q11. Trisomy or multisomy for 8q due to rearrangement or an isochromosome, and trisomy for 7q are also found on which is located the TCR β-chain receptor. The prognosis for T-PLL is poorer than in B-PLL.

Sezary cell leukaemia

This is a chronic T-cell proliferation which does not have a B-cell counterpart. It is also termed 'cutaneous T-cell lymphoma' which emphasizes the characteristic skin lesions and erythroderma due to infiltration with the 'mycosis fungoides' cells. In the blood they are referred to as Sezary cells which are relatively large with moderate cytoplasm and have a typically convoluted or cerebriform nuclear appearance. Marker studies show the phenotype associated with normal helper/inducer T lymphocytes (CD4+). Acid phosphatase activity is strong and β-glucuronidase shows strong granular activity. The PAS reaction is variable.

Table 13.11 summarizes the immunological and cytochemical characteristics of the chronic lymphoproliferative disorders.

Table 13.11 Immunological markers and cytochemical patterns in the chronic lymphoproliferative disorders

Disorder	*SmIg*	*CIg*	*CD4*	*CD8*	*Mo*	*DR*	*CD7*	*FMC7*	*PAS*	*ANBE*	*AP*	*β-Glu*
B-CLL	+/−	−	−	−	++	++	−	−	+	−	−	−
T-CLL	−	−	−	++	−	−	++	−	−	+ (loc)	+	+
B-PLL	++	−	−	−	+/−	++	−	++	+	−	−	−
T-PLL	−	−	+/−	+/−	−	−	++	−	−	+ (loc)	+	+
HCL	++	+/−	−	−	+/−	++	−	++	−	+ (cres)	++ (TRAP)	−
WM	+	+	−	−	+/−	++	−	+	+	−	−	+
Sezary	−	−	++	−	−	−	++	−	+/−	+ (loc)	++	++

loc, localized; cres, crescent.

Chronic myeloid leukaemia

The term chronic myeloid leukaemia (CML) was originally used to distinguish chronic leukaemias involving marrow-derived cells from those arising in lymphoid tissues [58]. CML is recognized to be a clonal disorder caused by mutation of a multipotent stem cell resulting in involvement of granulocytes, erythrocyte precursors, monocytes, megakaryocytes and some B lymphocytes.

The aetiology of CML is unknown. It is an acquired disorder and there is no evidence of familial predisposition. As in the acute leukaemias, the incidence of CML increased substantially among survivors of the atomic bomb explosions in Japan and there is a higher incidence among patients exposed to therapeutic doses of X-rays.

CML is characterized by discrete phases. A chronic phase lasts 2–5 years during which cell maturation and function can support normal haematological requirements and responds to certain regulatory controls. This is followed by an accelerated phase with increasing myelopoiesis and resistance to therapy and finally an acute phase of 6–12 months characterized by loss of differentiation, i.e. transformation to an 'acute blast cell' phase. Although the clonal defect affects all myeloid cell lines, chronic phase proliferation is almost always confined to the granulocytes, platelets and, sometimes, the monocytes.

The Philadelphia chromosome

The characteristic tiny G group chromosome discovered in 1960 and termed the Philadelphia (Ph) chromosome was shown to be a consistent finding in CML. The small chromosome was shown to be a shortened chromosome 22 and that it arose from a reciprocal transformation between chromosomes 9 and 22. It is now clear that the breakpoint on chromosome 22 consistently occurs within the same band (q11) and is termed the 'breakpoint cluster region' (bcr). The current terminology is for the entire gene to be designated BCR, within which there is a 'major breakpoint cluster region' (M-BCR) and the first intron of the gene is designated the 'minor breakpoint cluster region' (m-BCR) [59].

The Ableson proto-oncogene (c-ABL) is located on 9q and is translocated to 22q in Ph-positive CML with the reciprocal translocation of c-SIS from 22q to 9q. The classical Ph translocation is represented by t(9;22)(q34;q11). The combination of c-ABL with the remaining BCR results in a chimeric BCR-ABL protein with enhanced protein tyrosine kinase activity which might result in inappropriate or excessive signal transduction controlling cell division [60]. The precise breakpoint in the BCR determines the molecular variation in Ph-positive CML, AML and ALL [60–62].

The appearance of the Ph chromosome is not the cause of CML and the progression to the acute phase appears to be independent of BCR-ABL rearrangements. The presence of Ph is one stage in the multistep pathogenesis of CML [63].

Haematological classification of CML [58]

In over 90% of cases of CML the clinical and haematological features are remarkably uniform and about 90% have the Ph chromosome (Ph+). The

Ph-negative (Ph−) cases are divided into CML Ph− with rearranged BCR (BCR+), juvenile CML, chronic neutrophilic leukaemia, chronic myelomonocytic leukaemia and atypical CML. CML is therefore comprised of five subtypes:

1. Chronic granulocytic leukaemia (CGL) (95% of all CML; 90% Ph+, BCR+; 5% Ph−, BCR+).
2. Juvenile CML (extremely rare; Ph−, BCR−).
3. Chronic neutrophilic leukaemia (CNL) (extremely rare; Ph−, BCR−).
4. Chronic myelomonocytic leukaemia (CMML). CMML with low or normal leucocyte counts is classified as myelodysplastic syndrome (MDS). CMML with high leucocyte count is both myelodysplastic and myeloproliferative; Ph−, BCR−.
5. Atypical CML (aCML). Intermediate between CGL and CMML but has distinctive features. Ph−, mostly BCR−. Significance of few reported BCR+ uncertain. Markedly worse survival than CGL and probably worse than CMML.

Types 2, 3, 4 and 5 account for 5% of CML.

CGL, CMML, aCML and CNL can be diagnosed in the great majority of cases from the morphological profile of well stained blood films.

Chronic granulocytic leukaemia (CGL)

CGL typically presents with splenomegaly, marked leucocytosis, elevated platelet count and anaemia. The development of anaemia and splenomegaly correlates with the total leucocyte counts.

Blood changes in CGL

A study of 50 cases of Ph+ CML [64] showed consistent haematological features – the pattern of the differential granulocyte count, elevated mean platelet count, increase in basophils, a low percentage of monocytes and minimal dysplasia of the granulocyte series. It has been subsequently shown that there are no significant differences in the blood changes between Ph+ and Ph− CGL [58].

Haemoglobin

Values show a mild to moderate anaemia and the red cells are usually normocytic and normochromic. The haemoglobin concentration may be falsely high due to turbidity caused by the high leucocyte count and values of MCV obtained by electronic sizing may also be falsely high due to the inclusion of leucocyte volumes in the red-cell measurements.

Red-cell morphology

This is usually unremarkable though basophilic stippling is sometimes seen and nucleated red cells are almost always present.

Platelet count

Although normal or even low values may be found, platelet numbers are characteristically increased and may exceed 1000×10^9/l. Platelet anisocytosis with macrothrombocytes is usual.

Total leucocyte count
This is usually over 100 × 10^9/l and in all but the very earliest stages is over 20 × 10^9/l. Levels up to 600 × 10^9/l are not uncommon.

Differential leucocyte count and leucocyte morphology [58]
The types and appearances of the leucocytes are the major diagnostic features. The distribution of the granulocytes shows distinct peaks, the predominant cells being segmented neutrophils and neutrophil myelocytes. The highest proportion of myelocytes are found with the higher leucocyte counts and may exceed the proportion of segmented neutrophils. An absolute increase in basophils is an invariable finding and an eosinophilia is also found in the great majority of cases. An increase in basophils is found even when the leucocyte count is less than 20 × 10^9/l and must be regarded as an essential diagnostic feature. Blast cells and promyelocytes are almost always seen in small numbers but there is no 'hiatus' in maturation from myeloblast to myelocyte. The reason for the gap in maturation between myelocyte and semented neutrophil, i.e. the lower metamyelocyte count, is not clear. Although percentages are low, the absolute numbers of lymphocytes and monocytes are also increased in the majority of cases.

Bone-marrow appearances

If examined in isolation from the blood picture the bone-marrow appearances are not diagnostic. Hypercellularity with few fat spaces is a feature even in early cases. The predominant cell is the neutrophil myelocyte with increases in eosinophil and basophil precursors. Megakaryocytes are also increased.

Cytochemistry

Neutrophil alkaline phosphatase (NAP)
NAP activity in untreated CGL is very low or absent in contrast to the high scores associated with non-leukaemic neutrophil proliferations. Following treatment, the NAP activity usually rises to normal levels and may occasionally be elevated. Blast-cell transformation of CGL (*see* page 450) is sometimes associated with a marked increase in NAP activity. Measurement of NAP activity is therefore clearly of value in the diagnosis and further study of CGL but a low value is not pathognomic of the disorder. The mechanism for the decreased activity in untreated CGL has been intensively studied. The early misconception that the Ph chromosome was a 21 chromosome led to the suggestion that the long arms of chromosome 21 controlled NAP activity and this concept was supported by the fact that trisomy 21 (Down's syndrome) is associated with increased NAP activity. The recognition that the Ph chromosome was associated with chromosome 22 invalidated this argument. Furthermore the increase in activity following treatment occurs despite the persistence of the Ph chromosome. The reason for the low NAP in CGL is not clear. The number and ultrastructure of the enzyme-containing granules are normal. The low values may be due to decreased synthesis or increased degradation of the enzyme. The transfusion of CGL neutrophils with very low NAP activity into recipients with disorders associated with high NAP scores results in the infused neutrophils acquiring high NAP activity some 14–17 hours after transfusion. This observation has been interpreted as evidence for the presence of an extracellular factor.

Other cytochemical changes
Glycogen content of CGL neutrophils is lower than normal but is not readily recognizable by visual assessment of the PAS reaction. In contrast to the low NAP activity, peroxidase is often increased.

Additional features of CGL

Platelet function is usually abnormal. *In vitro* aggregation studies show absence of second-wave adrenaline-induced aggregation and impaired collagen aggregation, both due to storage-pool deficiency. There is also defective thrombin-induced aggregation due to a membrane defect involving thrombin receptors [65].

Neutrophil function in respect of mobilization, phagocytic index, hydrogen peroxide production and nitroblue tetrazolium dye reduction is impaired in most cases of untreated CGL [66, 67]. Neutrophil membrane alterations involving sialic acid or sialylated glycoprotein may affect granulocyte adhesion and migration [68].

Factor V deficiency appears to be a common feature of CGL [69].

Serum B12 and B12-binding capacity are increased in most cases of CGL due to the release of transcobalamin I from granulocytes. The levels are therefore related to the granulocyte mass and fall after reduction of the leucocyte count following treatment.

Ph-negative CGL

The 5% Ph– CGL with characteristic haematological changes and clinical course may be explained by one of a number of reasons. Technical failure, late appearance of Ph, disappearance and 'masked' translocations are possible causes.

Complex translocations involving a third chromosome in addition to 9 and 22 are found. Translocation between 9 and chromosomes other than 22, e.g. 8, 11 or Y may be associated with genes other than BCR activating the ABL gene.

Juvenile CML (JCML)

This very rare disorder is characterized by leucocytosis, hepatosplenomegaly and thrombocytopenia. It is Ph– BCR–, has a relatively short course of 1–2 years and terminates in blast cell transformation. Monocytes are usually increased and basophilia is not a feature. A consistent finding is an increase in Hb F levels. Although clearly a leukaemia by definition, the disorder could also be regarded as being within the spectrum of myelodysplastic syndromes (MDS).

Atypical CML (aCML)

Rare cases of CML which show distinctive though variable differences from typical CGL and with poorer prognosis have been described. Promyelocytes, myelocytes and metamyelocytes comprise 15% or more of the total leucocyte count and monocytes are over 3%. The absolute number of basophils is normal. Granulocyte dysplasia is a prominent feature.

Chronic neutrophil leukaemia (CNL) [70]

This very rare form of CML is characterized by persistent leucocytosis confined to the segmented neutrophils. Basophils are not increased and the platelet count may range from low to increased. The NAP score is elevated.

Chronic myelomonocytic leukaemia (CMML)

Persistent leucocytosis due to increases in neutrophils and monocytes, with or without dysplasia, is at present sufficient grounds for inclusion in the CML disorders. Immature granulocytes are typically less than 5% of leucocytes while monocytes are usually greater than 10%. There is no increase in basophils. The mean platelet count is low. Hyperplasia of granulocytes and monocytes with normal or low leucocyte counts can be classified with the myelodysplastic syndromes.

Chronic eosinophilic leukaemia (CEL) [71–73]

This is a very rare and distinct form of CML with parameters similar to CGL but is Ph−. The eosinophils show morphological abnormalities which include hypersegmentation, hypogranularity and asynchronous nuclear/cytoplasmic maturation. Chromosome analysis may be helpful in identifying the small proportion of patients who progress from 'idiopathic' hypereosinophilic syndrome to leukaemia [74].

Acute phase of CGL

Although 30% of cases of CGL die during the accelerated phase, the remaining 70% progress to an acute stage characterized by 'blast cell transformation' in which the leukaemic cells lose the capacity to mature normally. Acute phase CGL can involve different lineages – myeloid, T and B lymphoid, erythroid, megakaryocytic and even mast cells and basophil blasts [76]. Mixed lineage transformation may occur.

Difficulties in clinical management are associated with rising leucocyte counts, fall in Hb level and of platelet numbers. Additional morphological changes in the blood film may resemble myelofibrosis. The changes can progress to those indistinguishable from *de novo* acute leukaemia. There is no correlation with changes within the BCR-ABL gene which suggests that other factors are involved. Transformation is preceded or accompanied by additional chromosome abnormalities in about 80% of cases and specific abnormalities are associated with myeloid and lymphoid types. In order of frequency the additional changes are trisomy 8, 19, additional Ph and isochromosome i(17q) [77]. The translocation t(15;17) is associated with progression to M3 and i(17q) and t(3;21)(q26;q22) are restricted to myeloid transformation.

As additional chromosome changes may precede the blast-cell transformation, sequential chromosome analysis during the chronic phase should be standard practice in order that treatment may be modified or instituted.

Myelodysplastic syndromes

The concept of chronic disorders of haemopoiesis with a greater or lesser likelihood of progression to acute leukaemia has a long history. *Table 13.12* summarizes the reports and terminology leading to the general acceptance of 'myelodysplastic syndromes' (MDS).

Table 13.12 Terminology used prior to the acceptance of 'myelodysplastic syndromes'

Early isolated reports	1900–49
Pre-leukaemic anaemia	1949
Preleukaemia	1953
Subacute leukaemia	1953
Chronic refractory anaemia with ring sideroblasts	1956
Refractory normoblastic anaemia	1959
Smouldering leukaemia	1963
Oligoblastic leukaemia	1975
Dysmyelopoietic syndrome	1976
Haemopoietic dysplasia	1978
Pre-leukaemic syndrome	1978
Myelodysplasia	1982

The FAB group proposed that all the conditions listed in *Table 13.12* should be grouped under the term 'myelodysplastic syndrome'[78]. MDS has attracted in a few years an extensive literature and several comprehensive reviews[79–81]. For the laboratory haematologist the review of Hamblin and Oscier[82] is particularly useful. MDS is a clonal abnormality of a haemopoietic stem cell with a variety of haematological manifestations with varying degrees of ineffective haemopoiesis. The clonal definition of MDS is important because myeloid dysplasia can be found as temporary, reversible changes associated with drugs, deficiency states and alcohol abuse. Dysplastic changes are seen in AIDS[83] but unless a clonal origin can be demonstrated, should not be considered to be part of MDS.

The frequency of MDS has been variously reported to be similar to that of AML and to being six times more frequent[81]. It is essentially a disease of the elderly but MDS in children and young adults does occur and is usually associated with exposure to cytotoxic or mutagenic drug therapy or with ionizing radiation. Indeed, cases of MDS under the age of 60 are largely those treated for other malignancies.

The recognition that MDS can follow successful treatment for other malignancies has required comparisons between primary or *de novo* MDS (p-MDS) and secondary or treatment-related (t-MDS) disorders.

The aetiology of MDS is unknown and a single factor is unlikely, particularly in the context of the wide variation in presentation. Evidence for both single and multistep pathogenesis has been presented[84, 85].

Blood and bone-marrow abnormalities

The common feature is cytopenia or cytopenias involving more than one cell line. It is emphasized that only one cell line may show evidence of dysplasia and with a limited range of abnormalities.

Erythroid

Blood changes are those of dyserythropoiesis – oval macrocytes with anisocytosis, dimorphism, basophilic stippling, erythroblasts, low number of reticulocytes though occasionally polychromasia, Howell–Jolly bodies. The bone marrow usually shows erythroid hyperplasia, megaloblastic features, ring sideroblasts and cytoplasmic vacuolation. Exceptionally there may be multi-nuclearity, nuclear budding and karyorrhexis.

Leucocytes

The most common features are hypogranular or agranular neutrophils, 'pseudo' Pelger neutrophils[86], abnormal chromatin clumping[87], hypersegmentation, hypogranular eosinophils, neutrophils with multiple nuclear appendages including frequent 'drumsticks' in females. Monocytosis, sometimes with an abnormal horseshoe nucleus or elongated lobes, and promonocytes may be prominent. In the marrow, hypogranularity of granulocyte precursors, asynchronous myelocyte maturation, increased monocytes or promonocytes, increased myeloblasts with agranular (Type I) or granular (Type II) forms are the most common features.

Platelets

Micro-megakaryocytes[88], megakaryocyte nuclear fragments, cytoplasmic fragments/giant platelets and agranular forms are found. Micro-megakaryocytes with abnormal nuclear appearances are a feature of the marrow and megakaryoblasts may be identified.

The FAB classification of MDS [78]

Five types of MDS are defined:

1. *Refractory anaemia (RA)*. The blood picture shows reticulocytopenia, <1% blasts and dysplasia in one, two or three lineages. The bone marrow generally shows erythroid hyperplasia and/or dyserythropoiesis and <5% blasts.
2. *Refractory anaemia with ring sideroblasts (RA-S)*. The general features of RA but with ring sideroblasts representing >15% of erythroblasts in the bone marrow. A dimorphic red-cell picture in the blood film may be a feature.
3. *Refractory anaemia with excess of blasts (RAEB)*. As for RA with 5–20% type I or type II blasts in the marrow. The revised criteria for classification of AML[14] emphasized that if the percentage of blasts in the bone marrow is less than 30% of all nucleated cells or less than 30% of all non-erythroid cells, the diagnosis is MDS. Ring sideroblasts may also be found but the excess of blasts defines the category. Dyshaemopoiesis of granulocytes, erythroblasts and megakaryocytes is always present.
4. *RAEB in transformation (RAEB-T)*. Less than 5% blasts but with Auer rods in the blood. Marrow blasts 20–30% or as for RAEB with Auer rods.
5. *Chronic myelomonocytic leukaemia (CMML)*. The defining feature is $>1 \times 10^9/l$ monocytes in the blood. The bone marrow may show any of the above features + promonocytes.

Scoring systems to assess the qualitative and quantitative laboratory features have been recommended[89].

The proposed classification has not been without its critics[90, 91] and that prognosis was independent of leukaemic transformation[92] and apart from the number of blasts, the morphological features do not appear to form a useful basis for prognosis [93]. This has been confirmed [94, 95] with emphasis that deaths due to cytopenias are more common than transformation to acute leukaemia [95]. There are differences between the morphological findings in t-MDS and p-MDS [96]. Trilineage abnormalities are a feature of t-MDS and marked abnormalities of the erythroblasts are not uncommon. Bone-marrow cellularity is increased in only about 25% of cases. Basophil numbers in the blood and bone marrow may also be increased in about 25% of cases.

Cytogenetics

Using high-resolution banding techniques, abnormal karyotypes have been detected in 79% of cases of MDS [97] and in approximately 60% of patients with p-MDS. The MIC study group recommend that p-MDS should be differentiated from t-MDS [96].

In p-MDS the commonest abnormalities are monosomy 7, trisomy 8 and a variety of deletions particularly 5q− and 7q−, and reciprocal translocations t(1;3), t(2;11), t(6;9) and t(11;21). The 5q− syndrome [98] is associated with a specific variant of MDS – macrocytosis and non-lobulated megakaryocytes in females and are usually classified as RA or RARS with a low incidence of blast transformation. Monosomy 7 and 7q− are usually associated with very short survival. The deletion del(11q) is associated with RA-S. Changes in t-MDS tend to be multiple at diagnosis, but a few single changes have been described. As in p-MDS, del(5q−), del(7q−) and monosomy 5 or 7 are found. In a series of patients with t-MDS 98% had a clonal abnormality and 94% had abnormalities of chromosome 5 and/or 7 either alone or in combination with other changes. Xq13 is associated with RA-S and is associated with transformation to AML. The Ph chromosome is very rare in MDS.

Cytochemistry

Earlier reports of the simultaneous presence of specific and non-specific esterase activity in myeloid cells have been confirmed [99] but are not confined to clonal dysmyelopoeisis. The double-staining cells are granulocytes.

Lysozyme activity demonstrated by cytological technique or by assaying serum and urine levels, indicates a possible monocyte proliferation. Absent myeloperoxidase activity of subpopulations of neutrophils may be demonstrated and the pattern of cells in the peroxidase channel of the Technicon H1 system is particularly useful in this respect. The PAS reaction to demonstrate disordered carbohydrate metabolism of erythroblasts is helpful. Iron staining is essential for the recognition and differentiation of the MDS.

Cell markers

The application of MoAbs to the identification of blast cells in MDS follows that of the acute leukaemias. A particularly useful application is the study of biphenotypic leukaemias [100] and those that evolve from t-MDS [96].

Immunological aspects

The majority of patients with MDS have low lymphocyte counts due to reduction in T cells, primarily a decrease in helper/inducer (CD4) population though the suppressor/cytotoxic (CD8) subset is also reduced[101]. The association between activated T cells, interleukins and interferons may be relevant in the natural history of MDS.

Immunoglobulin abnormalities are common and both high and low levels are found[102]. In a small proportion of cases a monoclonal gammopathy is present and can be due to associated lymphoid or plasma cell neoplasm.

Defective neutrophil function is a common feature of MDS[103] and separately or in association with lymphocyte and immunoglobulin abnormalities may contribute to the high incidence of infection in MDS.

Other laboratory aspects

The features of dyserythropoiesis described in Chapter 12 can also be found in MDS. The majority (80%) show increased Hb F and unbalanced synthesis of globin chains may give rise to Hb H formation. Red-cell membrane abnormalities can result in positive sucrose lysis tests and *in vitro* lysis by high titre cold antibodies, probably due to abnormal complement binding of the cell membrane.

Non-leukaemic myeloproliferative disorders

The term ‘myeloproliferative disorder’ was used by Dameshek to encompass CML, primary proliferative polycythaemia (PPP), myelofibrosis (MF) and essential or primary thrombocythaemia (PT). These disorders have certain haematological similarities: bone-marrow hyperplasia, thrombocytosis, leucocytosis, increase in basophils and presence of immature granulocytes. The disorders are clonal proliferations arising from a pluripotent stem cell. However, unlike CML the other disorders do not show frankly leukaemic blood pictures and again unlike CML the progression to leukaemic blast cell transformation is not an inevitable or even frequent occurrence. CML has been described in the preceding section on chronic leukaemia. The other conditions are regarded as ‘non-leukaemic myeloproliferative disorders’.

Polycythaemia

What constitutes possible polycythaemia?

Polycythaemia is characterized by a raised PCV. The raised PCV increases whole-blood viscosity which is associated with a liability to develop vascular problems resulting in morbidity and mortality. It is accepted that an increased PCV warrants further investigation. The PCV value above which polycythaemia should be considered has been variously stated to be 0.500[104], 0.520[105] and even as high as 0.550[106]. More recently, the upper reference limit for PCV has been established as 0.500 for men and 0.450 for women[107]. In a study examining the relationship between red-cell mass (RCM), plasma volume (PV) and elevated PCV[108], values were >0.510 for men and >0.490 for women. In the large series of the Polycythaemia Vera Study Group[109], PCV of 0.500–0.510 was associated with an increased RCM in 15% of cases. Venous occlusive episodes are significantly more frequent at the 0.500 level[110].

It has been suggested that further studies should only be carried out when the PV is persistently increased on repeated measurements of samples collected under controlled conditions[107]. As the great majority of PCV values are nowadays obtained from automated instruments which compute the PCV from MCV measurement and red-cell count, accurate calibration of the instrument is essential. A spun microhaematocrit should be the arbiter when the value is borderline or as a confirmatory test.

What constitutes an increased RCM or lowered PV?

The expression of RCM and PV studies as ml/kg body weight lacks precision for the diagnosis of absolute polycythaemia, mainly due to the problem of interpretation in obese subjects due to the influence of relatively avascular adipose tissue. Determining lean body weight is not a practical alternative. The ICSH[111] recommended several formulae for predicting RCM and PV which are essentially based on height and weight taking into account sex differences. A significant increase in RCM is taken as >125% of predicted normal[122]. A significant decrease in PV is if its value is <80% of predicted normal[108]. A comprehensive study[108] concluded that predicting RCM and PV from height and weight by various formulae all gave similar results except at extremes of height and weight.

Classification of the causes of persistently increased PCV

1. Primary proliferative polycythaemia – erythropoietin independent.
2. Secondary polycythaemia due to increased erythropoietin production:
   (a) due to decreased blood oxygen saturation:
      (i) high altitude;
      (ii) chronic lung disease;
      (iii) heart disease;
      (iv) high oxygen-affinity haemoglobin; and
      (v) decreased erythrocyte 2,3-DPG level;
   (b) due to inappropriate erythropoietin production:
      (i) tumour (renal carcinoma, ovarian carcinoma, hepatoma etc.);
      (ii) renal abnormality (cysts, hydronephrosis, post-transplant).
3. Familial erythrocytosis with over-production of erythropoietin[113].
4. Idiopathic erythrocytosis[114].
5. Pseudopolycythaemia (relative, spurious, stress polycythaemia; Gaisbock's syndrome).

PPP, secondary polycythaemia and familial and idiopathic erythrocytosis are 'true' polycythaemias in that there is an increased RCM. Pseudopolycythaemias have a RCM <125% of normal and the increased PCV is due to a PV <80% of normal. However, elevation of RCM and reduction of PV within the normal range can together result in a persistent increase in PCV and may be associated with circulatory disturbance[107].

Note

As the haemoglobin and PCV are dependent on MCV as well as red-cell numbers, an elevated haemoglobin level and PCV may be due to an increased MCV rather than an erythrocytosis. For example, a normal red-cell count of $5.5 \times 10^{12}/l$ and a MCV of 88 fl will result in a normal PCV of 0.484; a normal red-cell count of $5.5 \times 10^{12}/l$ and a MCV of 100 fl will result in an increased PCV of 0.550. As the haemoglobin content of red cells is a function of MCV, the haemoglobin concentration would be similarly increased. The anomaly is further complicated by the fact that a normal red-cell count with increased MCV will also produce an increased RCM, the essential criterion of 'polycythaemia'. The increased RCM due to a normal red-cell count with a high MCV can give rise to the same clinical symptoms of an increased red-cell mass due to erythrocytosis with a normal MCV. Conversely erythrocytosis with a low MCV is a recognized presentation of primary polycythaemia, which could result in a normal RCM.

Primary proliferative polycythaemia

Proliferative polycythaemia (PPP) is characteristically a disease of the elderly, more than 90% of cases being over the age of 45. Palpable splenomegaly is found in 75% of patients at presentation. PPP is not the commonest cause of increased PCV and therefore the laboratory investigation and differential diagnosis must include recognition of other causes. The role of erythropoietin in the control of erythropoiesis and the low or normal level of erythropoietin in PPP is clear evidence of the autonomous nature of the red-cell proliferation.

Blood changes in PPP

Red-cell and plasma volume As discussed above the generally accepted criteria for the diagnosis of 'true' polycythaemia is a RCM >125% of predicted normal in both males and females. RCM must be measured, since although haemoglobin level, PCV and red-cell count reflect RCM they do not show good correlation. One reason for the poor correlation is variation in plasma volume in the presence of splenomegaly even though the average plasma volume does not differ from normal. The mean RCM in the PVSG series was 150% of normal with values up to 300%.

Red-cell morphology This is usually normocytic and normochromic but may be microcytic and hypochromic due to iron deficiency caused by chronic gastrointestinal blood loss which is probably exacerbated by platelet dysfunction (*see* page 457). A complication of PPP is the development of bone-marrow fibrosis possibly with extramedullary erythropoiesis and the presence of tear-drop poikilocytes, immature granulocytes and normoblasts and the picture may be indistinguishable from that of myelofibrosis.

The reticulocyte count expressed as a percentage is slightly increased in about 50% of patients and when expressed in absolute numbers is increased in the great majority of cases.

Platelets The platelet count is over $400 \times 10^9/l$ in about two-thirds of patients and may reach $1000 \times 10^9/l$ or even higher. The mean platelet diameter is slightly larger than normal. Additional abnormalities of giant forms, hypogranularity and megakaryocyte nuclei are seen when myelofibrosis supervenes.

Leucocytes The total leucocyte count is over $12 \times 10^9/l$ in about 40% of patients; levels up to $25 \times 10^9/l$ are not uncommon and may rarely reach $50 \times 10^9/l$ or even higher. The pattern of the differential count is an important aspect, with segmented neutrophils being predominant and only occasional metamyelocytes and myelocytes (cf. CGL, MF). An increase in the absolute number of basophils occurs in the majority of cases and is reflected by an increase in blood histamine levels over 10 mg/l in almost all patients. The NAP score is greater than 100 in 70% of patients but does not correlate with the total leucocyte count. Other biochemical findings which probably reflect increased granulocyte mass and turnover are increased serum levels of lysozyme, myeloperoxidase and lactoferrin. Of particular diagnostic interest is the increase in serum vitamin B_{12} level and unsaturated B_{12} binding capacity (UB_{12} BC); both are due to an increase in TCI. Levels of serum B_{12} over 900 ng/l and $UB_{12}BC$ over 2200 ng/l are considered to be useful secondary diagnostic criteria.

Bone-marrow appearances
The changes can only be recognized in sectioned material. Hypercellularity, reduced or absent fat spaces and an increase in megakaryocytes are typical appearances with about one-third of patients at presentation showing increased reticulin and evidence of fibrosis. Assessment of bone-marrow cellularity by 'point-counting', particularly using trephine material [115, 116], shows that cellularity >75% is characteristic of PPP. Cellularity in secondary polycythaemia and pseudopolycythaemia is usually <65%. Iron staining shows that in most patients there is reduced or absent iron stores which reflects the establishment of an increased red-cell mass or/and occult blood loss.

Chromosomes in PPP [117]
PPP is Ph negative though in the rare transformation to CML may become Ph positive. Almost 12% of cases at diagnosis have a clonal chromosome abnormality, the most common being an additional chromosome, + 8 or + 9. The deletion 20q−, though not specific for PPP, is not infrequent in untreated cases.

Platelet function
Paradoxically, in PPP there is a tendency to both thrombosis and haemorrhage. The thrombocytosis and increased blood viscosity can explain the thrombotic tendency and there is *in vitro* evidence of platelet hyperfunction in some myeloproliferative disorders [118]. Platelet aggregation responses, adhesiveness and PF3 availability are often subnormal in the myeloproliferative disorders but the data of some studies are conflicting. Biochemical studies of platelets have shown abnormal lipid peroxidation as judged by the production of malonyl dialdehyde [49].

Red cells containing Hb F (F-cells)
In a minority of cases F-cells may be demonstrated in the circulating blood by the Kleihauer technique or by the more sensitive method using labelled anti-Hb F. In about 10% of the patients in one study the number of F-cells was 30–45% and the Hb F was demonstrable biochemically.

Splenic red-cell volume
The demonstration of splenomegaly is important in differentiating primary and secondary polycythaemia. Apart from clinical examination, ultrasound and isotopic imaging procedures, the measurement of the splenic red-cell pool clearly distinguishes PPP from secondary polycythaemia [120].

Cell culture
In vitro culture of erythroid colonies in the absence and presence of erythropoietin (Epo) can help distinguish between PPP, secondary polycythaemia and idiopathic erythrocytosis [121, 122]. Epo-independent colony growth may also be useful in the diagnosis of PPP in patients without splenomegaly and with a normal splenic red-cell pool [123].

Other causes of polycythaemia

Secondary polycythaemia
Unlike PPP erythropoietin production is increased in secondary polycythaemia and is due either to tissue hypoxia (group 2(a) above) or to inappropriate erythropoietin production associated with tumours or renal ischaemia (group 2(b)). Heart and lung disease resulting in reduced arterial oxygen saturation is the commonest cause of polycythaemia and is recognized by clinical examination and measurement of arterial oxygen saturation. The secondary polycythaemias due to inappropriate Epo production are essentially a clinical rather than a laboratory problem other than establishing routine blood parameters and morphology and the increased RCM. Measurements of serum Epo levels obviously play an important role in investigation.

High-affinity haemoglobins
Of particular haematological interest are the rare inherited abnormal haemoglobins with increased oxygen affinity. Familial polycythaemia has been known for many years and the recognition of the high-affinity variant Hb Chesapeake [124] established an explanation for some cases of familial polycythaemia. Over 80 high-affinity variants have now been recognized, most of which are stable and are associated with polycythaemia. Some high-affinity variants do not have erythrocytosis which may in some instances be due to instability and chronic haemolysis.

When the pO_2 falls in the peripheral circulation a high-affinity haemoglobin will release less oxygen which will result in tissue hypoxia and the stimulation of Epo production with consequent erythrocytosis. The mechanisms by which the oxygen affinity of the abnormal haemoglobin is altered depend on the site of the amino-acid substitution. The equilibrium between the deoxy and oxy conformational states depends on the inter-chain contacts and it is therefore not surprising that about half of the high-affinity haemoglobins have a substitution in the contact areas and in particular the $\alpha_1\beta_2$ contact. Other sites affecting the deoxy conformation are the C-terminal residues and the 2,3-DPG binding sites of the β chain. Most of the remaining substitutions are in these areas of the polypeptide chain. The effect of substitutions in these areas of the haemoglobin molecule affect haem–haem interactions, the Bohr effect and the P_{50} value (pO_2 at 50% oxygen saturation).

High-affinity haemoglobins are best recognized by measuring the oxygen dissociation curve or by measuring the P_{50}. Electrophoresis on cellulose acetate at pH 8.6 and agar at acid pH or by isoelectric focusing will demonstrate only about two-thirds of the variants. Clearly the P_{50} measurement is the screening method of choice. A search for an abnormal haemologlobin and perhaps a family study is indicated in any polycythaemic patient with normal arterial oxygen saturation, without splenomegaly and no apparent secondary cause. The association between high-affinity haemoglobin and polycythaemia, and electrophoretic and functional data has been reviewed[125, 126].

Familial erythrocytosis with over-production of Epo
Genetically determined over-production of Epo, suggested as a cause of polycythaemia for some years, has been confirmed[113, 127].

Idiopathic erythrocytosis
Patients with unexplained persistently high PCV but not fulfilling the criteria of PPP have been termed 'idiopathic erythrocytosis' (IE). In one series[114], 40% of cases developed features of PPP within 6 years. The use of cell culture methods has shown that IE is a heterogenous polycythaemic grouping[128].

Investigation of polycythaemia

The differential diagnosis of the causes of polycythaemia will depend to some extent on the laboratory resources available. After the measurement of RCM to separate pseudo polycythaemia from the true polycythaemias the major problem is to identify PPP and to differentiate the causes of secondary polycythaemia. Arterial oxygen saturation can be used as the initial discriminator and a scheme for the investigation of a persistently raised PCV has been recommended[109]. Measurement of serum Epo levels by immunoradiometric (IRMA) or enzyme-linked immunoabsorbent (ELISA) assays is an alternative starting point.

Myelofibrosis

Myelofibrosis (MF) or myeloid metaplasia, is a clonal proliferative disorder characterized by anaemia, massive splenomegaly, extramedullary haemopoiesis (metaplasia), leucoerythroblastosis and collagenous fibrosis or sclerosis of the bone marrow. Although the haemopoietic cells can be shown to be monoclonal, marrow fibroblasts are not usually derived from the same clone which suggests that the fibrous replacement is a secondary reaction of normal stromal cells to some other abnormality. Bone-marrow fibrosis is found in many diseases, particularly PPP and other proliferative disorders but also in non-malignant disease[129], but clonal myelofibrosis has characteristic clinical and haematological features and is a specific syndrome.

Evidence has been presented that immune complexes play a role in the pathogenesis of MF[130, 131], but other reports have emphasized the probable role of platelets. Platelet-derived growth factor (PDGF) released from platelets or megakaryocytes stimulates fibroblasts to divide and secrete collagen[132]. Degradation of the newly formed collagen can be inhibited by simultaneous release of platelet factor 4 which inhibits collagenase[133]. Release of analogous factors from other cell lines can also result in collagen synthesis.

The disease occurs mainly in the middle-aged and elderly and has a chronic course with a 'short-lived' median survival of 2 years and a 'long-lived' group with a median survival of 10 years[134]. Acute leukaemia supervenes in 10–25% of cases.

The acute form of myelofibrosis (malignant myelosclerosis, acute myelodysplasia with myelofibrosis) is now classified as acute megakaryoblastic leukaemia (M7).

Blood findings

Anaemia is usual and may require regular blood transfusions. The anaemia is multifactorial – ineffective erythropoiesis, shortened red-cell survival, expanded plasma volume and red-cell pooling in the enlarged spleen are usual. Iron deficiency or folate deficiency may develop. The reticulocyte count reflects the degree of effective erythropoiesis. The platelet count may be normal or even elevated though thrombocytopenia is usual but does not correlate well with a clinical bleeding tendency.

Blood-film appearances
All cell lines show changes which together present a picture that is typical of myelofibrosis with extramedullary haemopoiesis. The *red cells* are usually normochromic with anisocytosis and poikilocytosis and in particular show the characteristic 'tear-drop' shapes. Basophilic stippling is often seen and polychromasia reflects a reticulocytosis. Additional features of hypochromia and macrocytosis may reflect the presence of iron or folate deficiency. Erythroblasts are almost always present and all stages of maturity may be seen.

The differential leucocyte count shows immature granulocytes including promyelocytes and myeloblasts which together with the circulating erythroblasts constitute the leucoerythroblastic picture (*see* page 412). Basophils and eosinophils are often present.

Giant platelets, many with abnormal granulation, are a typical feature and megakaryocyte nuclei can usually be found.

The picture as a whole is characteristic of myelofibrosis but occasionally there may be difficulties in differentiating myelofibrosis from early CGL. Myelofibrosis supervening on PPP may also cause problems in differential diagnosis. The NAP score is useful but not definitive; the majority of patients have normal or elevated values in contrast to the low or absent activity of CGL. A low score does not exclude a diagnosis of myelofibrosis.

Bone-marrow changes

Aspiration biopsy can be expected to result in a 'dry-tap' in about 50% of cases; this is most likely when the leucoerythroblastic picture has developed[135] and in association with moderate anaemia and lower leucocyte counts. Trephine biopsy will establish the diagnosis in the majority of cases by the demonstration of collagenous fibrosis with reticulum-cell and megakaryocytic hyperplasia. The histological patterns in MF have been categorized and shown to be associated with prognosis though their significance has been questioned[134].

Cytogenetics

Difficulty in obtaining cells from the fibrotic bone marrow has resulted in limited reports of cytogenetic findings. Assessment of prognosis in relation to abnormalities has been reported[136]. Translocations involving chromosome 1, trisomy 8, 5q−, 13q− and 20q− had the longest survival; presence of the Ph translocation, −7 and 7q− had the shortest survival; normal karyotype had an intermediate prognosis. Another report[137] concluded that cytogenetic abnormalities were not useful in assessing prognosis. No abnormality characteristic of MF has been demonstrated.

Biochemical findings

The biochemical findings associated with increased haemoglobin catabolism and cell destruction are to be expected because of the shortened red-cell survival and ineffective erythropoiesis (*see* page 403). The marked elevation of serum vitamin B_{12} and unsaturated B_{12} binding capacity found in PPP and CML are not found in myelofibrosis.

Radioistope studies in myelofibrosis

The pathophysiology of the anaemia of myelofibrosis is complex. Bone-marrow hyperplasia, extramedullary erythropoiesis in the spleen and/or liver, shortened red-cell life span, increased splenic red-cell pool, splenic destruction of red cells and increased plasma volume all contribute to the degree of anaemia which may be further complicated by haemorrhage. The contribution and interaction of each of the above aspects can be measured using radioisotope tracer techniques. Radio-iron studies will demonstrate the sites and degree of erythropoiesis and measure the degree of effective and ineffective erythropoiesis. Red-cell labelling with ^{51}Cr will measure red-cell life span, sites of sequestration and the splenic red-cell pool. Plasma volume must be measured by dilution of a plasma label rather than by calculation from the red cell and PCV.

Red-cell survival and sites of sequestration are measured by random labelling of autologous red cells followed by serial measurements of blood activity and external scintillation counting (*see* page 339). Red-cell survival shows a mean red-cell life span in the order of 20–40 days, i.e. moderately shortened, with the spleen being in part responsible for the increased destruction.

Measurement of the *splenic red-cell pool* by quantitative imaging may be performed at the commencement of the ^{51}Cr red-cell survival study[138]. Alternatively the RCM and splenic red-cell volume can be measured independently using ^{99m}Tc-labelled red cells. Grossly enlarged spleens may contain as much as 50% of the total red-cell volume.

Total plasma volume is invariably increased in myelofibrosis in the presence of splenomegaly. There is a correlation between plasma volume and spleen size. After splenectomy the plasma volume returns slowly to normal.

Ferrokinetic studies (*see* page 408). Plasma iron clearance and plasma iron turnover are increased in the majority of patients and in most instances reflect increased erythropoietic activity rather than iron depletion, but red-cell iron utilization is usually below normal showing that ineffective erythropoiesis is a feature of myelofibrosis. The typical pattern of *external scintillation counting* in myelofibrosis shows minimal take-up of radio-iron by the sacrum, rapid accumulation in the spleen or liver alone or in both organs, indicating the sites of erythropoiesis (*Figure 13.2*). Complex patterns of activity over the spleen can be interpreted as indicating extramedullary erythropoiesis, destruction and sequestration. In the terminal stages of myelofibrosis, patterns of activity resembling aplastic anaemia may be found (*see Figure 12.1*). Sacral activity may not represent the erythropoietic activity of the skeletal marrow as a whole. The short-lived isotope ^{52}Fe, if available, can be used for whole-body erythropoietic imaging. Erythro- and ferrokinetic studies are considered to be valuable in the diagnosis, prognosis and management of myelofibrosis[139].

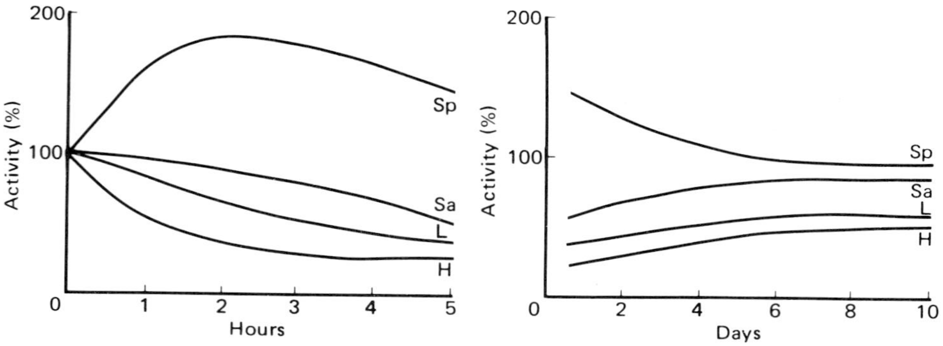

Figure 13.2 Surface counting patterns after intravenous injection of ^{59}Fe-labelled transferrin in a patient with myelofibrosis. Extramedullary erythropoiesis is demonstrated by the rapidly increasing spleen counts with little sacral activity. The activity in the spleen falls slowly in the following days but retains some activity, suggesting ineffective erythropoiesis in the spleen. Surface counting pattern in normal subjects is shown in *Figures 12.1(a)* and *12.3(a)*. H = heart; L = liver; Sa = sacrum; Sp = spleen

Essential or primary thrombocythaemia (PT)

Persistently raised platelet counts $>600 \times 10^9$/l without an apparent cause such as chronic haemorrhage, infection, malignancy, surgery or splenectomy, may be a manifestation of a clonal proliferation which is part of the spectrum of the non-leukaemic myeloproliferative disorders. The terminology may be confusing: 'essential' thrombocythaemia refers to a 'primary' abnormality; 'thrombocythaemia' infers a primary abnormality; 'thrombocytosis' is usually applied to the increased platelet counts secondary to other conditions.

Thrombocythaemia has been defined as platelet counts over 1000×10^9/l but this is an arbitrary figure and the clinical sequelae of thrombocythaemia, haemorrhage and thrombosis may be found when the count is less than 1000×10^9/l, and conversely levels over 1000×10^9/l are not always associated with haemorrhage and thrombosis.

While thrombocythaemia may be the only manifestation of marrow proliferation and be present for a number of years, transformation to PPP is recognized and an increased platelet count may be an early sign of CGL[140].

Transformation to acute leukaemia rarely occurs and may follow chemotherapy or radiotherapy with ^{32}P. Transformation to early T-ALL, M5[141] or leukaemia of mixed lineage including megakaryoblasts[142] has been described.

Blood findings

The platelet count is typically over 1000×10^9/l and may even reach 5000×10^9/l. Platelet morphology is abnormal with giant forms, and megakaryocyte nuclei are often present. As chronic haemorrhage is a major clinical complication, iron deficiency is common and the red cells are microcytic and hypochromic. The tendency of the platelets to block the microcirculation can result in splenic atrophy due to repeated infarction and the blood film will then show the typical features of absent splenic function: Howell–Jolly bodies, acanthocytes and target cells. Most cases have a neutrophil leucocytosis.

Bone-marrow appearances

There is a striking increase in megakaryocytes in a generally hypercellular marrow. The megakaryocytes are larger than normal with hyperlobulation of the nucleus. Reticulin is generally increased.

Cytogenetics

These have generally been unhelpful but 21q— has been described in five consecutive patients at the time of diagnosis[143].

Platelet function

Most cases show abnormal platelet function. Early studies were reported to show defective platelet contribution in tests requiring platelet factor 3, e.g. prothrombin consumption test, thromboplastin generation test. Additional abnormalities are found in response to the addition of ADP and/or adrenaline though response to collagen is variable. Spontaneous aggregation of stirred platelets may be demonstrated. As in the other myeloproliferative disorders, defects of lipid peroxidation may be present. Reduced levels of von Willebrand factor/ristocetin co-factor activity with the loss of large vWf multimers has been reported[144].

Differential diagnosis

As stated above the initial differentiation is from reactive thrombocytosis. Morphological and functional abnormalities are not a feature of thrombocytosis in general, but thrombocytosis following splenectomy may show morphological abnormalities and the picture would be further complicated by the red-cell changes of splenic atrophy. Estimation of serum LDH activity has been suggested as a means of differentiating thrombocythaemia and thrombocytosis, since LDH levels are elevated in thrombocythaemia[145].

After establishing that the increased platelet count is probably a primary proliferation, the problem is to exclude PPP with iron deficiency. Hypochromic anaemia with a red-cell count over 5×10^9/l would suggest PPP but interpretation of measurements of RCM in the presence of microcytosis can be difficult. Correction of RCM to allow for a reduced MCV may be helpful.

Splenic enlargement, growth of erythroid colonies, increased platelet distribution width, increased ATP:ADP platelet nucleotide ratio and clinical ischaemia have been used in a scoring system[146] to differentiate proliferative thrombocythaemia from reactive thrombocytosis.

Techniques in the investigation of the proliferative disorders

Cytochemical techniques

Cytochemical techniques have been used for many years in the study of blood and bone-marrow cells and have been the subject of reviews and textbooks[147–150]. The ICSH have published[151] recommended methods for enzyme cytochemistry for light microscopy of air-dried blood films and bone-marrow preparations and included the practical aspects and principles applied in the selection of the methods. For details of the biochemical and theoretical aspects of cytochemistry, reference[152] is recommended.

With most of the methods and particularly those that demonstrate enzyme activity, freshly fixed films made from fresh blood without added anticoagulant are preferable. Data regarding the influence of anticoagulant and storage of samples are given where available.

Some methods demand the use of reagents known or suspected to be carcinogens. As these substances are often unstable in solution, it is common practice to weigh the powder each time it is required. To reduce unnecessary exposure, bulk preparation and storage at −80°C or at 4°C dissolved in suitable solvents has been recommended[153, 154]. Additional precautions are the use of gloves, mask and a ventilated hood when weighing powders, no mouth pipetting and immediate cleaning of any spills.

The reactivity of different batches of substrates and couplers may vary and each batch should be tested and the optimum concentration determined.

Peroxidase (Px) reaction

Principle

Myeloperoxidase (MPx) catalyses the transfer of two electrons from the substrate to hydrogen peroxide with the production of oxidized substrate and water. The oxidized substrate is precipitated at the site of MPx activity as blue or brown granules as seen by light microscopy.

Blood samples

Blood samples in EDTA are suitable if films are made within 2 hours of collection. Unfixed films may be stored for up to 4 weeks, in the dark, at room temperature.

Reagents

The traditional substrate for MPx was benzidine. The regulations regarding the production and handling of benzidine and its derivatives make it impractical to expect its continued use. A variety of alternative substrates have been suggested including benzidine hydrochloride, *o*-tolidine, 2,7-fluorenediamine and 3-amino-9-ethylcarbazole, each of which are known carcinogens; 3,3-diaminobenzidine has been listed as hazardous. Hanker–Yates reagent (*p*-phenylenediamine and pyrocatechol) has been recommended and 4-chloro-l-naphthol has a low risk.

Diaminobenzidine method[151]

Reagents

(a) Fixative: 3% glutaraldehyde in 60% acetone. Mix 60 ml acetone in 40 ml distilled water. Add 4.3 ml of 70% glutaraldehyde (i.e. 12 ml of 25% glutaraldehyde). Keep in the freezer compartment of a refrigerator.
(b) 0.5 M Tris-HCl buffer pH 7.6: Tris-HCl base 1.818 g and Trizma base (Sigma) 0.417 g. Dissolve the bases in 300 ml distilled water.
(c) Substrate: 3,3′-diaminobenzidine (DAB). This is available in 10 mg vials (Sigma).
(d) 3% H_2O_2.

Incubation solution
Measure 10 mg of 3,3′-diaminobenzidine into a beaker, add 40 ml of buffer and then 0.13 ml of 3% H_2O_2. Alternatively, add 10 ml of buffer to a vial of DAB; mix thoroughly, empty into 0.13 ml of 3% H_2O_2.

Shake the mixture vigorously for 2–3 minutes; some black particles may remain. Filter rapidly into a Coplin jar.

Procedure
1. Fix films for 1 minute in the fixative kept in the freezer compartment of a refrigerator.
2. Rinse briefly in running tap water.
3. Place in the incubation mixture for 10 minutes at room temperature.
4. Rinse for 2 minutes in running tap water.
5. Counterstain in Mayer's haematoxylin for 5–10 minutes.
6. Rinse briefly in tap water and then air dry.

Results
Sites of peroxidase activity are golden brown colour. The advantage of this method is that the reaction product is formed slowly, and over-incubation with crystalline precipitate is not a problem. Although peroxidase activity decreases with age of the film, unfixed films will still contain demonstrable enzyme sites for 4 weeks. The method is particularly suitable for demonstrating Auer rods and Phi bodies when stained at pH 9.5.

3-Amino-9-ethylcarbazole method [151]

If the spread films contain much fat, immerse for 1 minute in diethyl ether and then dry in air; do not rinse.

Reagents
(a) Fixative: 10 ml 37% formaldehyde in 90 ml absolute ethyl alcohol. Store at room temperature.
(b) Incubation solution: Dissolve 10 mg of 3-amino-9-ethylcarbazole in 6 ml of dimethylsulphoxide. Add to 50 ml of 0.1 mol/l sodium barbitone-HCl buffer, pH 7.4. Add 0.5 ml of 0.3% H_2O_2.

Procedure
1. Fix in the fixative for 30 s at room temperature. Rinse briefly and air dry.
2. Place in the incubation mixture for 15 minutes at room temperature.
3. Wash in running water.
4. Counterstain in acid Mayer's haematoxylin for 15 minutes.
5. Mount in glycerine jelly.

Results
Cytochemical reaction product stains red; nuclei stain blue. Although not as sensitive as the DAB method for the study of leukaemic blasts, it is useful for the assessment of peroxidase-negative neutrophil populations in blood.

Interpretation

MPx is a lysosomal enzyme normally found in the azurophil granules of granulocytes and monocytes and in the specific granules of eosinophils, though eosinophil MPx is a distinct entity and is cyanide resistant. MPx activity may be demonstrated in myeloblasts which by light microscopy are devoid of granules. The reaction in myeloblasts is stronger and coarser than that of the finely granular appearance of the monocyte series: in the more primitive or undifferentiated monoblast, MPx is usually absent. Auer rods are MPx positive. The blasts of ALL are negative by light microscopy. Myeloperoxidase activity closely parallels Sudanophilia. Additional applications are in the demonstration of the absence of MPx in neutrophils in myelodysplasia, and in hereditary MPx deficiency.

Notes

The demonstration and localization of peroxidase activity by transmission electron microscopy in glutaraldehyde-fixed or unfixed cells using 3,3′-diaminobenzidine (DAB) as substrate is valuable for demonstrating activity that cannot be shown by light microscopy[155]. Of particular interest is the demonstration of a specific platelet peroxidase in megakaryoblasts and a peroxidase-like enzyme in hairy cells and in a small proportion of cases of apparent null-ALL[156].

Sudan Black B

Principle

Sudan Black B is an inert diazo dye with an affinity for polar phospholipids and sterols but the specificity of the reaction with blood and bone-marrow cells is uncertain. With the addition of phenol as a mordant there is a relationship to peroxidase activity, though some differences in the pattern of staining are seen. Two techniques are widely used: (1) Sudan Black in absolute ethanol with added phenol after formalin fixation; and (2) formal–ethanol fixation and a saturated solution of Sudan Black in 70% ethanol. The former technique is described[150].

Blood samples collected into EDTA are satisfactory. Sudanophilic material is stable in unfixed films for several days.

Reagents

(a) Fixative: 40% formaldehyde.
(b) Buffer: dissolve 16 g phenol in 30 ml ethanol. Add to an aqueous solution of 0.3% $Na_2HPO_4 12H_2O$.
(c) Stock solution Sudan Black B: dissolve 0.3 g Sudan Black B in 100 ml absolute ethanol.
(d) Working solution: mix 40 parts buffer and 60 parts stock stain, filter and use immediately.

Method

1. Fix air-dried films in formaldehyde vapour for 5–10 minutes.
2. Wash well in running tap water.
3. Stain for 60 minutes.
4. Wash in 70% ethanol and destain in further 70% ethanol to remove background stain deposit.

5. Wash in water.
6. Counterstain with Romanowsky stain or 1% methyl green or neutral red particularly when blast cell reactions may be weak.

Results
Sudanophilic material stains dark brown/black. Megakaryocytes, platelets, erythroblasts, plasma cells and lymphocytes are negative. Neutrophils and precursors are stongly positive. Eosinophils are positive with a characteristic appearance, basophils are variable. Myeloblast activity usually parallels peroxidase activity with a few positive granules. Monocytes tend to show fine granular staining. Positive cells are sometimes seen in ALL and for this reason it is recommended that both Sudan Black and peroxidase reactions are routinely performed in acute leukaemia.

Oil Red O

Blood samples
As for Sudan Black B.

Reagents
(a) Fixative: 40% formalin.
(b) Oil Red O: 2 g/l in propan-2-ol (isopropyl alcohol). Keeps indefinitely.
(c) Working stain: 60 ml stock solution and 40 ml distilled water
(d) 50% propan-2-ol.

Method
1. Fix air-dried films in formalin vapour for 15 minutes and wash briefly in 50% propan-2-ol.
2. Immerse in the stain for 30 minutes at room temperature and rinse in 50% propan-2-ol.
3. Counterstain with Romanowsky stain or haematoxylin.

Results
Oil-Red-O-positive material is orange.

Applications
The major application is in ALL. Coarse droplets are found in the cytoplasmic vacuoles of the blasts in L3 (Burkitt's type ALL) which are PAS-negative. In other types of ALL, Oil Red O and PAS-positive material are often present[157].

Periodic acid–Schiff (PAS) reaction

Principle
Periodic acid oxidizes 1–2 glycol groups to produce a dialdehyde which reacts with Schiff's leucobasic fuchsin to produce a magenta colour. A positive reaction is given by mono- and polysaccharides, glyco- and mucoproteins and cerebrosides. Over-oxidation may lead to false-negative results. Positivity in haemic cells is usually due to glycogen which can be distinguished from PAS-positive high-molecular-weight compounds by its sensitivity to salivary amylase (diastase) digestion.

Blood samples
Blood or marrow samples in EDTA are satisfactory. Films previously fixed in methanol or stained by Romanowsky are stable for many years. Previous Romanowsky staining must be completely removed by prolonged immersion and washing in absolute methanol.

Reagents
(a) Fixative: Absolute methanol.
(b) Periodic acid: 10 g/l, stores for months at 4°C in a dark bottle.
(c) Schiff's reagent: Dissolve 1 g basic fuchsin in 400 ml hot distilled water. Cool to 50°C and filter. Add 1 ml of thionyl chloride ($SOCl_2$) and stand in the dark for 12 hours. In a fume cupboard, add 2 g activated charcoal, shake and filter. Store in a dark bottle at 4°C.

Method
1. Films are fixed in methanol for 15 minutes, washed in running water and allowed to dry.
2. Control films for diastase digestion are exposed to diastase solution (1 g in 1 litre of 9 g/l NaCl) at room temperature for 60 minutes.
3. The slides are immersed in periodic acid for 10 minutes at room temperature.
4. Rinse in running water.
5. Counterstain with haematoxylin.

Results
Glycogen stains magenta and gives a negative reaction in diastase-treated films. Positivity may appear as a diffuse pale pink or deep magenta colour, show fine or coarse granulation, or 'block' positivity.

With normal haemic cells, myeloblasts are negative with diffuse positivity appearing with maturation, the mature neutrophil showing intense diffuse positivity. Other mature granulocytes show a diffusely positive cytoplasm and negative specific granules. Monocytes show fine, scattered positive granules. Erythroblasts are negative. Megakaryocytes show diffuse and scattered granular positivity; platelets are strongly positive. Lymphocytes contain a few discrete granules in 10–40% of cells with 1–2% showing clumped material.

In haematological disorders the pattern and amount of positive material can be quite abnormal. In dyserythropoietic states erythroblasts are often positive. Diffuse positivity is seen in moderate to severe iron deficiency, thalassaemia, sideroblastic anaemia, myelofibrosis, etc. Strong diffuse, granular or block positivity is often a feature of the disordered erythropoiesis in erythroleukaemia (M6). Myeloblasts may show diffuse or granular positivity and monocytic cells may show blocks of glycogen. In cALL, coarse granules or blocks are common but are infrequent in T-ALL. The PAS reaction is therefore of limited value in differentiating the cell lines involved in acute leukaemia.

In the chronic lymphoproliferative disorders, granular positivity is present in a majority of the lymphocytes in B-CLL and B-PLL while only a small number of positive cells are found in the rarer T-CLL. Strong diffuse or granular reactions are seen in HCL with weak or negative findings in Sezary cells as might be expected from their T-cell origin.

Feulgen reaction for DNA

Principle
Free pentose aldehyde groups are liberated from DNA by mild acid hydrolysis and are reacted with Schiff's reagent.

Blood samples
Blood samples in EDTA are satisfactory. Fixed films are stable almost indefinitely.

Reagents
(a) Fixative: methanol 85 ml; 40% formaldehyde 10 ml; glacial acetic acid 5 ml.
(b) 1 mol hydrochloric acid.
(c) Schiff's reagent (*see* PAS reaction, page 468).

Method
1. Air-dried films are fixed for 10 minutes.
2. Wash and immerse in HCl at 37°C for 1 hour.
3. After rinsing, the slides are placed in Schiff's reagent for 30 minutes.
4. Rinse and counterstain with Romanowsky stain.

Results
DNA is stained magenta; RNA does not react and therefore nucleoli appear as vacuoles with a stained rim. Inclusions of nuclear origin such as Howell–Jolly bodies show a positive reaction.

Applications
In routine morphology the reaction has little application other than the demonstration of nucleoli. The major application is in the quantitative measurement of DNA by microdensitometry in the study of cells in interphase.

Note
For quantitative microdensitometry a longer period of fixation and exposure to 5 mol/l HCl at room temperature produces more reproducible results.

Methyl green–pyronin for RNA [158]

Principle
Methyl green is specific for DNA and pyronin stains RNA. The specificity of the pyronin staining can be determined by abolishing the reaction by digestion with ribonuclease.

Blood samples
Blood samples in EDTA are satisfactory. Fixed films are stable indefinitely.

Reagents
(a) Fixative: 10 ml glacial acetic acid, 60 ml ethanol, 30 ml chloroform.
(b) Acetate–HCl buffer, pH 3.8: 50 ml 1 mol/l anhydrous sodium acetate, 42 ml 1 mol/l HCl, made up to 250 ml with distilled water.

(c) Staining solution: 4 ml 20 g/l methyl green, 6 ml 20 g/l pyronin Y, 2 ml absolute ethanol, made up to 100 ml with acetate–HCl buffer. The mixture is stable for 1 week.

The methyl green and pyronin solutions should be extracted repeatedly with chloroform until the chloroform phase is colourless.

Method

1. Air-dried films are fixed for 5 minutes, rinsed and allowed to dry.
2. Immerse the slides in staining solution for 45 seconds.
3. Rinse *briefly* and dry.

Applications

In general pyroninophilia follows the cytoplasmic basophilia of Romanowsky staining. Primitive haemic cells are therefore pyronin positive with decreasing intensity as the cells mature. The notable exception is the deeply basophilic, mature plasma cell which shows intense pyroninophilia reflecting RNA content associated with immunoglobulin synthesis. Reactive lymphocytes associated with autoimmune disorders and infection are also pyronin positive. Döhle bodies in toxic neutrophils and in the neutrophils in May–Hegglin anomaly, though not identical, contain RNA.

Azo-dye coupling techniques

Azo-dye coupling techniques are routinely used for the demonstration of phosphatases and esterases. Azo dyes are formed by the coupling of a diazonium salt with naphthol, or a naphthol derivative, liberated from a substrate by enzyme action, to form a brightly coloured insoluble azo dye. The insoluble complex precipitates at its point of reaction provided that the coupling rate is faster than the diffusion rate. As the coupling reaction is pH dependent, a technique must take into account the optimum pH of the enzyme and the optimum pH of the coupling reaction. If the pH is similar, 'point' or granular activity is found. If the reaction occurs at differing pH a 'diffuse' reaction is more likely. With some techniques the chosen pH is a compromise.

Methods of fixation are a compromise between cell adhesion to the slide, penetration of reagents and maintaining localization of enzyme activity, against denaturation of protein and variable inactivation of enzymes. Fixatives include methanol, ethanol, acetone and formaldehyde either singly or in combination. Cold fixation for as short a period as possible is the general rule.

Alkaline phosphatase

Choice of method

The ICSH recommend naphthol AS-BI phosphate/Fast violet B and the AS-MX phosphate/Fast Blue BB methods. The method of Rutenberg *et al.* [159] using naphthol-AS-phosphate and Fast Blue BB is mentioned as being quite satisfactory, is widely used and is described below. Delay in fixation of fresh blood films has a minimal effect on activity and the azo dye is stable.

Principle
In the presence of activating magnesium ions alkaline phosphatase hydrolyses naphthol-AS-phosphate at pH 9.1 and the liberated naphthol is coupled with the diazonium salt Fast Blue BB to form an insoluble blue precipitate.

Blood samples
Fresh air-dried films are preferred. Samples collected into EDTA show significant loss of activity after 30 minutes. Fixation of fresh films may be delayed at least 24 hours without significant loss of activity. Fixed films may be stored, packed tightly, at 4°C for at least 6 weeks, which permits the use of stored films for quality control.

Reagents
(a) Fixative: absolute methanol 90 ml, neutral formaldehyde 40%, 10 ml. It is essential to avoid using acidic formaldehyde which should therefore be stored over calcium carbonate. The fixative is stored and used at 4°C.
(b) Tris buffer, pH 9.1: Tris (hydroxymethyl) aminomethane (24.23 g/l), 250 ml; 1 mol/l HC1 5 ml. Make up to 1 litre with distilled water.
(c) Stock substrate: dissolve 30 mg naphthol-AS-phosphate sodium salt (Sigma) in 0.5 ml N,N-dimethylformamide, add 100 ml Tris buffer; stable at 4°C for several months.
(d) Fast Blue BB: Sigma, purified grade.
(e) Neutral red: 1 g/l aqueous solution.

Method
Fix air-dried films for 30 seconds at 4°C. Rinse in tap water and allow to dry. To 10 ml stock substrate, allowed to warm to room temperature, is added 10 mg Fast Blue BB. Stir to dissolve and filter, preferably directly on to the slides. The working solution *must be used within 4 minutes of preparation*. Flood slides with the working solution at room temperature for 15 minutes. Slides can be examined and scored without mounting for up to 8 hours, but some immersion oils will cause fading. A neutral mounting medium may be used.

Results
Alkaline phosphatase activity is indicated by bright blue granules. Activity in the blood is virtually confined to 'band' and segmented neutrophils. Monocytes, lymphocytes, erythroblasts, platelets, basophils and usually eosinophils are negative. In normal bone marrow, positivity is seen in reticuloendothelial cells and osteoblasts.

Scoring of neutrophil activity (NAP)
The intensity of staining and number of positive granules can be scored as follows:

0 = Negative or colourless.
1 = Faint diffuse positivity or occasional granules.
2 = Diffuse positivity with moderate number of granules.
3 = Strong positivity with numerous granules.
4 = Very strong positivity with numerous granules often obscuring the nucleus.

100 band or segmented neutrolphils are scored, giving a possible total of 0–400. Earlier neutrophils must not be included. A source of error is inadequate counterstaining and failure to identify and include neutrophils with no activity. The

scoring technique is obviously subjective, but reasonable correlation between different observers can be obtained.

Quality control should include films, previously fixed and stored, of known score. It is insufficient simply to use slides of 'normal' and 'increased' activity.

The normal range is 20–100, but each laboratory must determine its own normal reference range with their technique, reagents and scoring criteria.

Significance and application
The major use of the NAP is in the study of CGL and the non-leukaemic myeloproliferative disorders. Normal or high scores are found in PPP, MF and PT. A low score or absent activity is found in CGL. High scores are also found in infections, pregnancy, active Hodgkin's disease and in aplastic anaemia. Low scores are found in PNH. NAP scores are usually low in AML and normal or high in ALL but are of limited practical value partly because of the difficulty in identifying sufficient neutrophils for scoring.

Alkaline phosphatase activity other than in neutrophils may occasionally be seen in the blasts in AML and in the cells of lymphoproliferative disorders. In the latter case the activity may be that of N-alkaline phosphatase which differs from NAP in its substrate specificity (reviewed in reference [148]).

Acid phosphatase [151]

Choice of technique
The techniques for demonstrating acid phosphatase illustrate the compromise between optimum pH of enzyme activity (pH 5.0) and that of the coupling reaction; diazonium dyes react better at alkaline pH. Although the isoenzymes of acid phosphatase have differing substrate affinities, naphthol AS-BI phosphoric acid and AS-BI phosphate are the most suitable. Fast garnet GBC is a rapid and sensitive coupler and is suitable for demonstrating tartrate-resistant acid phosphatase (TRAP) activity in hairy-cell leukaemia.

Principle
Acid phosphatase hydrolyses naphthol AS-BI phosphoric acid at pH 5.0 and the liberated naphthol couples with fast garnet GBC to form a brick-red product.

Blood samples
Samples in EDTA appear to be satisfactory for 24 hours. Films may be stored for up to 2 weeks without prior fixation or cold storage.

Reagents
(a) Fixative: methanol-acetone mixture: Add 10 ml of methanol to 90 ml of 60% acetone in 0.03 mol/l citrate buffer. Adjust pH of this solution to 5.4 with 1 mol/l NaOH or HCl. Store at about 4°C. This fixative is stable for at least 1 month.
(b) Substrate solution: Dissolve 10 mg of naphthol AS-BI phosphoric acid in 0.5 ml of N-N′-dimethylformamide. Add 0.1 mol/l acetate buffer, pH 5.0 to a final volume of 10 ml. This solution is stable at about 4°C for 2 months.

(c) Incubation medium: Dissolve 5 mg of fast garnet GBC in 10 ml of substrate solution. Filter before use. Tartrate-containing medium is prepared by adding 75 mg/l L(+) tartaric acid and 5 mg of fast garnet GBC to 10 ml of substrate solution. Adjust pH of this solution to 5.0 with concentrated NaOH solution. Filter and use immediately.

Procedure
1. Fix smears with cold methanol-acetone mixture for 30 seconds. Wash briefly with distilled water. Air dry.
2. Incubate smears in incubating medium with or without tartaric acid at 37°C for 45 minutes.
3. Wash with water. Counterstain with Mayer's haemalum for 1–5 minutes.
4. Wash with water, dry and mount with glycerine jelly.

Results
Acid phosphatase activity is shown as a granular or diffuse brick-red precipitate.

Application and interpretation
Acid phosphatase is found in most mature and immature blood and bone-marrow cells. The distribution of the isoenzymes in normal cells is shown in *Table 13.13*. The activity in normal lymphocytes is weak with no clear difference between T and B cells.

Table 13.13 Distribution of isoenzymes of acid phosphatase in normal cells

	Isoenzyme			
Cell	*1*	*2*	*3*	*4*
Neutrophils	++	++	−	++
Lymphocytes	−	−	+	−
Monocytes	++	−	−	++
Platelets	−	−	+	−

Additional isoenzymes are found in Gaucher's disease (0), AML (3b) and most importantly in HCL (5). All isoenzymes are inhibited by the presence of tartrate with the exception of 5, which is typically but not consistently tartrate resistant (TRAP).

Although acid phosphatase in normal lymphocytes is of limited interest, in B-CLL activity is low while in the much less common T-CLL the majority of cells show block or granular positivity. Similarly in T-ALL the majority of blasts in most cases show localized paranuclear positivity. In HCL the reaction is stronger than in CLL and in the presence of tartrate the reaction is equally intense or even stronger. However, the TRAP reaction is now recognized as not being specific for HCL and acid phosphatase activity may be weak in some cases of HCL and may be inhibited by tartrate.

β-Glucuronidase

Principle
β-glucuronidase is an acid hydrolase present in most tissues and is located mainly in the lysosomes and other microsomal fractions. The enzyme hydrolyses naphthol AS-BI glucuronide at pH 5.0, and the liberated naphthol is coupled with hexazotized pararosaniline.

Blood samples
EDTA samples are satisfactory. Heparin is inhibitory. Activity decreases rapidly in unfixed films but they may be stored at −20°C for up to 2 years. Fixed films may be stored at 4°C.

Reagents
(a) Fixative: absolute methanol 70 ml; 40% formaldehyde 30 ml. Store at 4°C.
(b) Acetate buffer 0.2 mol/l, pH 5.2: acetic acid, 2.26 ml glacial acetic acid made up to 100 ml with distilled water. Sodium acetate solution, dissolve 3.3 g anhydrous sodium acetate in 100 ml water. Mix 14.8 ml diluted acetic acid and 35.2 ml sodium acetate solution and make up to 200 ml with distilled water.
(c) Substrate stock solution: dissolve 4 mg naphthol AS-BI glucuronide in 1 ml 0.05 mol/l sodium bicarbonate and make up to 100 ml with 0.2 mol/l acetate buffer, pH 5.
(d) Pararosaniline: 1 g pararosaniline hydrochloride (Sigma) in 20 ml distilled water; add 5 ml concentrated HCl. Store in the dark.
(e) Sodium nitrite: 40 g/l freshly prepared.
(f) Working solution: immediately before use add 0.3 ml pararosaniline to 0.3 ml sodium nitrite, leave 1 minute and add 10 ml stock substrate. Adjust to pH 5.2 with 1 mol/l NaOH if necessary and make up to 20 ml with distilled water. Filter before use.

Method
Fix films in formal–methanol for 60 seconds at 4°C, rinse and allow to dry. Immerse slides for 60 minutes in working solution at 37°C. Rinse in distilled water and counterstain with methyl green or aqueous haematoxylin.

Results
β-glucuronidase activity is shown by a red preciptate.

Note
After fixation some workers freeze the films for 60 minutes at −20°C.

Applications
β-glucuronidase activity closely parallels that of acid phosphatase but is weaker in HCL. The chronic T-cell proliferations, i.e. T-CLL and Sezary syndrome, show increased activity. Plasma cells in myeloma show strong activity.

Esterase activity

Esterases are a group of enzymes capable of hydrolysing a variety of aliphatic or aromatic esters at acid or neutral pH. Those with a preference for short-chain esters such as butyrate and acetate are termed 'non-specific esterases' (NSE) and are inhibited by fluoride. The esterase isoenzymes of granulocytes and mast cells hydrolyse naphthol AS-D chloracetate, are fluoride resistant, and are referred to as 'specific esterase' or chloracetate esterase (CE) activity. NSE activity of monocytes, megakaryocytes, lymphocytes and plasma cells is best demonstrated with α-naphthyl butyrate (ANB) and α-naphthyl acetate (ANA); ANB appears to be more selective for monocyte isoenzymes at pH 6.3 using hexazotized pararosaniline as coupler. ANB can also be used to demonstrate fluoride-resistant localized activity in a proportion of T lymphocytes and shows a pattern of activity in HCL which is considered to be characteristic. NSE activity is also found in megaloblasts and the erythroblasts in M6. CE is extremely stable and for blood films naphthol AS-D chloracetate with fast garnet GBC or new fuchsin as coupler gives good results.

For the differentiation of AML it is useful to demonstrate NSE and CE activities in the same film and a 'combined esterase' method can be used. The less stable NSE is stained first followed by the stable CE. Pararosaniline is used in the NSE reaction and Fast Blue BBN for CE to allow good colour contrast between monocytic and granulocytic cell lines. Alternatively, a single incubation method[160] can be used.

The esterase activity of mast cells can be specifically demonstrated using naphthol AS ε-aminocaproate as substrate[150].

Non-specific esterase reaction [151]

Alpha-naphthyl butyrate method

Reagents

(a) Fixative: buffered formal acetone, pH 6.6: Formaldehyde, 1 volume, 60% acetone in 0.1 mol/l phosphate buffer, pH 6.6, 2 volumes. Keep in the refrigerator at about 4°C.
(b) 100 mg α-naphthyl butyrate (20 mg/ml) in 5 ml ethylene glycol monoethyl ether. Store at 4°C.
(c) Add together 38 ml 0.066 mol/l phosphate buffer, pH 6.3; 0.2 ml hexazotized pararosaniline and 2 ml (40 mg) of the α-naphthyl butyrate solution. Filter before use.

Procedure

1. Fix smears in cold fixative for 30 seconds; wash and air dry.
2. Incubate in the mixed reagent for 45 minutes at room temperature. Rinse in water.
3. Counterstain with methyl green for 2 minutes. Rinse in water and air dry.
4. Mount in a synthetic mounting medium.

Results

Enzyme activity is seen as diffuse, dark-red staining in the cytoplasm of monocytes and histiocytes. Focal staining is a characteristic of T lymphocytes.

Chloracetate esterase reaction [148, 149]

New fuchsin method

Reagents

(a) Fixative: buffered formalin–acetone solution (*see* above).
(b) 4% sodium nitrite solution; freshly prepared.

(c) New fuchsin solution: dissolve 1 g of new fuchsin in 25 ml of 2 M hot hydrochloric acid. Allow to cool and then filter. Stable for 2 months. Allow the new fuchsin solution to react with an equal volume of 4% sodium nitrite for one minute immediately before use. This results in hexazotization.
(d) 1% methyl green solution.
(e) Naphthol-AS-D-chloracetate solution: dissolve 10 mg of naphthol-AS-D-chloracetate in 5.0 ml of N-N′-dimethylformamide. Store at about 4°C.

Procedure
1. Fix smears in cold buffered formalin–acetone for 30 seconds. Wash with distilled water and dry.
2. Incubate fixed smears at room temperature for 10 minutes in the following solution without filtering. Phosphate buffer (0.066 mol/l, pH 7.4), 9.5 ml; fresh hexazotized new fuchsin, 0.05 ml; naphthol-AS-D-chloracetate solution, 0.5 ml. Do not filter.
3. Wash with tap water.
4. Counterstain with methyl green solution for 2 minutes.
5. Rinse in tap water, dry, mount in synthetic mounting medium.

Results
Enzyme activity is seen as bright red granules in the cytoplasm of mast cells and neutrophilic granulocytes, including promyelocytes and many myeloblasts. An occasional monocyte may also be weakly positive.

Comments
All solutions except the fresh sodium nitrite solution are stable for at least 1 month after preparation. The sodium nitrite may be kept at 4°C for 1 week without affecting the cytochemical reaction for chloracetate esterase.

Combined esterase – double incubation method [148]

Reagents
(a) Fixative: buffered formalin–acetone pH 6.6 (*see* above).
(b) Hexazotized pararosaniline: mix equal volumes of pararosaniline and 4% sodium nitrite for 1 minute before use.
(c) Substrate 1: dissolve 100 mg α-naphthyl butyrate in 5 ml ethylene glycol monoethyl ether. Store at 4°C.
(d) Substrate 2: dissolve 10 mg naphthol-AS-D-chloracetate in 5 ml N-N-dimethylformamide. Store at 4°C.
(e) Phosphate buffer 0.066 M pH 6.6.
(f) Phosphate buffer 0.066 M pH 7.4.
(g) Fast Blue BBN.
(h) Mayer's haematoxylin.

Method
1. Fix films with cold formalin–acetone for 30 seconds. Wash with water.
2. Place in the following mixture, filtered before use, at RT for 30–60 minutes: buffer pH 6.6 38 ml; fresh hexazotized pararosaniline 0.4 ml; α-naphthyl butyrate solution 2 ml.
3. Rinse well in water.

4. Place in the second incubation solution at RT for 5–10 minutes consisting of: buffer pH 7.4 38 ml; Fast Blue BBN 40 mg; naphthol-AS-D-chloracetate 2 ml. This solution should NOT be filtered before use.
5. Rinse well in water.
6. Lightly counterstain with Mayer's haematoxylin.
7. Dry and mount with Permount mounting medium.

Result
Butyrate esterase activity is seen as a dark red precipitate in the cytoplasm on monocytes and histiocytes. Chloracetate esterase is seen as a blue granular precipitate in the cytoplasm of neutrophil granulocytes. Individual cells showing both butyrate and chloracetate esterase activities are not seen in normal preparations but are found in myelodysplasia and in hypergranular variants of promyelocytic leukaemia (M3).

Other cytochemical reactions
β-glucosaminidase activity shows very similar reactions to that of β-glucuronidase but is usually quite negative in B-cell proliferations.

Diaminopeptidase IV (DAPIV) has been used as a marker for CD4+ T-CLL and T-PLL [150].

Cell marker techniques

The development, production and availability of labelled monoclonal antibodies against a multiplicity of cellular antigens, together with the introduction of labels other than fluorochromes, has broadened the use of immunocytochemistry in leukaemia diagnosis and differentiation.

The requirement of harvesting 'mononuclear' and leukaemic cells from whole blood and reacting the cells in suspension or as cytospin preparations with fluorochrome-labelled antibody has been supplemented by the use of films of blood, bone marrow or biopsy imprints and of sectioned material, and the detection and localization of cell markers with enzyme-labelled antibodies. Additional methods use antibodies conjugated to colloidal gold particles and antibody-coated red cells or polyacrylamide beads.

Cell rosette methods using sheep and mouse red cells to detect T and B lymphocytes respectively have been largely superseded. The sheep-cell rosette, once the 'gold standard' for T-cell lineage does not detect the early thymocyte recognized by CD7. Although mouse-cell rosetting shows differences between B-cell proliferations, alternative markers of differentiation are available.

Immunofluorescence

First described in 1941, the fluorescent antibody or immunofluorescence (IF) technique is rapid but requires a fluorescence microscope or fluorescence-activated flow cytometer. Direct or one-stage reaction with antigen uses fluorochrome-conjugated primary antibodies. An indirect or two-stage procedure using unlabelled primary antibody followed by labelled second antibody against the primary antibody is more sensitive (*Figure 13.3*). Unfixed cells obtained by density gradient separation from red cells and granulocytes are reacted in tubes or

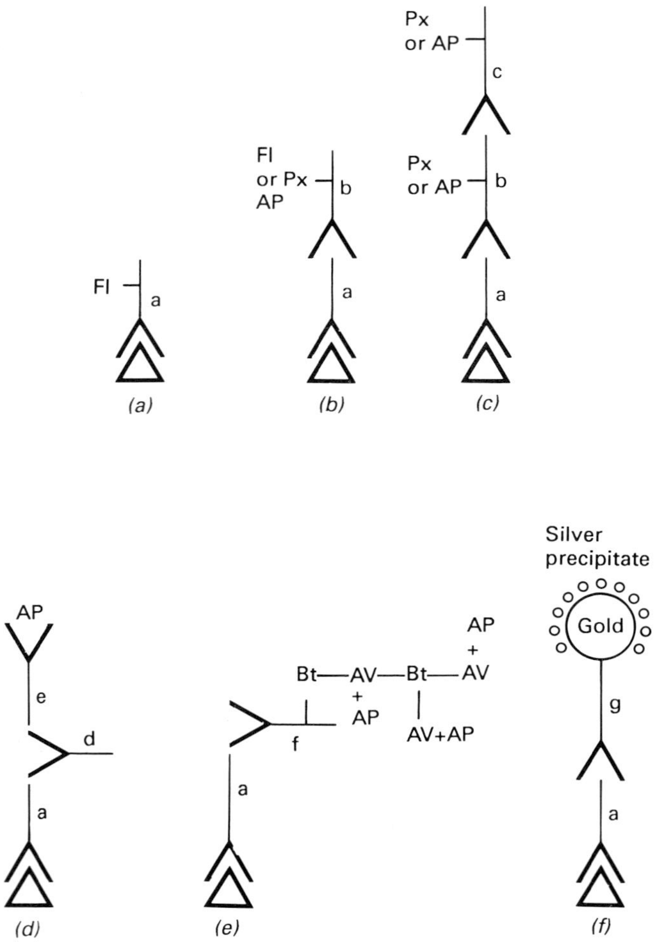

Figure 13.3 Immunocytochemical labelling techniques: (*a*) direct (IF); (*b*) indirect two-stage (IF, PAP); (*c*) indirect three-stage (Px, AP); (*d*) unlabelled antibody bridge (APAAP); (*e*) avidin–biotin complex method; (*f*)immunogold. Fl, Px, AP = label; a = mouse monoclonal antibody; b = labelled rabbit anti-mouse Ig; c = labelled swine anti-rabbit Ig; d = unlabelled rabbit anti-mouse Ig; e = mouse monoclonal anti-enzyme antibody; f = biotin-conjugated rabbit anti-mouse Ig; g = rabbit anti-mouse Ig coated gold particle

microtitre plates[161], transferred to a slide and sealed under a cover-slip. Using unfixed cells permits only surface antigens to be demonstrated. Fixation of cytospin preparations allows penetration of the cells by antibody and allows demonstration of cytoplasmic and nuclear components.

Although widely used, IF has disadvantages. Permanent preparations are not possible due to fading even using mounting medium containing polyvinyl alcohol. Cell morphology is poor. Advantages are the rapidity of the method and, by using additional fluorochromes, double-labelling is possible in the same cell preparation.

Non-specifically bound immunoglobulin on cells is removed by washing and Fc binding to membranes is overcome by using $F(ab')_2$ reagents prepared by pepsin digestion.

Immunoenzyme methods

This group of techniques uses enzyme labels conjugated to antibodies, enzyme–antienzyme complexes or enzyme-labelled avidin. Peroxidase and alkaline phosphatase are the most commonly used labels. Enzyme activity is demonstrated by suitable substrate or azo-coupling methods with consequent localized colour development detected by light microscopy.

Although the techniques take longer than IF, cell separation is not necessary, conventional light microscopy is used, the reaction product is stable and counterstaining permits morphological identification of the cell types. Furthermore, unstained films can retain their antigenic reactivity for up to 12 months at −20°C[162]. Because fixed preparations are used, membrane, cytoplasmic and nuclear antigens can be detected in contrast to using IF and cell suspensions.

Fixation is an important aspect of immunocytochemistry. An important advantage is visualization of cell morphology but those fixatives which best preserve morphology (formalin, methanol) usually destroy antigens and conversely fixatives that best preserve antigens (e.g. acetone) result in poor morphology. In practice, a compromise is reached by using methanol–acetone, buffered formalin–acetone or, most commonly, acetone–methanol–formalin in the proportions 19:19:2.

By combining two methods, e.g. peroxidase and alkaline phosphatase, two antigens can be demonstrated in the same film as the enzyme products will have different colours. Double staining is best visualized in separate populations of cells in the same preparation but the detection of two antigens in individual cells may result in masking of one label by the other. Double fluorochrome labelling and IF is superior to double labelling by immunoenzyme methods[163].

Peroxidase anti-peroxidase (PAP)

Originally described for use with sectioned material, the technique is used with haematological material by the two-stage or three-stage techniques (*Figure 13.3*) using horseradish peroxidase conjugated to antibody. Because granulocytes and their precursors, monocytes, erythroblasts and red cells contain endogenous peroxidase which can interfere with immunoperoxidase labelling, quenching with methanol/hydrogen peroxide is necessary but may cause denaturation of antigens. The use of rabbit–anti-mouse second antibody requires blocking of cross-reactivity with human immunoglobulins by incorporating human serum. Alkaline phosphatase can be used as the conjugated enzyme and endogenous alkaline phosphatase activity blocked by levamisole.

Alkaline phosphatase–anti-alkaline phosphatase (APAAP)

Probably the most widely used immunoenzymatic technique in haematology. The method is considered to be more sensitive than the PAP method[164]. Endogenous alkaline phosphatase in granulocytes and monocytes is labile and residual activity is blocked by levamisole without denaturing antigens while maintaining morphology. The azo-dye product using Fast Red or New Fuchsin is a vivid red and is readily seen. The method is a three-stage procedure using an unlabelled antibody bridge between the primary antibody and the monoclonal APAAP immune complex (*Figure 13.3*). Further enhancement of sensitivity can be achieved by extending the method to a five-stage technique[165] but then becomes laborious and time-consuming.

Avidin–biotin complex

Biotin is a water-soluble vitamin and many molecular structures including immunoglobulins can be labelled or biotinylated. Many biotin molecules can be bound to a single antibody molecule thus enhancing sensitivity, though steric hindrance must be avoided.

Avidin is a glycoprotein (MW 68 kD) obtained from egg-white which can be conjugated with many labels including peroxidase, alkaline phosphatase, gold, fluorochromes and ^{125}I. Avidin has a strong positive charge at neutral pH and binds non-specifically to negatively charged molecules, e.g. phospholipids, nucleic acids, which can result in non-specific staining. Streptavidin is extracted from *Streptomyces avidinii*, has a MW of 60 kD and shows less non-specific binding. The interaction between avidin/streptavidin and biotin shows much greater avidity than antibody–antigen reactions and is therefore very sensitive and rapid.

For immunocytochemistry, avidin or streptavidin is conjugated with either peroxidase or alkaline phosphatase. A three-stage avidin–biotin–alkaline phosphatase method (ABAP) has been described[166] with a sensitivity equal to that of the five-stage APAAP method and with minimal non-specificity. The method uses an unlabelled primary antibody, a biotinylated second antibody, avidin–alkaline phosphatase conjugate (*Figure 13.3*), naphthol AS MX phosphate and Fast Red TR as coupler.

Immunogold

Originally developed for localization and visualization of antigens by electron microscopy, the technique has been enhanced by the addition of silver precipitation which allows visualization by light microscopy[167]. Sensitivity is equal to or better than PAP and can be combined with IF to give triple marker capability. The reaction is stable and conventional Romanowsky staining can be used to provide maximum morphological detail.

Antibody-coated red cells

Antibodies can be attached to chromic chloride-treated red cells of various species[168]. The coated cells are then used in rosetting techniques to demonstrate surface markers. The method was originally used to demonstrate SmIg on lymphocytes. Although superseded by alternative methods of demonstrating surface markers, the coated red cells can be used in passive agglutination techniques for a variety of assays depending on the attached antibody and for antibody detection[169].

Automated immunofluorescence

The capability of examining large numbers of cells in respect of intensity of staining, size, cell granularity, double or triple labelling, etc. makes this the method of choice for large numbers of samples and particularly for lymphocyte subsets when the number of cells influences treatment, e.g. in HIV infection. Sample handling has improved by the facility of labelling cells in whole blood with red-cell lysis prior to counting.

Isolation of mononuclear cells on Ficoll–Isopaque

Principle

Anticoagulated diluted blood or bone marrow is layered on top of a mixture of Ficoll-Isopaque (FI) and centrifuged at 20°C. Erythrocytes and granulocytes sediment to the bottom. Lymphocytes, monocytes, mononuclear bone-marrow elements and leukaemic cells remain on the top of FI at the interface.

Materials

(a) Separation fluid: 10 parts Isopaque (33.9%, density 1.200 g/ml, Triosil, Vestric Ltd.) are mixed with 24 parts Ficoll 9% (Pharmacia). Final density is 1.077 g/ml.

(b) Blood is collected into lithium heparin (10 IU preservative-free heparin per ml blood). Collect bone marrow similarly and add 2–4 ml of Hanks TC-199.

(c) Phosphate-buffered saline (PBS): containing 1–2% bovine serum albumin.

Method

1. Dilute blood with PBS. If the nucleated cell count is under $20 \times 10^9/l$ dilute 1 in 2; if over $20 \times 10^9/l$ dilute 1 in 4.
2. Place 4 ml FI into a 14 ml tube and carefully layer-on 10 ml diluted blood without disturbing the interface.
3. Spin at 1800 rpm (400 *g*) for 25 minutes at 20°C (not at 4°C).
4. Discard the top portion of the supernatant and transfer the layer of leucocytes at the interface into another tube.
5. The suspension is diluted at least five times in PBS and centrifuged at 400 *g* (10 minutes at 20°C). Since this sample still contains some FI, loss of leucocytes occurs at lower speeds.
6. Remove supernatant, wash cells in 10 ml PBS and re-suspend in 2–5 ml PBS. Count the cells. Adjust the cell concentration to $1–2 \times 10^7$/ml with PBS.

Note

For analysing small samples polyethylene tubes (with caps, volume 1.5 ml) are used with 0.5 ml FI and 1.0 ml cell suspension. Tubes are spun for 1 minute at approximately 600 *g*.

Measurement of red-cell and plasma volume

Red-cell and plasma volume are measured by the dilution in the circulation of a measured amount of an intravenously injected red-cell or plasma marker. Early methods used dyes as plasma markers, e.g. Evans Blue or Vital Red, and red cells of different blood group as the red-cell marker. These methods have been superseded by radionuclide labelling.

The circulation should be regarded as an 'open' system in the sense that plasma labels leave the vasculature and red-cell distribution is in 'compartments' in the circulation or organs. These variables may be overcome by extrapolation if the rate of disappearance from the plasma is slow, and by delayed sampling to ensure complete mixing of the entire red-cell mass.

Plasma volume and total blood volume may be calculated from the measured red-cell volume or vice versa, by reference to the PCV and the ratio of venous haematocrit (H_v) to whole-body haematocrit (H_b). The procedure is not recommended when accurate measurements are required as the $H_v : H_b$ ratio has a relatively wide normal range. The measurement of red-cell volume and plasma volume should ideally be performed separately though simultaneously, and the total blood volume obtained by simple summation of the values.

Standard techniques for the measurement of red-cell and plasma volumes have been detailed by the ICSH[170, 171] who recommended ^{51}Cr or ^{99m}Tc as red-cell labels and ^{125}I-human serum albumin as the plasma label. Alternative isotopes can be used and will be briefly considered after the description of the standard techniques.

Measurement of red-cell volume (RCV)

The ICSH[170] described techniques using ^{51}Cr as sodium chromate and ^{32}P as sodium phosphate. ^{51}Cr has several advantages: the labelling procedure is straightforward, elution of the label is minimal during the period of study and the γ-emission can be readily differentiated from that of ^{125}I used as a plasma label. A disadvantage is that the lengthy survival of the labelled red cells and the relatively long half-life of ^{51}Cr make repeated measurements difficult. Various labelling procedures have been used but as measurement of red-cell volume may be followed by a red-cell survival study the procedure recommended for ^{51}Cr labelling for red-cell survival is recommended and for convenience is given again in detail.

Sequential blood volume estimations pose the problem that residual radioactivity may be present in subsequent blood samples and may contribute to the counting rate. It is necessary to select a radionuclide with an effective half-life such that the residual radioactivity is reduced between one estimation and the next to 1% or less of the preceding radioactivity. The residual radioactivity may then be neglected. Accordingly, ^{99m}Tc should be used for sequential measurements at short intervals. It is sometimes possible to use a different tracer for each estimation, selecting each so that the later measurements can be made independently of the earlier ones in mixed samples.

General preparations

All procedures are carried out using sterile technique and all solutions must be sterile and pyrogen free. As posture and muscular activity cause fluctuation in the PCV, the subject should be at rest and ideally recumbent for 15 minutes prior to the injection of the labelled cells. It is essential that the injection of the labelled cells is entirely intravenous.

Subsequent blood samples are collected into solid EDTA (1.5 mg/ml blood) or heparin (0.1 mg/ml blood). The proportions of EDTA and blood must be adhered to otherwise alterations of MCV and consequently of PCV may occur. Any calculation involving the PCV must use measurements corrected for trapped plasma (*see* page 108). The PCV derived from an electronic counter may be used provided that the instrument is accurately calibrated to allow for trapped plasma. The subject's own red cells should be used.

Technique using ^{51}Cr and washed cells

Blood is obtained by venepuncture and 10 volumes blood is added to 1.5 volumes 'NIH A' ACD solution (trisodium citrate dihydrate 22 *g*; citric acid 8 g; dextrose 25 g; water to 1 litre; sterilized by autoclaving at 126°C for 30 minutes; final pH 5.4). Centrifuge at 1000–1500 *g* for 5–10 minutes. Remove and discard the supernatant plasma, taking care not to remove any red cells. If the leucocyte count is greater than 25×10^9/l and/or the platelet count is greater than 500×10^9/l, remove and discard the buffy coat.

Add [^{51}Cr]sodium chromate solution (0.2 μCi (7.4 kBq)/kg body weight) slowly and with continuous gentle swirling. The amount of ^{51}Cr added should be as low as possible while consistent with the equipment used to measure the radioactivity of the samples and in any case limited to 0.5 μCi (18.5 kBq)/kg body weight. The specific activity of the ^{51}Cr should not be less than 20 mCi (740 MBq)/mg of chromium at the time of use. The added [^{51}Cr]sodium chromate should be in a volume of at least 0.2 ml, being diluted if necessary in isotonic sodium chloride. Incubate in a water bath at 37°C, for 15 minutes.

Wash the cells twice in 4–5 volumes isotonic sodium chloride. After the second wash there is generally less than 1% of the remaining radioactivity in the supernatant. Re-suspend and thoroughly mix the red cells in a sufficient volume of isotonic saline to allow injection of 10 ml or a lesser amount in children. When osmotic fragility is greatly increased, wash and re-suspend the red cells in 12 g/l sodium chloride. Set aside about 1.5 ml of the labelled red-cell suspension for preparation of a standard.

Administration of labelled cells

The amount of labelled cells injected must be accurately measured by volume, weight or radioactivity. The amount of labelled cells used in the preparation of the standard must also be determined precisely.

Measurement by volume is the easiest method and is satisfactory. The graduation and volume of disposable syringes show good precision and the calibration can be checked by filling the syringe to a mark with distilled water and the volume determined by expelling and weighing the water. Alternatively a syringe and needle is filled with labelled cell suspension and weighed (w_1), the contents of the syringe injected and the syringe and needle re-weighed (w_2). The weight (g) of blood injected is $w_1 - w_2$.

Preparation of standard

Add an aliquot of the labelled red-cell suspension, either 1 ml if the injected cells are measured by volume, or 1 g if measured by weight, to a 100 ml volumetric flask containing 0.4 g/l NH_4OH and fill to the mark. Deliver measured volumes of the diluted standard into duplicate counting tubes for radioactivity measurement.

Sampling
At 10 minutes and 20 minutes after injection take 5–10 ml blood from a vein other than that used for the injection. If mixing might be delayed, e.g. in patients with splenomegaly, a further sample should be taken at 60 minutes. Divide each sample into vials containing an appropriate amount of EDTA and determine the PCV of each aliquot. Lyse the remainder of the sample with saponin powder and deliver known volumes into counting vials.

Measurement of radioactivity
Using a well-type scintillation counter, count samples and standard to a coefficient of variation of less than 2%.

Calculation of results

$$\text{RCV (ml)} = \frac{\begin{matrix}\text{counting rate of}\\ \text{standard (cpm/ml)}\end{matrix} \times \begin{matrix}\text{dilution of}\\ \text{standard}\end{matrix} \times \begin{matrix}\text{volume of red}\\ \text{cells injected}\end{matrix} \times \begin{matrix}\text{PCV}\\ (H_v)\end{matrix}}{\text{counting rate of blood sample (cpm/ml)}}$$

Total blood volume (TBV) may be calculated by:

$$\text{TBV} = \text{RCV} \times \frac{1}{\text{PCV} \times 0.9}$$

The factor 0.9 represents the mean ratio of whole-body Hct to venous Hct (0.9:1) which may be incorrect in some patients, particularly those with splenomegaly, and therefore inaccurate results may be produced.

Technique using ^{99m}Tc [171]

Treatment of red cells with very small amounts of stannous ion before incubation with pertechnetate results in the subsequent binding of almost all of the added technetium, provided that essentially all of the plasma has been removed from the red cells before the addition of the stannous ion. This method also results in a more stable technetium label on the red cells, so that the rate of elution of technetium is less rapid than when technetium is added to the red cells before the stannous ion. It has been shown that optimal labelling is obtained when stannous chloride is used at a dose of about 0.015 μg stannous ion per ml of red cells. Accordingly, the following method is recommended.

Labelling
Take approximately 10 ml of blood into a container to which a few drops of liquid heparin have been added. Transfer exactly 5 ml of blood to another container to which 20 ml of saline have previously been added. Centrifuge the container and remove as much of the supernatant as possible to leave approximately 2 ml of packed red cells. Then add 0.015 μg of stannous ion per ml red cells. The necessary dilute solution of tin is prepared by a two-stage procedure as in the following examples.

Example 1. Weigh out 2 mg $SnCl_2.2H_2O$ and dissolve in 10 ml saline. Take it up into a syringe and pass through a 0.22 μm Millipore filter into an empty container.

Now transfer 1 ml into a 500 ml bottle of saline (as prepared for intravenous use; contents usually about 525 ml). After mixing, withdraw 0.2 ml to provide 0.03 μg stannous ion and add to the 2 ml packed red cells.

Example 2. Weigh out 2 mg $SnCl_2.2H_2O$ in 35 ml saline. Pass this solution through a 0.22 μm Millipore filter into an empty vial. Using a tuberculin syringe, transfer 0.25 ml of the filtered solution into a sealed 250 ml bottle of saline to provide a solution containing 0.15 μg stannous ion/ml. Using a tuberculin syringe, withdraw 0.2 ml to provide 0.03 μg stannous ion to be added to the 2 ml packed red cells.

The stannous chloride may be weighed out in advance, but the time between dissolving it and adding the dilute solution to the red cells should not exceed 10 minutes.

Commercially available kits now provide alternative methods for pretreating the red cells, e.g. with stannous pyrophosphate or citrate, and which avoid the necessity for fresh preparation on each occasion. The acceptability of any such kits must first be checked by comparison with the recommended method, especially taking account of fractional uptake of the ^{99m}Tc and its elution rate.

Five minutes after adding the tin, add 25 μCi (925 kBq) of freshly generated pertechnetate in approximately 0.2 ml saline to the red cells. Incubate for 5 minutes; then centrifuge and wash in cold saline and resuspend in a convenient volume of cold saline (e.g. approximately 25 ml to provide 20 ml suspension for injection and preparation of the standard). Reinject the patient as soon after preparation as possible, determining the amount injected as outlined in the chromium technique.

Preparation of standard

As described in the chromium technique.

Sampling

At 10 minutes after injection, collect blood from a vein other than that used for injection and add half to each of two specimen containers with anticoagulant. Measure the PCV on an aliquot of each sample. Dispense an appropriate volume into counting tubes. Where delayed mixing is suspected, another sample should be collected at 30 minutes and similarly treated.

Radioactivity measurements

Because of the short half-life of ^{99m}Tc, radioactivity has to be measured on the day of the test. The coefficient of variation attributable to counting statistics should not exceed 2%.

Calculation of results

Measurement is normally based on the 10 minute sample. The RCV is calculated using the formula given in the chromium method.

Although up to 2% of the radioactivity is eluted from the red cells in 30 minutes, it is not considered necessary to apply a correction factor to measurements calculated from the 10 minute and 30 minute samples; however, as the elution increases significantly with time, this method is not suitable for sampling at 60 minutes. If in cases where some delayed mixing is suspected, there is a significant difference between measurements at 10 and 30 minutes, the 30 minute measurement is likely to be more reliable and should be used for calculating the red-cell volume.

Expression of results

Blood volume studies are usually expressed in relation to body weight. The relationship between blood volume and body weight varies according to body composition. Blood volume studies show a slightly better correlation with lean body mass derived from height and weight. Various formulae have been put forward for obtaining blood volume reference values from height and weight or body surface area[108]. The relationship between height, weight and expected red-cell volume in males and females is shown in *Table 13.14*.

Table 13.14 The prediction of normal red-cell volume. The figures corresponding to the weight and height of the patient added together give the red-cell volume in ml [172]

Weight (kg)	*Males*	*Females*	*Height* (m)	*Males*	*Females*
30	519	171	1.45	496	729
35	606	200	1.50	537	811
40	692	228	1.55	578	893
45	779	257	1.60	619	975
50	865	285	1.65	660	1057
55	952	314	1.70	701	1139
60	1038	342	1.75	742	1221
65	1125	371	1.80	783	1303
70	1211	399	1.85	824	1385
75	1298	428	1.90	865	1467
80	1384	456	1.95	906	1549
85	1471	485	2.00	947	1631
90	1557	513			
95	1644	542			
100	1730	570			

Normal ranges

Adult males: 25–35 ml/kg (mean 30 ml/kg). Adult females: 20–30 ml/kg (mean 25 ml/kg).

Alternative red-cell labels

The disadvantage of ^{51}Cr when repeated measurements may be required has been mentioned above. ^{32}P has no advantages because of elution and the added difficulties in counting the β-emission. ^{113m}Indium is a γ-emitter with a half-life of 100 minutes, and with the lipophilic chelating agent acetylacetone the labelling procedure is simple. Elution *in vivo* is less than that of ^{99m}Tc. The results using ^{113m}In labelling are reported to be identical with those using ^{51}Cr, repeated measurements at short intervals are possible and the technique is considered to be generally superior to ^{51}Cr and ^{99m}Tc techniques for red-cell volume and the measurement of the splenic red-cell pool by quantitative imaging[173].

Measurement of plasma volume

All methods for measuring plasma volume are based on the labelling of a plasma protein fraction. Human serum albumin (HSA) is most commonly used despite its loss from the circulation. Labelling of plasma proteins of higher molecular weight would be an advantage, e.g. fibrinogen, transferrin or IgM. The albumin must be obtained from donors who are known to be HBsAg negative and HIV negative though albumin may be heat treated to inactivate HBsAg. Radioiodine-labelled HSA is used with ^{111}I, ^{125}I or ^{131}I as labels. The activity of the radioiodine can be readily measured in the presence of ^{51}Cr or ^{99m}Tc.

Method

The general preparation of the patient and the general comments for the measurement of red-cell volume apply to plasma volume estimation.

Collection and labelling of plasma

Heparinized plasma is separated by centrifugation and to approximately 7 ml is added 0.05 μCi (1.8 kBq)/kg body weight of radioiodine-labelled HSA. Alternatively, the radioiodine-labelled HSA may be added to a solution of 50 g/l HSA. Mix thoroughly.

Administration and sampling

Inject a known amount e.g. 5 ml intravenously. An aliquot is retained for preparation of the standard. Start a stop-watch at the mid-point of injection. At 10, 20 and 30 minutes collect 5 ml blood into EDTA from a vein other than that used for the injection. If multiple sampling is impractical collect one sample at 10 minutes.

Preparation and counting of samples and standard

The plasma of each sample is separated by centrifugation and duplicate measured amounts of each are transferred to tubes for counting. The standard is prepared by accurately diluting the labelled plasma 1 in 100 in saline. The activity is measured by counting in a well-type scintillation counter to a standard deviation of less than 2%.

Calculation of results

The activity of the plasma samples as cpm/ml are plotted against time of sampling on semi-log graph paper and the activity at zero time obtained by extrapolation. If only one sample was obtained at 10 minutes the activity is multiplied by 1.015 to correct for loss of the label during the 10-minute period.

$$\text{Plasma volume (PV)} = \frac{\begin{array}{c}\text{counting rate of}\\ \text{standard (cpm/ml)}\end{array} \times \begin{array}{c}\text{dilution of}\\ \text{standard}\end{array} \times \begin{array}{c}\text{volume of labelled}\\ \text{plasma injected}\end{array}}{\begin{array}{c}\text{counting rate of plasma sample corrected to zero time}\\ \text{(cpm/ml)}\end{array}}$$

$$\text{Total blood volume (TBV)} = \text{PV} \times \frac{1}{1 - (\text{PCV} \times 0.9)}$$

The limitations of a calculated TBV have been detailed above.

Normal ranges

Males and females: 35–45 ml/kg (mean 40 ml/kg). Expected plasma volume in relation to lean body mass derived from height and weight is given in *Table 13.15*.

Table 13.15 The prediction of normal plasma volume. The figures corresponding to the weight and height of the patient added together give the plasma volume in ml[172]

Weight (kg)	*Males*	*Females*	*Height* (m)	*Males*	*Females*
30	270	252	1.45	1728	1062
35	315	294	1.50	1846	1264
40	360	336	1.55	1965	1467
45	405	378	1.60	2083	1669
50	450	420	1.65	2202	1872
55	495	462	1.70	2320	2074
60	540	504	1.75	2439	2277
65	585	546	1.80	2557	2479
70	630	588	1.85	2676	2682
75	675	630	1.90	2794	2884
80	720	672	1.95	2913	3087
85	765	714	2.00	3031	3289
90	810	756			
95	855	798			
100	900	840			

Note

The liberation of radioiodine by the catabolism of HSA will result in radioiodine uptake by the thyroid which can be blocked by an oral dose of 30 mg potassium iodide daily for 3–4 weeks.

Estimation of TBV

TBV is derived from the sum of the values for red-cell volume and plasma volume or less satisfactorily by calculation from either estimation using a PCV corrected to whole-body haematocrit. The combined values of RCV and PV will approximate to the circulating TBV unless a significant proportion of the RCV is pooled in an organ, e.g. the spleen. An underestimation of TBV will also occur if the volume of leucocytes and platelets, which in health is very small, is markedly increased, as can occur in the proliferative disorders.

The simultaneous measurement of red-cell and plasma volume using different tracers is the best method of measuring TBV. The activities of the different isotopes may be measured in dual-channel counters using appropriate settings for each isotope. ^{51}Cr can be counted free from ^{125}I activity whereas some ^{51}Cr activity will be included in the ^{125}I channel, the ^{125}I activity being corrected by measuring the activity of a ^{51}Cr standard at the ^{125}I settings.

Measurement of the splenic red-cell pool

Early methods of estimating the volume of splenic red-cell pool were by determining the ratio of venous to whole-body haematocrit which increases in relation to the degree of splenomegaly, or by determining the difference in the red-cell volume from samples taken at 3 minutes and 20 minutes after injection of ^{51}Cr-labelled red cells; the difference is taken to represent the splenic red-cell pool. The latter approach underestimates the volume of the pool, because a proportion of labelled cells enters the spleen within the first 3 minutes and mixing is not necessarily complete at 20 minutes.

A direct measurement of splenic red-cell pool can be obtained by quantitative imaging using a double-headed rectilinear scanner following the injection of ^{99m}Tc or ^{113m}In-labelled red cells. Accurate measurement of splenic red-cell pool is now clearly outside the province of the haematology laboratory. The technique and its application have been described and reviewed [173–175]. Of particular interest in the diagnosis of PPP is an increased splenic red-cell pool even in the absence of splenomegaly which suggests a structural abnormality of the spleen that is not simply a function of the increased circulating red-cell mass [176].

Demonstration of reduced splenic function

Reduced or absent splenic function is reflected by abnormalities of blood-film morphology and by increased numbers of platelets and lymphocytes. Absent splenic function is usually due to surgical removal. Other causes are atrophy due to repeated infarcts as occurs in sickle-cell disease and primary thrombocythaemia, or the atrophy associated with coeliac disease and in inflammatory bowel disease. Other rare causes are congenital asplenia, splenic infiltration or after irradiation. Reduced splenic function is usually but not invariably associated with absence of the spleen or a reduced splenic volume as judged by imaging procedures [177].

Splenic function can be studied by the clearance from the circulation and uptake by the spleen of radioisotope-labelled damaged red cells [178], labelled intact platelets [179] or labelled sulphur colloid. Sulphur-colloid uptake reflects phagocytosis by the macrophages in the spleen and may be normal when the ‘trapping’ of damaged red cells shows reduced splenic function.

Normal red cells may be modified by a number of procedures which result in their rapid removal by the spleen. Sulphydryl inhibitors, antibody sensitization and heat damage have each been used. The rate of clearance from the circulation or uptake by the spleen can each be used as the measure of splenic function. Heat-damaged red cells labelled with ^{51}Cr or ^{99m}Tc have been widely used, ^{99m}Tc being particularly useful because of its short half-life and its excellent imaging properties which allows quantitative measurement of functioning splenic tissue although indium labelling may be superior [180]. The rate of clearance of heat-damaged red cells from the circulation is not a single function [181] and quantitative scanning has been considered the better measurement [182].

The technique described below uses heat-damaged red cells labelled with ^{99m}Tc by a post-tinning method and measurement of clearance from the circulation. It is slightly modified from the ^{99m}Tc labelling and heat-damage methods previously described [183].

Assessment of splenic function by clearance of ^{99m}Tc-labelled heat-damaged red cells

Principle

Autologous red cells are labelled with ^{99m}Tc, heated at 50°C and reinjected. Blood samples are collected and the clearance assessed by the time taken to reach 50% remaining activity, or, when clearance is slow, the percentage activity remaining after 20 minutes.

Method

10 ml of blood is collected into 1.5 ml ACD in a 30 ml *glass*, screw-capped container and centrifuged at 1500 *g* for 5 minutes. The plasma is removed aseptically with a syringe and needle and retained. Approximately 1.4 mCi (50 MBq) ^{99m}Tc as sodium pertechnetate is added to the packed red cells and allowed to stand for 5 minutes after gently mixing (the stated activity of ^{99m}Tc is to allow splenic imaging; if this is not to be performed 100 μCi (3.7 MBq) is sufficient). Add 80 μg (equivalent to 20 μg/ml cells) of stannous chloride, freshly prepared by dissolving 8 mg in 20 ml 9 g/l NaCl and filtering through a membrane (pore size 0.22 μm). Stand for 3 minutes. Wash three times with 9 g/l NaCl and heat for *exactly* 20 minutes at 50 ± 0.5°C. Resuspend by replacing the plasma. Reinject 5 ml of the re-suspended, labelled, heat-damaged red cells, starting a stop-watch at the mid-point of injection. After exactly 3 minutes a 5 ml blood sample is collected into EDTA from the opposite arm and further samples are similarly collected at 10, 20, 30, 60 and 120 minutes. A measured volume of each sample is counted after saponin lysis in a well-type scintillation counter, and the radioactivity of each sample is expressed as a percentage of the activity of the 3-minute sample.

Note

This method differs in that the cells are labelled and washed *before* heating to avoid manipulations after the cells are damaged.

Normal range

$T_{0.5}$ clearance = 10–17 minutes which compares well with previous measurements of 9–18 minutes[178]. When red-cell clearance is prolonged, measurement of half-clearance times is impractical and results can be expressed as percentage activity remaining at 20 minutes, which is 17.5–46.5% in normal subjects[184].

Non-invasive assessment of hyposplenism

The counting of erythrocytes with membrane abnormalities visible as 'pits' by phase-interference microscopy (pitted red cells) has been used as a simple method of assessing splenic function[185]. The technique correlates well with heat-damaged red-cell clearance rates and with measurement of splenic volume[186]. Normal subjects have less than 4% pitted cells, the great majority having less than 1%. In splenectomized patients the range is about 30–50%.

Erythropoietin assay

Erythropoietin (Epo) can be measured by *in vivo* and *in vitro* bioassays and by immunological techniques[187]. The *in vivo* biological activity of Epo preparations and test materials was most commonly assayed in mice rendered polycythaemic by exposure to reduced atmospheric pressure or red-cell hypertransfusion, the increased red-cell mass suppressing endogenous Epo production. The administration of exogenous Epo in test samples evokes an erythropoietic response measured by the uptake of radio-iron. However, the test is relatively insensitive, extremely laborious and time-consuming and cannot measure Epo levels in normal plasma without prior concentration.

In vitro bioassays include the use of suspension culture of fetal mouse liver cells and radio-iron incorporation into haem as the measure of Epo activity, and the formation of erythroid colonies on solid phase with the number of colonies being used for assessment of activity. The colony-forming technique has a much higher sensitivity than *in vivo* bioassays.

Following the isolation and purification of human urinary Epo in 1979 and the production of polyclonal antibodies, a number of radioimmunoassays (RIA) were developed[188, 189] together with haemagglutination inhibition assays (HAI). The cloning of Epo, production of recombinant human Epo (rhEpo) and the production of monoclonal antibodies to various epitopes of Epo[190], has allowed the development of enzyme-linked immunosorbent assay (ELISA) techniques[191]. RIA and ELISA techniques are capable of detecting 1 mIU of serum immunoreactive Epo (siEpo). All methods should be standardized against the 2nd International Reference Preparation of human urinary erythropoietin and expressed as milli-International Units/ml (mIU/ml).

In the investigation of polycythaemia, siEpo has a lower mean value in PPP than in secondary polycythaemia and normal controls but with considerable overlap of observed values. Determinations on a single sample may be misleading due to fluctuating levels in PPP[192] and diurnal variation in levels are found in normal subjects[193]. The assay may be most useful in identifying patients with secondary erythrocytosis due to inappropriate erythropoietin secretion[190]. Mean siEpo levels measured by RIA in normal subjects are in the order of 20–25 mIU/ml[192, 194] which overlap the values of PPP and secondary polycythaemia. In one series[195] 94% of patients with secondary polycythaemis had values >30 mIU/ml, in contrast to 92% of cases of PPP with values <30 mIU/ml.

Measurement of plasma vitamin B_{12}-binding capacity [196]

Principle

The total vitamin B_{12}-binding capacity (TBBC) of plasma is obtained by adding together the serum B_{12} concentration and the plasma unsaturated binding capacity (UBBC). Measurement of UBBC is simple and useful in the investigation of the chronic myeloproliferative disorders. Because of variable *in vitro* release of granulocyte transcobalamins into serum, blood should be collected into EDTA with 2 mg/ml sodium fluoride added.

Materials

[^{57}Co] vitamin B_{12} A vial containing 10 µCi (370 kBq)/ml of ^{57}Co with a specific activity of 15 µCi (555 kBq)/µg of B_{12} (equivalent to about 0.66 µg/l) is diluted in

100 ml water to give a stock solution of approximately 6.6 μg/ml. On the day of the assay it is further diluted to provide a working standard of 2000 ng/l.

Albumin-coated charcoal 2.5 g acid-washed activated charcoal (BDH) are suspended in 50 ml deionized water and 1.7 ml of 300 g/l bovine albumin in 50 ml deionized water added and well mixed. The suspension may be stored at 4°C for several days but is best prepared freshly on the day of the test.

Method

Three 10 ml conical centrifuge tubes are used and the test set up as shown in *Table 13.16*.

Table 13.16 Measurement of plasma vitamin B_{12}-binding capacity; figures in body of table are in ml

Substance	*Tube*		
	A (standard)	*B (control)*	*C (test)*
9 g/l NaCl	2.5	0.5	0
Plasma	0	0	0.5
^{57}Co-B_{12}	1.0	1.0	1.0
	Mix, stand at room temperature for 30 minutes		
Charcoal suspension	0	2.0	2.0
	Stand for 10 minutes and centrifuge at 1500 *g* for 10 minutes		

Transfer 3 ml of each supernatant, count radioactivity for 100 seconds and correct for background counts.

Calculation

$$\text{UBBC (ng/l)} = \frac{\text{C} - \text{B}}{\text{A}} \times \text{ng/l } ^{57}\text{Co-B}_{12}$$

If the UBBC is equal to or greater than the amount of ^{57}Co-B_{12} added the test is repeated after diluting the plasma with sodium chloride and the result multiplied by the plasma dilution.

Normal range

Serum = 600–2200 ng/l; fluoride-EDTA plasma = 505–1208 ng/l.

References

1. Moloney, W. C. (1987) Radiogenic leukaemia revisited. *Blood*, **70**, 905–8
2. Gardner, M. J., Snee, M. P., Hall, A. J. *et al.* (1990) Results of case-control study of leukaemia and lymphoma among young people near Sellafield nulcear plant in West Cumbria. *Br. Med. J.*, **300**, 423–9

3. Rinsky, R. A., Smith, A. B., Hornung, R. *et al.* (1987) Benzene and leukaemia. *N. Engl. J. Med.*, **316**, 1044–50
4. Jacobs, A. (1989) Benzene and leukaemia. *Br. J. Haematol.*, **72**, 119–21
5. Boros, L. and Bennett, J. M. (1984) The acute myeloid leukaemias. In *Haematology I. Leukaemias*. Butterworths International Medical Reviews (eds J. M. Goldman and H. D. Preisler) pp. 104–35. London: Butterworths
6. Chan, V. T. W. and McGee, J. O'D. (1987) Cellular oncogenes in neoplasia. *J. Clin. Pathol.*, **40**, 1055–6
7. Pierce, J. H., Alessandra, E. and Aaronson, S. A. (1986) Interaction of oncogenes with haemopoietic cells. *Clin. Haematol.*, **15**, 573–96
8. Bennett, J. M., Catovsky, D., Daniel, M.-T. *et al.* (1976) Proposals for the classification of the acute leukaemias. *Br. J. Haematol.*, **33**, 451–8
9. Bennett, J. M., Catovsky, D., Daniel, M.-T. *et al.* (1981) The morphological classification of acute lymphoblastic leukaemia: concordance among observers and clinical correlations. *Br. J. Haematol.*, **47**, 553–61
10. Golomb, H. M., Rowley, J. D., Vardiman, J. W., Testa, J. R. and Butler, A. (1980) 'Microgranular' acute promyelocytic leukaemia: a distinct clinical ultrastructural and cytogenetic entity. *Blood*, **55**, 253–9
11. Bennett, J. M., Catovsky, D., Daniel, M.-T. *et al.* (1980) A variant form (M3) of hypergranular promyelocytic leukaemia. *Br. J. Haematol.*, **44**, 169–70
12. Bennett, J. M., Catovsky, D., Daniel, M.-T. *et al.* (1985) Criteria for the diagnosis of acute megakaryoblastic lineage (M7). *Ann. Intern. Med.*, **103**, 460–2
13. Bennett, J. M., Catovsky, D., Daniel, M.-T. *et al.* (1982) Proposals for the classification of myelodysplastic syndromes. *Br. J. Haematol.*, **51**, 189–99
14. Bennett, J. M., Catovsky, D., Daniel, M.-T. *et al.* (1985) Proposed revised criteria for the classification of acute myeloid leukaemias. *Ann. Intern. Med.*, **103**, 626–9
15. Bloomfield, C. D. and Brunning, R. D. (1985) FAB M7: acute megakaryoblastic leukaemia – beyond morphology. *Ann. Intern. Med.*, **103**, 450–2
16. Bloomfield, C. D. and Brunning, R. D. (1985) The revised French-American-British classification of acute myeloid leukaemias: is new better? *Ann. Intern. Med.*, **103**, 614–16
17. Childs, C. C., Stass, S. A. and Bennett, J. M. (1986) The morphologic classification of acute lymphoblastic leukaemia in childhood. *Am. J. Clin. Pathol.*, **86**, 503–6
18. Lilleyman, J. S., Hann, I. M., Stevens, R. F., Eden, O. B. and Richards, S. M. (1986) French American British (FAB) morphological classification of childhood lymphoblastic leukaemia and its clinical importance. *J. Clin. Pathol.*, **39**, 998–1002
19. First MIC Cooperative Study Group (1986) Morphologic, immunologic and cytogenetic (MIC) working classification of acute lymphoblastic leukaemias. *Cancer Genet. Cytogenet.*, **23**, 189–97
20. First International Workshop of Chromosomes in Leukaemia (1978) Chromosomes in acute nonlymphocytic leukaemia. *Br. J. Haematol.*, **39**, 311–16
21. Testa, J. R., Golomb, H. M., Rowley, J. D., Vardiman, J. W. and Sweet, D. L. (1978) Hypergranular promyelocytic leukaemia (HPL). Cytogenetic and ultrastructural specificity. *Blood*, **52**, 272–80
22. Bain, B. J., Catovsky, D., O'Brien, M. *et al.* (1981) Megakaryoblastic leukaemia presenting as acute myelofibrosis – a study of four cases with platelet-peroxidase reaction. *Blood*, **52**, 206–13
23. Mohandes, E. El. and Hayhoe, F. G. J. (1983) 5-nucleotidase activity of megakaryoblasts in a case of acute megakaryoblastic leukaemia. *Br. J. Haematol.*, **53**, 523–6
24. Pombo de Oliveira, M. S., Gregory, C., Matutes, E., Parreira, A. and Catovsky, D. (1987) Cytochemical profile of megakaryoblastic leukaemia: a study with cytochemical methods, monoclonal antibodies and ultrastructural cytochemistry. *J. Clin. Pathol.*, **40**, 663–9
25. Coleman, M. S. and Hutton, J. J. (1981) Terminal transferase. In *Methods in Haematology* (ed. D. Catovsky), No. **2**. *The Leukaemic Cell*, pp. 203–19. London: Churchill Livingstone
26. Parreira, A., Pombo de Oliveira, M. S., Matutes, E. *et al.* (1988) Terminal deoxynucleotidyl transferase positive acute myeloid leukaemia: an association with immature myeloblastic leukaemia. *Br. J. Haematol.*, **69**, 219–24
27. Diamond, B. A., Yelton, D. E. and Scharff, M. D. (1981) Monoclonal antibodies. *N. Engl. J. Med.*, **304**, 1344–9

28. Knapp, W., Dorken, B., Rieber, P., Schmidt, R. E., Stein, H. and van den Borne, A. E. G. J. (1989) CD antigens 1989. *Blood*, **74**, 1448–50
29. Second MIC Cooperative Study Group (1988) Morphologic immunologic and cytogenetic (MIC) working classification of the acute myeloid leukaemias. *Br. J. Haematol.*, **68**, 487–94
30. Campos, L., Guyotat, D., Archimbaude, E. *et al.* (1989) Surface marker expression in adult acute myeloid leukaemia: correlation with initial characteristics, morphology and response to therapy. *Br. J. Haematol.*, **72**, 161–6
31. Wain, S. L. and Borowitz, M. J. (1987) Practical application of monoclonal antibodies to the diagnosis and classification of acute leukaemias. *Clin. Lab. Haematol.*, **9**, 221–44
32. Janossy, G., Coustan-Smith, E. and Campana, D. (1989) The reliability of cytoplasmic CD3 and CD22 antigen expression in the immunodiagnosis of acute leukaemia: a study of 500 cases. *Leukaemia*, **3**, 170–81
33. Flug, F., Pelicci, P.-G., Bonetti, F. *et al.* T-cell receptor gene rearrangements as markers of lineage and clonality in T-cell neoplasms. *Proc. Natl. Acad. Sci.*, **82**, 3460–4
34. Arnold, A., Cossman, J., Bakshi, A. *et al.* (1983) Immunoglobulin gene rearrangements as unique clonal markers in human lymphoid neoplasms. *N. Engl. J. Med.*, **309**, 1593–9
35. International Workshop on Chronic Lymphocytic Leukaemia (1981) Chronic lymphocytic leukaemia: Proposals for a revised prognostic staging system. *Br. J. Haematol.*, **48**, 365–7
36. Noel, P. and Kyle, R. A. (1987) Monoclonal proteins in chronic lymphocytic leukaemia. *Am. J. Clin. Pathol.*, **87**, 385–8
37. Catovsky, D., Lauria, F., Matutes, E. *et al* (1981) Increase in $T_\gamma$lymphocytes in B-cell chronic lymphocytic leukaemia. *Br. J. Haematol.*, **47**, 539–44
38. Han, T., Ozer, H., Sadamori, N. *et al.* (1984) Prognostic importance of cytogenetic abnormalities in patients with chronic lymphocytic leukaemia. *N. Engl. J. Med.*, **310**, 288–92
39. Melo, J. V., Catovsky, D. and Galton, D. A. (1986) The relationship between chronic lymphocytic leukaemia and prolymphocytic leukaemia. *Br. J. Haematol.*, **63**, 377–87
40. Sadamori, N., Han, T., Minowada, J. *et al.* (1983) Possible specific chromosome change in prolymphocytic leukaemia. *Blood*, **62**, 729–36
41. Cawley, J. C., Burns, G. F. and Hayhoe, F. G. J. (1980) *Hairy Cell Leukaemia*. Heidelberg: Springer
42. Burns, G. F. and Cawley, J.C. (1980) Hairy-cell leukaemia. *Clin. Lab. Haematol.*, **2**, 249–54
43. Cawley, J. C. and Worman, C. P. (1985) Hairy cell leukaemia. *Br. J. Haematol.*, **60**, 213–18
44. Hernandez, D., Cruz, C., Carnot, J., Dorticos, E. and Espinosa, E. (1978) Hairy-cell leukaemia of T-cell origin. *Br. J. Haematol.*, **38**, 504–6
45. Cawley, J. C., Burns, G. F., Nash, T. A., Higgy, K. E., Child, J. A. and Roberts, B. E. (1978) Hairy-cell leukaemia with T-cell features. *Blood*, **51**, 61–9
46. Naeim, F., Hoon, D. B. S., Cheng, L. *et al.* (1987) Reactivity of neoplastic cells of hairy cell leukaemia with antisera to S-100 protein. *Am. J. Clin. Pathol.*, **88**, 86–91
47. Sansoni, P., Rowden, G., Manara, G. C. *et al.* (1988) Immuno-electron microscopic demonstration of S-100 protein in hairy cell leukaemia cells. *Am. J. Clin. Pathol.*, **89**, 374–7
48. Hayhoe, F. G. J. and Neuman, Z. (1976) Cytology of myeloma cells. *J. Clin. Pathol.*, **29**, 916–22
49. Reed, M., McKenna, R. W., Bridges, R., Parkin, J., Frizzera, G. and Brunning, R. D. (1981) Morphologic manifestations of monoclonal gammopathies. *Am. J. Clin. Pathol.*, **76**, 8–23
50. Hayhoe, F. G. J. and Flemans, R. J. (1980) *An Atlas of Haematological Cytology*. London: Wolfe Medical Publications
51. Bataille, A. B., Durie, B. G. M., Sany, J. and Salmon, S. E. (1980) Myeloma bone marrow acid phosphatase staining: a correlative study of 38 patients. *Blood,* **55**, 802–5
52. Gould, J., Alexanian, R., Goodacre, A. *et al.* (1988) Plasma cell karyotype in multiple myeloma. *Blood*, **71**, 453–6
53. Sinclair, D., Sheehan, T., Parrot, D. M. V. and Stott, D. I. (1986) The incidence of monoclonal gammopathy in a population over 45 years old determined by isoelectric focusing. *Br. J. Haematol.*, **64**, 745–50
54. Pruzanski, W., Platts, M. E. and Ogryzlo, M. A. (1969) Leukaemic forms of immunocytic dyscrasia (plasma cell leukaemia). *Am. J. Med.*, **47**, 60–74

55. Catovsky, D. (1984) Chronic lymphocytic, prolymphocytic and hairy cell leukaemias. In *Haematology I. Leukaemias*. Butterworths International Medical Reviews (eds J. M. Goldman and H. D. Preisler), pp. 266–98. London: Butterworths
56. Foon, K. A. and Todd, R. F. (1986) Immunologic classification of leukaemia and lymphoma. *Blood*, **68**, 1–31
57. Brito-Babapulle, V., Pomfret, M., Matutes, E. and Catovsky, D. (1987) Cytogenetic studies of prolymphocytic leukaemia. II. T-cell prolymphocytic leukaemia. *Blood*, **70**, 926–31
58. Shepherd, P. C. A., Ganesan, T. S. and Galton, D. A. G. (1987) Haematological classification of the chronic myeloid leukaemias. *Clin. Haematol.*, **1**, 887–906
59. Goldman, J. M. (1987) Foreword. Chronic myeloid leukaemia. *Clin. Haematol.*, **1**, ix–x
60. Gale, R. P. and Cannani, E. (1985) The molecular biology of chronic myelogenous leukaemia. *Br. J. Haematd.*, **60**, 395–408
61. Goldman, J. M. (1987) The Philadelphia chromosome: from cytogenetics to oncogenes. *Br. J. Haematol.*, **66**, 435–6
62. Dreazen, O., Cannani, E. and Gale, R. P. (1988) Molecular biology of chronic myelogenous leukaemia. *Semin. Haematol.*, **26**, 35–49
63. Fialkow, P. J., Martin, P. J., Najfeld, V., Penfold, G. K., Jacobson, R. J. and Hansen, J. A. (1981) Evidence for a multistep pathogenesis of chronic granulocytic leukaemia. *Blood*, **58**, 158–63
64. Spiers, A. S. D., Bain, B. J. and Turner, J. E. (1977) The peripheral blood in chronic granulocytic leukaemia. *Scand. J. Haematol.*, **18**, 25–38
65. Ganguly, P., Sutherland, S. B. and Bradford, H. R. (1978) Defective binding of thrombin to platelets in myeloid leukaemia. *Br. J. Haematol.*, **39**, 599–605
66. Whittaker, J. A., Khurshid, M. and Hughes, H. R. (1974) Neutrophil function in chronic granulocytic leukaemia before and after busulphan treatment. *Br. J. Haematol.*, **28**, 541–9
67. El-Maallem, H. and Fletcher, J. (1979) Defective hydrogen peroxide production in chronic granulocytic leukaemia neutrophils. *Br. J. Haematol.*, **41**, 49–55
68. Taub, R. N., Baker, M. A. and Madyastha, K. R. (1980) Masking of neutrophil surface lectin-binding sites in chronic myelogenous leukaemia (CML). *Blood*, **55**, 294–8
69. Hasegawa, D. K., Bennett, A. J., Coccia, P. F. *et al.* (1980) Factor V deficiency in Philadelphia positive chronic myelogenous leukaemia. *Blood*, **56**, 585–95
70. You, W. and Weisbrot, I. M. (1979) Chronic neutrophilic leukaemia. Report of two cases and revision of literature. *Am. J. Clin. Pathol.*, **72**, 233–42
71. Zucker-Franklin, D. (1974) Eosinophil function and disorders. *Adv. Intern. Med.*, **19**, 1–25
72. Goldman, J. M., Najfeld, V. and Th'ng, K. H. (1975) Agar culture and chromosome analysis of eosinophil leukaemia. *J. Clin. Pathol.*, **28**, 956–61
73. Presentey, B., Jerushalmy, Z. and Mintz, U. (1979) Eosinophil leukaemia: morphological, cytochemical and electron microscopic studies. *J. Clin. Pathol.*, **32**, 261–71
74. Parreira, L., Tavares, D. E., Castro, J. *et al.* (1986) Chromosome and cell culture studies in eosinophilic leukaemia. *Br. J. Haematol.*, **62**, 659–69
75. Spiers, A. S. D. (1979) Metamorphosis of chronic granulocytic leukaemia: diagnosis, classification and management. *Br. J. Haematol.*, **41**, 1–7
76. Soler, J., O'Brien, M., Tavares, D. E. Castro, J. *et al.* (1985) Blast crisis of chronic granulocytic leukaemia with mast cell and basophil precursors. *Am. J. Clin. Pathol.*, **83**, 254–9
77. First International Workshop on Chromosomes in Leukaemia (1978) Chromosomes in Ph′-positive chronic granulocytic leukaemia. *Br. J. Haematol.*, **39**, 305–9
78. Bennett, J. M., Catovsky, D., Daniel, M. T. *et al.* (1982) Proposals for the classification of the myelodysplastic syndromes. *Br. J. Haematol.*, **51**, 189–99
79. Galton, D. A. G. (1984) The myelodysplastic syndromes. *Clin. Lab. Haematol.*, **6**, 99–112
80. Jacobs, A. (1985) Myelodysplastic syndrome: pathogenesis, functional abnormalities and clinical implications. *J. Clin. Pathol.*, **38**, 1201–17
81. Griffin, J. D. (ed.) (1986) Myelodysplastic syndromes. *Clin. Haematol.*, **15**, 909–1107
82. Hamblin, T. J. and Oscier, D. G. (1987) The myelodysplastic syndrome – a practical guide. *Haematol. Oncol.*, **5**, 19–34
83. Schneider, D. R. and Picker, L. J. (1985) Myelodysplasia in the acquired immune deficiency syndrome. *Am. J. Clin. Pathol.*, **84**, 14–52

84. Raskind, W. W., Tirumali, N., Jacobson, R., Singer, J. and Fialkow, P. J. (1984) Evidence for a multistep pathogenesis of a myelodysplastic syndrome. *Blood*, **63**, 1318–23
85. Dormer, P., Hershko, C., Voss, R. and Wilmanns, W. (1987) Myelodysplastic syndrome: evolution of overt leukaemia by one or several steps of transformation. *Br. J. Haematol.*, **67**, 141–6
86. Kuriyama, K., Tomanaga, M., Matsuo, I., Ginnai, I. and Ichimaru, M. (1986) Diagnostic significance of detecting pseudo-Pelger–Huet anomalies and micromegakaryocytes in myelodysplastic syndromes. *Br. J. Haematol.*, **63**, 665–9
87. Brizard, A., Huret, J. L., Lamotte, F. *et al.* (1989) Three cases of myelodysplastic-myeloproliferative disorder with abnormal chromatin clumping in granulocytes. *Br. J. Haematol.*, **72**, 294–5
88. Erber, W. N., Jacobs, A., Oscier, D. G., O'Hea, A. M. and Mason, D. Y. (1987) Circulating micromegakaryocytes in myelodysplasia. *J. Clin. Pathol.*, **40**, 1349–52
89. Mufti, G. J., Stevens, J. R., Oscier, D. G., Hamlin, T. J. and Machin, D. G. (1985) Myelodysplastic syndrome: a scoring system with prognostic significance. *Br. J. Haematol.*, **55**, 691–700
90. Spitzer, T. R. and Goldsmith, G. H. (1982) Myelodysplastic syndromes: is another classification necessary? *Br. J. Haematol.*, **52**, 343–4
91. Greenberg, P. and Bagby, G. (1983) Biologic rather than morphologic markers in myelodysplastic syndromes. *Br. J. Haematol.*, **53**, 532–4
92. Weisdorf, D. J., Oken, M. M., Johnson, G. J. and Rydell, R. E. (1983) Chronic myelodysplastic syndrome: short survival with or without evolution to acute leukaemia. *Br. J. Haematol.*, **55**, 691–700
93. May, S. J., Smith, S. A., Jacobs, A., Williams, A. and Bailey-Wood, R. (1985) The myelodysplastic syndrome: analysis of laboratory characteristics in relation to the FAB classification. *Br. J. Haematol.*, **59**, 311–19
94. Mufti, G. J., Stevens, J. R., Oscier, D. G., Hamblin, T. J. and Machin, D. (1985) Myelodysplastic syndrome: a scoring system with prognostic significance. *Br. J. Haematol.*, **59**, 425–33
95. Kerkhofs, H., Hermans, J., Haak, H. L. and Leeksma, C. H. W. (1987) Utility of the FAB classification for myelodysplastic syndromes: investigation of prognostic factors in 237 cases. *Br. J. Haematol.*, **65**, 73–81
96. Third MIC Cooperative Study Group (1988) Morphologic, immunologic and cytogenic (MIC) working classification of the primary dysplastic syndrome and therapy-related myelodysplasias and leukaemias. *Cancer Genet. Cytogenet.*, **32**, 1–10
97. Yunis, J. J., Rydell, R. E., Oken, M. M., Arnesen, M. A., Mayer, M. G. and Lobell, M. (1986) Refined chromosome analysis as an independent prognostic indicator in *de novo* myelodysplastic syndrome. *Blood*, **67**, 1721–30
98. Nimer, S. D. and Golde, D. W. (1987) The 5q− abnormality. *Blood*, **70**, 1750–62
99. Scott, C. S., Cahill, A., Bynoe, A. G. *et al.* (1983) Esterase cytochemistry in primary myelodysplasia and megaloblastic anaemia: demonstration of abnormal staining pattern associated with dysmyelopoiesis. *Br. J. Haematol.*, **55**, 411–18
100. Clarke, R. E., Hoyt, G. and Jacobs, A. (1985) Granulocyte and monocyte surface membrane markers in the myelodysplastic syndrome. *J. Clin. Pathol.* **38**, 301–4
101. Bynoe, A. G., Scott, C. S., Ford, P. and Roberts, B. E. (1983) Decreased T helper cells in the myelodysplastic syndrome. *Br. J. Haematol.*, **54**, 97–102
102. Economopoulos, T., Economidou, J., Giannipoulos, G. *et al.* (1985) Immune abnormalities in myelodysplastic syndrome. *Br. J. Haematol.*, **38**, 908–11
103. Martin, S., Baldock, S. C., Ghoneim, A. T. M. and Child, J. A. (1983) Defective neutrophil function and microbiocidal mechanisms in the myelodysplastic disorders. *J. Clin. Pathol.*, **36**, 1120–8
104. Pearson, T. C. (1980) Who should you treat for polycythaemia? *Br. J. Hosp. Med.*, **24**, 66–73
105. Gilbert, H. S. (1975) Definition, clinical features and diagnosis of polycythaemia vera. *Clin. Haematol.*, **4**, 263–90
106. Leblond, P. F. and Weed, R. I. (1975) The peripheral blood in polycythaemia and myelofibrosis. *Clin. Haematol.*, **4**, 353–71

107. Marsh, J. C. W., Liu Yin, J. A. and Lewis, S. M. (1987) Blood volume measurement in pseudo-polycythaemia – when and why? *Clin. Lab. Haematol.*, **9**, 115–22
108. Pearson, T. C. and Guthrie, D. L. (1984) The interpretation of measured red cell mass and plasma volume in patients with elevated PCV values. *Clin. Lab. Haematol.*, **6**, 207–17
109. Berlin, N. I. (1975) Diagnosis and classification of the polycythaemias. *Semin. Haematol.*, **12**, 339–51
110. Pearson, T. C. and Wetherley-Mein, G. (1978) Vascular occlusive episodes and venous haematocrit in primary proliferative polycythaemia. *Lancet*, **ii**, 1219–22
111. International Committee for Standardisation in Haematology (1980) Recommended methods for measurement of red-cell and plasma volume. *J. Nucl. Med.*, **21**, 793–800
112. Pearson, T. C., Glass, U. H. and Wetherley-Mein, G. (1978) Interpretation of measured red cell mass in the diagnosis of polycythaemia. *Scand. J. Haematol.*, **21**, 153–62
113. Hellmann, A., Rotoli, B., Cotes, P. M. and Luzzatto, L. (1983) Familial erythrocytosis with over production of erythropoietin. *Clin. Lab. Haematol.*, **5**, 335–42
114. Pearson, T. C. and Wetherley-Mein, G. (1979) The course and complications of idiopathic erythrocytosis, *Clin. Lab. Haematol.*, **1**, 189–96
115. Lucie, N. P. and Young, G. A. R. (1983) Marrow cellularity in the diagnosis of polycythaemia. *J. Clin. Pathol.*, **36**, 180–3
116. Sharp, R. A. and Ho-Yen, D. O. (1983) Marrow cellularity and polycythaemia. *J. Clin. Pathol.*, **36**, 836–7
117. Lawler, S. D. (1980) Cytogenetic studies in Philadelphia chromosome-negative myeloproliferative disorders, particularly polycythaemia rubra vera. *Clin. Haematol.*, **9**, 159–74
118. Okuma, M. and Uchino, H. (1979) Altered arachidonate metabolism by platelets in patients with myeloproliferative disorders. *Blood*, **54**, 1258–71
119. Keenan, J. P., Wharton, J., Shepherd, A. J. N. and Bellingham, A. J. (1977) Defective platelet lipid peroxidation in myeloproliferative disorders: a possible defect of prostaglandin synthesis. *Br. J. Haematol.*, **35**, 275–83
120. Bateman, S., Lewis, S. M., Nicholas, A. and Zaafran, A. (1978) Splenic red-cell pooling: a diagnostic feature in polycythaemia. *Br. J. Haematol.* **40**, 389–96
121. Eridani, S., Dudley, J. M., Sawyer, B. M. and Pearson, T. C. (1987) Erythropoietic colonies in a serum-free system: results in primary proliferative polycythaemia and thrombocythaemia. *Br. J. Haematol.*, **67**, 387–91
122. Reid, C. D. L., Fidler, J. and Kirk, A. (1988) Endogenous erythroid clones (EEC) in polycythaemia and their relationship to diagnosis and the response to treatment. *Br. J. Haematol.*, **68**, 395–400
123. Marsh, J. C. W., Hibbin, J. and Marsh, G. W. (1987) Primary proliferative polycythaemia without splenomegaly: a diagnostic problem. *Clin. Lab. Haematol.*, **9**, 123–8
124. Charache, S., Weatherall, D. G. and Clegg, J. B. (1966) Polycythaemia associated with a hemoglobinopathy. *J. Clin. Invest.*, **45**, 813–22
125. Bellingham, A. J. (1976) Haemoglobin with altered oxygen affinity. *Br. Med. Bull.*, **32**, 234–8
126. Stephens, A. D. (1977) Polycythaemia and high affinity haemoglobins. *Br. J. Haematol.*, **36**, 153–9
127. Kulkarni, V., Ritchey, K., Howard, D. and Daniak, N. (1985) Heterogeneity of erythropoietin-dependent erythrocytosis: case report in a child and synopsis of primary erythrocytosis syndrome. *Br. J. Haematol.*, **60**, 751–8
128. Eridani, S., Pearson, T. C., Sawyer, B., Batten, E. and Wetherley-Mein, G. (1983) Erythroid colony formation in primary proliferative polycythaemia, idiopathic erythrocytosis and secondary polycythaemia: sensitivity to erythropoietic stimulating factors. *Clin. Lab. Haematol.*, **5**, 121–9
129. McCarthy, D. M. (1985) Fibrosis of the bone marrow: content and causes. *Br. J. Haematol.*, **59**, 1–7
130. Caligaris Caprio, F., Vigliani, R., Novarino, A., Camussi, G., Campana, D. and Gavosto, F. (1981) Idiopathic myelofibrosis: a possible role for immune complexes in the pathogenesis of the bone marrow fibrosis. *Br. J. Haematol.*, **49**, 17–21
131. Rondeau, E., Solal-Celigny, D., Dhermy, M. *et al.* (1983) Immune disorders in agnogenic myeloid metaplasia: relations to myelofibrosis. *Br. J. Haematol.*, **53**, 467–75

132. Groopman, J. E. (1980) The pathogenesis of myelofibrosis in myeloproliferative disorders. *Ann. Intern. Med.*, **92**, 857–8
133. Casto-Malaspina, M., Rabellino, E. M., Yen, A., Nachman, R. L. and Moore, M. A. S. (1981) Human megakaryocyte stimulation of proliferation of bone marrow fibroblasts. *Blood*, **57**, 78–87
134. Manoharan, A. (1988) Myelofibrosis: prognostic factors and treatment. *Br. J. Haematol.*, **69**, 296–8
135. Takácsi-Nagi, L. and Gráf, F. (1975) Definition, clinical features and diagnosis of myelofibrosis. *Clin. Haematol.*, **4**, 291–308
136. Lawler, S. D. and Swansbury, G. J. (1985) Cytogenetic studies in myelofibrosis and related conditions. In *Myelofibrosis. Pathophysiology and Management* (ed. S. M. Lewis), pp. 167–94. New York: Marcel Dekker
137. Miller, J. B., Testa, J. R., Lingren, V. and Rowley, J. D. (1985) The pattern and clinical significance of karyotypic abnormalities in patients with idiopathic and postpolycythaemic myelofibrosis. *Cancer*, **55**, 582–91
138. Bowring, C. S. (1981) *Radionuclide Tracer Techniques in Haematology,* pp. 80–100. London: Butterworths
139. Szur, A. B. and Lewis, S. M. (1975) Iron kinetics. *Clin. Haematol.*, **4**, 407–25
140. Fitzgerald, P. H., McEwan, C., Fraser, J. and Beard, M. E. J. (1981) A complex Ph′ translocation in a patient with primary thrombocythaemia. *Br. J. Haematol.*, **47**, 571–5
141. O'Hea, A. M., Erber, W., O'Connor, N. T. J. and Bunch, C. (1986) Acute transformation of essential thrombocythaemia: report of two cases. *J. Clin. Pathol.*, **39**, 1296–8
142. Frei-Lahr, D., Barton, J. C., Hoffman, R., Burkett, L. L. and Prchal, J. T. (1984) Blastic transformation of essential thrombocythaemia: dual expression of myelomonocytic/megakaryoblastic phenotypes. *Blood*, **63**, 866–72
143. Zaccaria, A. and Tura, S. (1978) Chromosomal abnormality in primary thrombocythaemia. *N. Engl. J. Med.*, **298**, 1422–3
144. Fabris, F., Casonato, A., Grazia del Ben, M., de Marco, L. and Girolami, A. (1986) Abnormalities of von Willebrand factor in myeloproliferative disease: a relationship with bleeding diathesis. *Br. J. Haematol.*, **63**, 75–83
145. Budman, D. R., Lackner, H., Berczeller, P. and Silber, R. (1981) The diagnostic value of the serum lactic dehydrogenase determination in the evaluation of unexplained thrombocytosis. *Am. J. Clin. Pathol.*, **75**, 840–3
146. Dudley, J. M., Messinesy, M., Eridani, S. *et al.* (1989) Primary thrombocythaemia: a scoring system for positive diagnosis. *Br. J. Haematol.*, **71**, 331–5
147. Scott, C. S. (1978) Cytochemical applications in haematology with particular reference to acute leukaemias: a review. *Med. Lab. Sci.*, **35**, 111–36
148. Hayhoe, F. G. J. and Quaglino, D. (1980) *Haematological Cytochemistry*. London: Churchill Livingstone
149. Catovsky. D. (1980) Leucocyte enzymes in leukaemia. In *Topical Reviews in Haematology* (ed. S Roath), Vol. **1**, pp. 157–85. Bristol: Wright
150. Scott, C. S. (ed.) (1989) *Leukaemia Cytochemistry*. Chichester: Ellis Horwood
151. International Committee for Standardisation in Haematology (1985) Recommended methods for cytological procedures in haematology. *Clin. Lab. Haematol.*, **7**, 55–74
152. Janckila, A. J. and Elias, J. M. (1989) Biochemical and theoretical aspects of haematological cytochemistry. In *Leukaemic Cytochemistry* (ed. C. S. Scott), pp. 68–90. Chichester: Ellis Horwood
153. Friedman, B. C., Binder, N. E. and Weiner, R. S. (1976) Reduction of health risks in the preparation of the non-specific esterase stain (Letter). *Am. J. Clin. Pathol.*, **66**, 766
154. Marty. J. and Kjeldsberg, C. R. (1977) Health risks in preparation of esterase stain (Letter). *Am. J. Clin. Pathol.*, **68**, 93
155. Breton-Gorius, J., Gourdin, M. F. and Reyes, F. (1981) Ultrastructure of the leukaemic cells. In *Methods in Haematology* (ed. D. Catovsky), No. **2**. *The Leukaemic Cell*, pp. 87–128. London: Churchill Livingstone
156. Reiffers. J., Darmendrail, V., Larrue, J. *et al.* (1981) Ultrastructural cytochemical prospective study of adult acute lymphoblastic leukaemia. *Cancer*, **48**, 927–31

157. Flandrin, G. and Daniel, M. T. (1981) Cytochemistry in the classification of leukaemia. In *Methods in Haematology* (ed. D. Catovsky), No. **2**. *The Leukaemic Cell*, p. 42. London: Churchill Livingstone
158. Dimmock, V. (1977) Methyl-green pyronin staining of blood and bone marrow smears. *Med. Lab. Sci.*, **34**, 173–4
159. Rutenberg, A. M., Rosales, C. L. and Bennett, J. M. (1965) An improved histochemical method for the demonstration of leukocyte alkaline phosphatase activity: clinical application. *J. Lab. Clin. Med.*, **65**, 698–705
160. Swirsky, D. M. (1984) Single incubation double esterase cytochemical reaction using a single coupling reagent. *J. Clin. Pathol.*, **37**, 1187–90
161. Campana, D. and Janossy, G. (1986) Leukaemia diagnosis and testing of complement fixing antibodies for bone marrow purging in ALL. *Blood*, **68**, 1264–71
162. Erber, W. N., Mynheer, L. C. and Mason, D. Y. (1986) APAAP labelling of blood and bone marrow samples for phenotyping leukaemia. *Lancet*, **i**, 761–5
163. Erber, W. N. (1989) Applications of immunocytochemistry in leukaemia diagnosis. In *Leukaemia Cytochemistry* (ed. C. S. Scott), pp. 342–61. Chichester: Ellis Horwood
164. Cordell, J. L., Falini, B., Erber, W. N. *et al.* (1984) Immunoenzymatic labelling of monoclonal antibodies using immune complexes of alkaline phosphatase and monoclonal anti-alkaline phosphatase (APAAP). *J. Histochem. Cytochem.*, **32**, 219–29
165. Greaves, M. F., Bell, R., Amess, J. and Lister, T. A. (1983) ALL masquerading as AUL. *Leukaemia Res.*, **7**, 735–46
166. Mack, D., Couzens, S., Reardon, D. and Marcus, R. (1989) Rapid diagnosis of leukaemia: a three-stage immunophenotyping technique. *Med. Lab. Sci.*, **46**, 316–23
167. Holgate, C., Jackson, P., Cowen, P. and Bird, C. (1983) Immunogold-silver staining: a new method of immunostaining with enhanced sensitivity. *J. Histochem. Cytochem.*, **31**, 938–44
168. Coombs, R. R. A. and Wilson, A. B. (1982) Rosette-forming reactions. In *Clinical Aspects of Immunology*, 4th edn (eds P. Lachman and D. K. Peters), pp. 343–95. Oxford: Blackwell
169. Coombs, R. R. (1987) Harnessing the red cell for immunoassays. *Med. Lab. Sci.*, **44**, 66–72
170. International Committee for Standardisation in Haematology (ICSH) (1973) Standard techniques for the measurement of red-cell and plasma volume. *Br. J. Haematol.*, **25**, 801–14
171. International Committee for Standardisation in Haematology (1980) Recommended methods for measurement of red-cell and plasma volume. *J. Nucl. Med.*, **21**, 793–800
172. Bowring, C. S. (1981) *Radionuclide Tracer Techniques in Haematology*. London: Butterworths
173. Radia, R., Peters, A. M., Deenamode, M., Fitzpatrick, M. L. and Lewis, S. M. (1981) Measurement of red-cell volume and splenic red-cell pool using ^{113m}Indium. *Br. J. Haematol.*, **49**, 587–91
174. Najean, Y. and Cacchione, R. (1977) Blood volume in health and disease. *Clin. Haematol.*, **6**, 543–66
175. Pettit, J. E. (1977) Spleen function. *Clin. Haematol.*, **6**, 639–56
176. Bateman, S., Lewis, S. M., Nicholas, A. and Zaafran, A. (1978) Splenic red-cell pooling: a diagnostic feature in polycythaemia. *Br. J. Haematol.*, **40**, 389–96
177. Spencer, R. P. and Pearson, H. A. (1974) Splenic radiocolloid uptake in the presence of circulating Howell–Jolly bodies. *J. Nucl. Med.*, **15**, 294–5
178. Marsh, G. W., Lewis, S. M. and Szur, L. (1966) The use of ^{51}Cr-labelled heat-damaged red-cells to study splenic function. 1. Evaluation of method. *Br. J. Haematol.*, **12**, 161–6
179. Peters, A. M., Klonizakis, I., Lavender, J. P. and Lewis, S. M. (1980) Use of ^{111}Indium-labelled platelets to measure spleen function. *Br. J. Haematol.*, **46**, 587–6
180. Peters, A. M., Osman, S., Reavy, H. J., Chambers, B., Deenamode, M. and Lewis, S. M. (1986) Erythrocyte radiolabelling: *in vitro* comparison of chromium, technetium and indium in undamaged and heat damaged cells. *J. Clin. Pathol.*, **39**, 717–21
181. Peters, A. M., Ryan, P. F. J., Klonizakis, I., Elkon, K. B., Lewis, S. M. and Hughes, G. R. V. (1981) Analysis of heat-damaged erythrocyte clearance curves. *Br. J. Haematol.*, **49**, 581–6
182. Bowring, C. S., Glass, H. I. and Lewis, S. M. (1976) Rates of clearance by the spleen of heat-damaged erythrocytes. *J. Clin. Pathol.*, **29**, 852–4

183. Dacie, J. V. and Lewis, S. M. (1975) *Practical Haematology*, 5th edn., pp. 438–472. London: Churchill Livingstone
184. Robinson, P. J., Bullen, A. W., Hall, R., Brown, R. C., Baxter, P. and Losowsky, M. S. (1980) Splenic size and function in adult coeliac disease. *Br. J. Radiol.*, **53**, 532–7
185. Casper, J. T., Koethe, S., Rodey, G. E. and Thatcher, L. G. (1976) A new method for studying reticuloendothelial dysfunction in sickle-cell disease patients and its clinical application. A brief report. *Blood,* **47**, 183–8
186. Corazza, G. R., Bullen, A. W., Hall, R., Robinson, P. J. and Losowsky, M. S. (1981) A simple method of assessing splenic function in coeliac disease. *Clin. Sci.*, **60**, 109–13
187. Dunn, C. D. R. and Lange, R. D. (1980) Erythropoietin: assay and characterisation. In *Topical Reviews in Haematology* (ed. S. Roath), No. **1**, pp. 1–32. Bristol: Wright
188. Goldwasser, E. and Sherwood, J. B. (1981) Radioimmunoassay of erythropoietin. *Br. J. Haematol.*, **48**, 359–63
189. Sherwood, J. B. and Goldwasser, E. (1979) A radioimmunoassay for erythropoietin. *Blood*, **54**, 885–93
190. Goto, E. (1989) Characterisation and use of monclonal antibodies directed against human erythropoietin that recognize different antigenic determinants. *Blood*, **74**, 1415–23
191. Wognum, G. (1989) An enzyme-linked immunosorbent assay for erythropoietin using monoclonal antibodies, tetrameric immune complexes and substrate amplification. *Blood*, **74**, 622–8
192. Cotes, P. M., Dore, C. J., Liu Yin, J. A. *et al.* (1986) Determination of serum immunoreactive erythropoietin in the investigation of erythrocytosis. *N. Engl. J. Med.*, **315**, 283–7
193. Miller, M. E., Garcia, J. F., Cohen, R. A., Cronkite, E. P., Moccia, G. and Acevedo, J. (1981) Diurnal levels of immunoreactive erythropoietin in normal subjects and subjects with chronic lung disease. *Br. J. Haematol.*, **49**, 189
194. Garcia, J. F., Sherwood, J. B. and Goldwasser, E. (1979) Radioimmunoassay of erythropoietin. *Blood Cells*, **5**, 405–19
195. Koeffler, H. P. and Goldwasser, E. (1981) Erythropoietin radioimmunoassay in evaluating patients with polycythaemia. *Ann. Intern. Med*, **94**, 44–7
196. Dacie, J. V. and Lewis, S. M. (1975) *Practical Haematology*, 5th edn., pp. 493–5. London: Churchill Livingstone

Chapter 14

Haematology of infections

Infection in man is a common occurrence. Apparently healthy subjects may be infected by bacteria, rickettsia, viruses, fungi, protozoa or helminths. Patients with haematological disorders – such as aplastic anaemia, acute or chronic leukaemias, lymphomas and myeloma – and those receiving cytotoxic or immunosuppressive therapy are particularly susceptible to infection because of impaired cellular or humoral immune responses. Absence of splenic function due to surgical removal or splenic atrophy has a higher risk of systemic infection.

The haematological changes associated with infection may be negligible; they may have diagnostic, prognostic and therapeutic significance; or they may be severe and even life threatening. The changes may be confined to alteration in the numbers and morphology of the circulating leucocytes or may affect the bone marrow, lymphoid tissues or reticuloendothelial system. A haemolytic anaemia may be found due to a variety of mechanisms. Haemostatic failure may occur due to defective coagulation, increased fibrinolysis or thrombocytopenia. Increased concentrations of certain plasma proteins are commonly associated with infection, particularly C-reactive protein (CRP) haptoglobins, fibrinogen and the immunoglobulins. Iron depletion or overload influences susceptibility to bacterial infection[1]. The changes in plasma proteins are reflected by the ESR and plasma viscosity. A substantial part of the work of the routine haematology department is involved in the detection and monitoring of infections.

Blood changes

Cellular elements

Changes in the numbers of circulating leucocytes are a common feature of infection and represent the cellular response to chemotaxins or antigen stimulus. Extensive tables listing or summarizing the common changes in leucocytes have been compiled[2]. A normal or low leucocyte count does not exclude infection and is a frequent finding in septicaemia or overwhelming infection.

Neutrophils

Emphasis is often placed on the presence of an increase in circulating neutrophils ($>7.5 \times 10^9/l$). It is important to recognize that elevated neutrophil counts due to mobilization of the marginal neutrophil pool can readily be produced by physiological factors such as stress, emotion, physical activity, etc. and are due to vasodilatation and increased blood flow through capillaries which also occurs in the presence of a fever from whatever cause. The neutrophils from the marginal pool will have normal morphology. Of greater significance is the presence of immature granulocytes such as band forms, metamyelocytes and myelocytes which must represent increased release from the bone marrow. The presence of toxic granulation, vacuolation and Döhle bodies are important indications of infection (*Figure 14.1*). A neutrophil leucocytosis with increased bone-marrow production and release represents an effective response to infection, and systemic infections associated with a normal or low neutrophil count may represent a poor prognosis.

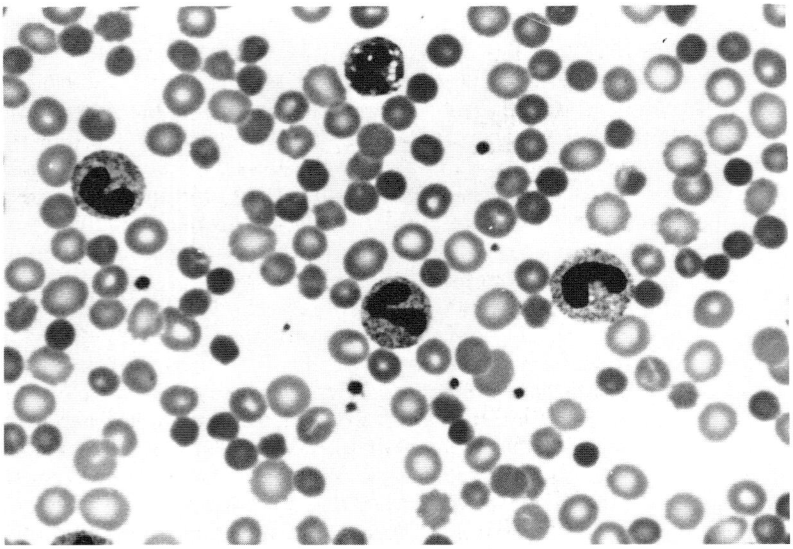

Figure 14.1 Blood film. Neutrophil changes in infection; shift to left, toxic granulation and vacuolation. The microspherocytes in this particular film suggest *Clostridium perfringens* infection. ×550

Severe bacterial infection will generally provoke a neutrophil leucocytosis irrespective of the organisms involved, though the Gram-positive, pyogenic (pus-forming) organisms such as staphylococci, pneumococci and streptococci tend to produce the highest neutrophil counts, whereas some Gram-negative organisms, for example *Salmonella* and *Brucella,* are associated with neutropenia. Viral infections are frequently associated with neutropenia.

In the pre-antibiotic era considerable attention was given to trends in the neutrophil count and in the maturity of the neutrophils. Schilling and Arneth counts, which are based on counting the neutrophil lobes and the presence of non-segmented neutrophils, were widely used as prognostic indicators and the term 'shift to the left' refers to the presence of immature granulocytes as judged by a Schilling count.

Eosinophils

In acute infections the eosinophils tend to disappear from the circulation and reappear as the infection subsides. A neutrophil leucocytosis and the presence of eosinophils suggests a physiological leucocytosis, but an important exception is streptococcal infections in which the eosinophils may not only be present but are often increased. The classic association with eosinophilia is parasitic infection due to helminths, or their larvae, in the gut, tissues and particularly in the blood. The condition known as tropical eosinophilia is recognized to be due to filarial infections.

Basophils

Because of their small number, an absence of basophils in a standard differential count is of little significance. An increase in basophils is said to be found in infections with pox viruses.

Monocytes

Monocytes may be increased in bacterial infections and particularly so when there is a diminished neutrophil response. As monocytes are associated with a response to an antigenic stimulus and in tissue reactions, they may be expected to be increased in chronic infections, such as tuberculosis, and in protozoal infections.

Lymphocytes

Acute bacterial infections are usually accompanied by a lymphopenia. A lymphocytosis ($>3.5 \times 10^9$/l) often accompanies virus infections and marked elevations are also seen in children with pertussis (whooping cough). Mild elevations may be found in chronic bacterial infections such as brucellosis and tuberculosis. A clear distinction must be made between an absolute lymphocytosis and a relative lymphocytosis due to a neutropenia.

The lymphocytosis in virus infections is often associated with morphological changes due to the immune response of the lymphocytes. The changes include increased size, a less dense nuclear chromatin, more copious cytoplasm and increased cytoplasmic basophilia. These appearances represent transformation of T and B lymphocytes and are particularly seen in infectious hepatitis, rubella and infectious mononucleosis (IM). In IM the appearances are of particular significance and the haematological features of IM are considered in detail elsewhere (*see* page 506). Morphological changes are also seen in brucellosis, toxoplasmosis and cytomegalovirus disease and may simulate those found in IM. Automated blood cell analysers routinely provide displays which analyse lymphocyte volume. The presence of 'large' lymphocytes (other than in proliferative disorders) is a sensitive, though non-specific indicator of acute viral infections[3].

Platelets

In chronic infections there may be a thrombocytosis ($>400 \times 10^9$/l) . In a study of platelet numbers in pulmonary tuberculosis there was a correlation between platelet numbers and the degree of inflammation[4]. Of greater importance is the occurrence of thrombocytopenia due to bone-marrow arrest, an immune mechanism associated with virus infection, or to bacterial products activating the coagulation pathway with resulting platelet consumption. The viral haemorrhagic fevers are invariably associated with thrombocytopenia[5]. Thrombocytopenia in most cases of necrotizing enterocolitis (NEC) in neonates is attributable to endotoxinaemia[6].

Erythrocytes
The anaemia of chronic infection has been considered in Chapter 9. A shortened red-cell survival is a feature of certain systemic infections. Release of haemolytic bacterial enzymes into the circulation, e.g. from *Clostridium perfringens* and in leptospirosis[7] can result in a frankly haemolytic picture; in other infections, e.g. streptococcal infection, the red-cell destruction is not morphologically obvious. Parasitization of red cells will result in their eventual destruction; malaria is the classic example (*see* page 514). A rare erythrocyte infection is babesiosis (piroplasmosis) which although common in animals is rare in man and is usually associated with absence of splenic function[8–10]. The term 'haemotropic bacteria'[11] has been applied to those micro-organisms with an affinity for red cells. *Bartonella bacilliformis* truly parasitizes the red cells but is restricted to a small geographical area in the Andes. Other organisms of uncertain taxonomy that adhere to the red-cell membrane have been reported occasionally[12, 13].

Autoimmune haemolysis secondary to virus or mycoplasma infections is an infrequent complication (*see* page 326) and the association of paroxysmal cold haemoglobinuria and syphilis is now very rarely seen. The anaemia of protozoal infections has an immune component.

Aplastic anaemia is a recognized sequel to virus infections such as measles, infectious mononucleosis and infective hepatitis. The mechanism of bone-marrow failure is assumed to be at the level of the common progenitor, or stem, cell. Aplastic episodes due to maturation arrest are more common and usually self-limiting. Of particular interest is the red-cell aplasia associated with B19 parvovirus infection. The aplastic episode is usually transient and in normal subjects is not clinically noticeable. In patients with haemolytic anaemia, who depend on adequate increased erythropoiesis, the sudden drop in circulating red cells may require transfusion support. Leucopenia and thrombocytopenia can also occur. Persistent infection in immunocompromised patients may result in chronic bone-marrow failure[14].

Plasma
Certain organisms are found in the plasma, and of particular haematological importance are the trypanosomes (*see* page 519) and microfilariae (*see* page 521).

Neonatal infections
The wide range of total leucocyte counts in neonates and the fall in neutrophils in the first 72 hours of life have led to statements that total and differential leucocyte counts are of little value in the diagnosis of neonatal infection. Certain aspects, however, require further consideration: (1) repeated neutrophil counts in the first 72 hours may show a rise rather than the expected fall; (2) immature neutrophil counts over 1000×10^{99}/l, (3) ratio of immature to total neutrophils >0.8[15]; (4) toxic granulation and vacuolation in severe infections; (5) profound neutropenia in overwhelming infections; and (6) eosinophils in severe infections. After 4 days the neutrophil count has well-established limits of $1.8–5.4 \times 10^9$/l[16]. Lymphocyte and monocyte numbers are of little value in the diagnosis of neonatal bacterial infections.

Intravascular coagulation in infections

Disseminated intravascular coagulation (DIC) may be caused by a wide variety of infectious diseases. It occurs more often in Gram-negative bacteraemia than in

Gram-positive infections. *Neisseria meningitidis* and Gram-negative bacilli are well recognized causes and endotoxins are the likely trigger. Gram-positive organisms such as streptococci and staphylococci can result in occlusive DIC with symmetrical gangrene.

The role of viral haemorrhagic agents in the pathogenesis of thrombocytopenia has been mentioned previously. DIC may also be demonstrated but is not invariably a feature.

Local or 'organ-specific' intravascular coagulation is associated with infection. The renal lesions of haemolytic uraemic syndrome (HUS) due to verotoxin-producing *E. coli* is the prime example [17, 18].

Absent splenic function and infections

Splenectomy or splenic atrophy leads to an increased risk of overwhelming infection and about half of the recorded cases are due to *Streptococcus pneumoniae*. These severe infections are usually accompanied by DIC. In the absence of splenic function, infection by exotic organisms not usually associated with systemic infection in humans can be found. Examples are *Babesia*, DF-2 and similar aerobic Gram-negative bacilli, *Campylobacter* and even unidentified organisms [12]. Infection may follow tick-bites or dog-bites. Clearly the recognition of the blood-film changes associated with loss of splenic function can be vital in patients with severe infections.

Cytochemistry

Cytochemical techniques for NAP activity and the nitro blue-tetrazolium (NBT) test have been used as screening tests and as supportive evidence for infection.

The NAP reaction has been claimed to be of value in distinguishing viral from bacterial infections and in differentiating painful sickle-cell crisis from bacterial infection. High scores are certainly found in subjects with localized and systemic infection but there is overlap with the scores of hospital patients without infection [19].

The NBT test has been widely advocated as an indication of bacterial infection [20]. The reaction depends on the phagocytosis of a tetrazolium–heparin–fibrinogen complex with reduction of the tetrazolium to form an insoluble formazan deposit. The test is therefore a measure of phagocytosis, membrane permeability and oxidative reduction, in stimulated neutrophils. The original technique [20] has been subjected to many modifications and the initial enthusiasm for the test as a valuable marker of bacterial infection has been tempered by numerous reports questioning the value of the NBT test in its original or modified forms [21–23]. The NBT test is of most value in the diagnosis of chronic granulomatous disease (CGD) in which neutrophils have defective bacterial killing, the affected children being susceptible to repeated infection. The interpretation of the test in bacterial infection requires a full knowledge of bacteriological studies, and the test should be performed in bacteriology departments.

The demonstration of chloracetate esterase and acid phosphatase activities of the primary lysosomes of neutrophils after endotoxin stimulation has been studied in parallel with NAP and NBT techniques [19]. Although the scores for each technique were often increased in individual patients, there was an overlap of results with those in control groups and the tests either singly or collectively were of limited value in the recognition of infection.

Toxic granulation of neutrophils has been identified as being the demonstration by azure dyes of the persistence of sulphated mucosubstance in the azurophilic granules and reflects abnormal neutrophil maturation in the presence of infection [24].

Infectious mononucleosis

IM is an acute illness which characteristically presents with sore throat, lymphadenopathy and fever. Splenomegaly is common and a skin rash and jaundice may be present. The infection occurs predominantly in the 15–25 years age group, though children and infants may be affected [25]. Very rarely cases may be seen in middle-aged or elderly subjects. The infection is endemic and cases are sporadic, though periods of higher incidence and 'clustering' are observed. IM is not highly infectious and members of the family of infected subjects are not usually affected which suggests transmission by intimate contact, saliva being the likely vehicle of transmission.

Rarely the infection is fatal and is due to haemorrhage, bone marrow damage and opportunistic infection. Aplastic anaemia is a rare complication.

Pathogenesis [26]

The causative organism is Epstein–Barr virus (EBV). This belongs to the herpes group and was first identified in cultured cells from biopsies of Burkitt's lymphoma. Antibodies to EBV are found in the serum of 90% of normal adult males, indicating a previous infection that confers immunity to further infection. IM in subjects previously seronegative for EBV antibody is accompanied by a rising titre of antibody to EBV, which then persists for many years. The presence of EBV can be detected in the saliva during the acute phase and apparently persists at a low level for life.

Blood picture

The total leucocyte count is increased in 70% of cases and an initial neutrophil leucocytosis is rapidly replaced with a predominance of 'mononuclear' cells, often with a neutropenia. This population of 'mononuclears' is made up of normal lymphocytes and monocytes and a variable proportion of atypical cells. The atypical cells are larger than normal lymphocytes, with a less dense nucleus which may be irregular and show nucleoli (*Figure 14.2*). The cytoplasm is more copious and basophilic and a few vacuoles may be seen. The basophilic cytoplasm tends to be a deeper shade at the periphery which is often irregular in outline (*Figure 14.3*). 'Hand-mirror' cells are reported as being significantly increased in the transformed T-cell population (*see* below) in IM [27]. Mild thrombocytopenia ($100–150 \times 10^9$/l) is not unusual and severe thrombocytopenia is occasionally found, with haemorrhages in the skin and mucous membranes. The thrombocytopenia is probably due to an immune mechanism [28, 29]. Red-cell morphology is usually unremarkable though autoagglutination is occasionally seen (*Figure 14.4*) and more rarely an overt haemolytic picture is present.

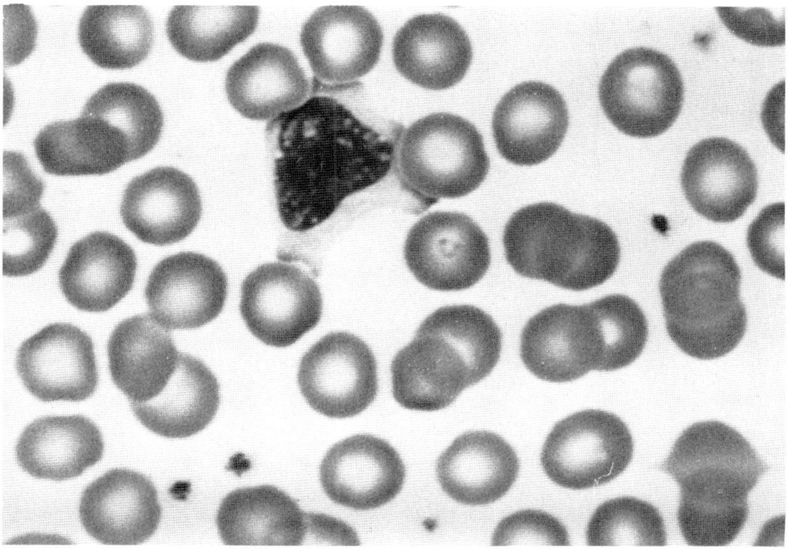

Figure 14.2 Blood film. Infectious mononucleosis. Atypical lymphocyte showing fine nuclear chromatin, suggestion of nucleoli, irregular shape and peripheral shading of the cytoplasm. ×1200

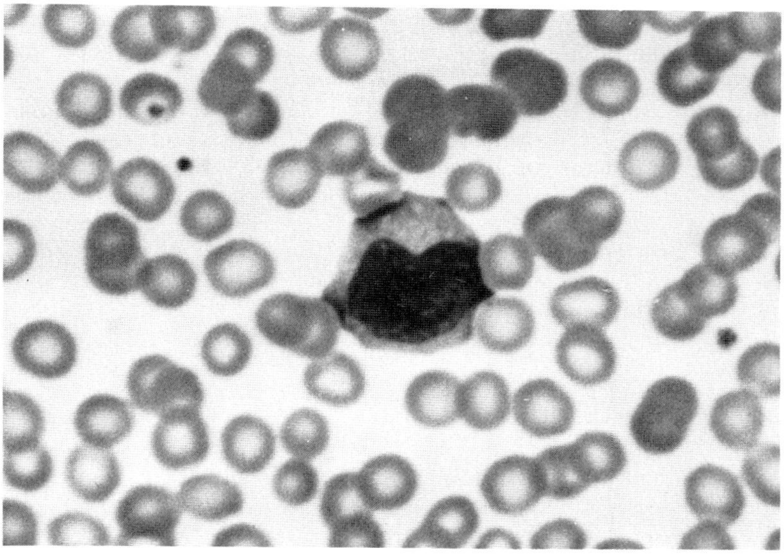

Figure 14.3 Blood film. Infectious mononucleosis. Atypical lymphocyte with 'monocytoid' features. ×825

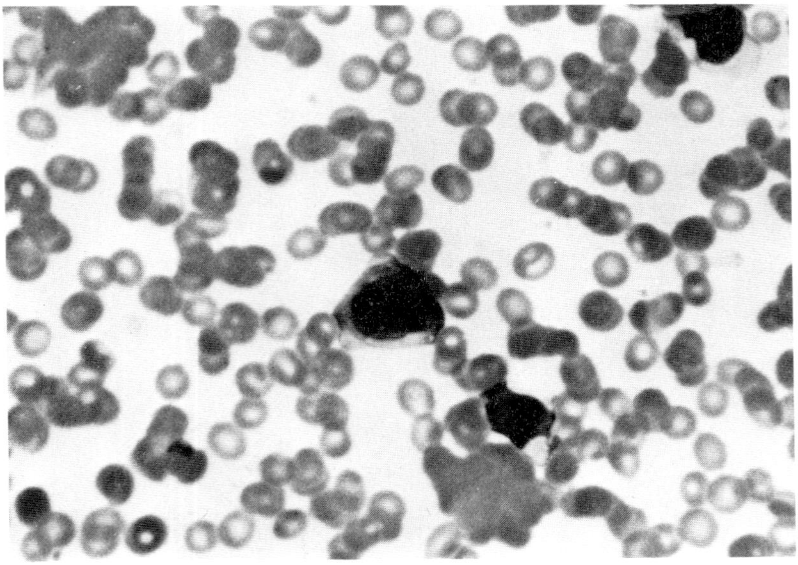

Figure 14.4 Blood film. Infectious mononucleosis associated with cold autoagglutination. ×550

Origin of the atypical cells

B lymphocytes have membrane receptors for EBV. This results in infection of the B lymphocytes, which proliferate and evoke a greater proliferative response and transformation of the T lymphocytes. The transformed T-lymphocyte population is cytotoxic for the infected B cells. The great majority of the atypical 'mononuclear' cells are therefore transformed T lymphocytes. The abnormal morphology persists for 1–2 weeks, though the predominance of lymphocytes persists for several weeks with minor morphological changes.

It is important to realize that the picture is not specific for IM, and that similar pictures may be seen in toxoplasmosis and cytomegalovirus infection which is not uncommon following transfusion of blood, particularly in immunosuppressed patients.

Serology

IM provokes the formation of a variety of antibodies which are not normally present. Of particular diagnostic importance is the production of heterophil antibody and antibodies to EBV.

Heterophil antibody in IM

In 1932 Paul and Bunnell described the presence of an anti-sheep red-cell agglutinin in the serum of patients with IM. Such an antibody is a heterophil antibody (defined in footnote to *Table 14.1*).

The 'sheep-cell agglutinin titre' or Paul–Bunnell test was used in the diagnosis of IM. The Paul–Bunnell titre is not specific for IM because the presence of heterophil antibody is not confined to IM; normal sera contain heterophil antibodies although usually in relatively low titre.

The heterophil antibody in normal serum is directed against an antigen widely distributed in nature and termed the Forssmann antigen. Furthermore, the therapeutic or prophylactic injection of antitoxins raised in horses (i.e. injection of horse serum) gives rise to the heterophil antibody of 'serum sickness'. *Table 14.1* shows the reactions of the heterophil antibody of IM, the Forssmann antibody and that of serum sickness, with cells from various animal species.

Table 14.1 Reactions of heterophil antibodies with red cells of various species

Species	*Heterophil antibody**		
	IM	*Forssmann*	*Serum sickness*
Sheep	+	+	+
Horse	+	+	+
Ox	+	−	+
Guinea-pig	−	+	+
Rat	−	−	−
Mouse	−	+	−
Rabbit	−	−	−
Human	−	−	−

Heterophil antibody is variously defined as:

1. Antibody that reacts with an antigen apparently unrelated to that stimulating the production of the antibody.
2. Antibody produced in a species by antigen of a second species and reacting with antigen of a third species.
3. Antibody produced in one species and reacting with antigen found in an unrelated species.

An absorption pattern using ox red cells and guinea-pig kidney cells forms the basis of the differential absorption test of Davidsohn and Walker described in 1935. This is based on the observations that the heterophil antibody of IM is absorbed by ox red cells but not by an emulsion of guinea-pig kidney cells, that the Forssmann antibody is absorbed by guinea-pig kidney (rich in Forssmann antigen) but not by ox cells, while the antibody of serum sickness is absorbed by both guinea-pig kidney and by ox cells. By common usage the Paul–Bunnell test is now accepted to include differential absorption using a tube technique.

Horse cells are more susceptible to agglutination than sheep cells and a slide test using formalized horse cells was claimed to be as sensitive and almost as specific as the standard differential Paul–Bunnell test[30]. By combining the sensitivity of the horse cells with the specificity of differential absorption, a slide differential absorption test was developed[31] and has formed the basis of commercial test kits for the heterophil antibody of IM.

Other approaches to the identification of the heterophil antibody have been the use of trypsinized ox cells, which permit agglutination by the IM antibody but are not agglutinated by Forssmann antibody, and an ox-cell haemolysis test requiring the presence of complement.

The heterophil antibody of IM is of IgM type, usually appears between the fifth and tenth days of illness, rises to its highest level in the second to third week and persists for some months, or occasionally for years [32]. The antibody may be found in conditions other than IM and has been reported in lymphoma, leukaemia and histiocytic medullary reticulosis [33], observations that are of relevance when considering the differential diagnosis and possible aetiology. The heterophil antibody does not react with EBV-specific antigens.

Persistently positive tests for IM heterophil antibody in the absence of clinical or haematological evidence of IM may be due to previous subclinical infection with persistence of antibody. In such cases the presence of antibody to the EBV is clearly helpful though a small number of subjects who are seronegative for EBV have been described [34].

Negative heterophil antibody tests in otherwise typical cases of IM have been reported. Negative serology for EBV in such cases virtually excludes a diagnosis of IM and further investigation for infections that can simulate IM should be pursued.

EBV serology

EBV-infected lymphocytes exhibit several 'new' antigens derived from the virus (*Table 14.2*). These antigens may be detected by immunofluorescence (IF), immunoblotting or ELISA.

Table 14.2 Epstein–Barr virus antigens in lymphocytes of IM

	Nucleus	*Cytoplasm*
Epstein–Barr nuclear antigen (EBNA)	+	–
Early antigen (diffuse) (EA-D)	+	+
Early antigen (restricted) (EA-R)	–	+
Viral capsid antigen (VCA)	–	+

In addition to heterophil antibody, serum from patients with IM contain IgM and IgG antibodies to EBNA and VCA antigens. The class of immunoglobulin present depends on the stage of the infection – incubation, acute or post phases.

1. Anti-EBNA IgM, anti-VCA IgM and heterophil Ab peak in the acute phase and decrease rapidly.
2. Anti-VCA IgG appears early and persists.
3. Anti-EBNA IgG appears much later in the course of the infection, indicates a previous infection and persists for life.
4. Anti-EBNA IgM is present in heterophil-negative cases of IM.

The patterns of antibody production and decline are summarized in *Figure 14.5*.

Anti-i

This antibody which typically reacts with the i antigen of cord red cells is found in the great majority of cases of uncomplicated IM and probably accounts for the cold-autoagglutination sometimes seen in blood films. The occasional cases of overt haemolytic anaemia in IM have been ascribed to the presence of high thermal

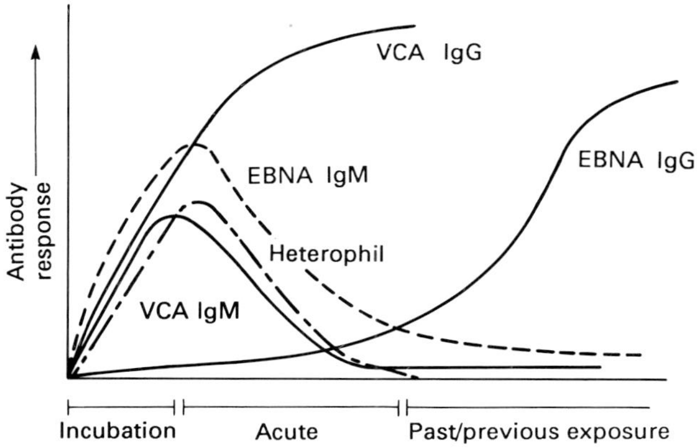

Figure 14.5 Patterns of antibody production and decline

amplitude (about 30°C) IgM anti-i. A further mechanism in which IgG anti-i reacts with an IgM anti-IgG has been postulated. Although both mechanisms can apparently produce haemolytic anaemia in IM, in some cases an additional mechanism is indicated [35].

Other antibodies

Antibodies with rheumatoid factor activity, anti-nuclear factor specificity and of Donath–Landsteiner type have been reported.

Laboratory diagnosis

Apart from the clinical symptoms, the diagnosis of IM depends on the blood picture and serology. Classically, in the vast majority of cases the serological diagnosis has been based on the demonstration of the heterophil antibody of IM.

As previously discussed, this depends on the demonstration of heterophil antibody which is not absorbed by guinea-pig kidney and is absorbed by ox red cells (*Table 14.3*).

The classic differential absorption tube test is read as a titre, but the level of antibody does not correlate with clinical severity or the changes in the blood film.

Table 14.3 Absorption patterns of heterophil antibodies of infectious mononucleosis (IM) and those of the Forssmann and serum-sickness antibodies

Antibody	*Absorbed by*	
	G-P kidney	*Ox cells*
IM	No	Yes
Forssmann	Yes	No
Serum-sickness	Yes	Yes

G-P = Guinea-pig.

Repeated titres during an infection may serve as an indication of the immune response but can only be compared if the indicator cells, sheep or horse, are carefully selected for similar reactivity in test to test. The sole criterion of a positive tube test is a significant difference between the titres of serum absorbed with guinea-pig kidney and with ox cells. A two-tube difference is considered significant. The tube test is a qualitative and not a quantitative test.

The slide or 'spot' tests are clearly qualitative and have been extensively compared with the classic tube test. They show excellent correlation [36]. Any disparity is towards unexplained positive results which may or may not be confirmed by the tube test. It is important that in any comparison between slide and tube tests, horse cells should be used in the tube test. Slide tests are rapid, simple and reliable and have replaced the standard tube test in the routine testing for IM heterophil antibody.

Slide agglutination test for heterophil antibody

Principle

Plasma or serum is absorbed by guinea-pig kidney suspension and with ox red-cell stroma by mixing on a slide, and unabsorbed antibody detected by the addition of fresh horse cells. The heterophil antibody of IM produces a characteristic pattern of agglutination.

Blood samples

Serum or plasma from blood collected into EDTA are equally satisfactory. The plasma must be free of cells and debris.

Reagents

Guinea-pig kidney emulsion The kidneys of several guinea-pigs are cut into small pieces, washed with isotonic saline solution to remove any blood and reduced to a fine pulp in a mortar or by using a homogenizer. Suspend the macerated tissue in isotonic saline to make a 10% v/v suspension and boil for 1 hour. Make up to the original volume with distilled water and add 2 g phenol/l as a preservative. The suspension will keep for at least 1 year at 4°C. The absorbing ability should be tested using sera known to contain Forssmann-type heterophil antibody.

Suspension of ox-cell stroma Washed ox red cells are lysed with distilled water and the red-cell stroma deposited by high-speed (about 10 000 *g*) centrifugation. Re-suspend in isotonic saline to produce a 10% v/v suspension as judged by microhaematocrit centrifugation. Add 2 g phenol/l. The suspension is potent for several years at 4°C. Absorption should be checked by testing with sera containing IM heterophil antibody.

Horse-cell suspension 20% suspension of horse blood in 31.3 g/l trisodium citrate. The cells will store for several months at 4°C if free of bacterial contamination. A broad-spectrum antibiotic may be added.

Method

Mark out two areas about 2.5 cm^2 on a glass tile. In the corner of each square deliver one drop (approximately 20 μl) of horse cells. To the centre of square '1', deliver one drop of guinea-pig kidney emulsion and in square '2' one drop of ox red-cell stroma. Add one drop of serum or plasma to each square and mix with an applicator by a standard technique, e.g. 10 circular motions in 15 seconds, and then blend in the horse cells. Start a stop-watch and *do not disturb the tile*. After exactly 1 minute observe for agglutination.

Interpretation

1. Heterophil antibody in normal serum is absorbed only by guinea-pig kidney suspension.
2. Heterophil antibody of serum sickness is absorbed both by ox cells and by guinea-pig kidney.
3. Heterophil antibody of IM is absorbed only by the ox-cell stroma. Therefore a *positive* result is when agglutination is stronger in square 1 than in square 2. A *negative* result shows:
   (a) no agglutination in either square;
   (b) stronger agglutination in square 2 than square 1; or
   (c) similar agglutination in both squares.

Notes

1. Known weak-positive and negative controls should be set up alongside each test or with each batch of tests.
2. The volumes of guinea-pig kidney, ox-cell stroma, serum and horse cells, while not critical, influence the sensitivity, absorption and ease of reading.
3. Guinea-pig kidney emulsion is available commercially.

Demonstration of antibodies to EBV

The demonstration of antibodies to EBV by IF has been the standard approach and can identify IgM and IgG antibodies. The method is time-consuming and usually involves titration to demonstrate rising or significant titres and to avoid false positives. Immunoblotting (Western blot) is specific, identifies the antibody class but is less sensitive than IF and is unsuitable for prompt diagnostic work.

An ELISA technique using a 20-amino acid synthetic peptide (p62) which is a glycine-arginine segment of an epitope of EBNA-1 has been described [37, 38]. The method allows recognition of both IgG and IgM anti-EBNA antibodies, thus differentiating between acute and previous EBV infection. The method has been made available in commercial form (Ortho Monolert®). Improved sensitivity and predictive value is considered to be the advantage over heterophil antibody tests.

Parasitic infections

Parasitic infections in man are acquired by insect bite, from polluted water whether by mouth or through the skin, and from contaminated or infected food. The haematological consequences can be fever, anaemia, organ enlargement, eosinophilia, altered plasma proteins and, in some instances, disturbance of the haemostatic mechanisms.

The parasites comprise two main groups, the protozoa and the helminths (worm or worm-like parasites). In addition arthropod parasitization of the skin, e.g. scabies, can cause an eosinophilia.

Protozoal infections

Malaria

The malarial parasite belongs to the sub-phylum Sporozoa, sub-class Haemosporidiae, family Plasmodiae and genus *Plasmodium*. Four species are pathogenic to man – *P. falciparum, P. vivax, P. malariae* and *P. ovale*. They have sexual and asexual cycles and are adapted to intracellular parasitization of fixed tissue cells of the RE system and the erythrocytes. Infection is acquired by the bite of certain species of mosquito of the genus *Anopheles* and, rarely but importantly, by the transfusion of parasitized blood or by placental transmission (congenital malaria).

Life cycle

The definitive host of the plasmodia is the mosquito and man is the intermediate host. The sexual cycle occurs exclusively in the mosquito (sporogony) and the asexual cycle in man (schizogony). The bite of an infected mosquito injects *sporozoites* into the circulation which migrate to the liver where schizogony takes place (exoerythrocytic cycle), with eventual release of *metacryptozoites* into the circulation which infect erythrocytes (erythrocytic cycle), at which stage the parasite is a *trophozoite* until division occurs to form a *schizont*. When mature the red cell containing the schizont distintegrates releasing *merozoites* to reinfect further red cells. Some merozoites return to the liver to start a new exoerythrocytic cycle. Some trophozoites do not divide but develop into male (micro-) or female (macro-) gametocytes which do not develop further in man. Male and female gametocytes taken into the stomach of a susceptible mosquito by feeding, unite to form a *zygote* (sexual cycle) which develops by division into an *oocyst* in which are formed sporozoites which are liberated into the salivary ducts from which they are injected into a susceptible human host to begin a new cycle.

Factors affecting Plasmodium parasitization of red cells [39–41]
Attachment of free forms of parasite to the red-cell membrane prior to invasion is necessary for certain *Plasmodium* species. *P. vivax* infection is not found in populations where the Duffy blood group Fy^-/Fy^- is commonest. Invasion of red cells by *P. falciparum* may depend on the sialoglycopeptide receptor glycophorin A, on the red-cell membrane. $Eu(a^-)$ red cells which lack glycophorin A show reduced infection by *P. falciparium*. 'Young' red cells are invaded preferentially by *P. vivax* and *P. ovale* and to a lesser extent by *P. falciparum*. Invasion is decreased in red cells containing Hb S but not by Hbs C and E or high levels of Hb F, nor in examples of α and β thalassaemia or G6PD deficiency.

Parasite growth and replication *within* red cells is reduced in the presence of elevated levels of Hb F, by the presence of Hb S at low oxygen tension, and in homozygous Hb C disease. The red cells of thalassaemia and G6PD deficiency may not support division of *P. falciparum* due to their sensitivity to oxidant stress.

Clinical aspects of significance in laboratory diagnosis
There is an incubation period between infection and appearance of the first symptoms which depends on the length of the exoerythrocytic cycle, periodicity and degree of parasitaemia. The major symptoms of malaria are fever and rigor and the intervals between paroxysms are related to the periodicity of schizogony of

Table 14.4 Clinical aspects of the various species of malarial parasite

Species	*Incubation period* (days)	*Schizogony* (hours)	*Periodicity* (days)	*Type of malaria**	*Relapse* (years)
P. falciparum	8–10	48	3	Malignant tertian	Very rare
P. vivax	10–15	48	3	Benign tertian	3
P. malariae	Up to 30	72	4	Quartan	Up to 20
P. ovale	10–15	48	3	Ovale tertian	3

* Tertian = every third day; quartan = every fourth day.

the *Plasmodium* species (*Table 14.4*). The paroxysms relate to the liberation of merozoites and toxic metabolic products into the circulation.

Malaria infection in non-endemic areas is most commonly found in patients who have recently visited areas where malaria is endemic. In the UK, travellers from the Indian subcontinent are most likely to have *P. vivax* infection, while *P. falciparum* is most often found in patients from west and west-central Africa[42].

Anaemia of malaria [43]

The anaemia associated with malaria infection is essentially haemolytic. The concept that red-cell destruction is limited to parasitized cells does not explain the degree of anaemia. Parasitized cells are destroyed by intravascular disintegration, extravascular phagocytosis and red-cell damage due to splenic 'pitting' of the parasites from infected cells. Immune haemolysis, ineffective erythropoiesis, hypersplenism and secondary folate deficiency are additional mechanisms of anaemia.

The immune mechanism is apparently due to the formation of IgG antibody against the parasites with non-specific attachment of the immune complexes to the red-cell membrane with complement activation and subsequent phagocytosis. A positive direct antiglobulin test due to IgG, with or without C3d, may be found in 50% of cases of *P. falciparum* infection but there is no correlation between severity of the anaemia and red cell-associated IgG[44, 45]. In severe *P. falciparum* infection gross intravascular haemolysis may occur with methaemalbumin formation and haemoglobinuria (blackwater fever).

Laboratory diagnosis

Blood samples

Samples may be taken at any stage of the schizogony cycle but from first principles certain points may be made. In acute and early infections, and in *P. ovale* and *P.malariae* infections, parasites may be very scanty. At the peak of the paroxysm schizonts are not expected to be found and only early trophozoite stages may be seen. Maximum entry of merozoites into red cells and more mature trophozoites may be expected 8–10 hours after the peak of pyrexia. In chronic infections, or when there is more than one cycle of parasite development, samples may be taken at any time and gametocytes, particularly of *P. vivax* (*Figure 14.6*) may be seen in apyrexial stages. Liberation of parasitized cells from capillaries and organs may be provoked by subcutaneous injection of adrenaline.

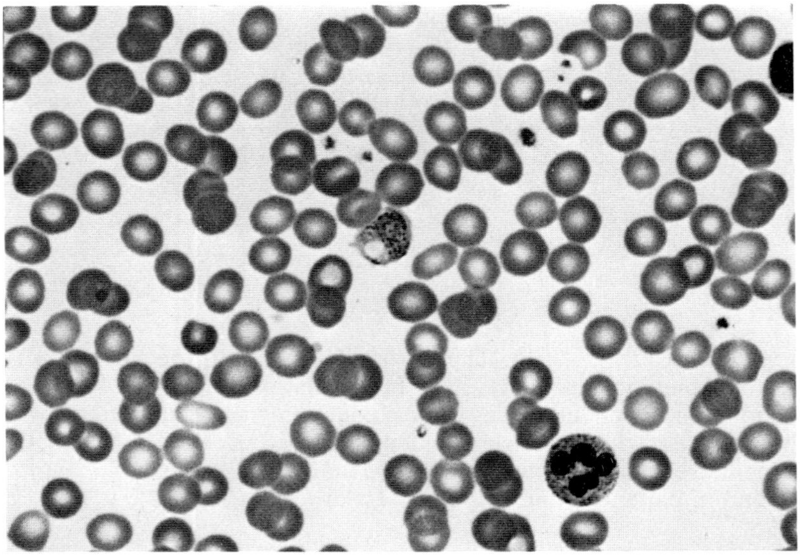

Figure 14.6 Blood film. Gametocyte of *Plasmodium vivax*. ×550

Preparation of blood films

Thin and thick films should be prepared. Thin films are conventionally prepared wedge films. For thick films a drop of blood is spread on a separate slide to cover an area of about 1 cm diameter, and of sufficient thickness to allow bold print to be seen. The thick film *must* be thoroughly dried to prevent flaking off during staining; 15 minutes at 37°C or 30 minutes gentle warming by a microscope lamp is recommended.

Staining of films

Thin films Conventionally stained blood films, though usually adequate, are not ideal for the demonstration of malaria parasites. At pH 6.8 basophilic staining is not sufficiently intense and Schüffner's dots (*see* below) are not readily seen. Leishman's stain (BDH) with buffer, pH 7.2, is recommended. Giemsa stain, diluted 1 in 10 with buffer, pH 7.2, is satisfactory after fixing the film in absolute methanol for 1 minute. If there is any problem with stain deposit the slide is stained, film-side down, in a dish and supported by glass capillaries.

Thick films The films are stained without fixing which allows elution of haemoglobin from the red cells. The film must be *perfectly dry*. Leishman or Giemsa stain, diluted 1 in 10 with buffer pH 7.2, is freshly prepared and the slide immersed for 30 minutes, rinsed with water and allowed to drain and dry. *Do not blot*. A final rinse in 9 g/l NaCl results in greater clarity.

Examination of blood films

Parasite density may be as low as 1 per 100 000 red cells which is equivalent to about one parasite per 400 oil immersion (× 50) fields which can take up to 1 hour to examine thoroughly. Five minutes examination of a thick film may be considered equivalent to 1 hour examination of a thin film. Trophozoites in thick films are more compact and lack clarity, and red-cell size and appearance cannot of course be seen. Schizonts and gametocytes can be readily identified. Considerable experience is required for species identification in thick films and descriptions of parasites apply to their appearances in thin films. Estimates of parasite density as number per 100 red cells is of clinical value; 4% is a severe infection and is associated with clinical complications such as renal failure, cerebral malaria, hepatic dysfunctions, pulmonary oedema and anaemia.

Fluorescent staining of malaria parasites [46]

Principle By acridine orange staining of nucleic acids, RNA shows a brilliant-red fluorescence while DNA fluoresces green. Plasmodia are rich in RNA and their bright fluorescence under ultraviolet light contrasts sharply with the dark background.

Reagents Phosphate buffer 0.66 mol/l, pH 6.4: 6.76 g KH_2PO_4, 2.37 g Na_2HPO_4 in 1 litre distilled water. Adjust to pH 6.4 if necessary. Working acridine orange solution: 0.01 g acridine orange in 1 litre buffer (1 g/l diluted 1 in 100 in buffer). Clearing solution: 16.5 g/l $CaCl_2$ (0.06 mol/l). Fixative: equal volumes of ethyl ether and ethanol. Ethanol solutions: 80, 70, and 50% ethanol.

Method Air-dried films are fixed for 15 minutes and rinsed successively in 80%, 70% and 50% ethanol and in two changes of buffer. The films are stained for 45 seconds in acridine orange, rinsed in buffer for 3 minutes and differentiated in clearing solution for 2–3 minutes with periodic agitation.

Examination Films are cover-slipped using buffer as mountant and examined immediately at × 100 magnification. All forms of plasmodia are easily seen and at × 500 magnification the different stages can be recognized. Gametocytes can be seen at × 40 magnification. Differentiation of species is not usually possible.

Notes
1. The fluorescence fades after about 5 minutes exposure to ultraviolet light, but films may be re-stained repeatedly.
2. A fall in pH below 6.4 results in a dull orange fluorescence. The pH of the stain should be checked.
3. The position of parasites in the film may be marked and the slides re-stained with Romanowsky stain for identification but they cannot be re-stained for fluorescence microscopy.
4. It is estimated that by low-power examination 100 times as many red cells may be scanned in any given period compared with conventional thin-film preparations.

Differentiation of Plasmodium species
The differentiating features of the plasmodia are the appearance of the trophozoites, the number of merozoites in the schizonts, whether the infected red cell is enlarged and the presence of Schüffner's dots. Differentiation by gametocyte is only possible with certainty in the case of the crescent-shaped forms of *P. falciparum*. The morphological features are summarized in *Table 14.5*.

Table 14.5 Differentiation of malaria parasites in blood

Stages	*P. falciparum*	*P. vivax*	*P. malariae*	*P. ovale*
Trophozoites:				
Ring forms	Diameter ⅙–½ of RBC of normal size. Older rings may be stippled (Maurer's dots). Cytoplasm fine. Marginal (accolé) forms, double chromatin dots and multiple parasites in a single cell may be seen. *Ring forms may be the only forms seen in the blood*	Diameter ⅓–½ of RBC of normal size. Indistinguishable when alone Cytoplasm thin and faintly stained. Pigment absent	Cytoplasm thick. Deeply stained. Pigment absent	Diameter ½ of RBC of normal size. Schüffner's dots common. Cytoplasm thick, deeply stained. Pigment absent
Growing forms	Not normally seen in blood	Red cell enlarged. Stippled. Parasite amoeboid, vacuolated	Red cell unaltered. Parasite compact or band-shaped with scattered dark granules	Red cell frequently oval, slightly enlarged with ragged margins. Stippled. Band forms rare. Scanty dark brown granules
Mature schizonts	If present are of serious prognostic significance. Number of merozoites >12. Red cell normal size	Red cell much enlarged. Schüffner's dots. Parasite fills cell. Number of merozoites >12. Loose mass of pigment	Red cell unaltered. Parasite fills cell completely. Merozoites <12	Red cell frequently oval. Stippled. Appearance as for *P. malariae*. Merozoites <12.
Gametocytes	Crescent shaped with central nucleus surrounded by dark granules of pigment	Red cell much enlarged. Schüffner's dots. Parasite large, round, fills cell. Pigment evenly distributed	Red cell unaltered. Parasite small, round, filling cell. Pigment scattered	Red cell normal or only slightly enlarged. Schüffner's dots. Similar to *P. malariae*
	Female: cytoplasm stains deep blue; nucleus small and compact Male: cytoplasm stains pale blue or reddish; nucleus large and diffuse			

Other blood changes

In acute malaria there is initially a neutrophil leucocytosis which is followed by a neutropenia due to reduction in circulating neutrophils, though the marginal pool is increased. Monocytes are often increased in number, show vacuolation and contain malarial pigment; erythrophagocytosis may be seen as a result of C3d on the red cells. The lymphocytes show transformation indicating an immune response. Eosinophilia may be seen in the convalescent period. Mild thrombocytopenia is commonly found and the platelet depression is inversely related to the degree of parasitaemia. Severe malaria may precipitate disseminated intravascular coagulation (DIC) with consumption of coagulation factors and platelets, fibrinolysis and increased fibrin degradation products (FDPs). Reports of elevated Hb A_2 levels have not been confirmed.

Serology

Malaria infection provokes a humoral response. The presence of antibody may only indicate a previous infection but can be useful in diagnosis if antimalarial therapy has been given before a blood sample is taken. Antibody may be detected by complement fixation, indirect immunofluorescence or enzyme-linked immunosorbent assay (ELISA).

Trypanosomiasis

The genus *Trypanosoma* are of the sub-phylum Mastigophora, class Zoomastigophora (flagellates) and are parasites of the blood and tissues. Several species are pathogenic to man: *T. rhodesiense* and *T. gambiense* cause African trypanosomiasis (sleeping sickness) which is transmitted by the blood-sucking fly *Glossina* (tsetse fly); *T. cruzi* is the cause of Chagas' disease, is confined to South America and is transmitted by blood-feeding bugs. Reproduction of trypanosomes is entirely asexual, with multiplication in the reservoir host (man and animals) and intermediate host (fly or bug).

The parasites enter the blood, lymphatics, and RES and central nervous system, but do not invade tissue cells, i.e. the parasites are free-living forms. After an incubation period of 10–21 days the motile flagellates can be found in the blood, lymph-node aspirate and, in the cerebral stage, in CSF. A moderate to severe haemolytic anaemia due to several mechanisms can develop and thrombocytopenia is usual and may be severe. DIC may supervene.

Laboratory diagnosis

Diagnosis is usually made by the demonstration of the parasites in blood and body fluids. The motile forms may be seen in wet preparations under a cover-slip, in stained thick films or in thin films if there are many parasites (*Figure 14.7*). The parasites may be concentrated by centrifuging whole blood in microhaematocrit tubes and examining the buffy layer. Morphological differentiation of *T. rhodesiense* and *T. gambiense* in blood is not possible. Serological diagnosis by the demonstration of antibody is useful in epidemiological surveys or in relatively asymptomatic stages. Trypanosomiasis is extremely infrequent in travellers to Europe.

Leishmaniasis

Leishmaniasis (kala-azar) involving the organs of the reticuloendothelial system is caused by *Leishmania donovani*. *Leishmania* are a genus of the same class as the *Trypanosoma* but the flagellate forms are only seen in the sandfly vector and in culture. In vertebrates only the intracellular leishmanial stage is seen. Many species of *Phlebotomus* (sandfly) act as vectors of *L. donovani* and the disease is therefore widespread throughout Asia, the Middle East, North Africa, Southern Europe and South and Central America. The life cycle in man is simple; the organism is

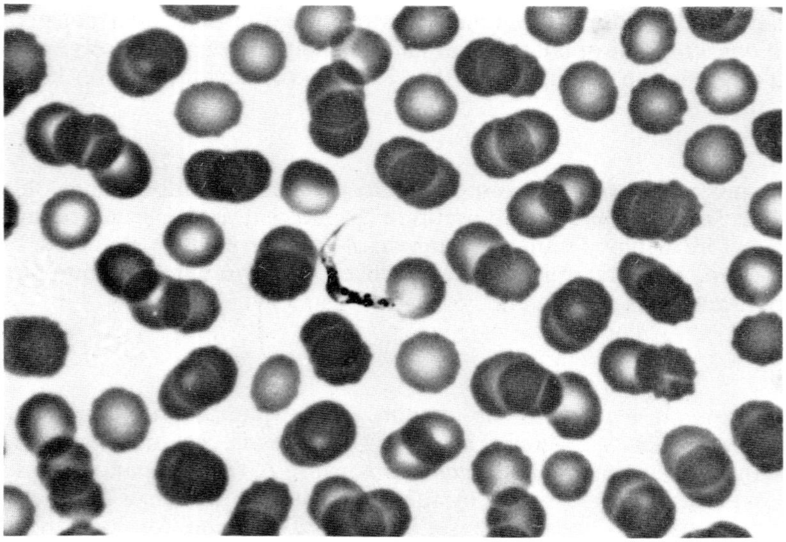

Figure 14.7 Blood film. Flagellated form of *Trypanosoma gambiense*. ×825

phagocytosed by reticuloendothelial macrophages in which it multiplies by simple binary fission with eventual cell disruption and infection of further cells.

The onset of the disease is insidious over a period of months and presents as hepatosplenomegaly, anaemia and pancytopenia but often with an absolute monocytosis. The pancytopenia is mainly due to hypersplenism though the anaemia is due to splenic pooling, an increase in plasma volume and reduced red-cell life span. Dyserythropoiesis and ineffective erythropoiesis have also been described.

Laboratory diagnosis

Diagnosis is by demonstration of the parasites. They are not present in blood, and bone-marrow aspiration is usually performed. The infected cells are sought in marrow films but are usually scanty. In spleen, liver and lymph-node biopsies the parasitized cells are more numerous. Tissue biopsies should be cultured. There is usually a marked increase in serum immunoglobulins and a decreased serum albumin, which together produce a marked increase in plasma viscosity and ESR. Serological diagnosis is of value.

Leishmania should be looked for in any patient with pancytopenia and hepatosplenomegaly who has resided or travelled in an endemic area during the previous 18 months.

Other protozoal infections

Babesiosis

Babesia are of the same sub-class as the plasmodia and were thought to be parasites only of cattle and dogs, with ticks as intermediate hosts or vectors. Scattered cases of human infection have been recognized, almost all being in splenectomized subjects in rural areas who were exposed to bites by cattle-infected ticks. The intraerythrocytic parasites are similar to the malarial trophozoite stages and heavy parasitaemia can be found.

Toxoplasmosis

Toxoplasmosis is an endemic infection in temperate climates and is acquired from domestic pets and some forms of wildlife. The organism is sporozoal with sexual and asexual life cycles. In the adult, infection is by the oral route and is often subclinical. It is of haematological interest because the clinical presentation can mimic IM – i.e. lymphadenopathy, neutropenia and atypical lymphocytes – but the heterophil antibody of IM is not formed. Congenital toxoplasmosis derived by placental transfer from the mother is more serious and is associated with jaundice, hepatosplenomegaly and failure to thrive, and can be fatal.

Diagnosis is usually serological by immunofluorescence, complement fixation, passive agglutination, or ELISA. The organism is highly infectious and appropriate precautions must be taken in handling infected tissues.

Helminths

Eosinophilia is the most constant haematological finding in helminth infections, which can be divided into filariasis, in which larvae (microfilaria) are found in the blood, and the worm infections mainly involving the intestine.

Filariasis

Filarial worms are nematodes (roundworms) and eight species are found in man but in only four species are the microfilariae commonly found in the blood. The adult worms reside in the lymphatic vessels and glands, connective tissues and body cavities. Infection is acquired by the bite of a variety of arthropods, and filarial infections are endemic throughout the warm zones of the world. The major symptoms due to the filaria whose larvae are found in the blood are obstruction of the lymphatics and migration in the subcutaneous tissues.

Microfilariae may be differentiated by: (1) periodicity; (2) the presence or absence of a sheath; (3) accurate measurement; (4) shape and appearance of head and tail; (5) manner of movement; and (6) appearance in stained preparations. *Table 14.6* summarizes the characteristics of the microfilariae found in the blood and their morphology, periodicity, vectors and geographical distribution.

Laboratory diagnosis

Blood samples are collected into anticoagulant. Specimens taken at any time may be examined for *Dipetalonema perstans* but the nocturnal periodicity of the other species demand that samples be taken during the night, and the period 10 p.m. to 2 a.m. is best. Some strains of microfilariae show subperiodicity and appear around midday. In EDTA samples at 37°C, the microfilariae will remain motile for many hours; if allowed to cool, motility diminishes but can be restored by warming to 37°C.

Microfilariae may be seen in conventional films if the infection is very heavy. Examination of a drop of blood under a cover-slip may reveal microfilariae, which

Table 14.6 Selected characteristics of the commoner filarial infections

Species	*Distribution*	*Vector*	*Tissues involved*	*Microfilariae*		
				Sheath	*Periodicity*	*Length* (μm)
Wucheria bancrofti	World-wide warm climate	Culex mosquito	Lymphatics	Yes	Nocturnal	250–300
Brugia malayi	Asia, Pacific	Mosquito spp.	Lymphatics	Yes	Nocturnal	170–300
Loa-loa	Tropical Africa, West Indies	*Chrysops* (biting fly)	Subcutaneous tissues	Yes	Diurnal	250–300
Dipetalonema perstans (acantho-cheilonema)	Tropical Africa, South America	*Culicoides* (midges, gnats)	Mesentery	No	None	200

can be located by the agitation of the suspended red cells by the motile larvae. A small amount of blood may be examined after centrifugation in a microhaematocrit tube, the section immediately above the red cells being expelled on to a slide and examined under a cover-slip. Higher recovery of parasites is obtained by examining larger volumes of blood.

Concentration by saponin lysis and centrifugation

Principle Anticoagulated blood is centrifuged to provide preliminary concentration, the red cells lysed with saponin, further centrifuged and the deposit examined.

Method Centrifuge blood anticoagulated with EDTA for 10 minutes at 800 *g*. The larger the amount of blood the greater the recovery of microfilaria. Discard the supernatant plasma and add 5 mg saponin for each ml of cells, mix gently and stand for 15 minutes. Centrifuge in a conical tube for 15 minutes at 1500 *g* and discard the supernatant. Make a series of wet preparations from the deposit and examine under a cover-slip for motile microfilaria. A dry film will show the microfilaria in a curved or coiled form. The addition of one drop of 1% acetic acid to a wet preparation will kill and straighten the microfilaria and allow details of morphology to be studied more readily. Dried films may be fixed and stained by Romanowsky stain or methylene blue.

Membrane filtration
Membrane filtration is the method of choice for demonstrating microfilariae [47]. Blood is passed through a membrane filter which allows the passage of red cells or red-cell stroma, leucocytes and platelets but retains the microfilariae. Lysed blood is necessary using Millipore filters while whole blood can be passed through Nuclepore membranes.

Nuclepore filtration [48] Blood collected into EDTA is drawn into a syringe and passed directly through a 5 μm pore, 25 mm Nuclepore polycarbonate filter in a suitable holder. The membrane is washed by passing successive volumes of saline until the washings are clear of blood. A syringeful of air is blown through the filter followed by 1 ml of methanol and a further volume of air. The membrane is removed from its holder and placed on a clean slide, allowed to dry and then stained with dilute Giemsa for 1 hour, rinsed rapidly with water, cleared with xylene and examined at × 100 magnification. The more slender microfilariae *D. perstans, Mansonella ozzardi* and *D. streptocerca* are recovered in greater numbers using a 3 μm pore filter.

Other helminth infections

Hookworm is one of the world's commonest infections and is usually acquired by the larvae penetrating the skin. The adult worms attach to the wall of the small bowel and can extract up to 0.15 ml blood daily which is clearly a significant blood loss when the worms are numerous. The blood picture is therefore typically one of chronic blood loss, i.e. hypochromic anaemia, and an eosinophilia.

Other intestinal nematodes, e.g. *Trichuris trichuria* (whipworm) may also cause significant blood loss.

The *Cestodes* (tapeworms) do not produce haematological changes other than eosinophilia, with the exception of the fish tapeworm *Diphyllobothrium latum* which may be associated with vitamin B_{12} deficiency (*see* page 277).

Immune deficiencies

Bacterial, viral, fungal and parasitic infections which are overwhelming, severe, slow to resolve or recurrent may be due to immune deficiency. Immunodeficiency may affect one or more aspects of the mechanisms of immunity – neutrophil/macrophage function[49] and defects in the humoral or cellular response of lymphocytes[49, 50].

Immune deficiency disorders can be classified as congenital/hereditary or acquired.

Congenital immune deficiencies

1. Neutrophils.
   (a) Quantitative:
      (i) Chronic neutropenia.
      (ii) Isoimmune neonatal neutropenia.
      (iii) Cyclic neutropenia.
      (iv) Schwachmann–Diamond syndrome.
   (b) Qualitative:
      (i) Impaired bacterial killing:
         (a) chronic granulomatous disease;
         (b) Chediak–Higashi syndrome;
         (c) myeloperoxidase deficiency;
         (d) Job's syndrome.
      (ii) Impaired chemotaxis:
         (a) abnormal complement;
         (b) lazy-leucocyte syndrome.
      (iii) Defective complement function.
      (iv) Defective opsonization.

2. Lymphocytes.
   (a) Predominant antibody defects:
      (i) X-linked agammaglobulinaemia.
      (ii) Autosomal recessive agammaglobulinaemia.
      (iii) IgA deficiency.
      (iv) kappa-chain deficiency.
      (v) Transient hypogammaglobulinaemia of infancy
      (vi) Immunodeficiency with predominant B-cell defect.
      (vii) Immunodeficiency with predominant regulatory T-cell disorder,
         (a) deficiency of helper T cells;
         (b) presence of activated suppressor T cells.
      (viii) Autoantibodies to B or T cells.
   (b) Predominant defects of cell-mediated immunity:
      (i) Combined immunodeficiency with predominant T-cell defect.
      (ii) Purine-nucleoside phosphorylase deficiency.
      (iii) Adenosine deaminase deficiency.
      (iv) Severe combined immunodeficiency:
         (a) reticular dysgenesis;
         (b) low T- and B-cell numbers;
         (c) low T-cell and normal B-cell numbers (Swiss type);
         (d) 'Bare-lymphocyte syndrome'.
3. Immunodeficiency associated with other defects.
   (a) Transcobalamin II deficiency.
   (b) Ataxia telangiectasia.
   (c) Third and fourth-pouch/arch (di George's) syndrome.

The immune deficiencies are clearly within the speciality of clinical immunology and the techniques of investigation those of the immunology laboratory, other than those aspects concerned with cell quantitation and abnormal leucocyte or platelet morphology, e.g. the Chediak–Higashi and Wiskott–Aldrich syndromes.

Acquired immune deficiencies

Acquired immunodeficiencies are found secondary to haematological disorders and simulate congenital defects. For example, in the proliferative diseases there are quantitative and qualitative disorders of neutrophils and humoral and cellular defects of lymphocytes. A unique disorder is the acquired immune deficiency syndrome (AIDS) in which infection *causes* immunodeficiency and *results* in haematological abnormalities.

Acquired immunodeficiency syndrome (AIDS)

The first reports of AIDS in 1981[52, 53] in homosexual men were followed by further reports of opportunistic infections and Kaposi's sarcoma in intravenous drug users, Haitians and haemophiliacs in 1982[54]. Epidemiological studies indicated an infectious agent transmitted by sexual intercourse or infected blood.

Human immunodeficiency virus (HIV), formerly called LAV (lymphadenopathy-associated virus) and HTLV III (human T-cell lymphotropic virus type III), was first reported in 1983 and the aetiological association with AIDS established in 1984. A second human retrovirus, HIV-2, appeared in West Africa and is also associated with AIDS.

Retroviruses, so called because there is a step 'backwards' in genetic information during their replication cycle, contain genes in single-stranded RNA which is converted into double-stranded DNA 'provirus' by the viral enzyme reverse transcriptase. The DNA provirus becomes inserted into chromosomal DNA of the host cell and establishes a persistent infection. HIV shows specificity for infection of certain cell types which exhibit the CD4 membrane antigen which acts as a cell surface receptor for HIV. CD4+ cells include helper/inducer T lymphocytes, monocytes, macrophages and possibly brain cells. The CD4 receptor specificity explains the pathogenesis of AIDS which affects the immune system, the gut and the brain[55]. Given the role of CD4+ T cells as inducers of both immunoglobulin production and cytotoxic CD8+ T cells and as the major source of IL-2 and other cytokines, this tropism explains many of the immunological manifestations of the disease.

Clinical features of AIDS

The US Centre for Disease Control (CDC) proposed a classification[56] for the staging of AIDS which is widely accepted:

Group I: Symptoms of acute viral infection; may exhibit the features of heterophil negative IM[57].
Group II: Asymptomatic, HIV seropositive infection.
Group III: Persistent generalized lymphadenopathy (PGL); at least 3 months lymphadenopathy affecting two or more extra-inguinal sites.
Group IV: (A): constitutional disease.
(B): neurological disease.
(C): secondary infectious disease.
(D): secondary cancers.
(E): other conditions.

AIDS-related complex (ARC) – Group III and Group IV A and B – is an additional grouping.

Infections associated with AIDS

1. Protozoa and helminths:
   Pneumocystis
   Toxoplamosis
   Cryptosporidiosis
   Strongyloidosis.
2. Fungal:
   Candidiasis
   Cryptococcus
3. Bacteria:
   Atypical mycobacteria.
4. Viral:
   Cytomegalovirus
   Herpes
   Leucoencephalopathy.

Haematological aspects of AIDS

Study of haematological parameters and changes in blood and bone marrow can be related to staging and progressive development of AIDS.

Lymphocyte sub-typing

Early studies with AIDS cases observed a decrease in both the proportion and numbers of CD4+ lymphocytes. The normal proportions of CD4+:CD8+ cells (helper : suppressor ratio) of >1.2:1 was shown to be reversed. More importantly, the *number* of CD4+ cells has been shown to be the best prognostic indicator of progression to full-blown AIDS. If $<0.4 \times 10^9$/l, there will probably be continued decline leading to the development of infections. A low CD4+ cell count cannot be used to diagnose HIV infection.

Total lymphocyte counts are not as good a prognostic indicator of progression of the disease. Absolute lymphopenia ($<1.5 \times 10^9$/l) is found in groups II, III and IV and may only decline sharply as a terminal event. Accurate counting of CD4+ cells is important and automated cytometry using monclonal antibodies is the method of choice.

Cytopenias [59–61]

Thrombocytopenia: incidence increases with staging and in group IV has been variously reported to occur in 30, 45 and 67% of cases and may be $<30 \times 10^9$/l. Neutropenia develops in 20–50% of group II and IV patients.

Lymphopenia: a count of $<0.8 \times 10^9$/l is reported in 10% of ARC and 50–75% of group IV cases.

The mechanisms of thrombocytopenia and neutropenia are, in part at least, due to autoimmune destruction [60, 62] and respond to treatment [63].

Anaemia [59]

Slight to moderate normocytic, normochromic anaemia is found in the majority of group IV patients. The mechanism of the anaemia, other than that due to bleeding, is generally agreed to be due to dyserythropoiesis and ineffective erythropoiesis. The role of autoimmune haemolysis is unclear. Although positive direct antiglobulin tests (DAT) have been reported in about 20% of group IV patients [59, 64], overt haemolysis was not considered to be a feature [59] and no positive DATs were found in another series [65]. Technical aspects may account for the discrepant reports.

Bone-marrow appearances

Hypercellularity and dysplasia of granulocyte, erythroid and megakaryocyte cell lines are features of the marrow in AIDS. Plasmacytosis and lymphoid aggregates are also consistently reported. Mycobacterial and fungal infections were found in about 20% of cases in one series [66].

Other findings

Anti-cardiolipin antibodies (23 of 28 patients) and anti-phospholipid antibodies (lupus anticoagulant) have been reported.

References

1. Barclay, R. (1985) The role of iron in infection. *Med. Lab. Sci.*, **42**, 166–77
2. Eastham, R. D. (1977) *Clinical Haematology*, 5th edn. Bristol: Wright
3. Nixon, D. F., Parsons, A. J. and Eglin, R. P. (1987) Routine full blood counts as indicators of acute viral infections *J. Clin. Pathol.*, **40**, 673–5
4. Baynes, R. D., Bothwell, T. H., Flax, *et al.* (1987) Reactive thrombocytosis in pulmonary tuberculosis. *J. Clin. Pathol.*, **40**, 676–9
5. Fisher-Hoch, S. P. (1983) The haemostatic defect in viral haemorrhagic fevers. *Br. J. Haematol.*, **55**, 565–71
6. Scheifele, D. W., Olson, E. M. and Pendray, M. R. (1985) Endoxinemia and thrombocytopenia during neonatal necrotizing enterocolitis. *Am. J. Clin. Pathol.*, **83**, 227–9
7. Trowbridge, A. A., Green, J. B., Bonnett, J. D., Shohet, S. B., Ponnappa, D. B. and McCoombs, W. B. (1981) Hemolytic anaemia associated with leptospirosis. Morphological and lipid studies. *Am. J. Clin. Pathol.*, **76**, 493–8
8. Lancet (1976). Human Babesiosis. *Lancet*, **i**, 1001–2
9. Entrican, J. H., Williams, H., Cook, I. A. *et al.* (1979) Babesiosis in man: a case from Scotland. *Br. Med. J.*, **ii**, 474
10. Cahill, K. M., Benach, J. L., Reich, I. M. *et al.* (1981) Red-cell exchange: treatment of babesiosis in a splenectomised patient. *Transfusion*, **21**, 193–8
11. Ristic, M. and Kreier, J. P. (1979) Hemotropic bacteria. *N. Engl. J. Med.*, **301**, 937–9
12. Archer, G. L., Coleman, P. H., Cole, R. M., Duma, R. J. and Johnston, C. L. (1979) Human infection from an unidentified erythrocyte-associated bacterium. *N. Engl. J. Med.*, **301**, 897–900
13. Clark, K. G. A. (1975) A basophilic micro-organism infecting human red-cells. *Br. J. Haematol.*, **29**, 301–4
14. Kurtzman, G. and Young, N. (1989) Viruses and bone marrow failure. *Clin. Haematol.*, **2**, 51–67
15. Christensen, R. D., Bradley, P. P. and Rothstein, G. (1981) The leucocyte left shift in clinical and experimental neonatal sepsis. *J. Paediatr.*, **98**, 101–5
16. Manroe, B. L., Weinberg, A. G., Rosenfeld, C. R and Browne, R. (1979) The neonatal blood count in health and disease. I. Reference values for neutrophilic cells. *J. Paediatr.*, **96**, 89–98
17. Cooke, R. P. D., Wells, F. E. and Rose, P. E. (1986) Laboratory management of haemolytic uraemic syndrome. *Med. Lab. Sci.*, **43**, 382–5
18. Rose, P. E. and Clark, A. J. B. (1989) Haematology of the haemolytic uraemic syndrome. *Blood Rev.* **3**, 136–40
19. Mackie, P. H., Mistry, D. K., Wozniak, J. T., Dodds, W. N., Geddes, A. M. and Stuart, J. (1979) Neutrophil cytochemistry in bacterial infection. *J. Clin. Pathol.*, **32**, 26–30
20. Park, B. H., Fikrig, S. M. and Smithwick, E. M. (1968) Infection and nitroblue–tetrazolium reduction by neutrophils, *Lancet*, **ii**, 532–4
21. Segal, A. W. (1974) Nitroblue–tetrazolium tests. *Lancet*, **ii**, 1248–52
22. Steigbigel, R. T., Johnson P. K. and Remington, J. S. (1974) The nitroblue–tetrazolium reduction test versus conventional hematology in the diagnosis of bacterial infection. *N. Engl. J. Med.*, **290**, 235–8
23. Gordon, P. A., Stuart, J., Lee, T. R., Breeze, G. R. and Pugh, R. N. H. (1975) The cytocentrifuge NBT test. *J. Clin. Pathol.*, **28**, 674–9
24. Schofield, K. P., Stone, P. C. W., Beddall, A. C. and Stuart, J. (1983) Quantitative cytochemistry of the toxic granulation blood neutrophil. *Br. J. Haematol.*, **53**, 15–22
25. Horwitz, C. A., Henle, W., Henle, G. *et al.* (1981) Clinical and laboratory evaluation of infants and children with Epstein–Barr virus-induced infectious mononucleosis: report of 32 patients (aged 10–48 months). *Blood*, **57**, 933–8
26. Eptein, M. A. and Achong, B. G. (1977) Pathogenesis of infectious mononucleosis. *Lancet*, **ii**, 1270–2
27. Thomas, W. J., Yasaka, K., Srong, D. M., Woodruff, C. M., Stass, S. A. and Schumacher, H. R. (1980) Hand-mirror lymphocytes in infectious mononucleosis. *Blood*, **55**, 925–30
28. Chanarin, I., James, D., Stafford, D. and Tidmarsh, E. (1977) Platelet autoimmunity. *Br. J. Haematol.*, **37**, 283–8

29. O'Brien, J. R. and Etherington, M. D. (1978) The platelets in glandular fever and idiopathic thrombocytopenic purpura. *Br. J. Haematol.*, **40**, 161–2
30. Hoff, G. and Bauer, S. (1965) A new rapid slide test for infectious mononucleosis. *J. Am. Med. Assoc.*, **194**, 351–3
31. Lee, C. L., Davidsohn, I. and Panczyszyn, O. (1968) Horse agglutinins in infectious mononucleosis. II, The spot test. *Am. J. Clin. Pathol.*, **49**, 12–18
32. British Medical Journal (1980) Tests for infectious mononucleosis. *Br. Med. J.*, **i**, 1153–4
33. Davson, J., Mallick, N. P., Lyon, R. L. and Geary, C. G.(1981) Heterophil antibody and histiocytic medullary reticulosis. *Clin. Lab. Haematol.*, **3**, 77–84
34. Horwitz, C. A., Henle, W., Henle, G., Hoffman, N. and Ward, P. C. J. (1979) Persistent falsely positive rapid tests for infectious mononucleosis. *Am. J. Clin. Pathol.*, **72**, 807–11
35. Wilkinson, L. S., Petz, L. D. and Garratty, G. (1973) Reappraisal of the role of anti-i in haemolytic anaemia in infectious mononucleosis. *Br. J. Haematol.*, **25**, 715–22
36. Seitandis, B. (1969) A comparison of the Monospot with the Paul–Bunnell test in infectious mononucleosis and other diseases. *J. Clin. Pathol.*, **22**, 321–3
37. Smith, R. S., Rhodes, G., Vaughan, J. H., Horwitz, C. A., Geltowsky, and Whalley, A. S. (1986) A synthetic peptide for detecting antibodies to Epstein–Barr virus nuclear antigen in sera from patients with infectious mononucleosis. *J. Infect. Dis.*, **154**, 885–9
38. Geltosky, J. E., Smith, R. S., Whalley, A. and Rhodes, G. (1987) Use of a synthetic peptide-based ELISA for the diagnosis of infectious mononucleosis and other diseases. *J. Clin. Lab. Anal.*, **1**, 153–62
39. Luzzatto, L. (1979) Genetics of red-cells and susceptibility to malaria. *Blood*, **54**, 961–76
40. Pasvol, G. and Weatherall, D. G. (1980) The red-cell and the malaria parasite. *Br. J. Haematol.*, **46**, 165–70
41. Nagel, R. L. and Roth, E. F. (1989) Malaria and red cell genetic defects. *Blood*, **74**, 1213–21
42. Ellis, C. J., Eykyn, S. J., Watkins, P., Bell, M. and Geddes, A. M. (1979) Malaria in Birmingham and a London teaching hospital. *Br. Med. J.*, **i**, 385–7
43. Fleming, A. J. (1981) Malaria and other parasitic diseases. *Clin. Haematol.*, **10**, 983–1011
44. Abdalla, S. H. (1986) Red cell associated IgG in patients suffering from *Plasmodium falciparum* malaria. *Br. J. Haematol.*, **62**, 13–19
45. Merry, A. H., Looareesuwan, S., Phillips, R. E. *et al.* (1986) Evidence against immune haemolysis in falciparum malaria in Thailand. *Br. J. Haematol.*, **64**, 187–94
46. Richards, D. F., Hunter, D. T. and Janis, B. (1969) Detection of Plasmodia by acridine orange stain. *Am. J. Clin. Pathol.*, **51**, 180–3
47. Ridley, D. S. (1974) The laboratory diagnosis of tropical diseases with special reference to Britain: a review. *J. Clin. Pathol.*, **27**, 435–44
48. Abaru, D. E. and Denham, D. A. (1976) A comparison of the efficiency of the Nuclepore and Millipore filtration systems for detecting microfilariae. *S. E. Asian J. Trop. Med. Pub. Hlth.*, **7**, 367–9
49. Malech, H. L. and Gallin, J. L. (1987) Current concepts: immunology – neutrophils in human diseases. *N. Engl. J. Med.*, **317**, 687–94
50. Rosen, F. S., Cooper, M. D. and Wedgewood, R. J. P. (1984) The primary immunodeficiencies (first of two parts). *N. Engl. J. Med.*, **311**, 235–42
51. Rosen, F. S., Cooper, M. D. and Wedgewood, R. J. P. (1984) The primary immunodeficiencies (second of two parts). *N. Engl. J. Med.*, **311**, 300–10
52. Friedman-Kien, M., Laubenstein, L., Marmot, M. *et al.* (1981) Kaposi's sarcoma and pneumocystis pneumonia among homosexual men – New York and California. *MMWR*, **30**, 305–8
53. Gottleib, M. S., Schroff, H. M., Schanker, J. D. *et al.* (1981) *Pneumocystis carinii* pneumonia and mucosal candidiasis in previously healthy homosexual men. Evidence for a new acquired immunodeficiency. *N. Engl. J. Med.*, **305**, 1425–30
54. CDC (1982) *Pneumocystis carinii* pneumonia among persons with haemophilia A. *MMWR*, **31**, 365–7
55. Weiss, R. A. (1987) Retroviruses and human disease. *J. Clin. Pathol.*, **40**, 1064–9
56. CDC. (1986) Classification system for the human T-lymphotropic/lymphadenopathy-associated virus infection. *MMWR*, **35**, 334–7

57. Steeper, T. A., Horwitz, C. A., Hanson, M. *et al.* (1988) Heterophil-negative mononucleosis-like illnesses with atypical lymphocytosis in patients undergoing seroconversion to the human immunodeficiency virus. *Am. J. Clin. Pathol.*, **89**, 169–74
58. Scadden, D. T., Zon, L.I. and Groopman, J. E. (1989) Pathophysiology and management of HIV-associated haematologic disorders. *Blood*, **74**, 1455–63
59. Zon, L. I., Arkin, C. and Groopman, J. E. (1987) Haematological manifestations of the human immunodeficiency virus (HIV). *Br. J. Haematol.*, **66**, 251–6
60. Murphy, M. F., Metcalfe, P., Waters, A. H. *et al.* (1987) Incidence and mechanism of neutropenia and thrombocytopenia in patients with human immunodeficiency virus infection. *Br. J. Haematol.*, **66**, 337–40
61. Mancuso, S., Perricone, R., Accurso, V. *et al.* (1989) Haematological findings in HIV infection. *Labmedica*, **6**, 27–9
62. van der Lelie, J., Lange, J. M. A., Vos, J. J. E. *et al.* (1987) Autoimmunity against blood cells in human immunodeficiency virus (HIV) infection. *Br. J. Haematol.*, **67**, 109–14
63. Oskenhendler, E., Bierling, P., Farcet, J.-P. *et al.* (1987) Response to therapy in 37 patients with HIV-related thrombocytopenia. *Br. J. Haematol.*, **66**, 491–5
64. Toy, P. T. C. Y., Reid, M. E. and Burns, M. (1985) Positive antiglobulin test associated with hyperglobulinaemia in acquired immunodeficiency syndrome (AIDS). *Am. J. Haematol.*, **19**, 145–50
65. Dosworth, H. and Wiener, E. (1988) Non-immune nature of anaemia in HIV infection. *Br. J. Haematol.*, **68**, 498–9
66. Namiki, T. S., Boone, D. C. and Meyer, P. R. (1987) A comparison of bone marrow findings in patients with acquired immunodeficiency syndrome (AIDS) and AIDS related conditions. *Haematol. Oncol.*, **5**, 99–106

Chapter 15

General methods for the investigation of haemostasis

Collection and handling of blood samples

It cannot be overstressed that reliable results of tests of haemostasis require the highest standard of sample collection and handling.

Ideally, samples should be collected by venepuncture with minimal stasis and trauma. A 20G or 21G needle allows rapid collection with minimal frothing due to excessive vacuum. Contact activation is minimized by use of plastic syringes.

Collection of samples from venous or arterial lines requires strict protocols to prevent contamination of the sample with heparin solution used to keep the line patent. First blood samples must be discarded, the precise volume being dependent on the length and internal bore of the line and the rate of collection. For the majority of investigations whole blood is collected into anticoagulant in polystyrene or polypropylene tubes. Borosilicate or soda-glass tubes must not be used. Evacuated glass tubes must be siliconized to prevent contact activation. Conventionally, nine volumes of blood are added to one volume of 0.109 M trisodium citrate dihydrate. For certain tests, dried citrate has been used [1] which avoids the problems of evaporation of the anticoagulant during storage, bacterial contamination, or loss of anticoagulant due to leakage or spillage. HEPES-buffered citrate (*see* page 533) is widely used to control the pH of the plasma and limit the loss of activity of labile factors. The proportion of nine volumes of blood to one volume of anticoagulant is appropriate for blood samples with PCV of 0.370–0.500 l/l. For blood samples with PCV outside this range the proportions of citrate and blood should be adjusted for two reasons:

1. Samples with differing PCV contain different amounts of plasma which if mixed with a fixed amount of citrate will result in over- or under-citration with variation in the concentration of ionized calcium. This affects not only coagulation tests [2], but also platelet aggregation responses [3].
2. Plasma will be variably diluted with citrate, thus affecting assay values, as can be seen in *Table 15.1*.

While the variations may be considered relatively small for diagnostic work, the differences can be significant when calculating recovery of infused materials and in research (for example into age and sex differences in the levels of coagulation factors).

Figure 15.1 [2] indicates the amounts of citrate to be made up to 2 ml, 5 ml and 10 ml total volumes, with blood of PCV between 0.150 and 0.850. Although

Table 15.1 The influence of added citrate on assay values

Volume of whole blood (ml)	*PCV*	*Plasma content* (ml)	*With 1 ml citrate* (ml)	*Final plasma concentration* (%)
9.0	0.660	3.0	4.0	75
9.0	0.500	4.5	5.5	82
9.0	0.300	6.3	7.3	86
9.0	0.200	7.2	8.2	88

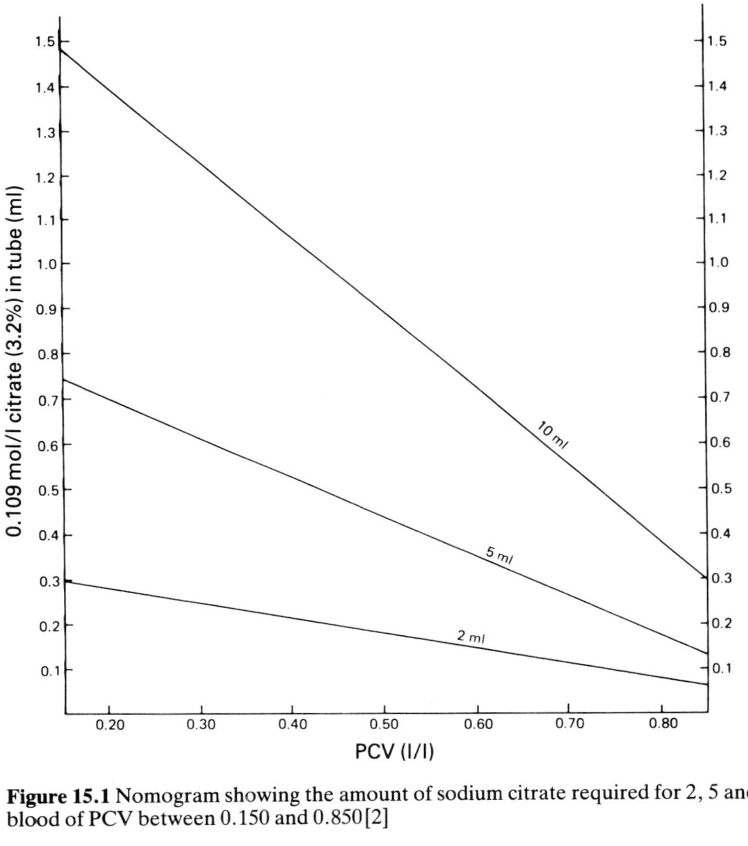

Figure 15.1 Nomogram showing the amount of sodium citrate required for 2, 5 and 10 ml volumes with blood of PCV between 0.150 and 0.850[2]

essentially designed for ensuring the correct proportion of citrate to plasma to maintain a constant concentration of ionized calcium, it also ensures constant plasma dilution.

Samples collected other than by laboratory staff should be examined carefully for clots and fibrin strands and to ensure that the tube has not been over- or underfilled with blood which would alter the blood: citrate ratio.

Separation of plasma

Platelet-rich plasma (PRP)

Citrated whole blood in a plastic tube is centrifuged at 170 *g* for 10 minutes and the supernatant PRP transferred to a further tube avoiding contact with glass. If necessary store at *room temperature* in a capped tube.

Platelet-poor plasma (PPP)

Citrated whole blood or PRP is centrifuged at 2700 *g* for 10 minutes at room temperature and the supernatant PPP transferred to clean polystyrene tubes using a plastic pipette. For fibrinolytic studies blood should be collected into cold citrate solution and *immediately* placed in melting ice. The plasma should be separated after centrifugation at 4°C.

Non-contacted plasma

PRP or PPP is collected as above again using *plastic* pipettes throughout. Non-contacted plasma should not at any stage be exposed to glass activation and should be tested with a minimum of delay. A certain amount of 'dilution–activation' by the anticoagulant will take place but can be ignored if tests are performed soon after collection. If delay is inevitable, whole blood should be anticoagulated with one-fiftieth volume of 0.532 mol/l (156 g/l) trisodium citrate dihydrate.

Serum

1 ml aliquots of blood are placed in 75 × 10 mm glass tubes and incubated at 37°C for 4 hours and then kept at 4°C overnight before separation to allow stabilization of activated factors and the decay of labile intermediate products.

Storage of platelet-poor plasma and serum

Samples to be tested within 4 hours should be kept in melting ice (1°C) or in a 'cold block'. Short-term storage of test plasmas should be at −20°C; for long-term storage, freezing at −70°C or freeze-drying is necessary, particularly for reference preparations.

Cold storage in glass tubes results in activation of factor VII mediated by activation of contact factors. In particular, samples for one-stage prothrombin time tests should not be stored in the cold. Polypropylene tubes largely prevent cold-activation of the prothrombin time.

Special collection procedures and handling requirements of samples for specific tests are described in the appropriate methods.

Significant changes in haemostatic activity can take place during transit of samples to or between laboratories. In certain instances, e.g. studies of fibrinolysis, delay in testing invalidates laboratory findings, while in other situations, e.g. inhibitor assay, samples sent through the post are acceptable. Delay in testing can result in significant loss of activity of labile factors, e.g. factors VIII and V, while conversely progressive activation of other factors, e.g. factor VII and contact factors, can occur.

The problem of samples for the control of oral anticoagulant therapy sent by post from outlying clinics and health centres can be overcome by collecting into liquid citrate in plastic containers. Slight changes in the one-stage prothrombin time are found but the differences are not significant [4].

For other investigations, separation and freezing of PPP and same-day transportation in solid CO_2 (dry ice) in an insulated container is satisfactory, but for periods greater than 24 hours freeze-drying may be the only satisfactory alternative.

Preparation of reagents

Distilled water

Distilled water is recommended for the preparation of all reagents. Deionized water may contain organic substances and, in particular, proteins can interfere with some reactions. Glass distilled water is preferable to that from metal stills and should be freshly prepared.

Trisodium citrate solution

Trisodium citrate dihydrate ($Na_3C_6H_5O_7.2H_2O$, molecular weight 294.10) is used as a 0.109 mol/l (32 g/l) solution in distilled water. The addition of the hydrogen-ion buffer N-2-hydroxyethylpiperazine-N′-2-ethanesulphonic acid (HEPES) to the sodium citrate solution at a concentration of 50 g/l maintains the pH of the anticoagulated plasma at 7.35 and improves the stability both of fresh and of lyophilized plasma. Citric acid-citrate-HEPES is reported to be more effective in preserving factors V and VIII:C[5]. Although there have been suggestions to the contrary, the use of HEPES at the above concentration is also suitable for platelet aggregation studies. Citrate solutions can support bacterial growth and should be checked for contamination.

Calcium chloride

Solutions of calcium chloride are best prepared by diluting a stock 1 mol/l solution which can be obtained commercially. Solid anhydrous calcium chloride is deliquescent and must be stored in a desiccator. The hexahydrate form may be used to prepare a stock 1 mol/l solution by dissolving 219.08 g in 1 litre glass-distilled water; 0.025 mol/l solution is prepared by diluting 25 ml 1 mol/l solution to 1 litre with distilled water. It is normal practice to maintain a working volume of calcium chloride solution at 37°C in the water bath but it must be changed frequently to prevent contamination or significant loss by evaporation. The practice of 'topping-up' the working solution is to be discouraged.

Imidazole (glyoxaline) buffer, pH 7.3

Dissolve 3.5 g imidazole and 5.85 g sodium chloride in approximately 500 ml distilled water. Add 186 ml 0.1 mol/l hydrochloric acid and make up to 1 litre with distilled water. Check with a pH meter. The reagent is stable at 4°C and at room temperature.

Kaolin suspension

Light kaolin is suspended in isotonic sodium chloride to a final concentration of 5 g/l. The suspension is generally stable at 4°C but may deteriorate unexpectedly. Re-suspend thoroughly before use.

Aluminium hydroxide suspension

1 g aluminium hydroxide (moist gel) is suspended in 4 ml of distilled water and is stable indefinitely if stored at 4°C.

Aluminium hydroxide adsorbed plasma

0.1 ml aluminium hydroxide suspension is added to 1 ml plasma and incubated at 37°C in a water bath for 3 minutes and centrifuged. The adsorption removes factors II, VII, IX and X thus leaving factors I, V, VIII:C, XI and XII. The one-stage prothrombin time of the adsorbed plasma should be between 60 and 240 seconds. Further adsorption will totally remove factors II, VII, IX and X but also results in alteration of factor VIII:C activity and some loss of factor XI.

Sodium oxalate solution

Factor V is particularly unstable in oxalated plasma and incubation at 37°C for 24 hours results in a marked depletion of factor V. 13.4 g sodium oxalate is dissolved in 1 litre distilled water. The solution is stable. Nine volumes of blood are mixed with one volume of sodium oxalate solution.

Celite-absorbed plasma (factor XI-deficient)

Add 6 mg of celite 512 (Johns Manville) to 1 ml non-contacted plasma (*see* page 532) and incubate at 37°C for 10 minutes, keeping the celite in suspension. Centrifuge twice at 1500 *g* for 10 minutes. Incubate the plasma at 37°C for 24 hours in a stoppered tube. Plastic or siliconed tubes and pipettes must be used throughout.

Brain products

Rabbit brain is obtained within 24 hours of death. Remove the meninges and superficial blood vessels *completely* and discard the cerebellum. Wash thoroughly in running tap water followed by distilled water to remove any traces of blood. Cut into sections and drain on filter paper.

Saline extract of brain for one-stage prothrombin time

Macerate the brain using an electric mixer for about 60 seconds and add 1500 ml phenol saline warmed to 45°C (1500 ml distilled water, 13.5 g sodium chloride, 7.5 g phenol) and continue the maceration for a further 60 seconds. Leave at 37°C for 30 minutes and then decant into sterile glass containers and leave overnight at 4°C. Centrifuge at 1800 *g* for 30 minutes. Aspirate the supernatant and add to it a one-tenth volume of the fine top layer of sediment. Store in sterile containers for about 2 weeks to stabilize and to allow any bacterial contamination to become apparent.

Prepare dilutions of the saline extract, e.g. 1 in 2, 1 in 4, 1 in 8, etc. and test by the one-stage prothrombin time using pooled normal plasma. Select the optimum dilution, i.e. the lowest dilution giving the shortest prothrombin time and dilute the neat extract accordingly with phenol–saline. Distribute in 10 ml amounts and store at 4°C. Do not freeze.

Acetone-extracted dried brain

Place about 100 g washed brain in a large mortar and cover with acetone. Mash with a pestle for about 2 minutes. Decant the acetone, replace with fresh acetone and continue macerating, decanting and replacing with fresh acetone until the residual material is granular and has lost its 'soapy' feel. Spread the granular material on a large filter paper and allow to dry at room temperature. Store the dried brain in containers with pierced lids in an evacuated desiccator.

Acetone-dried brain may be used for the one-stage prothrombin time by extracting 0.5 g in 10 ml saline with shaking and incubating for 30 minutes at 37°C. Saline brain extracts have virtually replaced the use of acetone-dried brain in the one-stage prothrombin time test.

Platelet substitute (Bell and Alton)

Platelet substitutes (partial thromboplastins) are used in the partial thromboplastin time, activated partial thromboplastin time, and other methods involving the intrinsic coagulation system.

Weigh 1 g acetone-dried brain and add 20 ml acetone. Mix continuously for 2 hours, centrifuge at 1500 *g* for 5 minutes and discard the supernatant. Add 20 ml chloroform and mix for a further 2 hours. Filter through a Whatman No. 1 paper and collect the filtrate into a wide-mouthed container. Evaporate the chloroform using a stream of warm air. Add 10 ml of normal saline to the residue and emulsify. This step is difficult, and prolonged mixing and agitation for up to 48 hours may be necessary.

Standardization
Prepare dilutions of the emulsion in saline (1 in 10, 1 in 20, 1 in 50, 1 in 100, 1 in 200 and 1 in 500). The optimum dilution will vary for each method and should be selected by determining the minimum clotting time using pooled normal plasma while retaining the ability to detect *mild* defects in the intrinsic pathway.

Phospholipid extract of brain

The chloroform extract of acetone-dried brain (*see* above) is relatively crude material and is generally far too active to use in two-stage techniques for the assay of factors VIII:C and IX. The brain residue remaining after chloroform extraction may be used as a starting material for further extraction using petroleum ether; alternatively, the original acetone-dried material may be extracted.

Equipment

It is remarkable that the investigation of haemostatic function can mostly be performed with a minimum of simple equipment: a water bath at 37 ± 0.5°C, stop-watches, pipettes, test tubes and racks.

Pipettes

Although there has been a move in recent years to the use of automatic pipettes with disposable plastic tips or of the 'positive-displacement' type, there is still a place for the use of graduated pipettes of the straight-bore capillary type for use with a teat, and calibrated 'to deliver' volumes of 0.1, 0.2 and 0.5 ml. When repeated measurements of reagents or plasma are necessary a separate pipette should be reserved for each reagent.

Test tubes

Soda-glass tubes 75 × 10 mm or 12 mm are used for all end-point determinations. They should be regarded as disposable, as plasma factors adsorbed on to glass surfaces are extremely difficult to remove. Scratched tubes should be avoided.

Stop-watches

Multiple stop-watches are needed for certain methods and their accuracy should be checked and not simply accepted. It is possible to make measurements to intervals of less than 1 second and the watches should therefore be graduated at intervals of 0.2 seconds.

Instrumentation and automation [6]

Laboratory assessment of haemostatic function developed and became established by the use of manual techniques with visual end-point assessment of clot formation or lysis and of platelet aggregation. As in other areas of laboratory haematology the use of instruments for quantitation, to detect test end-points and to study reaction kinetics has been extended to haemostasis testing. Not only have the basic procedures for the detection and timing of fibrin formation and the rate and degree of platelet aggregation been adapted to instrumentation, but additional methods using chromogenic substrates, antibodies, radioisotopes, enzyme labels and biochemical analysis are only possible by the use of instrumentation. Automation of methods allows greater throughput, improved precision by standardization of sample and reagent handling and by microprocessor handling of data. In many instances instrumentation and automation is based on the principles and equipment used in clinical chemistry, particularly for those reactions which are based on colorimetric, fluorometric or turbidometric measurement.

As the great majority of tests performed in routine laboratories are based on the time taken for clot formation, many instruments have been developed which detect the sol-gel end-point or the change in turbidity associated with fibrin formation. Various methods of end-point detection are used – photo-optical, mechanical, electromechanical, optical-mechanical. It is emphasized that different methods of end-point detection can give different 'clotting' times and therefore the results from different instruments are not necessarily comparable and that manual techniques largely remain the reference methods. Certain techniques, e.g. Clauss method for fibrinogen determination, were developed using instrument end-point detection and may not be transferable to manual/visual techniques. Instruments may only be reliable using specific reagents, usually the manufacturer's own product!

In summary, many manual methods can be transferred to semi- or fully-automated instruments and certain methods are dependent on the availability of appropriate instrumentation. Precision is improved and increased accuracy is possible. In general, the potential throughput of automated systems is far greater than the workload of most diagnostic laboratories. Careful cost analysis rarely shows economies and must be balanced against speed of results, convenience and the reduced requirement for technical expertise.

Tests of coagulation function

Principle

Equal volumes of citrated PPP and brain thromboplastin are warmed to 37°C, recalcified with calcium chloride and the time taken for fibrin to form is recorded. With each test or batch of tests, control times using a normal pooled plasma are determined. The test is used to demonstrate deficiencies of factors of the extrinsic system, i.e. factors I, II, V, VII and X, and the presence of inhibitors.

Method

1. Sufficient brain thromboplastin is warmed to 37°C prior to testing.
2. 0.1 ml of normal pooled plasma and 0.1 ml of thromboplastin are pipetted into a 75 × 10 mm glass tube and allowed to warm to 37°C (one minute).
3. Add 0.1 ml pre-warmed 0.025 mol/l $CaCl_2$ and start a stop-watch. Gently mix the contents of the tube and after 10 seconds gently tilt the tube back and forth through 90 degrees until the fibrin clot is formed and immediately stop the watch. The time recorded in seconds is the prothrombin time. The normal plasma is tested in triplicate and the mean time is the prothrombin time control value.
4. The procedure is repeated twice with the test plasma and the duplicate times compared. Clotting times in the 12–15 second range should agree within 1 second; times around 30 seconds should agree within 2 seconds.

Expression of results

For the investigation of acquired or inherited deficiencies, it is sufficient to compare the control and test values, e.g. control time = 12 seconds, patient's time 20 seconds, or 20/12. For the control of oral anticoagulant therapy the results are expressed as the International Normalized Ratio (page 676).

Significance of the results

A satisfactory thromboplastin preparation should give control values of 12 ± 1 second. There is a good case for including with each batch of tests an abnormal control with a prolonged prothrombin time.

The method is not equally sensitive to deficiencies of individual factors; it is most sensitive to factor VII and least sensitive to factors II and I. Factor I has to be severely depleted to cause significant prolongation of the prothrombin time and is associated with wispy fibrin formation. Mild deficiencies of factor II may not be apparent using the standard test and even moderate deficiencies, e.g. 10% of normal activity, may only result in a 3 or 4 second prolongation of the prothrombin time.

The significance of slightly prolonged times (2–3 seconds) can be studied by diluting the control and test plasmas and noting any divergence in prothrombin times, for example:

(A)	*Neat plasma*	*1 in 2*	*1 in 3*	*1 in 4*
Control(s)	12	14	19	26
Test(s)	14	16	22	29

Conclusion – The slightly abnormal prothrombin time is not due to factor deficiency.

(B)	*Neat plasma*	*1 in 2*	*1 in 3*	*1 in 4*
Control(s)	12	14	19	26
Test(s)	14	18	30	50

Conclusion – Deficient plasma; progressive dilution enhances the defect.

The principle and technique of progressive dilution may be applied to other tests.

Note
The ICSH and ICTH (International Committee on Thrombosis and Haemostasis) have published a reference technique for the one-stage prothrombin time on human blood [7].

Thrombotest technique

Principle

The Thrombotest reagent is formulated to be sensitive to the vitamin K-dependent factors of the extrinsic system (II, VII, X), factor IX and protein induced by vitamin K antagonist (PIVKA) proteins. It uses a bovine brain thromboplastin, with added bovine factor V to exclude variations in factor V activity in test plasma, and a cephalin preparation (partial thromboplastin) to reflect the activity of the intrinsic system. The two thromboplastin components are suitably diluted so that the activities of the intrinsic and extrinsic systems both contribute to thrombin formation and the fibrin end-point.

Method A – using capillary blood

The reagent is reconstituted as described by the manufacturers using the requisite amount of *distilled water*. 0.25 ml of reagent is pipetted into a glass tube 75 × 12 mm and warmed at 37°C for at least 3 minutes but no longer than 60 minutes. From a skin incision, the first 0.5 ml is measured in a capillary pipette and immediately delivered into the reagent at 37°C and a stop-watch started. The blood and reagent are quickly mixed and left undisturbed at 37°C for 30 seconds. The tube is then tilted through 90 degrees repeatedly and the clotting time noted.

The percentage 'Thrombotest activity' is calculated from the lower curve of the calibration graph supplied by the manufacturer with each batch of reagent.

Method B – using venous blood

The reagent is reconstituted as instructed by the manufacturer with the requisite amount of 3.2 mmol/l calcium chloride solution. Venous blood collected into one-tenth volume of 0.106 mol/l trisodium citrate dihydrate (31.3 g/l) and 0.05 ml of the whole blood is added to 0.25 ml of previously warmed reagent and the clotting time determined as above. The percentage Thrombotest activity is calculated from the upper curve of the calibration graph.

With each method correction should be made for variation in PCV.

Application of the method

Although the technique is designed for the control of oral anticoagulant therapy and does not have an apparent advantage over the use of a standardized saline extract of human brain adapted for use with capillary blood, Thrombotest can be used as a convenient reagent for screening for the activity of the liver-dependent factors in neonates or patients in whom clean venepuncture is difficult. An additional use is in distinguishing CRM^+ subjects with hereditary factor IX deficiency (*see* page 599).

Partial thromboplastin time (PTT)

Principle

The PTT is a development of the now outdated plasma recalcification time test in which the platelet activity was an undesirable variable and which is standardized in the PTT by the use of a partial thromboplastin (cephalin, platelet substitute) and PPP. Equal volumes of PPP, partial thromboplastin and calcium chloride are reacted at 37°C and the time taken for fibrin formation is the PTT.

Reagents

Control PPP, patient's PPP, partial thromboplastin (cephalin, e.g. Bell and Alton's platelet substitute at optimum dilution), 0.025 mol/l calcium chloride.

Method

Pre-warm sufficient partial thromboplastin and calcium chloride solution in separate tubes in the water bath at 37°C. Pipette 0.1 ml of plasma into a 75 × 10 mm glass tube and warm for 2 minutes. Add 0.1 ml partial thromboplastin followed by 0.1 ml of calcium chloride and start a stop-watch. Briefly mix and allow to stand for about 40 seconds undisturbed in the water bath, then remove from the bath, wipe the tube dry and tilt back and forth through 90 degrees until fibrin clot forms. Stop the watch. The test is repeated with both control and test plasmas; the duplicate times should be within 5 seconds. The average time is the PTT.

Normal range

This is largely dependent on the activity of the partial thromboplastin but should be in the order of 45–70 seconds. Each laboratory should determine its own normal range using a series of plasmas from healthy subjects.

Interpretation

The PTT may be expected to be prolonged by:

1. Defects in the intrinsic system – factors VIII:C, IX, XI, XII and other contact factors.
2. Defects in the 'common' coagulation pathway – factors X, V, II and I.
3. Inhibitory action – inhibitors to specific factors, high levels of fibrin degradation products, the presence of heparin.

The test is most sensitive to deficiencies in the intrinsic system, and in the presence of a normal one-stage prothrombin time clearly indicates an intrinsic system defect.

The test is capable of demonstrating deficiencies below 30% of normal activity except for platelet factor 3, factor XIII and factor VII. The sensitivity of the test is particularly influenced by the source of partial thromboplastin; some lack sensitivity to mild deficiencies.

Notes

1. The test may be used as a basis for correction studies (*see* below and page 541).
2. The test is influenced by variable contact activation of the plasma.
3. The wide normal range of about 25 seconds reduces sensitivity to mild defects.

Activated partial thromboplastin time (APTT)

Principle

The APTT is a development of the PTT in that the variable of contact activation is eliminated by the addition of an activator to obtain full contact activation. This results in shortening of the PTT and narrowing of the normal range. A variety of activators have been recommended: solid particulate materials such as silica, kaolin, celite and bentonite; or soluble activator, e.g. ellagic acid. It should not be assumed that all activators give comparable results. In the method described below PPP is exposed to kaolin activation for a predetermined period in the presence of a partial thromboplastin and recalcified. The time taken for fibrin formation is the kaolin–cephalin clotting time (KCCT).

Reagents

Control PPP, test PPP, light kaolin 5 mg/ml (*see* page 534), partial thromboplastin (cephalin, e.g. Bell and Alton's platelet substitute) and 0.025 mol/l calcium chloride.

Method

0.1 ml of plasma is pipetted into a 75 × 10 mm glass tube and warmed to 37°C in the water bath for 2 minutes. 0.1 ml of thoroughly suspended kaolin and 0.1 ml partial thromboplastin are added and maintained at 37°C while keeping the kaolin in suspension by occasional mixing. The mixture is incubated for 2 minutes (*see* note 1) and recalcified with 0.1 ml pre-warmed calcium chloride solution and a stop-watch started. The tube is left undisturbed for 25 seconds and then tilted at intervals through 90 degrees and the time for fibrin formation is noted. The test is performed twice with control and test plasmas; the duplicate times should be within 3 seconds. The average of the duplicate times is the KCCT.

Normal range

As with the PTT, this is dependent upon the source of the partial thromboplastin in addition to the activator used and the activation time. It is generally in the order of 30–42 seconds. Each laboratory should determine its own normal range with the reagents in use and the selected activation period.

Interpretation

The specificity of the KCCT is identical with the PTT (*see* above) but its sensitivity is greater because it is less variable and has a narrower normal range. With a suitable partial thromboplastin and good technique, levels of clotting factors of the intrinsic system below 40% can be detected.

Notes

1. The minimum time for maximum activation must be determined by experiment.
2. A prolonged KCCT should be repeated with an activation time of 10 minutes. A shortening of the KCCT after extended activation is a characteristic of prekallikrein deficiency.
3. Soluble activators such as ellagic acid are used, particularly for automated instruments which use photometry to detect the end-point when particulate activators can be unsuitable. Soluble activators also overcome the problem of sedimentation of particulate activators in automated systems, but the sensitivity of ellagic acid activation to prekallikrein deficiency has been questioned[8].
4. The KCCT can be used for correction studies.
5. The use of HEPES-citrate as anticoagulant results in a further narrowing of the normal range.

Correction tests using the kaolin–cephalin time or the one-stage prothrombin time

Principle

Correction studies usually take the form of the addition to the test plasma of a small proportion of normal plasma, plasma fraction or serum. The pattern of correction of the prolonged KCCT or one-stage PT can clearly identify a factor deficiency or narrow the possibilities to two or three factors.

The alternative approach of adding the test plasma to plasmas known to be deficient in a single factor depends on the availability of six or more deficient plasmas and, with the exception of using the relatively widely available plasmas with factors VIII:C, IX or XI deficiency (the last being prepared *in vitro*), this approach is not generally practicable unless commercial sources are used.

Reagents

Normal citrated plasma, aluminium hydroxide adsorbed plasma (*see* page 534) and aged serum (*see* page 532), '24-hour-37°C' oxalated plasma (*Table 15.2*).

Table 15.2 Reagents used for correction studies

Reagent	*Factor content*
Normal plasma	All plasma coagulation factors
$Al(OH)_3$ adsorbed plasma	I, V, VIII:C, XI, XII
Aged serum	VII, X, XI, XII, IX
'24-hour-37°C' oxalated plasma	All except V

Method

To four parts of test plasma are added one part of normal plasma, adsorbed plasma and serum in separate tubes. These proportions should not be exceeded; some workers use nine parts of test plasma to one part of added reagent. Standard KCCT or one-stage PT tests are performed with aliquots of each mixture.

Interpretation

The patterns of correction for each test with different plasma deficiencies are shown in *Tables 15.3* and *15.4*. A suggested factor deficiency must be confirmed by specific factor assay. The assessment of 'significant correction' is sometimes difficult, particularly when there are multiple deficiencies – e.g. in severe liver disease or in lack of vitamin-K activity.

Russell's viper venom clotting time

Principle

The venom of *Vipera russelli* acts as a thromboplastin by a direct action on factor X. A prolonged Russell's viper venom (RVV) time therefore suggests a deficiency of factor X, V, II or I. The main application of the test is the investigation of a prolonged one-stage PT which is corrected by normal plasma and aged serum, i.e. due to factor VII or X deficiency.

Reagents

Normal control plasma, 0.025 mol/l $CaCl_2$ solution, RVV and Bell and Alton's platelet substitute.

Method

RVV is diluted in platelet substitute to give a clotting time of about 15 seconds with normal plasma, the dilution is usually about 1 in 100 000. 0.2 ml normal plasma is pipetted into a 75 × 12 mm tube together with 0.2 ml RVV/platelet substitute and warmed to 37°C. 0.2 ml of pre-warmed calcium chloride is added and the clotting time noted. The procedure is repeated with the test plasma.

An abnormal RVV time excludes a single deficiency of factor VII. A prolonged time in the context of previous correction studies suggests factor X deficiency, but hereditary factor X deficiencies show considerable heterogeneity and the RVV time must not be considered in isolation from factor X assays using different systems, or from immunological studies.

Table 15.3 Correction studies applied to a prolonged prothrombin time

Addition of one-fifth volume of					
Normal plasma	*Adsorbed normal plasma*	*Aged serum*	*Oxalated plasma*	*Factor(s) deficient*	*Further tests*
C	C	NC	C	I	Fibrinogen assay
C	NC	NC	C	II	Factor assay
C	C	NC	NC	V	Factor assay
C	NC	C	C	VII, X	RVV time Factor assay
NC	NC	NC	NC	Inhibitor	Protamine neutralization Reptilase time

C = Correction; NC = no correction; RVV = Russell's viper venom.

Table 15.4 Correction studies applied to a prolonged activated partial thromboplastin time with normal prothrombin time

Addition of one-fifth volume of				
Normal plasma	*Aged serum*	*Adsorbed plasma*	*Factor(s) deficient*	*Further tests*
C	C	C	XII, XI	Correction with specific deficient plasmas Factor assay
C	C	NC	IX	Factor assay
C	NC	C	VIII:C	Factor assay
NC	NC	NC	Inhibitor ? heparin ? specific inhibitor	TCT Protamine neutralization Inhibitor assay

C = Correction; NC = no correction; TCT = plasma thrombin clotting time.

Thrombin clotting time

Principle

The thrombin clotting time is a rapid screening test for the conversion of fibrinogen to fibrin. Thrombin is added to plasma and the time taken for fibrin formation is the thrombin clotting time.

Reagents

Test PPP, control normal PPP, imidazole buffer, pH 7.3 (*see* page 533) and thrombin solution.

Thrombin solution A working solution of thrombin giving a TCT of 13–15 seconds with the control normal plasma, usually 4–5 units/ml. The thrombin solution is freshly prepared each day and kept at 4°C in a polystyrene tube.

Method

0.1 ml of plasma and 0.1 ml of buffer are mixed in a 75 × 10 mm glass tube and warmed to 37°C. 0.1 ml of thrombin is added, a stop-watch started and the time taken for fibrin to form is noted. Perform the test in duplicate; the mean time is the thrombin clotting time.

Normal TCT

Normal TCT is within 2 seconds of the time for the control plasma.

Interpretation

The TCT maybe prolonged due to:

1. Concentration of plasma fibrinogen less than 1 g/l.
2. The presence of high-molecular-weight forms of FDP.
3. The presence of heparin or heparin-like inhibitor.
4. Paraproteins interfering with fibrin polymerization.
5. Most dysfibrinogens (acquired or inherited).

A *shortened* TCT has been described in inherited dysfibrinogenaemia.

Notes

1. Some workers recommend performing the test at room temperature. Warming and maintaining the thrombin at 37°C is certainly not recommended.
2. The volume of buffer is incorporated to allow substitution in correction studies e.g. with protamine sulphate or normal plasma.
3. The TCT of 13–15 seconds with normal plasma is to ensure maximum sensitivity consistent with reproducibility.
4. Reconstitution or dilution of the thrombin in 0.025 mol/l calcium chloride (calcium-thrombin reagent) results in shorter TCT with normal plasma and is useful when investigating dysfibrinogenaemia.

Reptilase clotting time

Certain snake venoms and bacterial enzymes have a thrombin-like activity and initiate the conversion of fibrinogen to fibrin. They are useful laboratory reagents because, unlike thrombin, their activity is not inhibited by heparin.

A fraction of the venom of *Bothrops atrox* is available commercially as Reptilase (Pentapharm) and Atroxin (Sigma) and is widely used. The venom of *Bothrops jararaca* (Sigma) can be used as an alternative and is reported to be more sensitive to the presence of FDPs than Reptilase. Certain commercial sources may be sensitive to heparin. Thrombin-coagulase (Boehringer) is an activated bacterial coagulase and is apparently particularly sensitive for the detection of the dysfibrinogenaemia of liver disease.

Principle

The reagent is added to citrated plasma to convert fibrinogen to fibrin by a proteolytic action similar to, but not identical with, that of thrombin. The time taken for fibrin formation is the Reptilase clotting time.

Reagents

Control normal plasma, test plasma and Reptilase.

Reptilase The lyophilized venom is reconstituted as directed. The reagent is stable for 4 weeks at 4°C.

Method

To 0.2 ml control plasma warmed to 37°C is added 0.1 ml pre-warmed Reptilase and the clotting time noted. The test is repeated and the mean value taken as the control time which is usually 15–18 seconds. The test is repeated in duplicate using the test plasma, the mean time being the Reptilase clotting time.

Interpretation

Prolonged times are obtained in the same circumstances as the TCT, with the exception of the presence of heparin, that is:

1. At concentrations of fibrinogen less than 1 g/l.
2. In the presence of FDPs.
3. In the presence of paraproteins.
4. In the presence of most dysfibrinogens.

The test is therefore particularly useful in the investigation of fibrinogen–fibrin conversion, in patients on heparin and in the further investigation of an unexplained prolonged TCT, and the reagent can also be used as a substitute for thrombin in the Clauss technique for measuring fibrinogen, provided an appropriate standard curve is prepared.

Urea solubility test for factor XIII activity

Principle

Fibrin cross-linked by the action of factor XIII is insoluble in urea and weak acid solutions. In the absence of factor XIII activity a fibrin clot will dissolve within 1 hour.

Reagents

5 mol/l urea (300 g/l), 0.025 mol/l calcium chloride and normal plasma.

Method

Normal and test plasmas are set up as shown in *Table 15.5*. 0.2 ml aliquots from each tube are recalcified with 0.2 ml calcium chloride in 75 × 12 mm tube and incubated at 37°C until fibrin is formed and incubation is then continued for a further 30 minutes. 5 ml of 5 mol/l urea is added to each tube and the clot suspended. Incubate at 37°C examining at intervals for up to 24 hours.

Table 15.5 Arrangement of normal and test plasma solutions in urea solubility test for factor XIII activity

	Tube		
Plasma	1	2	3
Normal	10	–	1
Test	–	10	9

Interpretation

The normal plasma clot will remain for over 24 hours. In the absence of factor XIII activity the clot in tube 2 will dissolve within 1 hour. In factor XIII *deficiency* the small amount of plasma in tube 3 will completely correct the clot solubility while in the presence of *inhibitor* of factor XIII the clot will dissolve.

Notes

1. The plasmas must be clotted by the addition of calcium chloride and not by thrombin; calcium ions are essential for factor XIII activity.
2. High levels of fibrin monomer can impair clot stability and result in partial solubility.

Thromboplastin generation screening test (Hick's–Pitney test)

Principle

Diluted plasma with added platelet substitute is recalcified at 37°C (incubation mixture or 'first stage'). At timed intervals, aliquots of the incubation mixture are added to substrate normal plasma with the further addition of calcium chloride and the clotting time of the substrate plasma noted (second stage). This 'two-stage' technique follows the generation of factor Xa in the incubation mixture which is reflected by the clotting times of the substrate plasma. The technique is performed using normal and test plasmas and the *minimum* clotting times and the *rate of shortening* of the substrate clotting times compared. The use of diluted plasma increases the sensitivity for mild defects and is considered to be more sensitive than one-stage APTT tests.

Interpretation

Using a normal plasma the substrate clotting time quickly shortens to a plateau at about 8–10 seconds, which eventually lengthens as the factor Xa in the incubation mixture decays. If the test plasma fails to achieve minimum clotting times within 2 seconds of those obtained with the normal plasma, a deficiency is suggested; or if the test plasma takes much longer to achieve the same minimum clotting times as the normal plasma this also indicates a defect in factor Xa (thromboplastin) generation.

An abnormal thromboplastin screening test is found in deficiencies of the contact factors, factors IX, VIII:C, X and V. It is not affected by deficiencies of factors VII, II and I. Inhibitors of intrinsic thromboplastin formation will also produce abnormal results. The test, although sensitive, is non-specific and abnormal results should be followed by a thromboplastin generation test (*see* below), specific factor assays, or both.

The method has been superseded by specific factor assays.

Thromboplastin generation test (Biggs and Douglas)

Principle

The thromboplastin generation test (TGT) is a two-stage technique to demonstrate factor Xa formation in an incubation mixture containing diluted aluminium hydroxide adsorbed plasma, diluted serum, platelet substitute and calcium. By substituting adsorbed plasma and serum test fractions, defective thromboplastin generation can be ascribed to specific factors if the results are considered in association with the results of a one-stage prothrombin time.

Interpretation

The possible findings are summarized in *Table 15.6.* When the results are interpreted in conjunction with the one-stage prothrombin time, single factor deficiencies of V, VIII, IX and X can be identified and a typical pattern is obtained in factor XI, XII or other contact-factor deficiencies. Circulating anticoagulants also show a characteristic pattern of results. The presumptive diagnosis indicated by the TGT should be confirmed by factor assay. Rare examples of combined hereditary deficiencies – particularly of factors V and VIII – may be encountered.

The method has been superseded by specific factor assays.

Table 15.6 Interpretation of the patterns of results of the thromboplastin generation test in conjunction with the one-stage prothrombin time (PT)

	*Mixtures**				
Test plasma + Test serum	*Test plasma + Normal serum*	*Normal plasma + Test serum*	*Possible defects*	*One-stage PT*	*Defect in thromboplastin generation*
Normal	–	–	None	–	None
Abnormal	Normal	Normal	XI, XII, contact factor	Normal	XI, XII, contact factor
Abnormal	Abnormal	Normal	V, VIII:C	Normal	VIII:C
				Abnormal	V
Abnormal	Normal	Abnormal	IX, X	Normal	IX
				Abnormal	X
Abnormal	Abnormal	Abnormal	Circulating inhibitor	–	Inhibitor

* Mixtures also include platelet substitute and calcium chloride.

Assay methods

A satisfactory bioassay method should fulfil the following criteria:

Specificity A system in which the activity being assayed is the rate limiting factor.

Sensitivity The lowest concentration of activity producing a response in the assay system.

Good discrimination The ability to differentiate small differences in factor activity.

Specificity and *sensitivity* depend on the biological characteristics of the assay system; *discrimination* is dependent on:

1. *Precision* of the method, which influences the *accuracy* of the assay even when replicate assays are performed.
2. Dose–responsiveness of the assay system; the dose response is the relationship between *clotting times* and the *dose* (concentration or activity) and is shown by the *slope* of the standard graph (*Figure 15.2*).

Discrimination varies directly with the slope of the graph, i.e. an assay system producing a 'flat' slope will need a greater change in activity to produce a significant change in response (change in clotting time) than an assay system with a 'steep' slope; therefore a steep slope provides better discrimination.

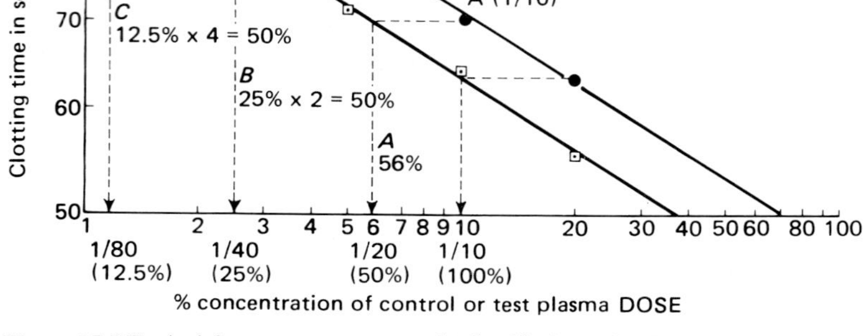

Figure 15.2 Typical dose–response curve obtained in factor VIII:C assay procedures. Assay values for dilutions of patient plasma (A, B, C) were 56, 50 and 50%, respectively

Dose–response curve The dose–response curve is constrained within certain limits because clotting is not instantaneous even with very high levels of activity and because absence of activity still results in a finite clotting time, resulting in a reversed 'S' or sigmoid curve (*Figure 15.3*). However, in specific, sensitive and

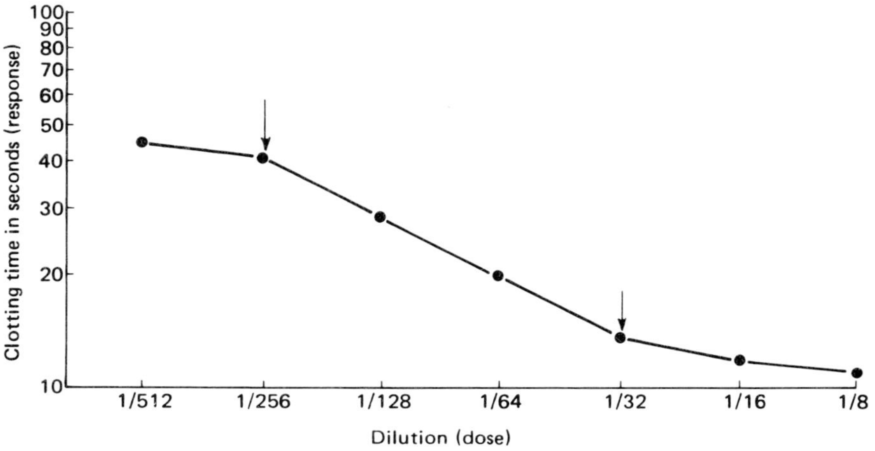

Figure 15.3 A dose–response curve prepared from a range of plasma dilutions, showing a reversed 'S' or sigmoid shape. Dilutions between 1/32 and 1/256 show linearity and discrimination and are used for assay procedures

discriminatory assay systems there is a linear intermediate section which is used in assay calculations. To obtain a linear plot transformation of data is usually necessary, e.g. log/log, log/linear or reciprocal plots.

Parallelism of assay graphs When several dilutions of standard and test preparations with different activities are assayed under identical conditions, the linear sections of the dose–response graphs should be parallel. This is an essential requirement for a valid assay; the horizontal distance between the graphs reflects the difference in activity. If the graphs are not parallel the dose–response graphs of the standard and test preparations show different discrimination.

Assay 'drift' The activity of the components of a bioassay system may show change of activity during the assay procedure resulting in progressive change in clotting times or 'drift'. To control drift it is recommended that:

1. Working dilutions are prepared immediately prior to testing.
2. Duplicate dilutions are tested in a balanced order, e.g. A→B→C→C→B→A.
3. Stable reagents are used.
4. Unnecessary delay during the assay procedure is avoided.

To summarize:

1. Select a wide range of dilutions without losing sensitivity.
2. Select dilutions likely to produce a linear dose–response.
3. Use a balanced order of testing to allow for 'drift'.
4. Check linearity.
5. Confirm parallelism of standard and test graphs.
6. The precision of the assay procedure at different levels of activity should be determined.

Factor II, V, VII and X assays based on the one-stage prothrombin time

Principle

The prothrombin time of plasma is prolonged in proportion to decreasing concentrations of factors II, V, VII or X. When a range of dilutions of a plasma standard are added to a plasma totally deficient in a *single factor,* the resulting prothrombin times show a linear relationship to factor concentration when plotted on double-log graph paper. The activity of the factor in the test plasma can be determined by comparing the corrective effect of dilutions of the test plasma on the clotting times of the deficient plasma by reference to the standard graph.

Reagents

Reference plasma, test plasma, brain thromboplastin, 0.025 mol/l calcium chloride and factor-deficient plasma.

Factor-deficient plasma This is obtained from patients severely deficient in a single factor and is available commercially. In the case of factors V and VII, artificially depleted plasma may be prepared. Factor V-deficient plasma is prepared by incubating oxalated plasma under sterile conditions for up to 72 hours or until the one-stage prothrombin time is in excess of 90 seconds; incubation for longer than 72 hours is undesirable due to loss of activity other than factor V. Factor VII-deficient plasma can be prepared by repeated adsorption with aluminium hydroxide which removes factors II, VII and X, and factors II and X replaced by adding sufficient 'prothrombin-complex concentrate' (factor IX concentrate) to restore the levels of factors II and X to normal.

Method

Standard calibration graph Prepare a range of dilutions of the standard plasma in imidazole buffer, e.g. 1 in 10, 1 in 20, 1 in 50, 1 in 100 (further dilutions may be necessary if test activity is very low). To 0.1 ml of each dilution add 0.1 ml deficient plasma and 0.1 ml thromboplastin and warm to 37°C. Add 0.1 ml calcium chloride and note the clotting times. Repeat the tests but in reverse sequence, i.e. A, B, C, C, B, A. Plot the clotting times against dilution on double-log graph paper, taking the 1 in 10 dilution to be equivalent to 100% normal activity (1 unit/ml plasma). A linear plot should be obtained.

Assay of test plasma Prepare a series of dilutions of the test plasma in imidazole buffer over a range that is varied depending upon the expected level of activity – e.g. in severe deficiency 1 in 2, 1 in 5 and 1 in 10; in moderate deficiency 1 in 5, 1 in 10 and 1 in 20; or, if activity is expected to be in the normal range, the same dilutions as for the standard plasma. Each dilution is tested as above and the results plotted. A linear graph should be obtained which is *parallel* to the standard graph (*see* page 549). The clotting times of the test dilutions are converted to factor activity by extrapolation to the standard curve and the result corrected for dilution factor if necessary, e.g. if the clotting time of the 1 in 10 dilution of test plasma is equivalent to 20% activity in the standard graph, the assay level is 20% of normal activity (0.2 units/ml); or, if the 1 in 5 dilution is equivalent to 20% activity in the standard graph, the assay level is 20% divided by 2 or 10% of normal activity (0.1 units/ml).

Alternative method for the assay of factor II using Taipan snake venom

Principle

The venom of *Oxyuranus scuttelatus* (Taipan venom) can convert prothrombin to thrombin without the involvement of other coagulation factors other than the presence of phospholipid. The amount of thrombin formed is proportional to the concentration of prothrombin present and is measured by the clotting time of added fibrinogen.

Reagents

1. Reference plasma.
2. Test PPP.
3. Taipan venom diluted 1 in 200 000 and mixed with an equal volume of 0.025 mol/l calcium chloride.
4. Phospholipid (platelet substitute) at optimum dilution.
5. Imidazole buffer, pH 7.3.
6. Citrated normal plasma adsorbed twice with aluminium hydroxide as a source of prothrombin-free fibrinogen.

Method

Prepare dilution of the standard plasma 1 in 10, 1 in 20, 1 in 50, 1 in 100 and 1 in 200 in imidazole buffer. To 0.1 ml of each dilution of standard plasma add 0.1 ml adsorbed plasma, 0.1 ml phospholipid and warm to 37°C. Add 0.2 ml of venom/$CaCl_2$ mixture and record the clotting time. Repeat the test in reversed order, and take the mean of the duplicate times. Prepare dilutions of the test plasma, 1 in 2 and 1 in 5 if the level of factor II is expected to be low, or 1 in 10 and 1 in 20 if within the normal range. Plot the results of the dilutions of the reference plasma as clotting times against reciprocal of dilution on linear (arithmetic) graph paper; a straight line should be obtained.

For each of the clotting times of the dilutions of the test plasma, read off the equivalent dilution of the standard plasma, convert to percentage activity and multiply by the test dilution, e.g. the clotting time of the 1 in 10 test dilution is equivalent to a 1 in 50 standard dilution or 2% activity multiplied by 10 (test dilution) = 20% activity (0.2 units/ml) (*Figure 15.4*). Convert each test result separately and average the activities obtained.

Two-stage prothrombin assay

Principle

Plasma is recalcified in the presence of brain thromboplastin (as in the one-stage prothrombin time test) and the thrombin generated is measured by sub-sampling at intervals into a second tube containing fibrinogen. The resulting clotting times are converted into thrombin units by reference to a thrombin–fibrinogen calibration graph. The activity of thrombin is plotted against time on linear graph paper and the area under the graph is assumed to represent the amount of prothrombin present in the plasma sample. An alternative method of interpretation is to plot the reciprocal of the fibrinogen clotting times against time.

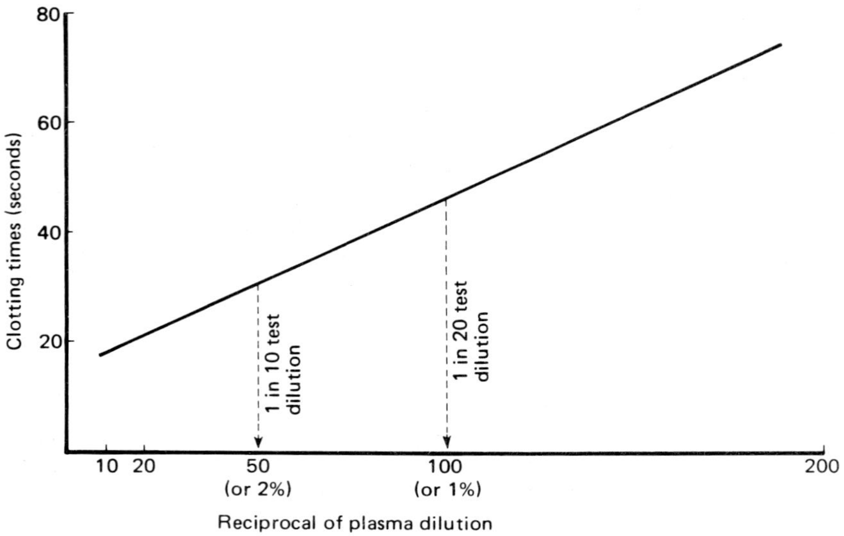

Figure 15.4 Taipan venom assay of factor II. A linear plot is obtained when dilutions of standard plasma are plotted against clotting time on arithmetic graph paper. The clotting times of dilutions of test plasma are converted to percentage activity and multiplied by the dilution factor. In the example shown the factor II assay = 20% (0.2 units/ml plasma)

Reagents

1. Brain thromboplastin diluted to give a one-stage prothrombin time of 30–45 seconds with normal plasma.
2. 0.025 mol/l calcium chloride.
3. Fibrinogen solution (approximately 4 g/dl).
4. Reference plasma.
5. Citrated test plasma.

Method

Add 0.2 ml fibrinogen solution to each of a series of 75 × 10 mm glass tubes and warm to 37°C. In a 75 × 12 mm tube pipette 0.4 ml standard plasma and 0.4 ml dilute thromboplastin. Allow to warm to 37°C and add 0.4 ml pre-warmed calcium chloride and start a stop-watch (it is advisable to insert an applicator or plastic rod into the mixture at this stage to facilitate removal of the expressed clot). At 1 minute after recalcification and at 1-minute intervals thereafter sub-sample 0.1 ml of the incubation mixture into a tube containing fibrinogen and note the clotting times using a separate stop-watch. Continue sub-sampling until the fibrinogen clotting times are in excess of 180 seconds. Repeat the procedure using the test plasma.

Analysis of results

Method A On linear paper, plot the reciprocal of the fibrinogen clotting times on the ordinate against time of sub-sampling on the abscissa.

Method B The fibrinogen clotting times are converted to thrombin units by reference to a thrombin–fibrinogen reference graph prepared by adding a range of dilutions of thrombin (1, 2, 5, 10, 15, 20 and 25 units/ml) to fibrinogen solution. The concentration of fibrinogen must be the same as used in the test and the volumes of thrombin and fibrinogen the same, i.e. 0.1 ml thrombin to 0.2 ml fibrinogen. Using linear graph paper, thrombin units are plotted on the ordinate against fibrinogen clotting times on the abscissa; a hyperbolic curve will result. Alternatively the thrombin units are plotted against the reciprocal of the fibrinogen clotting times to obtain a straight-line graph until thrombin is present in excess; the graph does not pass through zero due to the delay in fibrin formation irrespective of the concentration of thrombin.

Interpretation
Representative graphs of the production and decay of thrombin activity are shown in *Figure 15.5*. With normal plasma (plot 'A') there is a rapid rise in thrombin concentration (x) to a peak (y) which represents equilibrium between thrombin production and destruction, followed by a decay curve (z). In any comparison

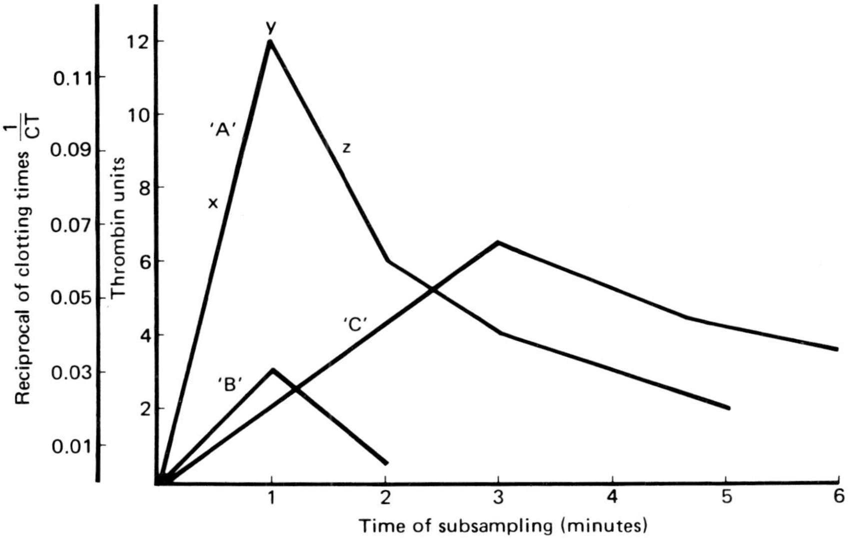

Figure 15.5 Representative graphs of results of two-stage prothrombin time tests. For interpretation, *see* text

between normal and test plasmas it is assumed that antithrombin activity is similar in each sample. In plasma deficient only in factor II (plot 'B'), the general shape is similar to that of normal plasma but less thrombin is formed. In deficiencies of those factors promoting conversion of prothrombin to thrombin, the rate of thrombin formation is slower (plot 'C').

Calculation of prothrombin concentration
The amount of prothrombin in the test plasma relative to the standard plasma can be calculated from (1) the *height* of the test graph compared with the *height* of the

standard graph; or (2) by the *areas* enclosed by the graphs, which can be measured by counting squares, by the use of a planimeter, or simply by cutting out the graph paper enclosed by the graphs and weighing.

Normal range 60–170% of normal activity.

Alternative method for the assay of factor X

Principle
Russell's viper venom (RVV) converts factor X to Xa in the absence of any other coagulation factors. Charcoal-filtered bovine plasma is depleted of factors VII and X but retains fibrinogen, factor V and prothrombin. If dilutions of plasma are added to charcoal-filtered bovine plasma in the presence of RVV and phospholipid, factor X is the rate-limiting factor and the system can be used as a specific assay for factor X.

Reagents
1. Charcoal-filtered bovine plasma (Diagnostic Reagents, UK).
2. RVV diluted 1 in 150 000 in platelet substitute at optimum concentration.
3. Imidazole buffer, pH 7.3.
4. Reference plasma.
5. Citrated test PPP.
6. Calcium chloride, 0.025 mol/l.

Method
Prepare dilutions of the standard and test plasmas 1 in 10, 1 in 30, 1 in 100 and 1 in 200 in imidazole buffer and place on melting ice. In glass tubes mix 0.1 ml plasma dilution and 0.1 ml absorbed bovine plasma and warm to 37°C. Add 0.1 ml RVV/phospholipid and after *exactly* 30 seconds recalcify with 0.1 ml calcium chloride and record the clotting time. Repeat the procedure with each dilution, testing the standard dilutions in duplicate in a balanced order. Plot clotting times against plasma concentration on double-log graph paper. Linear and parallel lines should be obtained within the range 100–1% activity.

Reference range 50–200% of normal activity.

Notes
1. Factor X can also be assayed using chromogenic substrates.
2. In patients with congenital deficiency of factor X different levels of activity may be recorded depending on the assay method used due to heterogeneity of the factor X molecule; in investigating congenital deficiencies it is recommended that more than one assay technique is used.

One-stage assays of factors VIII:C, IX, XI, XII, prekallikrein and HMWK factor based on the activated partial thromboplastin time

The APTT of plasma deficient in factors VIII:C, IX, XI, XII, prekallikrein or HMWK is prolonged. When a dilution of a standard or test plasma is added to a plasma totally deficient in a single factor the degree of correction of the prolonged time is proportional to the factor activity in the added plasma and linear plots can be obtained using log/log graph paper (*see Figure 15.2*).

One-stage assay of factor VIII:C

Principle Factor VIII:C is rate limiting when dilutions of a standard or test plasma are added to plasma totally deficient in VIII:C activity when tested by the APTT. The log of clotting times is linearly related to the log of concentration and the system can therefore be used to assay factor VIII:C (*see Figure 15.2*).

Reagents
1. Imidazole buffer, pH 7.3.
2. Platelet substitute at optimum dilution.
3. Kaolin suspension, 5 g/l.
4. Calcium chloride, 0.025 mol/l.
5. Factor VIII:C deficient (0%) plasma.
6. Citrated test PPP.
7. Plasma with factor VIII:C activity calibrated in International Units (IU) against a reference preparation.

Method Prepare dilutions of standard and test plasmas in buffer, 1 in 10 (100%), 1 in 30 (33%), 1 in 100 (10%). In glass, 75 × 10 mm, tubes pipette 0.1 ml factor VIII:C deficient plasma, 0.1 ml plasma dilution, 0.1 ml platelet substitute and allow to warm to 37°C, and add 0.1 ml well-mixed kaolin. Mix the contents of the tube and leave for 5 minutes, mixing gently at 1 minute intervals. Add 0.1 ml calcium chloride and record the clotting time. Repeat with all dilutions in duplicate in a balanced order.

Calculation Using two-cycle log/log paper plot the dilutions of standard (factor concentration) on the x axis (abscissa) and the clotting times on the y axis (ordinate) and draw a line through the points; a straight line should be obtained. Similarly plot the clotting times of the dilutions of test plasma against dilution. Again draw a line through the points which should be linear and *parallel* to the standard graph. Draw a horizontal line from each point of the test plasma to intersect the standard graph and at the point of intersection drop a perpendicular to the x axis and read off the concentration of clotting factor. Record the value for each dilution and multiply by the dilution factor e.g. 1 in 30 multiply by three, 1 in 100 multiply by 10, and average the values. Multiply the average value obtained by the value of the assayed value of the standard plasma to obtain the assay value for the test plasma (*see Figure 15.2*).

Notes
1. Prepare dilutions in plastic tubes to prevent activation or adsorption.
2. Test all dilutions within 5 minutes of preparation.
3. Make all dilutions separately; double diluting is not a satisfactory technique.
4. By staggering the times of the addition of the kaolin it is possible to shorten the overall time for the assay by testing three tubes simultaneously using separate stop-watches.
5. A ‘blank’ should be tested incorporating all reagents other than the dilution of plasma.

6. Plasma dilutions are added to substrate plasma which is deficient in the factor being assayed but has all other factors present.
7. Disadvantages: 0% activity plasma is required and the procedures are time consuming and may be affected by minute traces of thrombin.
8. Advantages: simple methodology and reagents include commercial products, and the assay system can easily be automated.

One-stage factor IX assay

Principle Factor IX activity is rate limiting in the APTT when dilutions of standard or test plasma are added to factor IX deficient (0%) plasma. The system can therefore be used to assay factor IX activity.

Reagents The reagents are those used in the one-stage assay of factor VIII:C with the exception that factor IX deficient plasma is substituted for factor VIII deficient plasma and that the plasma is calibrated against a factor IX reference preparation.

Method The method is identical with that for factor VIII:C assay.

Calculation As for factor VIII:C assay.

Notes
1. It is important that all plasmas are collected and handled without any contact activation.
2. Clotting times are usually longer than those in the factor VIII:C assay.
3. A two-stage assay method is available for assaying factor IX in concentrates. Some problems exist with the two-stage assay of factor IX which are difficult to overcome.

One-stage assay of factor XI

Principle Factor XI clotting activity is rate limiting when dilutions of *non-contacted* plasma are added to severely depleted plasma and the mixture tested by the APTT. The system can therefore be used to assay factor XI.

Reagents The reagents are the same as those used for the one-stage assay of factor VIII:C with the exception of the special requirements for handling the plasma samples.

Factor XI deficient plasma (0%) from a patient who has not been transfused with plasma for at least 3 weeks. Commercial sources are available.

Standard plasma. Fresh citrated human plasma from at least six normal donors. The blood should be collected into 19 g/dl trisodium citrate (1/50th volume) using plastic tubes and siliconized needles. Throughout processing of the samples care must be taken to avoid any form of surface activation.

Test plasma should be handled as for the standard plasmas.

Method As for the one-stage assay of factor VIII:C. Dilutions of plasma *must* be made in *plastic* tubes.

Calculation As for factor VIII:C assay.

Notes
1. The factor XI molecule is readily adsorbed to glass surfaces which can lead to loss of activity especially with the standard plasma.
2. The assay must be performed as soon as possible after collection of samples.

One-stage assay of factor XII

The assay is carried out in the same way as for factor XI assay though substituting factor XII deficient plasma for factor XI deficient plasma. Again, avoid contact activation. It may be necessary to extend the range of dilutions to 1 in 400 to obtain a sensitive linear portion of the dose–response curve.

One-stage assays of prekallikrein and high molecular weight kininogen

Factor-deficient plasmas are available commercially. The procedures and precautions are those of the assay for factor XI, with the additional problem of progressive shortening of the APTT by prolonged contact with kaolin. It is recommended that the kaolin activation time be reduced to 2 minutes to obtain greater sensitivity. Assay techniques using chromogenic substrate are available.

Chromogenic substrate method for the assay of prekallikrein

Principle The principle is as shown in *Figure 15.6*. The amount of *p*NA liberated is measured at 405 nm and is proportional to kallikrein activity which is dependent on the prekallikrein concentration.

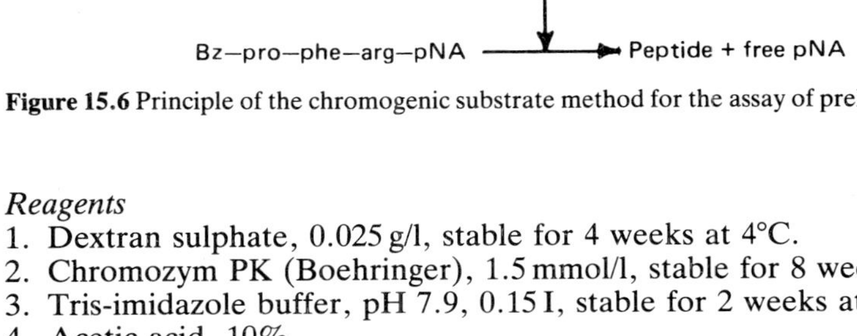

Figure 15.6 Principle of the chromogenic substrate method for the assay of prekallikrein

Reagents
1. Dextran sulphate, 0.025 g/l, stable for 4 weeks at 4°C.
2. Chromozym PK (Boehringer), 1.5 mmol/l, stable for 8 weeks at 4°C.
3. Tris-imidazole buffer, pH 7.9, 0.15 I, stable for 2 weeks at 4°C.
4. Acetic acid, 10%.
5. Citrated test PPP – keep at room temperature and assay within 4 hours, or store at −20°C for up to 6 months. Use plastic tubes and avoid contact activation.

Method To activate prekallikrein, pipette 0.1 ml plasma and 0.1 ml dextran sulphate into a plastic tube and place in melting ice for exactly 7 minutes and assay immediately.

For kinetic measurement warm the buffer and Chromozym PK to 37°C and pipette 1.5 ml buffer and 0.5 ml substrate into a 1 cm cuvette and warm for a further 1 minute. Add 0.02 ml activated plasma, mix well and read or record absorbance (A) at 405 nm for 3 minutes. Plasma kallikrein activity = ΔA min^{-1} × 19.4 units/ml plasma. For end-point measurement proceed as above and after exactly 3 minutes incubation at 37°C add 0.4 ml acetic acid and read absorbance at 405 nm. With each test or batch of tests run a reagent blank consisting of 1.5 ml buffer, 0.5 ml Chromozym, 0.4 ml acetic acid and 0.02 ml dextran sulphate. Deduct the blank absorbance from the test reading. Plasma kallikrein activity = difference in absorbance × 23.3 units/ml plasma.

Reference range 0.6–1.6 units/ml plasma.

Notes

1. Complete activation of prekallikrein will take place only if the factor XII level is over 50% of normal activity.
2. For greater economy the volumes given above may be reduced proportionately and readings taken using microcuvettes.

Two-stage assay of factor VIII:C

Principle

The method is based on the thromboplastin generation test and consists of testing dilutions of adsorbed standard and test plasmas in two stages (*Figure 15.7*).

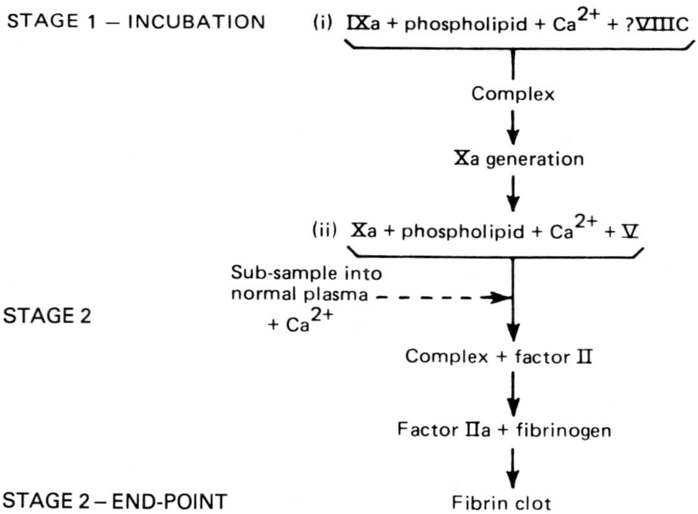

Figure 15.7 Two-stage assay of factor VIII:C

The first-stage incubation mixture contains the factors necessary for Xa generation. The rate-limiting factor is the factor VIII:C activity. Subsequent Xa generation is proportional to the activity of factor VIII:C. In the second stage the clotting time of the substrate plasma is proportional to the Xa→IIa→fibrin reaction and is therefore proportional to the amount of factor VIII:C in the incubation mixture.

Reagents

1. Citrate–saline – five parts 9 g/l sodium chloride and one part 32 g/l trisodium citrate.
2. Aluminium hydroxide suspension 1 g moist gel in 4 ml distilled water.
3. Calcium chloride, 0.025 mol/l and 0.05 mol/l solutions.
4. Substrate plasma – normal citrated plasma (a single donor is satisfactory).
5. Phospholipid at optimum dilution.
6. Serum – freeze-dried normal serum reconstituted in imidazole buffer. The reconstituted serum may require activation by incubating at 37°C for 2 hours.
7. Factor V – diluted bovine plasma.
8. Standard plasma, calibrated against a factor VIII:C reference preparation.
9. Test plasma, collected into HEPES-citrate (*see* page 533).

Method Adsorb the standard and test plasmas with aluminium hydroxide (*see* page 534). Dilute the adsorbed plasma with citrate saline; the range of dilutions will depend on the activity of the reagents in the assay but should be selected to give clotting times within the range 18–35 seconds. The dilutions should be prepared fresh and tested within 5 minutes. Dilutions of 1 in 64, 1 in 128 and 1 in 256 are suggested (*see Figure 15.3*).

Incubation mixture. Pipette 0.1 ml volumes of factor V, phospholipid and serum into each of six tubes to allow for two assays of three dilutions each (standard and test). To the first tube add 0.1 ml of the highest dilution of standard plasma, place in the water bath and start a stop-watch. After 1 minute recalcify with 0.1 ml 0.05 mol/l calcium chloride. During the second minute add 0.1 ml of the second dilution of standard plasma to a second tube and recalcify. Repeat the procedure with the lowest dilution of standard plasma. Continue with the dilutions of test plasma, recalcifying at 4, 5 and 6 minutes.

Testing the formed thromboplastin. Into 12 tubes pipette 0.2 ml 0.025 mol/l calcium chloride and at 10 minutes place six tubes in the water bath. At 12 minutes place 6 ml substrate plasma in the water bath to warm. To test the incubation mixtures at 15 and 21 minutes the following procedure is adopted:

> at 14 minutes 40 seconds remove 0.1 ml from the first incubation tube and add to one of the tubes containing calcium chloride, mix well and at 15 minutes add 0.2 ml substrate plasma and record the clotting time. Repeat at 1-minute intervals with each of the incubation mixtures until each tube has been tested once (20 minutes). At 21 minutes start again at the first incubation tube and repeat the procedure (21–27 minutes).

Plot the values on two-cycle log/log paper to ensure that they produce a linear plot. Adjust the dilutions if necessary before repeating the test procedure in the opposite order to obtain duplicate clotting times. Average the values and plot the clotting times of the standard and test dilutions. It is recommended that an 'in-house' standard be included in the assay and that the procedure is repeated with the standard plasma at the end of the assay as a control of 'drift'.

Calculations

These are as for the one-stage factor VIII:C assay (*see Figure 15.2*).

Notes

1. The two-stage assay is preferred for testing concentrates, or plasma when 'activated' clotting factors are present – e.g. in DIC.
2. Samples are adsorbed with aluminium hydroxide or barium sulphate in order to remove factors II, VII, IX and X.
3. The reagent mixture provides 'activated' IX, V and X.
4. Sub-sampling takes place when Xa generation is maximized and has plateaued.
5. Disadvantages include complexity of the technique.
6. Advantages are that totally deficient plasma is not required, and there is improved precision.
7. Modified two-stage assays using substrate plasma that has been treated with ion-exchange resins facilitate automation of the methods and eliminate sub-sampling.

Detection of inhibitors using the kaolin–cephalin time or the one-stage prothrombin time

Principle

Varied proportions of test and normal plasmas are mixed and incubated at 37°C and aliquots of the mixtures tested by the KCCT and/or one-stage PT to demonstrate: (1) the failure of normal plasma to correct a prolonged time; and (2) the ability of test plasma to prolong the clotting time of normal plasma.

Method

Normal and test plasma are mixed in the proportions shown in *Table 15.7.*

Table 15.7 Proportions of normal and test plasma

	Tube				
Plasma	*1*	*2*	*3*	*4*	*5*
Normal	10	8	5	2	0
Test	0	2	5	8	10

After 5 minutes incubation at 37°C, 0.1 ml aliquots of each mixture are tested by the KCCT or one-stage PT as appropriate. The procedure is repeated after 2 hours incubation even if the first tests clearly show inhibition.

Interpretation

Tube 1 will show the baseline time of normal plasma and tube 5 the initial prolonged time. Any extension of the time for tube 2 beyond 1 or 2 seconds in the PT or 5 seconds in the KCCT must be considered as evidence of inhibition by the presence of the test plasma. Failure of tube 4 to show significant correction of the time for tube 5 is evidence of inhibition. The results of tube 3 may be equivocal depending upon the activity of the inhibitor. The effect of inhibitors that react immediately (heparin, factor IX inhibitor, SLE inhibitor) can be expected to be apparent after 5 minutes incubation; progressive inhibitors, e.g. against factor VIII:C, show a progressive effect over a period of incubation.

The further characterization and assay of inhibitors is considered further in Chapters 16 and 17.

Measurement of plasma fibrinogen

Introduction

Fibrinogen has the highest concentration of all the plasma coagulation factors and many methods have been described for its quantitation. The methods are of three types: (1) based on the formation of fibrin by the action of thrombin or snake venoms; (2) physicochemical methods; and (3) immunological techniques.

Fibrin formation

1. Collection of fibrin and measurement by:
   (a) Weight.
   (b) Colorimetry – Folin and Ciocalteau's reagent, Biuret reagent.
   (c) Nitrogen content – Kjeldahl technique.
2. Based on thrombin clotting time – Clauss technique.
3. Plasma-fibrinogen titre.
4. Clot turbidity – Ellis and Stransky technique.

Comment

Methods based on fibrin formation generally measure functional fibrinogen. Some fulfil the requirement for a rapid result – e.g. Clauss technique, fibrinogen titre, clot turbidity and, to a lesser extent, clot weight. The colorimetric methods and nitrogen determination are time consuming, though the Folin and Ciocalteau (Ratnoff and Menzie) technique is accepted as a reference method for plasma fibrinogen. All methods based on fibrin formation underestimate fibrinogen by about 10% due to loss of fibrinopeptides. Thrombin clotting methods can be influenced by the presence of heparin, fibrinogen–fibrin degradation products (particularly the high molecular weight forms) and by dysfibrinogenaemia.

Physicochemical methods

1. Salting-out – ammonium sulphate, sodium sulphite.
2. Electrophoresis – quantitative, qualitative.
3. Heating – plasma, whole blood.

Comment

Physicochemical methods measure total fibrinogen and may not reflect functional activity. The methods based on heat denaturation of fibrinogen are rapid but may include high molecular weight degradation products. Salting-out using sodium sulphite is claimed not to measure degradation products. Zone electrophoresis and densitometric scanning is semi-quantitative unless total plasma proteins are measured.

Immunological methods

1. Passive agglutination (PA):
   (a) Latex particles – direct PA, reversed inhibition PA.
   (b) Haemagglutination inhibition.

2. Immunodiffusion:
   (a) Radial immunodiffusion.
   (b) Quantitative immunoelectrophoresis – Laurell technique.

Comment

Immunological methods for fibrinogen measure not only total fibrinogen but molecules with immunological identity, i.e. degradation products. Passive agglutination techniques can be adapted to provide quantitation and are rapid, but do not measure functional activity and suffer from interference by degradation products. Immunological measurements can be useful in identifying dysfibrinogens by the discrepancy between functional and total fibrinogen measurements.

Choice of method

The choice of method for measuring plasma fibrinogen is determined largely by clinical circumstances – research or diagnosis, degree of urgency, possible presence of heparin, FDPs or fibrinolytic activity, and the presence of dysfibrinogenaemia. No single technique is satisfactory for all situations or requirements. Three methods are recommended from which one or more can be chosen to satisfy most clinical requirements.

Blood samples for measurement of fibrinogen

Although citrated plasma is used for the majority of coagulation factor assays, for fibrinogen a solid anticoagulant is satisfactory and avoids dilution of the plasma. Dry sodium citrate can be used but plasma from samples collected into EDTA are entirely suitable. In the presence of fibrinolytic activity blood samples should be collected into anticoagulant containing EACA to a final concentration of 10 mg/ml blood to prevent *in vitro* fibrinogen degradation; a comparison of values with and without EACA can be informative.

Reference plasmas

The stated fibrinogen content of reconstituted reference plasmas refers to actual fibrinogen content and therefore the fibrinogen content of citrated plasma samples is underestimated because of dilution by the anticoagulant. Reference ranges for healthy subjects will depend on the choice of liquid or solid anticoagulants.

Plasma fibrinogen – thrombin clotting time method (Clauss) [9]

Principle

A rapid technique based on the principle that the thrombin clotting time of plasma is inversely related to fibrinogen concentration. The use of diluted plasma and a relatively high concentration of thrombin results in little interference by FDPs or heparin unless present in large amounts. The thrombin clotting time of test plasma is converted to fibrinogen concentration by the use of a calibration curve derived from a range of fibrinogen concentrations clotted by a fixed concentration of thrombin.

Several modifications of the original Clauss technique have been published using different buffers, slightly different pHs, and with thrombin concentrations varying between 20 and 100 NIH units/ml.

Reagents

1. Imidazole buffer, pH 7.3.
2. Bovine thrombin, 100 NIH units/ml.
3. Standard plasma of known fibrinogen content (commercially available, or determined by replicate analysis of plasma by the Ratnoff and Menzie technique).
4. Control normal plasma, stored at −20°C.
5. Test PPP.

Method

Preparation of standard graph
A range of dilutions of the standard plasma are prepared in buffer. Dilutions of 1 in 5, 1 in 10, 1 in 20 and 1 in 40 are usually adequate but if the test sample has a very low or high fibrinogen content, lower or higher dilutions of the standard plasma may be necessary. 0.2 ml of each dilution is warmed to 37°C, 0.1 ml thrombin added and the clotting times recorded. Duplicate measurements are made. Using log/log graph paper, thrombin clotting times are plotted against the fibrinogen content (g/l) of each dilution; a linear plot is usual. A new graph should be prepared whenever a new batch of thrombin is introduced. Multiple clotting times of the control plasma are determined and the mean value ±2 SD should be obtained with the control plasma when each test or batch of tests is performed.

Test

The test plasma is diluted 1 in 10 in buffer and duplicate thrombin clotting times obtained. Plasma fibrinogen value is derived by extrapolation of the mean of the duplicate values from the standard graph.

Reference range 1.7–4 g/l.

Notes

1. The thrombin solution is stable in a polystyrene tube at 4°C for 24 hours.
2. If the value of the test plasma is outside the limits of the standard graph it is preferable, though not essential, to extend the standard graph rather than vary the dilution of the test plasma.
3. The major causes of erroneous results are:
   (a) Inaccurate dilution.
   (b) Loss of thrombin activity.
   (c) Determination of the end-point.
4. Plasma heparin levels over 0.5 units/ml give falsely low fibrinogen values.
5. Dysfibrinogenaemia can result in delayed rate of conversion of fibrinogen to fibrin and therefore show discrepancy between thrombin *time* assays, and the Ratnoff and Menzie, physicochemical and immunological methods.

6. The method is designed for use with clot end-point instruments. Manual end-point time is poor in the presence of low fibrinogen levels.

Plasma fibrinogen: turbimetric method (modified from Ellis and Stransky [10])

Principle

Diluted plasma is clotted by thrombin and the increase in turbidity due to fibrin formation is measured at 300 nm using an ultraviolet spectrophotometer. The resultant turbidity of normal fibrinogen is proportional to the fibrinogen concentration of the plasma. The technique described below is a further modification of a rapid method based on that of Ellis and Stransky.

Reagents

1. Barbitone–saline buffer, 0.1 mol/l, pH 7.2: 2.93 g sodium chloride and 5.71 g sodium diethyl barbiturate are dissolved in about 900 ml distilled water and titrated to pH 7.2 with 1 mol/l HCl (about 22.5 ml). The volume is made up to 1 litre with distilled water.
2. Calcium chloride: 3.38 mol/l.
3. Thrombin: 50 units of lyophilized thrombin are reconstituted with 1 ml diluent and 1 ml 3.38 mol/l calcium chloride is added. The calcium–thrombin solution is stable for 24 hours at 4°C in a plastic container.
4. Test plasma: platelet-poor EDTA plasma (1.5 mg/ml).

Method

0.5 ml plasma is diluted with 5.5 ml buffer and 3 ml measured into a 1 cm silica cuvette; the remaining 3 ml is decanted into a second cuvette and is used as a 'blank'. The test and blank cuvettes are adjusted to zero absorbance at a fixed wavelength of 300 nm. 15 μl of calcium–thrombin reagent is added carefully to the test cuvette and mixed rapidly while avoiding bubbles, quickly replaced in the spectrophotometer, and the recorder started. Change in turbidity is followed for 10 minutes by which time the traces of most plasmas will have reached a plateau. In the presence of dysfibrinogens the increase in turbidity may be slower and the reaction should be followed until a plateau is reached.

Calculation

From experimental studies there is a linear relationship between fibrinogen concentration and absorbance, and from regression data using plasma of known fibrinogen content plasma fibrinogen concentration is derived from:

$$A_{300}\ 10' \times 270 + 16 (\text{g/l}),$$

where 16 is the intercept of the slope of the regression data.

Notes

1. The technique is rapid and can easily be completed within 30 minutes.
2. The method not only provides a rapid result but from the shape of the

spectrophotometer trace the rate of fibrin polymerization can be followed which allows recognition of dysfibrinogens.
3. The addition of protamine sulphate to the diluted plasma allows measurement of fibrinogen in the presence of heparin.
4. In the presence of fibrinolysis a fall in turbidity may be seen.
5. Although a simpler spectrophotometer may be used, the facility of recording changes in turbidity can reveal additional important information.

Plasma fibrinogen: clot collection method (modified Ratnoff and Menzie [11])

Principle

A measured volume of plasma is clotted with thrombin, the resulting fibrin collected and the tyrosine content determined colorimetrically using Folin and Ciocalteau's reagent by reference to a standard tyrosine curve.

Reagents

1. Plasma: platelet-poor EDTA plasma (1.5 mg/ml blood).
2. Glass beads: 0.5 mm diameter.
3. Thrombin solution: 100 units/ml in 0.025 mol/l calcium chloride, freshly prepared.
4. Sodium chloride: 0.15 mol/l.
5. Sodium hydroxide: 0.25 mol/l.
6. Sodium carbonate: 200 g/l.
7. Folin and Ciocalteau's reagent.
8. L-tyrosine: 20 mg in 100 ml 0.1 mol/l HCl. Stable at 4°C.

Method

Into a glass centrifuge tube containing about 1 ml of glass beads, pipette 0.2 ml plasma, 5 ml sodium chloride solution and 0.5 ml thrombin. Stopper the tube and twirl and rotate the tube gently until fibrin is formed and is caught up by the beads. Leave for a further 10 minutes and again rotate gently. Centrifuge at 700 *g* for 5 minutes, decant the supernatant ensuring that no fibrin or beads are lost, and wash the beads and adherent fibrin twice with sodium chloride solution, centrifuging between and after the final wash. Add 1 ml sodium hydroxide solution to the washed fibrin and beads and place in boiling water for 10 minutes, covering the tubes with foil or with metal caps. Allow to cool, add 7 ml distilled water and 3 ml sodium carbonate solution, mix and add 1 ml Folin and Ciocalteau's reagent with further rapid mixing. Stand for 20 minutes to allow colour development and read in a spectrophotometer at 650 nm against a blank prepared as above but with the omission of the plasma.

Tyrosine standard The standard solution is prepared by mixing 0.2 ml tyrosine standard, 1 ml sodium hydroxide, 6.8 ml distilled water, 3 ml sodium carbonate and 1 ml Folin and Ciocalteau reagent. A standard 'blank' is prepared by omitting the tyrosine and using 7 ml water. The absorbance of the standard is read at 650 nm against the blank.

Calculation

A factor of 11.7 is used to convert liberated tyrosine to fibrinogen:

$$\text{Fibrinogen (g/l)} = \frac{A^{650}\ \text{test}}{A^{650}\ \text{standard}} \times \text{volume standard (ml)} \times$$

$$\text{concentration of standard (g/l)} \times \frac{1}{\text{volume plasma (ml)}} \times 11.7$$

$$\text{or}\ \frac{A^{650}\ \text{test}}{A^{650}\ \text{standard}} \times 0.2 \times 0.2 \times \frac{1}{0.2} \times 11.7 = \frac{A^{650}\ \text{test}}{A^{650}\ \text{standard}} \times 2.34$$

Reference range 1.7–4.0 g/l.

Notes

1. The major sources of error are:
   (a) Loss of fibrin during collection or washing.
   (b) Contamination with serum by incomplete washing.
   (c) The presence of fibrin split products.
2. The volume of 0.2 ml plasma is suitable for results in the normal range; for lower fibrinogen levels 0.5 ml plasma can be used with adjustment to the calculation. Some workers use 1.0 ml plasma.
3. Although time consuming the technique is generally regarded as a reference method and is to be preferred when accurate measurements are required.
4. Some methods dilute the plasma in 10 ml sodium chloride but the larger volume makes it more difficult to handle the formed fibrin.
5. Thrombin is expensive and the concentration and volume used above is a compromise between using a small volume of 1000 units/ml or a larger volume of a weaker thrombin solution.

Tests for fibrinolytic activity

Fibrinolytic investigations are performed mainly to study:

1. 'Normal' fibrinolytic activity.
2. Reduced fibrinolytic activity (perhaps predisposing to thrombotic phenomena, *see* Chapter 17).
3. Increased, but subclinical, fibrinolytic activity.
4. Marked fibrinolytic activity often associated with intravascular coagulation and serious haemorrhagic problems.

Many methods have been recommended, ranging from very sensitive techniques to the relatively insensitive, and from time-consuming procedures (which are of little value in urgent clinical situations) to rapid methods more suited to providing urgent diagnostic information. Ideally, precise information regarding the presence of plasminogen activators, the level of plasminogen, and the presence of plasmin would be of value but in urgent situations an overall assessment using the end-point of fibrin lysis may be the only possibility. Long end-point methods such as whole-blood clot lysis (normally over 48 hours), dilute whole-blood clot lysis (normally over 2 hours) clearly have limitations; a further difficulty is that if the patient's plasma has a fibrinogen level less than 0.5 g/l it may be difficult or impossible to see fibrin formation, or to detect fibrinolysis when using methods employing whole blood. The methods for investigating fibrinolysis described below are a compromise between the requirement for specific, sensitive assays for individual components of the fibrinolytic pathway and the products of fibrin degradation, and the requirement for valid data in a short time.

Collection and handling of blood samples for studies of fibrinolytic activity

1. Samples must be collected with a minimum of trauma and circulatory stasis. If possible a tourniquet should not be used and skin cleansing kept to a minimum as brisk rubbing can release plasminogen activators from the vascular endothelium.
2. Ideally samples should be collected into tubes containing sodium citrate cooled to 4°C.
3. Samples should be centrifuged at 4°C at 2000 *g* for 20 minutes to obtain platelet-free plasma, transferred to plastic tubes at 4°C using a plastic pipette and stored on melting ice.
4. Tests should be commenced within 30 minutes of collection if possible, due to the extreme lability of plasminogen activators and free plasmin.

Fibrinogen titre [12]

Principle

Serial dilutions of plasma are clotted with thrombin and the highest dilution containing a fibrin clot is the fibrinogen titre. The technique is often supplemented by testing in the presence of ε-amino-caproic-acid (EACA) and protamine sulphate as indicators of fibrinolysis and the presence of fibrin(ogen) degradation products, respectively.

Reagents

1. Imidazole buffer, pH 7.3 (*see* page 533).
2. Thrombin, 20 units/ml (keep at 4°C in a plastic tube).
3. EACA, 1 mg/ml in imidazole buffer.
4. Protamine sulphate, 0.2 mg/ml in imidazole buffer.
5. PPP.

Method

Three rows of seven 75 × 12 mm tubes are set up and doubling dilutions of plasma from 1 in 2 to 1 in 128 in 0.5 ml amounts are prepared in buffer (row 1), in EACA–buffer (row 2) and protamine sulphate–buffer (row 3). The dilutions are warmed to 37°C and 0.1 ml thrombin is added to each tube with *immediate* gentle mixing and then left undisturbed for 15 minutes. Starting at the lowest dilutions of each row, the tubes are *gently* tilted and the presence of fibrin noted. Rough handling of the tubes will result in a wispy fibrin clot contracting to pin-head size which can easily be overlooked. The end-point dilution of each row is noted and the tubes left at 37°C and examined gently at intervals for evidence of clot lysis.

Interpretation

The normal fibrinogen titre in row 1 after 15 minutes is 1 in 64 or greater; 1 in 32 is a border-line value. A titre of 1 in 16 or less indicates fibrinogen depletion. In the absence of fibrinolysis or FDPs the titre of rows 2 and 3 should be similar (±1 tube difference) to that of row 1. Absence of fibrin formation indicates very severe depletion, the presence of fibrinolysis, or both. A higher titre (two tubes or more) in row 2 indicates fibrinolysis and represents the 'true' fibrinogen titre but if fibrinogen is absent it is of course not possible to demonstrate fibrinolysis.

In certain circumstances a 'prozone' effect may be found in which no fibrin is formed at low dilutions but appears at higher dilutions. This is usually due to the presence of heparin the effect of which is diluted out. If heparin is responsible, the prozone effect is not apparent in row 3 (heparin neutralized by the protamine sulphate). A higher titre in row 3 is also found in the presence of high concentrations of FDPs which inhibit thrombin activity and fibrin formation in row 1. Extended incubation and observation of the tubes for up to 24 hours may demonstrate slow fibrinolysis.

Notes

1. The major causes of inaccuracy are:
   (a) In the preparation of the doubling dilutions which are notoriously inaccurate if technique is poor.
   (b) The handling of the tubes and the detection of the fibrin end-point. Quality assessment trials have demonstrated the unreliability of the fibrinogen titre as an indicator of fibrinogen concentration in the hands of different workers and for fibrinogen measurement alone the test is not recommended.
2. If there is delay in testing (over 20 minutes) when the blood or plasma has not been maintained at 4°C, fibrinolytic activity may not be demonstrated.

Euglobulin lysis time [13]

Principle

The euglobulin fraction of plasma contains those plasma proteins that precipitate when plasma is diluted in acidified aqueous solution. The euglobulin fraction contains plasminogen activators, plasminogen, plasmin, fibrinogen and fast-acting t-PA inhibitor but leaves most of the inhibitors of plasminogen activator in solution. The precipitate is redissolved and clotted and the time taken for complete lysis of the fibrin is the euglobulin lysis time (ELT). The absence of fibrinolytic inhibitors results in a more rapid normal lysis time than methods using whole or diluted blood (or plasma).

Reagents

1. Citrated PPP, collected as described on page 532.
2. Acetic acid, 0.026 mol/l.

3. Barbitone–saline buffer, pH 7.38, 0.01 mol/l, sodium diethyl barbiturate 11.75 g, NaCl 14.67 g, 0.1 mol/l HCl 430 ml, distilled water to 2 litres.
4. Thrombin, 2 units/ml, freshly prepared.

Method

Add 1 ml plasma to 9 ml acetic acid at 4°C in a centrifuge tube. The pH should be 5.9–6.0. Mix and stand 30 minutes at 4°C to precipitate the euglobulins. Centrifuge at 2000 *g* for 5 minutes, preferably at 4°C. Discard the supernatant and invert to drain. Re-suspend and dissolve the precipitate in 1 ml barbitone–saline buffer. Incubate at 37°C for 10 minutes and add 0.5 ml thrombin solution and note the time of clot formation. Inspect at intervals for complete clot lysis.

Normal lysis time 150–300 minutes.

Interpretation

In hyperfibrinolysis the clot may lyse in less than 150 minutes; lysis times of under 30 minutes are of pathological significance.

Notes

1. A useful modification is to divide the redissolved euglobulin fraction into two 0.5 ml amounts after addition of the thrombin and take the average lysis times as the ELT.
2. If the plasma fibrinogen is very low due to pathological or therapeutic depletion only a wispy clot or no clot will form. Fibrinogen may be added (1 ml of a 200 mg/l solution) before the addition of the thrombin, or the euglobulin fraction may be tested on fibrin plates (*see* below).
3. Lysis depends on adequate concentrations of plasminogen and fibrinogen. In the presence of low plasminogen levels normal or even extended ELTs may be found even in the presence of increased plasminogen activators.
4. Fibrinolytic activity of the euglobulin fraction is more stable than in whole blood but the test should be performed within 2 hours of separating the euglobulin fraction.
5. PPP must be used.
6. The test is particularly sensitive to variations in technique, pH, ionic strength and temperature; each laboratory should establish its own normal range, rigidly following the technique.
7. The test may be performed on patients treated with heparin; heparin is not precipitated with the euglobulin fraction.
8. Lysis of the fibrin clot may be followed photometrically if a temperature of 37°C can be maintained. Platelet aggregometers with chart recorders can be used and purpose-designed instruments are available.

Lysis of fibrin plates

Principle

Fibrin gels are prepared in Petri dishes by clotting fibrinogen solutions with thrombin. Small measured volumes of plasma or plasma fractions are spotted on to the gels and incubated at 37°C. The diameter of the zones of lysis show correlation with fibrinolytic activity. By using plasminogen-rich and plasminogen-free fibrinogen preparations, the activity of plasminogen activator + plasmin and plasmin alone can be studied.

Demonstration of the combined activities of plasminogen activator and plasmin [14]

Reagents

1. Barbitone–HCl buffer, pH 7.8, ionic strength 0.15 – sodium diethyl barbiturate, 0.05 mol/l; NaCl, 0.093 mol/l; $CaCl_2$, 1.66 mmol/l; $MgCl_2$, 0.69 mmol/l; adjust to pH 7.8 with HCl.
2. Plasminogen-rich fibrinogen (Kabi, Stockholm) – reconstitute and store at −20°C. Dilute in buffer to give final fibrinogen concentration of 1 g/l and ionic strength 0.15.
3. Thrombin solution, 20 units/ml – dilute in 0.15 mol/l NaCl immediately before use and keep on melting ice.
4. Patient's PPP or euglobulin fraction prepared as for the euglobulin lysis time.

Method

Pipette 0.2 ml thrombin and 6 ml fibrinogen solution into a 100 mm diameter, flat-bottomed Petri dish. Swirl gently to mix, avoiding bubble formation, and allow to stand on a level surface at room temperature for 30 minutes. Accurately pipette three, 30 μl volumes of test and control preparations on to the fibrin gel at spaced intervals and incubate at 37°C for 18 hours in a level position. Measure the horizontal and perpendicular diameters of each area of lysis and express fibrinolytic activity as a mean of the six diameters of each preparation.

Interpretation

Average diameter of lysis of the normal control is 10–15 mm. Zones greater than 15 mm indicate increased plasminogen activator/plasmin activity. Plasmin activity can be measured by testing on plasminogen-free fibrin plates.

Notes

1. There is a linear correlation between area of lysis and log ELT.
2. In addition to using a control euglobulin fraction to check reactivity of the plates, urokinase can be used.
3. Some methods incorporate agarose into the fibrin plate to produce a firmer gel.
4. Clearly, the results depend on the method of preparing the euglobulin fractions, and laboratories should determine their own reference range.
5. Proteases other than plasmin can cause lysis.
6. Avoid bacterial contamination of reagents.

Demonstration of plasmin activity using heated fibrin plates

Plasminogen-free fibrin plates can be prepared from plasminogen-free fibrinogen. It is more usual to heat the fibrin plates prepared as described above to destroy plasminogen activity.

Glass Petri dishes must be used. Plates are prepared as described above and heated in an oven at 80°C for 45 minutes. Allow to cool with the lid removed to prevent condensation. The samples are applied as described above and the diameter of the zones of lysis compared with those obtained with the unheated plates. The activities of plasmin and plasminogen activator separately can be deduced.

Notes

1. If available, plasminogen-free fibrinogen is to be preferred due to the reduced sensitivity of heated fibrin to the action of plasmin.
2. Heated and unheated plates may be prepared and stored in sealed plastic envelopes at 4°C but they lose activity with time.

Demonstration of fibrin(ogen) degradation products (FDPs)

The demonstration of the degradation products of native fibrinogen and fibrin (early and late fibrin monomer (FM), fragments X, Y, D, E; *see* page 70) is widely accepted as evidence of *in vivo* lysis of fibrinogen and fibrin. The pioneering techniques did not differentiate between the degradation products of fibrinogen and fibrin. The recognition that cross-linked fragments, notably D-dimer, are obtained from the lysis of fibrin and the availability of antibody reacting only with the dimeric form, allows assessment of *fibrin*olysis. FDPs may be demonstrated indirectly by their effect on coagulation tests, e.g. prolongation of the thrombin clotting time and Reptilase clotting time of plasma, by immunological techniques and by the ability of FDPs to clump suspensions of certain strains of staphylococci.

The thrombin and Reptilase clotting times are prolonged due to the antithrombin and antipolymerization properties of the high molecular weight degradation products, but are also affected by the plasma fibrinogen concentration. Nevertheless, they are useful tests in the general investigation of fibrinolytic states.

Immunological techniques are more specific but it is important to recognize that different techniques are sensitive, to a greater or lesser extent, to the different degradation products depending on the specificity(ies) of the antibody or antibodies. Passive agglutination tests are widely used, particularly when rapid results are required. *Table 15.8* summarizes the specificity and sensitivity of some

Table 15.8 Specificity and sensitivity of passive agglutination tests and the staphylococcal clumping test (SCT) to the various degradation products of fibrin and fibrinogen

	Degradation product				
Method	*Fibrin monomer (FM)*	*X and Y*	*D*	*E*	*D-dimer*
SCT	+++	+	–	–	–
Direct agglutination of latex coated with anti-D and E	±	±	++	++	–
Direct agglutination of latex coated with anti-D dimer	–	–	–	–	++
Inhibition tests using fibrinogen-coated latex and anti-fibrinogen serum	++	+	+	+	–
Tanned red-cell haemagglutination inhibition (TRCHAI)	++	+	+	+	–

commonly used passive agglutination tests and the staphylococcal clumping test (SCT) [15] and shows that the direct agglutination and agglutination–inhibition techniques differ in sensitivity to the early and late degradation products and that the SCT is sensitive to the early products. It also implies that quantitation of total FDPs is not absolute because the varying fragments have varying reactivity with antibody. Furthermore, the early degradation products may be partially complexed with fibrin and removed from the serum.

Technique protocols for direct agglutination and agglutination–inhibition passive agglutination procedures will be described.

Direct latex agglutination test

Principle

Antisera are raised to highly purified preparations of human fibrinogen D and E or E alone. After absorption the specific antibody (or antibodies) are used to coat a suspension of latex particles in glycine–saline buffer. Monoclonal antibodies are available. The sensitivity of the latex reagent is adjusted so that in the presence of FDP concentrations of 2 mg/l (fibrinogen equivalent) or greater, the latex particles clump to produce macroscopic agglutination.

Blood samples

Blood is collected with a minimum of trauma into a tube containing approximately 3600 units of soybean trypsin inhibitor or alternatively 10 mg of EACA, and 20 NIH units of thrombin and left at room temperature or at 37°C for 30 minutes. Coagulation must be complete, hence the use of thrombin, and *in vitro* fibrinolysis is prevented by the inhibitor of fibrinolysis. The serum is separated and can be stored at −20°C if desired. If the blood fails to clot due to the presence of heparin it can be clotted by the addition of 40 μl Reptilase and allowed to stand for a further 30 minutes.

Reagents

1. Antibody-coated latex: latex suspension coated with antibody to be sensitive to 2 mg/l FDP (some preparations are adjusted to a sensitivity of 3 mg/l). Preparations are available commercially. (Thrombo–Wellcotest, Wellcome Reagents, Beckenham, UK).
2. Glycine–saline buffer, pH 8.2: 0.15 mol/l NaCl, 0.1 mol/l glycine, 0.0025 mol/l NaOH. Adjust to pH 8.2 with Na_2CO_3 if necessary. Add 0.2 g/l sodium azide.
3. Control sera: ideally, serum known to give positive and negative reactions should be tested alongside each test sample or with each batch.

Method

Serum is diluted 1 in 5 in glycine buffer and one drop placed on a clean glass slide. One drop of re-suspended latex is added and mixed with an applicator. The slide is rocked gently for exactly 2 minutes and the presence or absence of agglutination noted.

As the serum is diluted 1 in 5 and the latex suspension is sensitive to 2 mg/l FDP, a *negative* result indicates that there is less than 10 mg/l FDP in the serum. A *positive* result indicates that FDPs are present in a concentration of 10 mg/l or greater.

It is normal practice to use the test as a semi-quantitative method by testing serial dilutions of serum, the highest giving a positive result indicating the concentration of FDP (reciprocal of dilution × 2, e.g. if the highest dilution showing agglutination is 1 in 40 then FDP concentration = 80 mg/l).

Normal levels of FDP

Less than 10 mg/l. The additional manipulation of adding Reptilase may result in a slightly higher normal range.

Interpretation

The normal levels of FDP are probably the results of physiological fibrin degradation. Slight increases up to 20 or even 40 mg/l can be found in a wide variety of conditions, including post-surgery, post-partum, blood in body cavities, pulmonary embolus, etc. Levels over 100 mg/l are good evidence of systemic fibrinolysis though in the very early stages the late products of fibrin degradation may not have appeared. FDP levels should be interpreted in association with other parameters of coagulation, fibrinolysis and platelet numbers.

Latex agglutination–inhibition test for fibrin(ogen) degradation products [16]

Principle

Serum is mixed with antifibrinogen serum suitably diluted so as to be neutralized by the presence of 2 mg/l (fibrinogen equivalent) of FDP. Fibrinogen-coated latex is added and absence of agglutination indicates the presence of FDPs at a concentration of 2 mg/l or greater. The test may be made semi-quantitative by testing further dilutions of serum.

Blood samples

These are as for the direct agglutination test.

Reagents

1. Fibrinogen-coated latex.
2. Albumin–glycine buffered saline, pH 8.2 – buffered saline containing 0.1 mol/l glycine and 2% v/v bovine albumin.
3. Antifibrinogen serum – suitably diluted to be sensitive to a concentration of 2 mg/l fibrinogen.

Method

Serum is diluted 1 in 5 in albumin–glycine buffer and one drop placed on a clean slide. Add one drop of antifibrinogen serum and mix with an applicator and leave for 2 minutes. Add one drop of latex suspension, mix and rock gently for 2 minutes and observe for agglutination over a black background. Absence of agglutination is a *positive* reaction indicating the presence of FDP at a concentration of 10 mg/l or more (reciprocal of serum dilution × 2). Presence of agglutination is a *negative* reaction indicating that the antifibrinogen serum has not been neutralized by FDP in the serum dilution.

Normal levels of FDP Less than 10 mg/l.

Interpretation

As for the direct agglutination test. It is claimed that the inhibition technique gives fewer false-positive results than the direct method.

Direct latex agglutination for cross-linked FDP (XLFDP) [17]

Principle

The principle is identical to that of the direct agglutination test described previously, the latex particles being coated with monoclonal antibody to the D-dimer fragment of lysed fibrin. As there is no cross-reaction with native fibrinogen there is no requirement for the use of serum which eliminates the variables of collection and *in vitro* fibrinolysis. Plasma from blood collected into EDTA is ideal and into citrate is satisfactory if the dilution effect is taken into consideration.

Reagents

The test is available in kit form as Dimertest, Porton Products Ltd, Salisbury, Wiltshire, UK.

Method

The manufacturer's protocol is followed which essentially follows the procedure previously described. Undiluted and, if appropriate, serially diluted plasmas are tested. Agglutination is observed when the sample has XLFDP >200 μg/l. Quantitation is achieved by multiplying the reciprocal of the highest dilution showing dilution by 200 to give a value in μg/l.

Interpretation

Plasma levels in normal subjects are <200 μg/l. Increased levels are only found after lysis of cross-linked fibrin and indicate activation and subsequent lysis of *in vivo* coagulation. Levels are not increased in primary fibrinolytic states. The test is extremely sensitive to *in vivo* coagulation and elevated levels are found in most situations when there has been extravasation of blood, e.g. post-surgery, trauma, intramuscular or intra-articular haemorrhages. Elevated XLFDPs are therefore not necessarily evidence of pathological fibrinolysis unless very high levels are found, in which cases conventional methods for detection of FDPs are usually positive.

The major application may well be in the diagnosis or monitoring of thrombosis and in distinguishing between the disordered haemostasis of liver disease due to diminished synthesis of coagulation factors or the presence of fibrinolysis.

Demonstration of soluble fibrin monomer complexes

Introduction

Fibrin monomer formed by the action of thrombin on fibrinogen *in vivo* binds to fibrinogen or FDPs to form soluble fibrin monomer complexes (SFMC). Physicochemical manipulations such as exposure to cold, to strongly basic substances such as protamine sulphate, or to dilute ethanol, cause dissociation of the complexes thus allowing the fibrin monomer to polymerize to form a gel or fibrin strands. Such procedures are known as *paracoagulation tests* which, if reliable, would represent important evidence of *in vivo* intravascular coagulation. The major difficulties are in defining a positive reaction and in sensitivity and specificity; false positives are a particular problem. Nevertheless, the tests can provide evidence of early DIC before the production of late (low molecular weight) products of fibrin degradation.

Serial dilution protamine sulphate test (SDPS test) [18]

Principle

Protamine sulphate induces dissociation of SFMC and the insoluble fibrin monomer forms a gel or strands of fibrin which are specific for fibrin monomer and *fibrin* degradation products, and do not occur with fibrinogen or fibrinogen products. The preparation of a range of concentrations of protamine sulphate is to ensure an optimum concentration of protamine, and does not represent a quantitative procedure.

Reagents

1. Test plasma – nine volumes of blood collected into one volume of sodium citrate with aprotinin added to a final concentration of 100 KIE units/ml. Centrifuge at room temperature to obtain PPP. A clean venepuncture with a minimum of stasis is essential.
2. Control plasma from a healthy donor is collected as described above.
3. Protamine sulphate – dissolve protamine sulphate in 0.15 mol/l NaCl to a concentration of 1 g/dl. Store at 4°C for up to 7 days. Immediately before use make doubling dilutions in 0.15 mol/l NaCl from 1 in 5 to 1 in 80.

Method

Into each of a series of five 75 × 12 mm glass tubes containing 0.2 ml plasma, add 0.2 ml of a dilution of protamine sulphate to give final concentrations of 1000, 500, 250, 125 and 62.5 μg/ml. The tubes are gently shaken and left at room temperature for 30 minutes and then examined against a dark background. The appearances may be scored as follows: +++(gelation); ++(fibrin strands); +(coarse precipitate); ±(fine precipitate); and −(clear). Only gelation and fibrin strands are considered positive reactions; coarse precipitate is a negative result.

Interpretation

The test is sensitive to about 100 mg/l FDP and 20 mg/l fibrin monomer complexes. FDPs are normally precipitated by high protamine concentrations and fibrin monomer complexes form strands only with low protamine concentrations. Normal plasmas produce a coarse precipitate at dilutions of 1 in 10 or 1 in 5. As fibrin*ogen* degradation products do not form a gel with protamine sulphate it is possible to distinguish between fibrinolysis and fibrinogenolysis.

Notes

1. The test must be performed within 1 hour of blood collection as fibrin monomer complexes are unstable and precipitate in plasma on standing.
2. Not all sources of protamine sulphate are suitable for this test.
3. The practice of cooling blood samples and centrifuging at 4°C is inconsistent with the known instability of SFMC at low temperatures. Frozen samples are unsuitable.

Ethanol gelation test [19]

Principle

Fibrin monomers and small soluble fibrin polymers in plasma precipitate in the presence of low concentrations of ethanol.

Reagents

1. Plasma samples: collect samples as for the SDPS test. Samples must be obtained with the minimum of circulatory stasis by a clean venepuncture and tested without delay.
2. Ethanol: mix equal volumes of of absolute (96%) ethanol and distilled water.

Method

Into a glass tube 75 × 12 mm at 37°C is pipetted 0.5 ml plasma and after warming for 3 minutes, 0.15 ml ethanol is added, mixed and left at 37°C. After exactly 10 minutes the tube is examined for gel or fibrin strand formation. The test is positive only if gel or distinct strands are formed. A granular precipitate is a negative result.

Notes

1. The test must be performed within 1 hour of blood collection as fibrin monomer complexes are unstable and precipitate in plasma on standing.
2. The practice of cooling blood samples and centrifuging at 4°C is inconsistent with the known instability of SFMC at low temperatures. Frozen samples are unsuitable.
3. The test is less sensitive, but possibly more specific, than the SDPS test.

Plasminogen assay using chromogenic substrate

Principle

Excess streptokinase is added to plasma to form a streptokinase–plasminogen complex with amidolytic activity which is measured by the addition of a chromogenic substrate, the liberated *p*-nitroaniline being determined by an end-point technique. Under the above conditions the assay is insensitive to inhibitors.

Reagents

1. Chromozym PL (Boerhinger) 1 mmol/l in distilled water (1.2 μmol/l ampoule reconstituted with 1.2 ml distilled water).
2. Imidazole buffer, pH 7.3.
3. Streptokinase (Kabi) 10 000 units/ml, stored at −20°C.
4. Glacial acetic acid.
5. Standard plasma.
6. Citrated PPP.

Method

Standard plasma is diluted 1 in 10, 1 in 15, 1 in 20 and 1 in 40 in buffer and designated as equivalent to 1.0, 0.75, 0.5, and 0.25 units/ml plasminogen activity. Each dilution is made independently using 0.1 ml volumes of plasma. Dilute the test plasma 1 in 10 in buffer. Warm to 37°C; place 0.1 ml of each dilution in a plastic tube. At T_0 add 0.1 ml streptokinase to the first tube and at 10-second intervals add 0.1 ml streptokinase to the remaining tubes, mixing each tube after the addition of the streptokinase. Up to 17 tubes may be tested in one test run. Incubate at 37°C. At 3 minutes add 0.1 ml of Chromozym PL to the first tube, mix, and add to subsequent tubes at 10-second intervals. At 6 minutes add 0.1 ml acetic acid to the first tube to stop the reaction and to subsequent tubes at 10-second intervals. Add 1.5 ml distilled water to each tube. The colour will be stable for several hours. Read the absorption of each standard dilution and the test dilution at 405 nm against a reagent blank consisting of volumes of all reagents as above, substituting 0.1 ml buffer for the plasma dilution. Plot dilutions of plasma (plasminogen concentration) against absorbance using linear graph paper and convert the absorbance of the test dilution to plasminogen concentration from the standard graph.

Reference range 0.8–1.2 units/ml.

Tests of platelet function

Bleeding time

The technique of choice is one based on the Ivy method but in situations where this is not practicable, the Duke method can be used. Other methods are not recommended.

Template bleeding time (Ivy)

Principle

The bleeding time is the interval between making a small incision on the forearm and cessation of bleeding. The procedure has been standardized by the use of a mechanical device that permits an incision of precise dimensions by means of a template. A device is available commercially (Simplate, General Diagnostics).

Method

Wrap a sphygmomanometer cuff around the upper arm and inflate to a pressure of 40 mmHg. Maintain this pressure throughout the test. Cleanse and dry an area on the anterior surface of the forearm. The area should be free of scar tissue and superficial veins. The incision is made over the pronator muscles by placing the template firmly on the skin – *do not press* – and making the incision. Start a stop-watch. After 15 seconds and at similar subsequent intervals absorb the flow of blood with a filter paper *without touching the edge of the wound.* Continue soaking up the blood until the filter paper no longer stains. Stop the watch and record the bleeding time. There is usually no value in pursuing the test longer than 20 minutes. Continued bleeding can be arrested by pressure over the incision. Similar results are obtained from the medial aspect of the calf[20].

Reference values

Children – less than 8 minutes. Adults – less than 6 minutes. It is important that each laboratory should establish its own normal range, which will depend on whether a lateral or longitudinal incision is made, and the precise determination of the end-point.

Interpretation

The bleeding time is a measure of the effectiveness of haemostasis in small blood vessels and is dependent on platelet function and vascular integrity.

Prolonged bleeding may be found in inherited disorders of platelet function such as von Willebrand's disease, Bernard–Soulier syndrome, Glanzmann's disease, storage-pool disease, etc., in acquired platelet dysfunction in uraemia, dysproteinaemia, myeloproliferative disorders, etc. and in thrombocytopenia when the platelet count is less than 75×10^9/l. Prolonged bleeding times are also associated with deficiency of factor I and also, variably, of factor V and factor VIII:C[21]. In addition the effect of drugs on platelet function is a common cause of a prolonged bleeding time.

Applications of the bleeding time test

1. Screening test for platelet disorders and in the prediction of the risk of bleeding in various haemorrhagic states.
2. Monitoring the antithrombotic effect of drugs which impair platelet function.
3. Monitoring the effect of platelet transfusions in thrombocytopenic subjects.

Aspirin tolerance test [22]

Principle

Duplicate bleeding times are performed before and 2 hours after the ingestion of 600 mg aspirin. The effect of aspirin persists for the life span of the platelets (approximately 10 days) and prolongs the bleeding time in normal individuals. In subjects with abnormal platelets or intrinsic clotting defects the influence of aspirin is much greater compared with the effect in normal individuals.

Method

1. Perform a bleeding time in duplicate. Record the average bleeding time.
2. Administer two tablets of aspirin (600 mg) to the patient and perform a bleeding time 2 hours later.
3. Report the average bleeding times before and after ingestion of aspirin.
4. Positive results – bleeding time increased at least two-fold.

Interpretation

The aspirin tolerance test appears to be primarily sensitive to impairment of prostaglandin metabolism in platelet function. In patients with disorders of intrinsic coagulation, the influence of aspirin is greatly enhanced by several orders of magnitude as compared with normal individuals. When both the prostaglandin-dependent mechanism and the ability to produce thrombin is impaired, a markedly exaggerated bleeding time is produced. A similar response is seen in patients with von Willebrand's disease.

Platelet aggregation studies [23]

Principle

To induce platelet clumping in stirred PRP by the addition of various aggregating agents, monitoring the changes in light transmission using a platelet aggregometer and analysis of results by comparison with normal platelet responses; or by (1) percentage aggregation, (2) percentage aggregation over unit time, (3) analysis of slope, and (4) analysis of shape of slope (*Figure 15.8*).

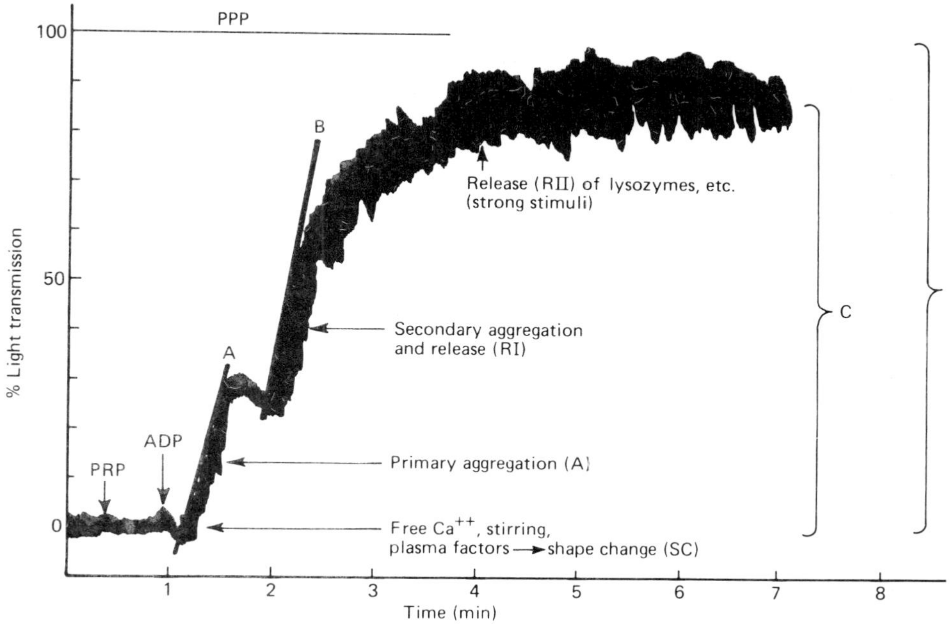

Figure 15.8 Some of the variables used to identify and measure platelet aggregation responses to ADP (3 μmol/l). A typical response is usually SC → A → RI → RII. (A) = Slope of primary aggregation ($mm.s^{-1}$); (B) = slope of secondary aggregation; (C) = maximum aggregation (%); (D) = maximum light transmission; PPP = platelet-poor plasma; PRP = platelet rich plasma

Reagents

1. ADP (Sigma Grade III) – 10 mM solution on saline. Store at −20°C in suitable small aliquots. Dilute stock solution to prepare 100, 50, 25, 10 and 5 µM solutions in saline and keep on ice.
2. Collagen (Hormon-Chemie, Munchen) – 1 mg/ml stored at 4°C. Prepare 40 µg/ml and 10 µg/ml solutions in buffer supplied. Keep on ice.
3. Adrenaline (Sigma) – 1 mg/ml (5.5 mM). Store at −20°C. Prepare 100, 50 and 10 µM solutions in saline. Keep on ice.
4. Arachidonate (Sigma) – 15 mM solution in distilled water. Store at −20°C. Thaw for use and keep on ice.
5. Ristocetin (Lundbeck) – 15 mg/ml in saline. Store at −20°C for 1 month.
6. Bovine fibrinogen – dissolve in saline to give 20 mg/ml. Prepare fresh.

Platelet-rich plasma

For blood samples with PCV in the range 0.350–0.500 l/l add nine volumes of blood to one volume of 0.109 M trisodium citrate. Platelet aggregation responses are sensitive to residual free calcium concentration and proportions of blood to anticoagulant should be adjusted according to PCV (*see* page 530). Centrifuge at 170 *g* for 10 minutes, remove the platelet-rich plasma and store at room temperature in a capped tube. Adjust the platelet count to approximately 200×10^9/l with autologous PPP.

Method

Tests are performed in stirred plasma at 37°C. The precise details of setting up and operating the aggregometer and recorder clearly vary according to the instrument used.

For all responses one volume of reagent (agonist) is added to nine volumes of prewarmed PRP. All responses are related to the *final concentration* of agonist, i.e. one-tenth of reagent concentration.

Terminology of the assessment of platelet aggregation responses (*Figure 15.8*)

Baseline The oscillating trace pattern on zero transmission or maximum absorption which represents discoid platelets polarizing the light passing through the unaggregated platelet suspension.

Lag phase The time taken from the addition of the aggregating agent until the platelets change shape and commence aggregation.

Shape change The change of the platelet from discoid to spherical form.

Primary aggregation The first phase of aggregation following addition of ADP or adrenaline.

Primary aggregation with disaggregation First-phase aggregation followed by disaggregation and return to baseline. No irreversible second-phase aggregation.

Single secondary response As seen in the response to collagen, i.e. a 90-second lag phase then a secondary response.

Biphasic response Response to ADP, adrenaline etc., showing primary phase aggregation followed by irreversible second-phase aggregation.

No response Less than 10% response to aggregating agents.

Slope of aggregation Rate of reaction expressed in $mm.s^{-1}$.

Maximum aggregation response Maximum change in optical density, i.e. maximum OD change – initial OD = maximum aggregation.

Aggregation threshold The lowest concentration of an aggregating agent necessary to produce a biphasic response, *or* the lowest concentration of collagen or arachidonate necessary to produce a maximum aggregation response over 50%.

Controls Normal subjects of the same sex with no drug ingestion during the previous 10 days. Controls should be tested before and after the test plasma using the same conditions and reagents.

Demonstration of decreased platelet aggregation responses

Aggregation responses are measured as follows.

ADP Demonstration of biphasic threshold, i.e. that concentration which produces greater than 50% biphasic aggregation using final ADP concentrations between 1 and 10 μmol/l. Normal biphasic threshold: 1–3 μmol/l.

Adrenaline As for ADP, but use 3 μmol/l, 10 μmol/l and 30 μmol/l final concentrations. Normal biphasic threshold: less than 3 μmol/l.

Collagen Determine threshold concentration, i.e. that producing greater than 50% irreversible aggregation using 2 μg/ml and 4 μg/ml final concentrations. Normal threshold: less than 2 μg/ml.

Arachidonate One concentration only, 1.5 mmol/l final concentration. Normal threshold, less than 1.5 mmol/l.

Ristocetin 1.5 mg/ml and 0.5 mg/ml final concentration. Normal threshold, >1 mg/ml.

Demonstration of platelet hyperaggregation: spontaneous platelet aggregation (SPA)

Principle

Platelet aggregation is usually performed with PRP with the platelet count adjusted to 200×10^9/l. Tests for spontaneous platelet agregation (SPA) are initially performed without adjustment of the platelet count, the PRP being stirred in an aggregometer for 10 minutes without addition of an aggregating reagent. If spontaneous aggregation occurs the test is repeated after adjustment of the platelet count.

Method

Without adjustment of the platelet count PRP is stirred in an aggregometer for 10 minutes and spontaneous aggregation recorded.

Interpretation

Positive results are frequently observed when the platelet count is over 900×10^9/l, i.e. in thrombocytosis or thrombocythaemia, and is usually simply due to the high platelet count; repeat testing after adjusting the count to 200×10^9/l usually results in a negative result. Other disorders – for example, diabetes, vascular disease and some forms of renal disease – may show positive SPA at normal platelet counts.

Increased sensitivity to aggregation by ADP (and other inducers)

Method

Add 1 μmol/l final concentration of ADP to adjusted PRP. A primary response with disaggregation is normally seen. If a biphasic response is produced, use 0.5, 0.2 and 0.1 μmol/l final concentrations of ADP until only a primary response is produced and record the lowest concentration of ADP producing a biphasic pattern.

Notes on platelet aggregation techniques

1. Expression of results:
   (a) Aggregation threshold is a rapid method of assessing aggregation and many abnormalities can be detected using this approach.
   (b) Maximum aggregation response is a quantitative method of interpreting aggregation patterns.
   (c) Slope of aggregation (V_{max}) is measured from the early slope of the aggregation trace and is not therefore suitable for abnormalities of second-phase aggregation.
2. The range of drugs known to affect platelet aggregation responses is now very wide. Interpretation of responses may be difficult or even impossible if continued medication is essential.
3. The speed of stirring, and the size of the stirrer when applicable, has a marked effect on aggregation responses and must be standardized.
4. With very low platelet counts it is virtually impossible to obtain meaningful aggregation traces.
5. Storage of PRP results in loss of dissolved carbon dioxide and a rise in pH with an increase in minimum threshold concentration. HEPES buffer, 5 g/dl trisodium citrate, will maintain the pH at 7.4 without interfering with aggregation responses.
6. Response of normal platelets to adrenaline is variable and it is difficult to define an abnormal response.

7. Lipaemic samples reduce the relative difference in OD of PRP and PPP and thus reduce sensitivity.
8. Samples stored or transported at 4°C may show spontaneous aggregation. Storage at room temperature is preferable.

Interpretation of platelet aggregation patterns

Representative patterns of normal platelets are shown in *Figure 15.9.*

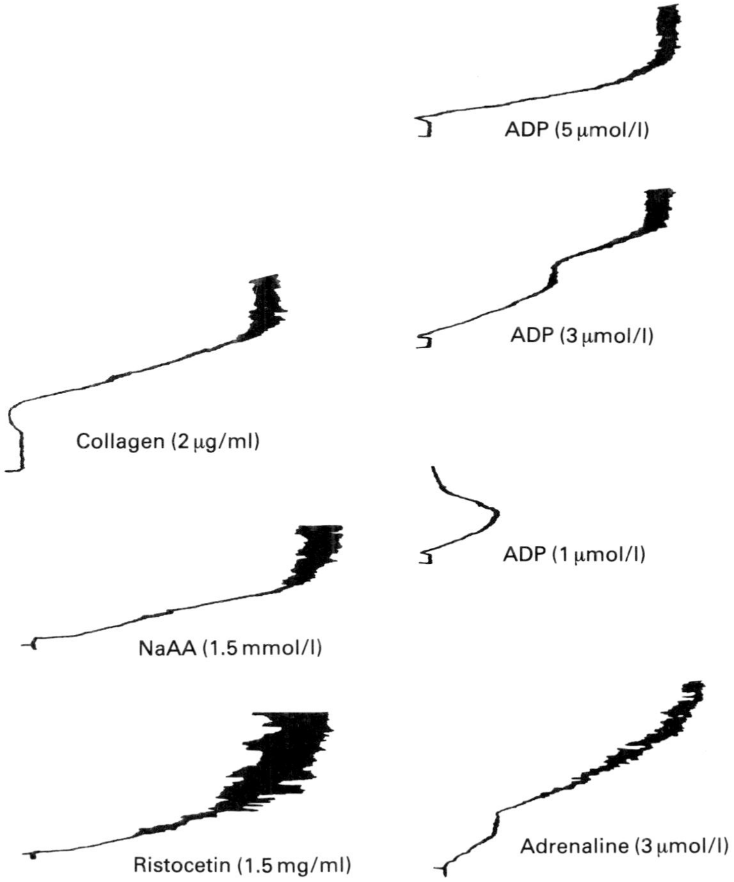

Figure 15.9 Aggregation responses of normal platelets to commonly used agonists

Whole blood platelet aggregation

It is accepted that aggregation of platelets in plasma in the absence of red cells and leucocytes is non-physiological. Furthermore, centrifugation may lead to selective loss of more dense platelets.

To overcome these objections, aggregometry of platelets in whole blood has been studied by an impedance technique which measures the progressive increase of electrical impedance between two electrodes as platelets adhere and aggregate on the electrodes in stirred whole blood[24]. The method has been mainly used for pharmacological studies and appears to offer little to diagnostic work.

Quality control and standardization

The general aims and principles of quality control described in Chapter 4 apply to the coagulation laboratory. Internal quality control programmes and external quality assessment schemes have resulted in considerable improvement in the reliability of coagulation testing.

Standardization of coagulation testing

A major contribution to standardization of results has been the establishment and availability of standards and reference preparations under the auspices of the Expert Committee on Biological Standardisation (ECBS) of the World Health Organisation (WHO).

Biological materials such as coagulation factors and the reagents used in testing cannot be completely characterized by physical and chemical methods and 'standard' preparations are made available with assigned potency generally determined on the basis of international collaborative studies. A standard is intended for use in the estimation of potency (activity) of test samples by direct comparison in suitable test systems. The preparations are mainly used in biological test systems though values obtained by immunoassay methods are also provided. Materials available fall into several groups.

An *International Standard* is a preparation to which an *International Unit* (IU) of activity has been assigned usually as a specified biological activity of a defined amount of the International Standard. In coagulation testing this is usually translated into IU/ml of plasma. *International Reference Preparations* have been assigned IU values prior to 1986 and although preparations may still be available, the term is no longer applied by the WHO.

In addition to international standards and reference preparations, national standards and reference preparations have been prepared and are currently available, e.g. in the UK – British Standards, Working Standards and Reference Reagents. The continued preparation of 'national standards' clearly complicates the concept of international standardization and these are no longer being assigned values.

An important contribution of International Standards, in addition to laboratory diagnosis and monitoring, is the assignment of potency to coagulation factor concentrates for therapeutic use.

The range of International Standards for coagulation factors currently includes factor VIII:C, vWf:Ag, vWf:R:CoF in plasma; II, VII, IX and X in plasma; human factor VIII:C in concentrate; ATIII, plasmin, prekallikrein and protein C in plasma; β-thromboglobulin and platelet factor 4. Preparations for either therapeutic or laboratory use include heparin, protamine, ancrod, streptokinase, urokinase, t-PA and thrombin. Additionally, there are preparations which have no official status such as XLFDPs, plasminogen and plasminogen activator inhibitor (National Institute for Biological Standards and Control (NIBSC), Hertfordshire, UK).

International Standards are intended to last for 10 years before replacement. Although they are freely available to the public sector so that assays can be directly compared with the Standard, the massive volume of testing makes it inappropriate to use the Standard preparation routinely. It is usual to use 'secondary standards' for routine testing either prepared 'in-house' or obtained from commercial sources.

Secondary standards

Whenever possible a secondary plasma standard should be assigned a potency value by reference to an International Standard after repeated testing. The secondary standard may be a pool of plasmas or a single plasma.

Assays of factors for which an International Standard is not available are usually ascribed a value as 'percentage of normal activity' with 100% taken to be 'mean normal activity'. This value can only be applied to the activity of a large pool of normal plasmas and it has been demonstrated that at least 100 plasmas from normal subjects must be pooled to give values of '100% normal activity'. This is clearly impractical and uneconomical as an in-house procedure. Preparations from commercial sources or national organizations are therefore appropriate.

Control plasmas

All procedures, whether single tests or test batches, should include the testing of one or more 'control' plasmas. These preparations are prepared from either sufficient quantity of a single plasma or from a pool of plasmas. Values are assigned to the control by repeated testing under standardized conditions and confidence limits determined by standard statistical methods. The control may be a reconstituted lyophilized preparation or plasma stored frozen in suitable aliquots, preferably at −70°C. The mean value and confidence limits are assigned *after* reconstitution or thawing.

Control plasmas are used in screening tests where the values are determined in seconds, e.g. PT, APTT, TCT, etc. or in assays when potency has been determined in IU/ml or '% normal activity'. A range of control plasmas can be used to monitor results both in the normal and abnormal ranges.

Screening tests have reference ranges which reflect individual variation. A mean value for the determination may be obtained by calculating the geometric mean of 20 plasmas from normal individuals.

The relationship between standard, reference and control preparations is summarized in *Figure 15.10*.

Quality control of the proficiency of individuals

To assess the proficiency of an individual it is necessary to collect the control values of each member of staff performing *routine* procedures. The analytical values that an individual has obtained is kept as a daily log. Assessment of the accuracy and precision of individual performance is then possible over a single day or for an extended period. If outside acceptable limits, the technique of the individual should be reviewed. This procedure should apply to all staff without exception. Staff should have ready access to the information.

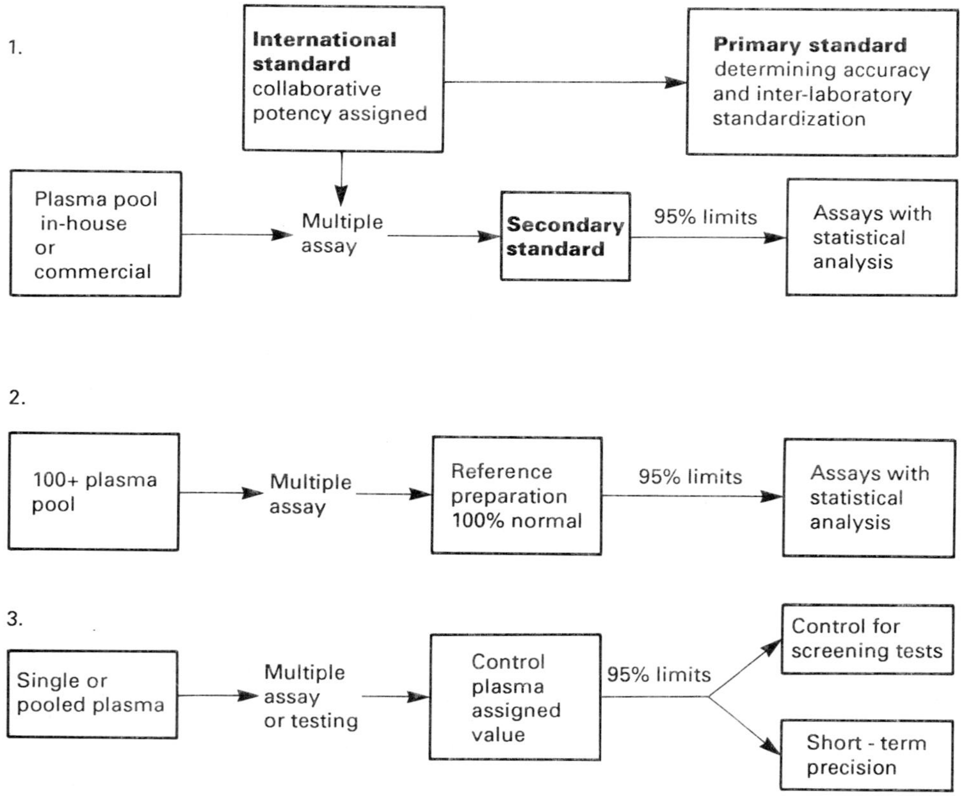

Figure 15.10 The relationship between standard, reference and control proparations

Instrumentation control

An instrument log should be kept with a record of daily or periodic checks. Problems that occur and are resolved should be recorded. All automatic pipettes should be frequently checked for accuracy. Instruments should be the object of in-house maintenance or have service contracts. Checks on the temperature of water baths and refrigerators should be made daily.

External quality assessment

The first aim of standardization is achieved by internal quality control. As with other haematological parameters, most laboratories take part in proficiency trials, both regional and national. In some instances the participation is voluntary but in others it may be mandatory to obtain 'registration' or licensing of the laboratory.

The aims of 'proficiency trials' are: (1) to relate and compare results from a laboratory with those produced in others; (2) to improve the reliability and accuracy of tests performed in individual laboratories (sometimes recommending methods or supplying standardized reagents); (3) to identify unsatisfactory performance; and (4) to achieve a high standard of performance over an extended period.

International standardization

International co-operation is the final level at which quality assurance in coagulation through standardization of methods and reagents is attempted. Since the early 1970s expert panels have been set up by the International Committee on Thrombosis and Haemostasis (ICTH) and the International Committee for Standardization in Haematology (ICSH).

Reference ranges for parameters of haemostasis

Probably in no other area of haematology is there greater variation than in the levels of haemostatic factors. This is due to physiological factors such as age, sex, blood group association and hormonal factors, particularly in pregnancy. Environmental aspects such as smoking, diet and stress also influence factor levels. Relatively minor inflammation and infections can also result in significant alterations in measurable factor levels. Reference values for adult males and non-pregnant females are reasonably well established though differences in methodology and choice of reagents may result in significantly different ranges of activity.

Haemostatic parameters in the neonate are particularly difficult to interpret. Neonatal haemostasis is normally compromised in comparison with children and adults and comprehensive data of the results of screening tests are available for premature [25] and full-term [26] babies and specific factor activities of older infants [27]. These data are particularly important because of the incidence of both acquired and congenital abnormalities of haemostasis which present at these ages. Listing the results of screening tests in neonates is not necessarily helpful due to

Table 15.9 Reference ranges of commonly measured factors. Adult ranges are expressed as IU/ml or units/ml of reference plasma. Trends in pregnancy are expressed as change from base value; NS = no significant trend. Activity in full-term neonates is expressed as percentage change from adult values

	Adult	*Pregnancy*	*Neonate*
Fibrinogen	1.7–4.0 g/l	× 4	NS
Factor II	0.6–1.7	NS	30–60
V	0.7–1.5	NS	35–110
VII	0.6–1.6	× 3	30–105
VIIIC:	0.5–1.5	× 5	40–180
vWf	0.5–1.5	× 10	40–200
IX	0.55–1.5	NS	20–90
X	0.6–1.25	NS	10–70
XI	0.55–1.5	× 0.5	20–65
XII	0.55–1.4	NS	20–90
XIII	0.5–1.5	× 0.5	30–130
Prekallikrein	0.6–1.6	?	20–70
ATIII	0.8–1.2	NS	40–100
Protein C	0.65–1.5	NS	25–75
Protein S	0.65–1.5	× 0.5	25–75

variations in reagents and techniques. Each laboratory should determine its own reference range under local conditions of testing.

In pregnancy, changes in factor activities associated with thrombotic tendencies and in the study of possible carrier status for inherited disorders, can make investigation of these aspects difficult to interpret. *Table 15.9* lists adult reference ranges for commonly determined haemostatic parameters and indicates the variation found in full-term neonates and trends in pregnancy.

References

1. Hoctor, D., Bottomley, J., Hyde, K. *et al.* (1981) Comparison of liquid and dried sodium citrate as the anticoagulant for Thrombotest and prothrombin time estimation. *J. Clin. Pathol.*, **34**, 902–5
2. Ingram, G. I. C. and Hills, M. (1976) The prothrombin time test; effect of varying citrate concentration. *Thromb. Haemost.*, **36**, 230–6
3. Kelton, J. G., Powers, P., Julian, J. *et al.* (1980) Sex related differences in platelet aggregation: influence of haematocrit. *Blood*, **56**, 38–41
4. Ramsay, D. M., Robertson, E. P. and MacArthur, E. (1977) Comparison of anticoagulants for preservation of prothrombin time specimens. *J. Clin. Pathol.*, **30**, 766–9
5. Godfrey, R., Rhymes, I. L., Bidwell, E. and Barrowcliffe, T. W. (1975) The buffering of anticoagulants for blood coagulation. *Thromb. Diath. Haemorrh.*, **34**, 879–82
6. Entwistle, M. B. P. (1988) Automation in haemostasis. In *Critical Factors in Haemostasis* (eds C. E. Williams, P. E. Short, A. J. George and M. B. P. Entwistle), pp. 244–281. Chichester: Ellis Harwood
7. Ingram, G. I. C. and Hills, M. (1976) International Committee Communications. Reference method for the one-stage prothrombin time test on human blood. *Thromb. Haemost.*, **36**, 237–8
8. Entes, K., Laduca, F. M. and Tourbaf, K. D. (1981) Fletcher factor deficiency, source of variation of the activated partial thromboplastin time test. *Am. J. Clin. Pathol.*, **75**, 626–8
9. von Clauss, A. (1957) Gerinnungsphysiologische scnell methode zur bestimmung des fibrinogens. *Acta Haematol.*, **17**, 237–46
10. Ellis, B. and Stransky, A. (1961) A quick and accurate method for the determination of fibrinogen in plasma. *J. Lab. Clin. Med.*, **58**, 477–88
11. Ratnoff, O. D. and Menzie, C. (1951) A new method for the determination of fibrinogen in small samples of plasma. *J. Lab. Clin. Med.*, **37**, 316–20
12. Giddings, J. C. and Bloom, A. L. (1968) A study of two methods for estimating plasma fibrinogen and the effect of epsilon aminocaproic acid and protamine. *J. Clin. Pathol.*, **24**, 467–71
13. Nilsson, I. M., Hedner, U. and Pandolfi, M. (1978) Measurement of fibrinolytic activities. In *Fibrinolytics and Antifibrinolytics* (ed. F. Markwardt), pp. 107–34. Berlin: Springer-Verlag
14. Lowe, G. D. O. and Prentice, C. R. M. (1980) The laboratory investigation of fibrinolysis. In *Blood Coagulation and Haemostasis* (ed. J. M. Thomson), 2nd edn., pp. 245–9. Edinburgh: Churchill Livingstone
15. Hawiger, J., Niewiarowski, S., Gurewich, V. and Thomas, D. P. (1970) Measurement of fibrinogen and fibrin degradation products in serum by staphylococcal clumping test. *J. Lab. Clin. Med.*, **175**, 93–108
16. Allington, M. J. (1971) Detection of fibrin(ogen) degradation products by a latex clumping method. *Scand. J. Haematol.* (*Suppl.*), **13**, 115–19
17. Whitaker, A. N., Elms, M. J., Masci, P. P. *et al.* (1984) Measurement of cross-linked fibrin derivatives in plasma: an immunoassay using monoclonal antibodies. *J. Clin. Pathol.*, **37**, 882–7
18. Donati, M. B. (1980) The laboratory diagnosis of acquired defects of haemostasis. In *Blood Coagulation and Haemostasis* (ed. J. M. Thomson), 2nd edn., pp. 192–3. Edinburgh: Churchill Livingstone
19. Breen, F. A. and Tullis, J. L. (1968) Ethanol gelation: a rapid screening test for intravascular coagulation. *Ann. Intern. Med.*, **69**, 1197–207
20. Hertzendorf, L. R., Stehling, L., Kirec, A. S. and Davey, F. R. (1987) Comparison of bleeding times performed on the arm and leg. *Am. J. Clin. Pathol.*, **87**, 393–6

21. Smith, P. S., Baglini, R. and Meissner, G. F. (1985) The prolonged bleeding time in haemophilia A: comparison of two measuring technics and clinical associations. *Am. J. Clin. Pathol.,* **83**, 211–15
22. Mielke, C. H. Jr, Kaneshiro, M. M., Maher, J. A. *et al.* (1969) The standardised normal Ivy bleeding time and its prolongation by aspirin. *Blood,* **34**, 204–15
23. British Society for Haematology (1988) Guideline on platelet function testing. *J. Clin. Pathol.,* **41**, 1322–30
24. Mackie, I. J., Jones, R. and Machin, S. J. (1984) Platelet impedance aggregation in whole blood and its inhibition by anti-platelet drugs. *J. Clin. Pathol.,* **37**, 874–8
25. Dube, B., Dube, R. K., Kolindewala, J. K. *et al.* (1986) Hemostatic parameters in newborn – I. Effect of gestation and rate of intrauterine growth. *Thromb. Haemost.,* **55**, 47–50
26. Kolindewala, J. K., Dube, B., Bhargava, V. *et al.* (1986) Hemostatic parameters in newborn – II. Sequential study during the first four weeks of life. *Thromb. Haemost.,* **55**, 51–3
27. Andrew, M., Paes, B., Milner, R. *et al.* (1987) Development of the human coagulation system in the full term infant. *Blood,* **70**, 165–72

Chapter 16

Haemorrhagic disorders

Haemorrhagic disorders may be inherited or acquired and may involve one or more of the mechanisms that maintain normal haemostasis – blood vessels, platelets, coagulation factors, fibrinolysis and the inhibitory mechanisms. The commonest of the inherited disorders, haemophilia A (factor VIII deficiency), occurs infrequently while acquired disorders are common and if the detectable, acquired abnormalities of platelet function due to drugs are included, it is likely that at any one time many of the population have an acquired bleeding tendency, though of minor clinical significance.

Haemorrhagic disorders are usually recognized by prolonged or repeated bleeding, often at more than one site, and may occur spontaneously or follow accidental or surgical trauma. In the very young or in the possible event of an acquired haemorrhagic disorder a first episode of bleeding could be significant. Occasionally a mild or subclinical disorder may be found by routine screening tests or by the chance observation of delay or absence of clot formation in a blood sample. A family history of bleeding points to a hereditary disorder but even severe inherited abnormalities may present without any family history because of the recessive inheritance of many defects and the occurrence of new mutations.

Hereditary coagulation disorders

Hereditary coagulation disorders are deficiency states caused by the lack of activity of a single coagulation factor, though very rarely several factors may be involved. A single deficiency allows the differentiation between a hereditary and acquired defect as the latter usually involves two or more coagulation factors. Lack of activity of a coagulation factor may be due to: (1) a quantitative defect due to decreased or absent synthesis and release of a factor; or (2) a qualitative defect due to the production and release of an abnormal coagulation factor. *Table 16.1* summarizes the plasma coagulation factors, their related deficiency states, pattern of inheritance and simple screening tests used in detection. Haemophilia A, (factor VIII:C deficiency) together with von Willebrand's disease and haemophilia B (factor IX deficiency), accounts for 95% of all hereditary coagulation deficiency states; the remaining 5% of disorders (including those of platelets) are clearly a diverse group of abnormalities.

Table 16.1 Disorders of coagulation factors

Factor	*Synonyms*	*Deficiency state*	*Inheritance pattern*	*Abnormal tests*
I	Fibrinogen	Afibrinogenaemia Dysfibrinogenaemia	Autosomal recessive Autosomal dominant	BT, PT APTT, TCT PT, APTT, TCT
II	Prothrombin	Hypoprothrombinaemia Dysprothrombinaemia	Autosomal recessive Autosomal recessive (?)	PT, APTT PT, APTT
III	Tissue thromboplastin	None		
IV	Calcium	None		
V	Accelerator globulin (proaccelerin)	Factor V deficiency†	Autosomal recessive	PT, APTT, BT (prolonged in 1/3)
VII	Proconvertin	Factor VII deficiency‡	Autosomal recessive	PT
VIII: C	Antihaemophilic factor	Classic haemophilia (haemophilia A)‡ von Willebrand's disease	X-linked recessive Autosomal dominant	APTT BT, APTT
IX	Plasma thromboplastin component	Haemophila B (Christmas disease)‡	X-linked recessive	APTT
X	Stuart factor	Factor X deficiency‡	Autosomal recessive	PT, APTT
XI	Plasma thromboplastin antecedent	Factor XI deficiency	Autosomal recessive	APTT
XII*	Hageman factor	Factor XII deficiency*	Autosomal recessive	APTT
Prekallikrein (PK)	Fletcher factor	Prekallikrein deficiency*	Autosomal recessive	APTT
High molecular weight kininogen (HMWK)	Fitzgerald factor	HMWK deficiency*	Autosomal recessive	APTT
XIII	Fibrin stabilizing factor	Factor XIII deficiency‡	Autosomal recessive	Clot solubility increased in 5 mol/l urea

BT = Bleeding time; PT = prothrombin time; APTT = activated partial thromboplastin time; TCT = thrombin clotting time.
* No clinical symptoms.
† Genetic heterogeneity suggested by variable levels of factor V activity.
‡ Genetic heterogeneity identified with some patients showing 'true' deficiency of factor synthesis while other patients have abnormal molecular structure incapable of supporting procoagulant activity yet present in antigenically normal quantity.

The 'haemophilias'

Originally the term haemophilia referred to a bleeding disorder characterized by X-linked inheritance and severe bleeding manifestations, including haemarthroses. In 1952 it was recognized that two kinds of sex-linked haemophilia exist which are indistinguishable clinically but can be clearly differentiated by laboratory tests and are termed haemophilia A (factor VIII:C deficiency, classic haemophilia) and haemophilia B (factor IX deficiency, Christmas disease).

Another hereditary disorder involving the factor VIII molecule is von Willebrand's disease (vWD) which differs from haemophilia A by its autosomal dominant inheritance, different pattern of bleeding and the results of laboratory tests, but typically both disorders are deficient in coagulation activity of factor VIII:C. These observations suggested that factor VIII is composed of two functional molecules.

Haemophilia A

Haemophilia A results from a deficiency of factor VIII:C. Typically, only males will be bleeders, although rarely a female carrier will have a mild to moderate bleeding diathesis. Sons of affected males will be normal and all the daughters will be carriers. Thus the disorder will appear to 'skip generations', as only some of the male offspring of female carriers will be bleeders (*Figure 16.1*). The absence of a characteristic family history does not exclude haemophilia A.

Haemophilia A occurs in all degrees of severity corresponding to the level of factor VIII:C in the affected persons. *Severely affected* patients have less than 1% factor VIII:C activity and intermittently have spontaneous haemorrhages, especially into large joints and muscles. Symptoms may begin at birth with bleeding from the umbilical cord, although this does not occur frequently. At around 9 months of age easy bruising may be noted, and when the child begins to walk, haemarthroses and muscle haematomas begin to be a problem. Haematuria is common. Bleeding into the central nervous system may occur either spontaneously or after trauma, and results in a life-threatening situation. Affected patients also have a marked tendency to bleed after minimal trauma. The introduction of factor VIII:C concentrates revolutionized the treatment of severe haemophilia A.

Moderately affected patients have approximately 1–5% factor VIII:C activity. Spontaneous haemorrhage occurs much less frequently, but haemorrhage usually occurs after trauma of even minor degree. *Mildly affected* patients have greater than 5–10% factor VIII:C activity and generally bleed only after significant injury.

Molecular defect in haemophilia A

Although termed factor VIII deficiency, haemophilia A may not be the result of an absence or reduction of the factor VIII protein but due to an abnormal molecule with reduced VIII:C activity. This concept of functional molecular abnormality rather than quantitative reduction applies to 'deficiencies' of all procoagulant proteins.

Molecular variants of haemophilia A were recognized by the ability of certain plasmas from haemophilia A patients to neutralize inhibitors of VIII:C[1] and therefore to contain 'cross-reacting material' (CRM). Inhibitor neutralization tests give variable results depending on the source of the homologous inhibitor. Even when monoclonal antibodies are used in more sensitive immunological methods,

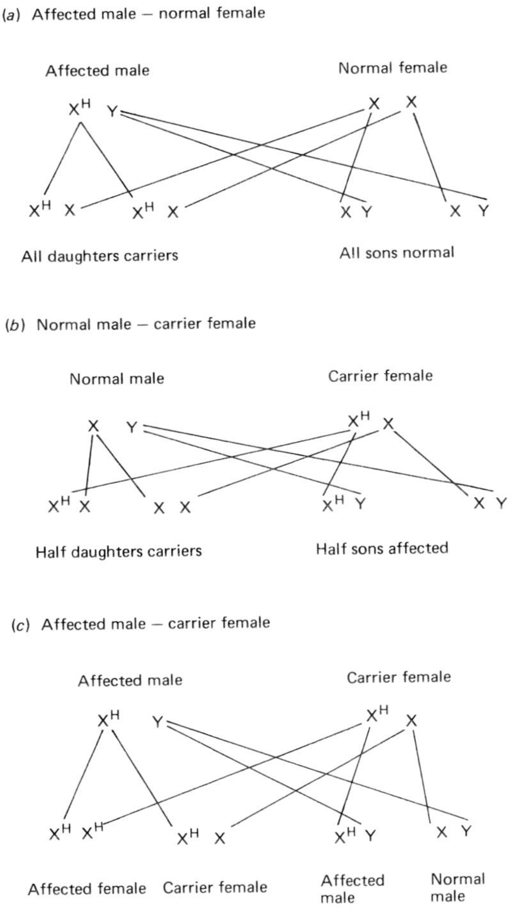

Figure 16.1 Inheritance of haemophilia A and B.

variable results are obtained which to some extent depend on methodological variables. Nevertheless, the concept of CRM^+ and CRM^- individuals is accepted. DNA technology has identified gene deletions, point mutation or insertions as molecular defects in haemophilia A [2, 3].

Carriers of haemophilia A

The majority of carriers of haemophilia A are asymptomatic. They have, on average, half the level of factor VIII:C found in normal females but activity may range from 10% to over 100%. This wide range of values is due to the 'Lyonization effect' which results in the random inactivation of one of the X chromosomes in females; inactivation of the normal X chromosome results in low levels of factor VIII:C whereas inactivation of the X chromosome carrying the haemophilia A defect usually results in a normal factor VIII:C

Measuring VIII:C levels alone is therefore an unreliable method of identifying carriers. A more effective approach to identifying carrier status is based on the observation that the ratio of VIII:C to vWf:Ag (formerly VIIIRAg) is decreased in the carrier state [4,5]. On average the VIII:C/vWf:Ag ratio is 1.0 in normal women and 0.5 in obligate carriers. A ratio of <0.7 is widely quoted as indicating carrier status but each centre should determine its own criterion. Variables which influence the VIII:C/vWf:Ag ratio include age, blood group, testing *during* pregnancy, infection, inflammation and oral contraception. In those families where the molecular defect has been identified, DNA studies can recognize the female carrier.

Diagnosis of haemophilia A

The diagnosis of haemophilia A is easy in patients with severe haemophilia A. These patients generally present with (1) a sex-linked disease; (2) 'spontaneous' haemorrhage, leading to crippling joint problems; (3) prolonged activated partial thromboplastin time (APTT); (4) low VIII:C activity; (5) normal bleeding time; and (6) normal vWf:Ag and ristocetin co-factor activity vWf (RiCoF).

It can be more difficult to diagnose *mild* haemophilia A due to limitations in laboratory testing. A satisfactory APTT method and technique will be sensitive to levels of VIII:C below 0.45 units/ml which can be confirmed by accurate VIII:C assay. Differentiation must be made between haemophilia A and the von Willebrand syndrome and it is emphasized that a low VIII:C level and a normal bleeding time *do not* allow a diagnosis of mild haemophilia A (*Table 16.2*).

Table 16.2 Laboratory differences between haemophilia A and von Willebrand's disease

Variable	*Haemophilia A*	*von Willebrand's disease*
Inheritance	Sex linked	Autosomal dominant
Factor VIII: C	Low	Low to nearly normal (variable)
Bleeding time	Normal	Normal or prolonged (variable)
Ristocetin aggregation of platelets	Normal	Normal, reduced or enhanced
vWf: Ag	Normal to high	Low to normal
De novo synthesis of factor VIII: C after plasma or cryoprecipitate infusion	No	Yes
Platelet retention in glass bead columns	Normal	Decreased

Factor VIII inhibitors

Factor VIII inhibitors arise in 5–10% of patients with severe haemophilia A (rarely in patients with mild to moderate haemophilia) as a result of antigenic stimulus by infused factor VIII and are more rarely acquired by patients with an unrelated disorder (*see* page 618). The inhibitors are antibodies ($IgG_4\kappa$) and, unusually, appear to be monoclonal [6]. They interact with factor VIII in a reaction which is time, pH and temperature dependent.

Factor VIII antibodies do not always appear in multi-transfused haemophiliacs and are independent of the presence of cross-reacting material (CRM^+) or the type and structure of the infused material (cryopecipitate, concentrate or plasma). It is not therefore possible to predict the development of antibodies, and before surgery patients with haemophilia A (and B) should be screened for the presence of inhibitors.

Kinetics of the inhibitor The kinetics of the interaction with the factor VIII molecule are variable and complex and in addition to being temperature and time dependent there are two types of antigen–antibody reaction. First, where the reaction displays second-order kinetics in which there is an initial rapid loss of VIII:C activity followed by a plateau occurring between 2 and 4 hours which may be caused by the formation of stable antigen–antibody complexes. Secondly, a more complex type of reaction where, following the rapid loss of VIII:C activity, there is a continuing slow decline rather than a plateau. The antigen–antibody complexes here are dissociable and weaker reacting. After initial sensitization, further exposure to factor VIII can produce a rise in the factor VIII antibody titre. The increase in antibody titre begins 3–7 days after the antigenic stimulus, peaks in 10–20 days and then declines or stabilizes over the following months. Those patients whose antibodies react in this manner are said to be *high responders*, whereas those who demonstrate little or no response are *low responders*. Patients have been described who have developed antibodies after repeated exposure to factor VIII over a long period and were initially *low responders* and remained low responders.

Laboratory diagnosis In a patient with haemophilia A inhibitory activity may be detected by mixing the patient's plasma with normal plasma and performing an APTT test on the mixture. The inhibitors in the patient's plasma will result in a prolonged APTT, usually at least 30 seconds longer than the control instead of showing the expected correction. Immediate testing may not detect the inhibitor, especially if the inhibitor is present in low titre; the mixture of normal plasma and the patient's plasma should be incubated for up to 2 hours at 37°C. The inhibitor to VIII:C can be assayed by methods based on the ability of the inhibitor to neutralize VIII:C and expressed in units, the value of which vary according to the method used. It can be shown that the inhibitor specifically neutralizes VIII:C. Experiments have shown that the inhibitors to VIII:C not only inhibit VIII:C but may have a slight effect on von Willebrand factor (vWf) activity.

von Willebrand's disease (vWD)

In 1926 von Willebrand described a bleeding disorder inherited as an autosomal dominant characteristic with variable penetrance and expression and the most consistent laboratory finding was a prolonged bleeding time. In contrast to haemophilia A, bleeding in this condition is variable and mainly affects the skin and mucosa (epistaxis, increased bruising, menorrhagia, gastrointestinal haemorrhage). Bleeding during and after surgical procedures, especially dental extractions, is very common, though haemarthroses are rare. It was subsequently shown that most patients with vWD have a deficiency of VIII:C, but the level may vary from being undetectable to normal. The VIII:C activities in male patients with haemophilia A are reasonably constant but the VIII:C activity in a given patient with vWD frequently alters, e.g. in pregnancy.

Because of the prolonged bleeding time and the fact that platelet adhesiveness is often decreased in vWD, a primary platelet defect was first suspected as the cause of the bleeding disorder. It is now recognized that the defect appears to be due to a quantitative or qualitative 'deficiency' in the VIII/vWf molecule which possesses not only coagulant activity and antigenic identity, but also an activity required for the aggregation of platelets to the subendothelium. The activity of the molecule related to platelet function is termed the von Willebrand factor (vWf). The bimolecular VIII/vWf complex has therefore two roles in haemostasis – the VIII protein related to the coagulation pathway and the vWf protein to platelet function (*Figure 16.2*).

It is now clear that vWD is heterogeneous in respect of severity, laboratory findings and response to therapy. The term *von Willebrand syndrome* is probably more appropriate.

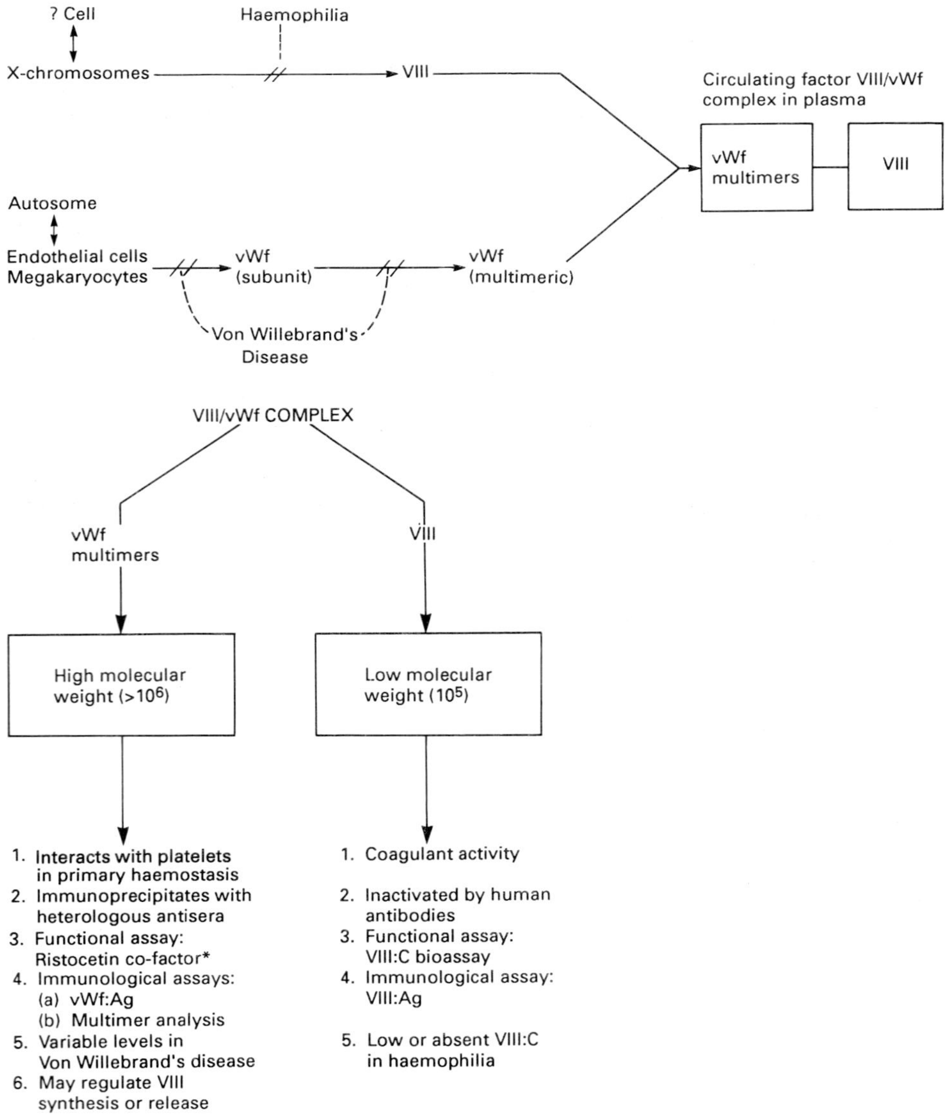

Figure 16.2 The interrelationships of the VIII/vWf complex; *does not entirely represent functional activity of vWf

Diagnosis of von Willebrand disease (vWD)

In contrast to haemophilia A, vWD has abnormal platelet function and generally prolonged bleeding time due to abnormality of the vWf protein. In classical vWD, VIII:C is reduced which may cause confusion with haemophilia A but, in contrast to haemophilia A, vWf:Ag is also reduced. The observation [7] that aggregation of the patient's platelets following the addition of the antibiotic ristocetin is defective in typical vWD has been developed into a direct platelet aggregation test using the patient's platelets and into an assay of the activity of vWf in plasma (ristocetin co-factor activity, vWf:RiCoF). The RiCoF assay does not completely or necessarily reflect functional vWf activity.

The high molecular weight vWf:Ag consists of 'higher' and 'lower' molecular weight multimers and variations in the multimeric composition give rise to the heterogeneity of vWD [8]. It is emphasized, however, that the commonest forms of vWD are associated with a reduction in the total amount of vWf:Ag or absence of the largest multimers. Other variants are very rare.

The analysis of the multimer composition of vWf is a complex procedure which is difficult to standardize. The simpler method of two-dimensional crossed immunoelectrophoresis (2DCIE) allows the recognition of abnormal multimer composition and thus identification of vWD variants. The diagnosis of vWD and its variants depends upon clinical presentation, pattern of inheritance, platelet count and bleeding time, assay of VIII:C and vWf:Ag and 2DCIE supported by direct ristocetin aggregation, and the plasma vWf:RiCoF assay.

A unique aspect of typical vWD is the response to infusion of normal plasma. The initial rise in VIII:C is followed by a sustained or further increase in VIII:C. This is in contrast to the 8–12 hour half-life of VIII:C in haemophilia A. Improved methods in diagnosis have made this contribution to diagnosis unnecessary but the phenomenon can still be of relevance in therapeutic protocols in selected patients.

The administration of the vasopressin analogue desamino-8-D-arginine vasopressin (DDAVP) produces a rapid rise in VIII and vWf and is used in the treatment of mild haemophilia A and vWD. However, contraindications or uncertainties in its use in the treatment of particular vWD variants make the classification and identification of vWD and its variants an important laboratory function.

Classification of vWD

A preliminary classification into types I (typical), II and III is shown in *Table 16.3*. The essential differences are that type I has low vWf:Ag with normal 2DCIE; type II has normal vWf:Ag with abnormal 2DCIE; and type III has undetectable vWf:Ag.

Table 16.3 Preliminary classification of vWD

Type	*Bleeding time*	*VIII: C*	*vWf: Ag*	*vWf: RiCoF*	*2DCIE*
I (typical)	↑	↓	↓	↓	Normal pattern
II	↑	N or ↓	N	↓	Abnormal
III (severe homozygote)	↑	↓	↓ ↓	↓ ↓	Not demonstrable

N = Normal. For other abbreviations see text.

Type II vWD is further divided by the additional use of direct, low concentration ristocetin platelet aggregation (DRiPA) and multimer analysis of plasma (*Table 16.4*). Types IIE, F, G and H have been described[9] based on further abnormalities of multimer patterns.

Table 16.4 Further classification of vWD variants

Type	*VIII: C*	*vWf: Ag*	*DRiPA*	*RiCoF*	*2DCIE*	*Multimer analysis*
I	↓	↓	↓	↓	N	Normal pattern, reduced amount
IIA	N or ↓	N or ↓	↓	↓ ↓	A	Large and intermediate absent; abnormal triplet
IIB	N or ↓	N or ↓	↑ ↑	N or ↓	A	Large absent; normal triplet
IIC	N or ↓	N or ↓	–	↓	DP	Large absent; smallest increased
IID	N	N	–	↓	–	Abnormal pattern on 3% agarose

N = Normal; A = absent; DP = double peak. For other abbreviations see text.

Type I vWD is the commonest form and accounts for up to 70% of cases. On the basis of multimeric analysis otherwise typical type I cases have been described which respond variably to administration of DDAVP[10]. A 'pseudo-' or 'platelet-type' of vWD has been described which resembles type IIB with enhanced DRiPA, and absent large multimers in plasma which are present in platelets. Adminstration of normal plasma may induce thrombocytopenia. Thrombocytopenia is also a consequence of administering DDAVP to type IIB which emphasizes the importance of classification into type I and type II forms.

Antibodies to vWf[11] In a small proportion of patients with severe vWD, antibodies directed against the vWf activity of the molecule but not directly affecting VIII:C activity may develop, probably as the result of treatment as occurs in haemophilia A. Antibody may be demonstrated by mixing experiments using the patient's plasma, normal platelet-rich plasma and direct ristocetin aggregation or by RiCoF assay. Antibody to vWf may also occur in patients who do not have vWD (*see* page 619).

Haemophilia B

Haemophilia B (factor IX deficiency, Christmas disease, hereditary factor IX deficiency) is due to a deficiency of factor IX. The bleeding manifestations vary from severe to mild and are identical with those of haemophilia A and it is also inherited as an X-linked disorder. Like the latter, haemophilia B results in a prolonged APTT. It is differentiated from haemophilia A by laboratory testing.

As in haemophilia A molecular variants are found[12, 13] and, indeed, the concept of CRM^+ and CRM^- defects was first established in patients with haemophilia B. Unlike haemophilia A, however, only a minority have undetectable factor IX antigen (CRM^-), many having reduced levels of antigen (CRM^R). Subsequent studies have demonstrated marked heterogeneity of haemophilia B, at least 35 point mutations and 17 types of deletion having been identified. Unlike haemophilia A, there is good correlation between complete or partial deletion of the factor IX gene and the production of inhibitors following infusion of factor IX.

One group of variants of particular relevance to laboratory investigation and diagnosis are those having a prolonged one-stage prothrombin time using bovine thromboplastin and a normal value using human or rabbit sources of thromboplastin. This type of variant is designated haemophilia B_M, the subscript being derived from the name of the index patient. It has been shown subsequently that approximately 15% of cases of haemophilia B react abnormally with bovine thromboplastin, usually by means of the Thrombotest reagent which incorporates bovine thromboplastin. Abnormal Thrombotest results are only found in CRM^+ patients and are considered to be due to the abnormal molecule having an abnormal reaction with, or inhibiting the action of, the thromboplastin.

CRM status and the reaction with bovine thromboplastin allows phenotypic classification into three groups. Type I has low IX activity, normal antigen and variable reaction with bovine thromboplastin; type II has low activity, intermediate or reduced antigen (CRM^R) and normal reaction with bovine thromboplastin; and type III has low activity, low antigen (CRM^-) and normal reaction with bovine thromboplastin.

Intermediate or slight abnormalities with bovine thromboplastin require careful interpretation and exclusion of lowered factor VII, factor X and/or factor II as possible causes.

Factor IX inhibitors

Approximately 2–10% of patients with haemophilia B develop inhibitors. Unlike factor VIII antibodies the inhibitors of factor IX are stable over a wide range of pH and temperature, they are found in the IgG fraction, and the interaction of factor IX with its inhibitor is virtually immediate rather than time dependent.

Carriers of haemophilia B

The low and high molecular weight structure of the VIII/vWf complex is not found with factor IX. In carriers of CRM^+ haemophilia B the ratio of IX antigen:IX clotting activity is higher than normal and determination of IX antigen in CRM^- carriers may also be of value. Overall the use of IX antigen:activity ratios in discriminant function analysis may be evaluated with up to 80% certainty.

In families with haemophilia B_M and increased bovine thromboplastin prothrombin times, carriers may be found to have increased prothrombin times[14]. Intragenic sequence variation may be demonstrated by restriction fragment length polymorphisms (RFLPs) and in families showing segregation for haemophilia B successful diagnosis can be made in 89% of families. More recently, the direct sequencing of genomic DNA, mismatch detection and direct detection of factor IX mutations allows carrier detection in a wider range of individuals[13].

'Contact factor' deficiencies

Although a deficiency of any of the factors which comprise the 'contact system' (XII and XI, prekallikrein and HMWK) can result in marked prolongation of the APTT, only factor XI deficiency is associated with a significant bleeding disorder. The importance of identifying deficiencies in factor XII, prekallikrein and HMWK lies in distinguishing them from other causes of a prolonged APTT in the presence of a normal one-stage prothrombin time, i.e. factors XI, IX and VIII, which require accurate diagnosis and appropriate treatment.

Factor XI deficiency

Factor XI deficiency was first recognized in 1953. It is inherited as an autosomal, incompletely recessive trait. Both homozygotes and heterozygotes may have increased bleeding, although the former have more severe symptoms. The incidence of this deficiency is highest in Ashkenazi Jews.

Bleeding in factor XI is usually mild even in apparently severe deficiencies, and most commonly seen are bruising, epistaxis and menorrhagia. Haemarthrosis is rare. Bleeding, which may be delayed, commonly follows dental extraction and surgery.

Factor XI deficiency can be suspected on the basis of a prolonged APTT, mild bleeding, and autosomal inheritance. It can further be distinguished from factor VIII and IX deficiencies by mixing experiments and specific factor assay. An important aspect of the investigation of contact factor deficiencies is that a defect can correct by storage of plasma and that the defects in prekallikrein and HMWK are corrected by a short exposure to the contact activator ellagic acid, and by extended incubation with kaolin.

Deficiencies of other factors

Factor X deficiency

Deficiency of factor X is a rare disorder discovered in 1957 and is inherited as an autosomal recessive trait and has a heterozygous frequency of about one in 500 persons. The most common bleeding manifestations are epistaxis, haematoma, menorrhagia and post-partum haemorrhage. Haemarthrosis may occur but rarely results in crippling arthropathy. Factor X deficiency classically results in a prolongation of both the prothrombin time and APTT with a normal thrombin clotting time. This pattern is also seen in factor V and II deficiency, and to distinguish between deficiencies of these factors specific assays are required.

Molecular variants of factor X deficiency have been confirmed in which factor X antigenic activity, as measured by its ability to neutralize heterologous antibody, is normal, while its clotting activity is deficient, e.g. factor X Friuli. This is analogous to the CRM status in haemophilia A and B. The Russell's viper venom time (RVV) is usually abnormal but not necessarily so in patients with molecular variants. By combining CRM status with the results of the RVV time, at least five types of factor X deficiency have been suggested[15]. The later introduction of amidolytic assays of factor X has revealed further heterogeneity and at least 12 patterns of results have been demonstrated[16].

Factor VII deficiency

Factor VII deficiency is inherited as an autosomal recessive trait with a homozygous frequency of about two per million individuals. Bleeding manifestations are most commonly epistaxis, gingival bleeding (especially after dental extraction), subcutaneous haemorrhages and menorrhagia. Bleeding from other sites including joints may occur. The severity of post-surgical bleeding varies considerably and may not correlate with the level of factor VII coagulant activity. Remarkably, thromboembolic complications may occur. Carriers of factor VII deficiency may have excessive bruising, epistaxis and postoperative bleeding[17]. Factor VII deficiency is the only deficiency that results in an isolated prolongation of the prothrombin time and the diagnosis is confirmed by specific factor VII assays.

Genetic variants of factor VII have been reported (e.g. factor VII Padua, factor VII Verona) which display discrepancies of antigenic and clotting activity, i.e. CRM^-, CRM^R and CRM^+ indicating genetic heterogeneity of factor VII. As with the factor IX_M variant, reaction of factor VII variants with thromboplastins of different species results in different levels of activity[18]. Activity:antigen ratios can be used to identify carriers of factor VII deficiency[19].

Factor V deficiency

Factor V deficiency is a rare disorder transmitted as an autosomal recessive trait in which only the homozygotes have bleeding manifestations. Severity of bleeding varies greatly but is usually mild and manifested by epistaxis, easy bruising, menorrhagia and post-surgical bleeding. In severely affected patients gastrointestinal and central nervous system bleeding may occur. The carriers are relatively easy to identify, as they have approximately one half the normal plasma level of factor V. Carrier identification by specific factor assay is indeed generally possible in all the coagulation disorders characterized by autosomal recessive inheritance. Factor V deficiency results in both a prolonged PT and APTT. The bleeding time is prolonged in approximately one-third of the patients. A specific assay of factor V is required for accurate diagnosis. Molecular variants have been described.

Factor II (prothrombin) deficiency

Deficiency of factor II is rare and inherited as an autosomal recessive trait. Bleeding manifestations generally correlate with the level of functional prothrombin, being insignificant with levels around 50% and potentially life threatening with levels less than 2%. Severely affected patients may show post-partum haemorrhage, menorrhagia and haemorrhage after surgery, or trauma. Haemarthrosis is unusual. The PT and APTT are often only slightly prolonged and a specific prothrombin assay is required to make the diagnosis.

At least 20 variants of the prothrombin molecule have been identified in the last 20 years (dysprothrombins). All but one have shown high antigen:activity ratios. Characterization has been based on the reaction of prothrombin with various snake venoms and staphylocoagulase and by two-dimensional crossed immunoelectrophoresis[20]. Point mutations have been identified in a few instances.

Disorders of fibrinogen

Hereditary afibrinogenaemia and hypofibrinogenaemia

The *absence* of fibrinogen is rare and is inherited as an autosomal recessive; affected subjects are homozygous for the abnormality. The clinical effects are a mild to moderate haemorrhagic defect which is present at birth. Bleeding from the umbilicus and following circumcision may be severe. Bruising, haematomas, epistaxis and haemorrhage after dental extraction are common, and wound healing is often defective. For reasons that are not entirely clear and despite the complete incoagulability of the blood, patients may go for long periods without spontaneous haemorrhages and in general have less disability than patients with severe haemophilia A or B. Fibrinogen appears to be absent by both chemical and immunological methods. The bleeding time is prolonged in about 50% of patients. In hypofibrinogenaemia the patient appears to be heterozygous for the defect though low fibrinogen levels are found in some examples of hereditary dysfibrinogenaemia.

Laboratory findings are:

1. Low or absent levels of fibrinogen.
2. Abnormal coagulation tests which rely on end-point fibrin formation.
3. Abnormal platelet function corrected by fibrinogen.

Hereditary dysfibrinogenaemias [21]

Dysfibrinogenaemia is characterized by a qualitative abnormality of the fibrinogen molecule. Although commonly an acquired abnormality (*see* page 614), at least 75 specific inherited abnormalities have been reported. The variants are identified by the name of the investigating centre, e.g. fibrinogen Oslo, Amsterdam, Tokyo, etc. and apparent geographic clusters represent centres of investigation rather than racial distribution.

Over half the reported cases or families are asymptomatic, in about one-third there is a mild bleeding tendency and in about 30 variants there is an association with thrombosis, thrombocytopenia and/or spontaneous abortion.

Dysfibrinogenaemia is usually recognized by chance during the course of routine laboratory testing. By far the commonest findings are prolongation of the thrombin clotting time and the Reptilase time, though a few variants have a normal or even shortened thrombin time (*Table 16.5*). Modifications of the thrombin clotting time, such as the presence of Ca^{2+} or protamine or the adjustment of pH, may correct or modify the clotting time.

Table 16.5 Dysfibrinogenaemia associated with a normal or shortened thrombin clotting time

Type	*Laboratory findings*	*Clinical findings*
Oklahoma	Defective, cross-linking, factor XIII 50% of normal. Abnormal tryptic digestion of fibrinogen	Bleeding
Oslo I	Shortened thrombin time	Recurrent venous thromboembolism
Tokyo	Defective cross-linking. Abnormal plasmin degradation products	Bleeding

By far the commonest results of dysfibrinogenaemia are delayed fibrinopeptide release and/or polymerization of fibrin monomer. Fibrinopeptides A or B, or both, may show defective release with consequent delay in monomer polymerization. Polymerization may be impaired even in the presence of normal fibrinopeptide formation. Abnormal fibrin cross-linking or increased sensitivity to fibrinolysis may contribute to a bleeding tendency. *Table 16.6* shows examples of dysfibrinogens with impaired fibrinopeptide release.

The molecular abnormalities are mainly point mutations in the $A\alpha$, $B\beta$ or γ chains or more rarely due to deletions or extensions.

Laboratory investigations of fibrinogen abnormalities Laboratory data in patients with hereditary dysfibrinogenaemia may include one or more of the following:

1. Prolonged TCT with other clotting parameters normal (or near normal). *A prolonged TCT is the most common laboratory finding.*
2. Prolonged TCT with long APTT, PT or both, but specific factor assays, other than fibrinogen, are normal.
3. Prolonged TCT and prolonged Reptilase time.
4. Low fibrinogen concentration as measured by clotting (functional) assay and low, normal or high fibrinogen (antigen) levels.
5. Abnormal fibrinogen polymerization rate as measured by clotting diluted plasma and monitoring the change in optical density in a spectrophotometer at 350 nm.
6. Presence of increased FDP in serum in the absence of other indications of disseminated intravascular coagulation (DIC) or activation of the fibrinolytic system.
7. Abnormal fibrinogen immunoelectrophoresis.
8. Presence of a similar fibrinogen defect in other relatives (evidence of hereditary abnormality).

Table 16.6 Examples of dysfibrinogenaemia with impaired fibrinopeptide release

Fibrinogen	*Abnormal release of fibrinopeptide*	*Fibrin polymerization*	*Clinical effect*	*Molecular defect*
Baltimore	FpA	Slow	Bleeding, thrombosis	α Polymer defect
Bethesda I	FpA + B	Normal	Bleeding	–
Madrid III	FpB	Normal	None	↑ Catabolism
New Orleans	FpA + B (A slower)	Normal	Bleeding	–
Detroit	FpB	Slow	Bleeding	$A\alpha^{19}$(Arg→ Ser)

Factor XIII deficiency [22]

At least 140 cases of factor XIII deficiency have been reported since the first description in 1960. Although the early reported cases were all males, inheritance is almost always autosomal recessive and sex distribution is almost equal. Clinical manifestations include a characteristic history of umbilical bleeding *after* birth, easy bruising, haematoma formation, poor wound healing and delayed bleeding after surgery. Intracranial bleeding is reported in about one-third of cases and is a major cause of death before the age of 16 years. The pattern of bleeding is therefore similar to that found in afibrinogenaemia.

Routine coagulation tests, platelet count and morphology are normal. Plasma fibrin clots formed in the presence of thrombin and Ca^{2+} are normally insoluble in 5 M urea for many hours; in hereditary XIII deficiency the clot will dissolve in 30 minutes. Only very low levels of factor XIII are necessary to produce fibrin cross-linking. Levels over 2% are sufficient to render the clot insoluble *in vitro* and to maintain haemostasis *in vivo*. Diagnosis of factor XIII deficiency cannot therefore be made after infusion of even small quantities of plasma; at least 8 weeks should elapse before attempting diagnosis by clot solubility methods.

The molecular defect in inherited factor XIII deficiency is mainly the absence of the 'a-chain' (A subunit) with low normal levels of 'b-chain' (S subunit). A much less common defect is absence of both 'a' and 'b' chains which may be inherited as an autosomal incomplete recessive as very low levels of 'b-chain' are found in heterozygotes.

The formation of inhibitors after infusion of plasma or factor XIII concentrates is extremely unlikely; only one possible unconfirmed example has been described.

Combined factor deficiencies [23]

Leaving aside the statistically possible, simultaneous inheritance of two rare recessive genes, particular combined congenital factor deficiencies resulting from a 'common gene abnormality' have been strongly suggested by family studies. The most frequent combined deficiency is that of factors V and VIII, of which over 87 cases in 57 unrelated families have been reported. The deficiency of each factor is generally mild (5–25% of normal), and there have been notable associated congenital abnormalities (e.g. syndactylism, retardation). It is important therefore to assay for both factors in situations where there is ostensibly mild deficiency of either factor, particularly if there are associated congenital malformations, and because replacement therapy should be chosen to correct both deficiencies. Suggestions that the apparent combined deficiency of factors V and VIII may be due to a defect of protein C inhibitor have now been disproved. In a number of cases there have been features of vWD [24].

Inherited combined deficiency of factors VII and X has been noted in conjunction with familial carotid-body tumours. Congential combined deficiency of factors VII and VIII has been reported. Two unrelated patients have been reported with combined congenital deficiency of all the vitamin K-dependent factors (II, VII, IX and X).

Other rare inherited 'coagulation' disorders

Mutation of antitrypsin to antithrombin

A severe and fatal haemorrhagic disorder has been reported [25, 26] in which a single amino acid substitution converted the elastase inhibitor α-antitrypsin to antithrombin III with consequent non-physiological inhibition of thrombin and other serine proteases. Laboratory investigations revealed prolongation of bleeding, clotting, partial thromboplastin, prothrombin and thrombin times. The mutant inhibitor did not require heparin for its activity. The only useful treatment was exchange transfusion.

Hereditary deficiency of α_2-antiplasmin

There have been at least five reports of individuals with homozygous α_2-antiplasmin deficiency [27, 28]. Clinical signs include epistaxis, bleeding after trauma and spontaneous haemarthroses. Laboratory findings show no abnormality of coagulation, inhibitor and platelet function tests. The results of initial investigation therefore resemble factor XIII deficiency. Tests of fibrinolysis show shortened euglobulin lysis time and increased FDPs. Functional and immunological tests for α_2-antiplasmin show absence or low levels. Heterozygotes with levels around 60% of normal may exhibit a mild haemorrhagic disorder. Haemorrhagic episodes are effectively treated with the fibrinolytic inhibitor tranexamic acid, which is also effective in prophylaxis.

Treatment of inherited coagulation defects

The management of life-long coagulation defects requires a comprehensive, co-ordinated programme to give the patient the maximum opportunity for a normal, productive life. The prevention or treatment of bleeding episodes is based essentially on replacement of the deficient factor by infusion of plasma concentrates and in recent years the increased availability of factor concentrates has dramatically improved the management of the haemophilic patient. Effective replacement therapy does, however, require an accurate assessment of the type and severity of the defect, knowledge of the physiological characteristics of the deficient factor and its availability and potency in plasma and plasma concentrates.

Types of therapeutic agents (*Table 16.7*)

Fresh frozen plasma (FFP) was introduced as a means of replacing the missing clotting factors in 1950 and remained the primary agent for treatment of haemophilia for nearly two decades. The effectiveness of FFP transfusions is limited by the large volumes needed to raise clotting factors to haemostatic levels. The cardiovascular system cannot accommodate the volumes of plasma needed to reach levels above 25–30% and such levels are not adequate to control moderate or severe haemorrhage or to provide haemostasis for surgery. Effective treatment became a reality with the development of concentrates of coagulation factors. With

Table 16.7 Therapeutic materials available for treatment of coagulation deficiencies

Deficiency state	*Deficient factor*	*Therapeutic materials*	In vivo *half-life*
Afibrinogenaemia	Fibrinogen	Cryoprecipitate, fibrinogen concentrates, FFP	4–5 days
Hypoprothrombinaemia	Prothrombin	FFP, cryo-removed plasma, prothrombin complex concentrate	60–80 hours
Factor V deficiency	V	Cryo-removed plasma, FFP	36 hours
Factor VII deficiency	VII	Cryo-removed plasma, FFP, prothrombin complex	3–4 hours
Haemophilia A	VIII	Factor VIII concentrate, cryoprecipitate, FFP	12 hours
von Willebrand's disease	VIII, vWf	Cryoprecipitate, FFP	*See* text
Haemophilia B	IX	Prothrombin complex concentrate, cryo-removed plasma, FFP	24 hours
Factor X deficiency	X	Cryo-removed plasma, prothrombin complex concentrate, FFP	40 hours
Factor XI deficiency	XI	FFP	1–2 days
Factor XIII deficiency	XIII	FFP, factor XIII concentrates	6–8 days

FFP = fresh frozen plasma

high-potency, low-volume concentrates, factor levels of 100% or more can be attained, severe bleeding episodes controlled and major surgery performed without excessive bleeding. Concentrates are an effective and convenient product for home therapy. Factor VIII concentrates are available as cryoprecipitated factor VIII and as fractionated plasma in lyophilized form. Cryoprecipitate can be prepared to yield 10-fold plasma concentrations.

Lyophilized concentrates are of two types:

1. Intermediate potency and purity preparations, which are similar in concentration to cryoprecipitate and contain about 10 units/ml (one unit of factor VIII equals that amount present in 1 ml of fresh, pooled normal human plasma).
2. High-potency and purity concentrates which are 30–40 times concentrated and have about 25 units factor VIII/ml.

Factor IX concentrates are available as 'prothrombin complex' concentrates, which also contain prothrombin and factors VII and X; the factor IX concentration is about 15–20 units/ml, a unit being defined as for factor VIII.

There are advantages and disadvantages of each type of concentrate. Cryoprecipitate must be stored deep-frozen to retain its potency, a significant obstacle to its use in home transfusion, whereas the lyophilized factor VIII or IX concentrates can be stored in the refrigerator or even at room temperature. One disadvantage of cryoprecipitate is its variable potency. Cryoprecipitate is prepared from single donors and the potency of each bag depends upon the initial factor VIII level of the plasma and the loss of activity during processing. On average, each bag should contain about 80–100 units of factor VIII. However, bags with as little as 50 units or less and as much as 300 units can be produced.

Lyophilized concentrates are prepared from large pools of FFP, and the concentration of factor in each batch is assigned which allows rational calculation of dosage.

The major advantage of cryoprecipitate and disadvantage of the lyophilized concentrates is the use of single-donor versus pooled plasma. Transfusion of blood products carries the risk of transmitting viral infections, and concentrates prepared from large plasma pools may pose a greater threat than single units of plasma or cryoprecipitate.

Administration and dosage

Plasma and concentrates are given intravenously. The amounts to be given depend upon the patient's plasma volume, the potency of the preparation and the plasma level of factor VIII or IX required. The maximum amount of *plasma* which can be infused without inducing circulatory overload is 15–20 ml/kg body weight in an adult and 10–15 ml/kg in a child, which is only sufficient to raise the VIII or IX level to about 25–30% of normal activity. With concentrates, however, volume considerations are not a limiting factor and high levels can be attained.

Dosage calculations are based on the definition of a 'unit' of factor activity. In the past one unit of activity of a coagulation factor was defined as that activity in 1 ml of average normal plasma collected for testing in the laboratory by mixing one part of sodium citrate as anticoagulant with nine volumes of blood. However, the activity of normal plasma pools vary appreciably due to the fact that the activity of normal plasma, for example in the case of factor VIII:C, varies from 50 to 150% of average normal and therefore the size of the plasma pool makes a difference, as does the method of storage; some pools are frozen in small volumes and others are partially purified and freeze-dried. In order to resolve these differences, international standard or reference plasmas have been prepared for a range of factors.

The patient's plasma volume is estimated and the number of units that must be added to the volume to raise the factor concentration to the desired level is calculated. In mild and moderately deficient patients who have an initial factor level, the 'starting level' must be subtracted from the desired level to obtain the actual increase needed; in severe haemophiliacs with levels of 1% or less, the desired rise is obviously equal to the desired level. Units to be given = desired rise (units/ml) × plasma volume (ml).

The patient's plasma volume can be estimated; in adults, the blood volume is usually about 70 ml/kg body weight in the male and 63 ml/kg in the female. In children the blood volume is approximately 75 ml/kg. When the PCV is in the normal range, the plasma volume may be estimated directly as 4% (adults) or 5% (children) of the body weight, or more simply 40–50 ml/kg. Another arbitrary calculation which can be used in a normally proportioned patient with normal PCV is that one unit of factor VIII/kg will give a 2% rise in factor VIII concentration. With factor IX, however, one unit/kg results in only about 1% rise in factor IX activity, i.e. there is a *lower recovery*.

The factor levels necessary for haemostasis in different types of bleeding episodes depend on many variables, including the site, type and degree of injury, the rate of bleeding and the duration of bleeding prior to treatment. In general, replacement of the deficient factor to a level of 30% of normal activity is usually sufficient to control moderately severe bleeding. Treatment of more severe haemorrhages requires higher levels and/or repeated or sustained replacement therapy, i.e. every 12 hours. Haemostatic levels are maintained for long periods by repeated infusions at regular intervals. When intermittent injections are used, an initial 'loading' dosage is given to raise the level to approximately twice the minimum level desired, and then further doses (equal to one-half the loading dose) are given at intervals. The dosage frequency is determined by the rate of disappearance of the factor from the plasma.

Both factor VIII and factor IX show biphasic exponential disappearance curves (*Figure 16.3*). The rapid, first phase of disappearance represents (1) the combined effects of equilibration of the clotting factor between the intra- and extravascular fluid; and (2) the loss of activity of the factor. The more gradual, second-phase disappearance represents only the rate of catabolism of the molecule after equilibrium has been reached. Numerous studies of the disappearance of VIII:C activity after infusions of plasma, Cohn fraction 1, cryoprecipitate, intermediate and high-potency concentrates and concentrates of animal factor VIII have produced similar findings – a first-phase disappearance rate of 5–7 hours, and a second-phase disappearance rate of about 12 hours. Factor IX has a more rapid first-phase disappearance rate (1.5–4 hours) and a longer second-phase half-life (variously estimated at 18–40 hours, with the majority of studies centering around 24 hours). Some haemophilia A patients are infused at shorter intervals to allow for saturation of the extravascular compartment, followed by 12-hourly doses to maintain levels above the desired minimum.

The same protocol is followed with factor IX-deficient patients, despite the longer second-phase half-life, as the very rapid first-phase disappearance results in a fall in factor IX concentration to only about 40% of the initial level of 12 hours

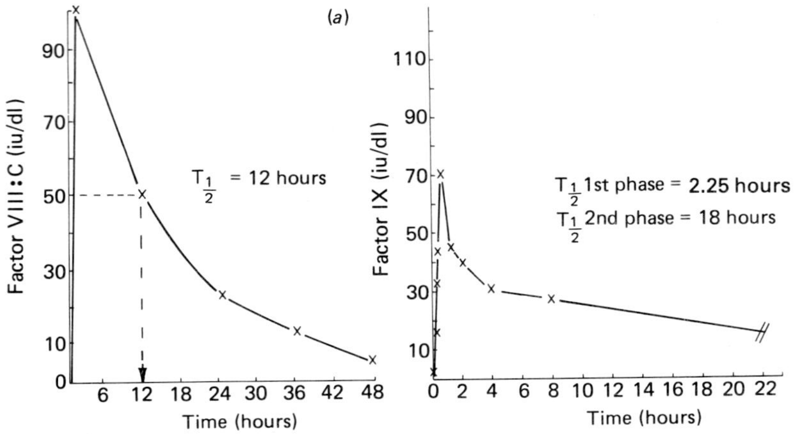

Figure 16.3 (*a*) The fall in factor VIII: C activity *in vivo* after an infusion of factor VIII. (*b*) The fall in factor IX activity after an infusion of factor IX concentrate. Note the short first-phase fall. This may be due to factor IXa being present in the preparation. If so it would be removed by natural inhibitors, e.g. ATIII

after a single injection as is found with factor VIII (*Figure 16.3*) and repeated infusions for several days are required for saturation of the extravascular compartment. Only when therapy is to be continued beyond 4–5 days can there be a change to 24-hourly doses. The desired factor VIII or IX level can also be maintained by continuous infusion of concentrate.

Home treatment

Prior to the development of concentrates, the limited use and effectiveness of plasma transfusion led to delayed treatment and joint deformities which may be irreversible. The introduction of concentrates has made treatment both effective and convenient.

Home transfusion treatment programmes have been shown to reduce absence from school or work by 70%, the frequency and length of hospitalization by 85%, the number of out-patient visits by 76% and the cost of treatment by 50%. Most importantly early adequate treatment by home transfusion may retard or prevent the development and/or progression of crippling joint changes. Early treatment of bleeding episodes may also help other consequences of haemophilia. The reduced absence from school or work results in better education and training and consequently greater employment opportunities, and it may relieve some of the social and economic pressures on haemophiliacs. The greater freedom and ability to live relatively normal lives may help to relieve the emotional stress in haemophiliacs and their families.

Use of vasopressin analogues in the treatment of mild haemophilia and vWD

Although coagulation factor replacement is the method of choice in the control of haemorrhage in deficiency states, alternative approaches are available. The intravenous or intranasal administration of a synthetic vasopressin, deamino-d-arginine vasopressin (DDAVP), to normal subjects and patients with mild factor VIII:C deficiency or vWD results in a measurable rise in the plasma level of the factor VIII complex. DDAVP apparently stimulates vascular endothelial cells to release part of the factor VIII molecule and, incidentally, plasminogen activator. In severe factor VIII:C deficiency there is no rise in plasma factor VIII:C following the administration of DDAVP.

Treatment of patients with antibodies directed against factor VIII

The development of antibodies to factor VIII complicates replacement therapy. Despite the heterogeneity of these antibodies their activity can be summarized as having:

1. Specificity within the factor VIII complex and directed mainly against VIII:C.
2. Differences in specificity to VIII:C from other species, e.g. less active against porcine VIII:C than human VIII:C.
3. Specificity within the coagulation system.

The presence of VIII antibodies results in inhibition or neutralization of VIII:C activity and often results in standard regimens of replacement therapy being totally ineffective. Available approaches to treating patients with VIII antibodies are:

1. Factor VIII concentrates in high dosage.
2. 'Prothrombin complex' concentrates.
3. Factor VIIa.
4. Porcine factor VIII.
5. Plasmapheresis in combination with factor VIII therapy.
6. Immunosuppressive therapy.

Factor VIII concentrates in high dosage

The success of this approach depends on the level of inhibitor and whether the patient is a 'low' or 'high' responder. Levels of inhibitor below 5 Bethesda units/ml plasma can be neutralized by large amounts of factor VIII. If the patient is a 'low' reponder a rise in inhibitor over 5 units/ml would not be expected and factor VIII therapy should be continued. In a 'high' responder a rise in inhibitor level will occur around the fifth day of treatment, although effective haemostasis may have been established by that time.

'Prothrombin complex' concentrates

Concentrates are available containing variable amounts of factors II, VII, IX and X. Two types are available: non-activated (Konyne, Proplex) and activated[29] (FEIBA, Autoplex). The mechanism by which the factor VIII inhibitor activity is 'bypassed' is not fully understood but probably results in Xa formation.

Factor VIIa preparations

Purified VIIa was shown to control bleeding in haemophilia A patients with inhibitors[30]. Studies with recombinant factor VIIa (rVIIa) have provided evidence that VIIa can activate factor X in the absence of tissue factor (TF)[31].

Porcine factor VIII

Early preparations of factor VIII from animal sources were associated with adverse reactions: anaphylaxis, strongly antigenic and thrombocytopenia due to the presence of a 'platelet aggregating factor'. Polyelectrolyte-purified porcine factor VIII (Hyate) preparation appears to have overcome some problems and is useful when an antibody does not cross-react with porcine material.

Other therapeutic approaches
Plasmapheresis combined with high-dose factor VIII:C is usually reserved for patients resistant to other therapies and immunosuppressive therapy is also not a treatment of choice. The long-term administration of frequent small doses of factor VIII is claimed to induce immune tolerance in some patients.

Acquired coagulation defects

Acquired defects in the haemostatic mechanism can occur in individuals who have no history of bleeding. The defect, usually of an 'acute' nature, may involve platelets, coagulation factors and/or fibrinolysis.

Clinical conditions associated with acquired coagulation defects include:

1. Intravascular coagulation, either disseminated (DIC) or localized.
2. Liver disease.
3. Blood disorders.
4. Malignant and non-malignant proliferations.
5. Pregnancy.
6. Renal disease.
7. Dysproteinaemias.
8. Acquired inhibitors to coagulation factors.
9. Coagulation problems of the new-born.
10. Drug-associated conditions.
11. Surgical procedures or trauma.

Disseminated intravascular coagulation syndrome (DIC)

DIC is defined as a disorder in which there is systemic activation of the coagulation cascade. Thrombin is generated resulting in consumption of clotting factors and platelets and possible activation of the fibrinolytic mechanism.

Pathogenesis

DIC itself is not a primary event, but occurs as a result of conditions that 'trigger' the process:

1. Tissue activation. Tissue factor enters the circulation and in association with factor VII activates the coagulation process. This mechanism is associated with surgery, chemotherapy, malignancy, obstetric problems, trauma and snake venoms.
2. Damage to the vascular endothelium and exposure of collagen. This is associated with shock, bacterial infection or antigen–antibody complexes and may result in activation of the fibrinolytic pathway (plasmin, complement, kallikrein).
3. Reduced hepatic clearance of activated factors by the liver. The reticuloendothelial system and the liver are responsible for the rapid uptake and clearance of 'activated' products. In liver disease this mechanism fails, and, with the simultaneous failure of the synthesis of the liver-dependent factors, levels fall and the natural inhibitory factors such as antithrombin III (ATIII) and antiplasmin can be overwhelmed and the haemostatic balance disturbed.

Diagnosis of DIC

DIC is diagnosed by a combination of the following criteria:

1. Clinical and laboratory changes indicating activated products in the plasma resulting in disordered coagulation.
2. Clinical conditions associated with DIC.
3. Secondary fibrinolysis.

Laboratory diagnosis of DIC

There is no single test available to make the diagnosis of DIC. This is because of the complex interrelationships between the various components of the coagulation process, and because thrombin cannot usually be measured directly. Only the indirect effects of thrombin can be observed, such as:

1. Decreased levels of coagulation factors (VIII:C, V, I) due to utilization and destruction.
2. Intermediate products from the prothrombin molecule will yield a prothrombin peptide which can react with factors Xa, V and phospholipid in the prothrombin complex yielding more thrombin and amplifying the system further.
3. The sequence thrombin + fibrinogen → fibrin causes hypofibrinogenaemia due to fibrin formation.
4. Thrombin may potentiate platelet aggregation and the release reaction, resulting in thrombocytopenia and acquired storage-pool defects.
5. Factor XIII may be depleted.
6. The plasminogen → plasmin pathway (via factor XIIa) may be activated, resulting in reduced plasminogen, fibrinolysis and production of monomers which may inhibit polymerization and form circulating soluble complexes with fibrinogen or FDPs.

DIC screening tests

1. PT: prolonged due to reduced levels of factors V, II and I.
2. Thrombin time: prolonged due to reduced fibrinogen or increase in FDPs (NB: the effect of heparin therapy must be excluded).
3. APTT: prolonged due to decrease in factors VIII, II, V and I.
4. Reptilase time: prolonged in combination with a prolonged thrombin time. A normal result suggests heparin effect. If both tests are abnormal hypofibrinogenaemia, dysfibrinogenaemia or FDPs may be found.
5. Plasma fibrinogen: quantitation helps to decide the treatment and severity of DIC.
6. Paracoagulation tests (ethanol gelation): indicate circulating fibrin monomers.
7. FDP screen.
8. Platelet count: *very senstitive* indicator of DIC; thrombocytopenia seen in the majority of cases.
9. Blood film: morphological changes of microangiopathic haemolytic anaemia due to vessel occlusion with fibrin may be seen in *some* examples of DIC, notably in thrombotic thrombocytopenic purpura (TTP) and in association with mucin-secreting adenocarcinoma.

Other tests include factor assays, measurement of ATIII, tissue activators and fibrinolytic activity.

Clinical manifestations of DIC

1. Generalized oozing from more than one site.
2. Local haemorrhage.
3. Petechiae/purpura.
4. Thrombotic/embolic episodes.

Note that as well as 'acute' DIC, a 'chronic' state can occur when a balanced state is present between rate of synthesis and rate of degradation of clotting factors.

Problems associated with DIC screening

1. Factor levels may not fall to a level which will produce an abnormal test result.
2. High levels of FDPs may not necessarily prolong clotting tests.
3. Screening tests for fibrinogen may not be sufficiently sensitive.
4. Initial levels of factor I, VIII (as acute-phase proteins) may be raised, e.g. postoperatively or in pregnancy, and consumption may only produce a 'normal' level.
5. A *fall* in FDPs may indicate consumption of fibrinogen and fibrinogen depletion.
6. Distinguishing between primary and secondary fibrinolysis.
7. Complications due to the transfusion of stored blood which is depleted in VIII:C and V.

'Intravascular coagulation' is not necessarily 'disseminated'. Apart from venous and arterial thrombus formation, fibrin deposition may be localized or 'organ-specific', e.g. the fibrin deposition in haemolytic uraemic syndrome and other renal diseases, and intravascular coagulation in haemangiomas and dissecting aneurysms, are reflected by increased fibrinogen turnover and increased FDPs often with a reduced platelet count and red-cell fragmentation.

Primary fibrinolysis

Fibrinolysis, the removal of formed fibrin clots, is a continuous physiological process mediated by plasmin. Fibrinolysis may be *primary* or *secondary* (as in DIC) and when increased can cause bleeding.

The main cause of bleeding associated with excessive fibrinolysis relates to:

1. Plasmin destroying factors V, VIII:C and fibrinogen.
2. Plasmin→fibrin→fibrinolysis→FDPs→inhibition of platelet function and blood coagulation.

The underlying cause may be (1) excess circulating activator (as in carcinoma of prostate), tissue anoxia or surgery; (2) reduced clearance of plasminogen activator; (3) leukaemic processes releasing cellular proteolytic enzymes. *Table 16.8* summarizes the main differences between the two disorders and it is essential that primary or secondary fibrinolysis is accurately identified as there are differences in treatment.

Coagulation abnormalities in liver disease

Coagulation abnormalities occur in 85% of patients with hepatocellular disease.

Table 16.8 Coagulation factors and components of the fibrinolytic system in disseminated intravascular coagulation (A) and primary fibrinolysis (B)

Factor/component	*A*	*B*
Fibrinogen	Low	Low
Factor II	Low	Normal
Factor V	Low	Low
Factors VII, X	Normal	Normal
Factor VIII:C	Low	Low
Thrombin clotting time	Prolonged	Prolonged
Plasminogen	Normal to low	Low
Plasminogen activator	Absent	Present (?)
Plasmin inhibitor	Normal	Low
Fibrin(ogen) degradation products	Present	Present
Antithrombin III	Low	Normal

Bleeding complications are seen in 15% of these patients. Abnormalities are usually the result of one or more of the following:

1. Decreased synthesis of clotting factors.
2. Increased utilization of clotting factors.
3. Production of abnormal clotting factors.
4. Platelet abnormalities.

The patterns of clotting abnormalities seen in liver disease are not specific for any single clinical cause.

Vitamin K-dependent factors in liver disease

Vitamin K-dependent factors are often diminished in liver disease. In cirrhosis and hepatitis it is common to find decreased levels of factors VII (half-life 4–5 hours), followed by prothrombin (half-life 72 hours), factor IX (half-life 20–24 hours) and factor X (half-life 40–45 hours). Mechanisms other than half-life must operate in determining the levels of these factors in liver disease. The prothrombin time and specific factor VII assays correlate with the level of serum albumin (a measure of hepatic synthesis) but not the bromosulphophthalein (BSP) retention test (which assesses hepatic excretory function). Factor VII levels of less than 8% of normal carry the worst prognosis for patients with advanced liver disease. Lowered levels of the vitamin K-dependent factors are noted earlier in liver disease than are the other coagulation factors, but do not necessarily indicate a poor prognosis.

Vitamin K deficiency can cause a decrease in factors II, VII, IX and X and can mimic the coagulation abnormalities in liver disease. Therefore, vitamin K deficiency secondary to diet, malabsorption, surreptitious or therapeutic warfarin ingestion, or the administration of broad-spectrum antibiotics must be excluded as a cause of reduced factors II, VII, IX and X activity.

Isolated acquired deficiencies of single clotting factors, i.e. prothrombin, factor VII and factor X have been reported in liver disease; factor X has been reduced in association with amyloidosis and factor VII deficiency has been noted in congenital hyperbilirubinaemia (Gilbert, Dubin–Johnson and Rotor syndromes).

Acquired hypofibrinogenaemia

In acute or chronic liver disease there may be reduced circulating levels of plasma fibrinogen. Laboratory findings may show:

1. Reduced fibrinogen levels.
2. Increased fibrinolysis.
3. Reduced half-life of fibrinogen.
4. DIC.

Acquired dysfibrinogenaemias [32]

In acute or chronic liver disease there may be an associated dysfibrinogenaemia characterized by prolonged thrombin and Reptilase clotting times and an unusually translucent clot due to the formation and release into the circulation of abnormal fibrinogen molecules with altered sialic acid residues. The severity of the disease can be correlated with appearance of the dysfibrinogen, and with even temporary recovery normal fibrinogen synthesis is re-established.

Although the concentration of normal and abnormal fibrinogen may be elevated in liver disease, the biological half-life of fibrinogen, as measured by disappearance of radiolabelled fibrinogen, is shortened. This may be a consequence of excess sialic acid residues and diminished galactose content noted in several abnormal fibrinogens. The structurally abnormal fibrinogen found in liver disease shows abnormal fibrin monomer polymerization.

Other non-vitamin K-dependent factors

Factor VIII:C activity is increased in liver disease even when there is advanced hepatic insufficiency. This clinical observation favours the existence of extrahepatic sites of VIII:C formation. In some patients with fulminant hepatic failure, VIII:C activity has been observed to be subnormal, suggesting the presence of concurrent consumption of factor VIII due to DIC, fibrinolysis or both. A low VIII:C level is a sign of serious and perhaps fatal liver disease.

Factor V levels are frequently decreased in liver disease and are usually an indication of serious hepatocellular damage. Decreased levels of factor XIII, ATIII and other factors produced in the hepatocyte are also found, presumably because of decreased synthesis and/or increased utilization of these factors. Factor XII level has also been reported to be decreased and together with factor V used as an indicator for liver transplantation.

DIC in liver disease

DIC and secondary fibrinolysis occur when 'thromboplastic' substances from hepatic cellular necrosis are released into the circulation. These events lead to the generation of thrombin and other activated factors, which the damaged liver is unable to clear from the blood. The generation of thrombin is the central event in DIC and accounts for the laboratory phenomena that are found in liver disease when DIC develops. *Table 16.9* outlines the theoretical sequence of events that occur when DIC accompanies hepatic disease.

Circulating thrombin leads to the generation of fibrin and consumption of fibrinogen; factors II, V, VIII:C and XIII; platelets; plasminogen and

Table 16.9 Disseminated intravascular coagulation in liver diseases

Trigger mechanisms
(A) Release of hepatic 'thromboplastic' substances
(B) Impaired hepatic clearance of coagulant factors

Primary events
(A) Generation of prothrombin activator:
Utilization of V and VIII:C
(B) Conversion of prothrombin to thrombin:
Utilization of prothrombin
(C) Actions of thrombin:
- (1) Destruction of factors V and VIII:C
- (2) Conversion of fibrinogen to fibrin monomer:
Utilization of fibrinogen
- (3) Activation of factor XIII:
Utilization of factor XIII
- (4) Platelet aggregation and formation of platelet thrombi
- (5) Conversion of plasminogen to plasmin (?):
Utilization of plasminogen
- (6) Complexes with antithrombin:
Utilization of antithrombin

Secondary events
(A) Secondary fibrinolysis:
- (1) Proteolysis of fibrinogen and fibrin with formation of degradation products X, Y, D and E:
  - (a) Fragment X–(i) clottable with thrombin, delayed polymerization
  - (b) Fragment Y–(i) inhibits fibrin polymerization; (ii) interferes with platelet function
  - (c) Fragment D–(i) inhibits fibrin polymerization; (ii) inhibits platelet aggregation
  - (d) Fragment E–(i) inhibits platelet aggregation
- (2) Degradation of factors V and VIII:C
- (3) Plasmin–antiplasmin complex:
Utilization of antiplasmin

(B) Effects of circulating fibrin monomer:
- (1) Complex with fibrinogen:
Formation of soluble fibrin monomer complexes
- (2) Complex with fibrin(ogen) degradation products:
Formation of soluble fibrin monomer complexes

antithrombin. Fibrin degradation products as well as soluble fibrin monomer complexes are present in the serum and can be detected by appropriate tests. Although these changes are typical of DIC, they can also be seen in liver disease without a consumptive process. For example, diminishing clotting factor levels could also be explained by several concurrent events such as decreased synthesis of clotting factors and inhibitors.

Several approaches have been used to distinguish DIC from diminished synthesis of clotting factors secondary to hepatic insufficiency. For example, heparin has been administered to patients with liver disease, and in some cases this has resulted in amelioration of thrombocytopenia and hypofibrinogenaemia, decrease of the fractional and total catabolic rate of fibrinogen and increase of the half-life of ^{125}I-labelled fibrinogen. These types of studies suggest that in some cases of liver disease, consumption of clotting factors partially accounts for the decreased factor levels. Measurement by radioimmunoassay of fibrinopeptide A has also been used to distinguish DIC of liver disease from the diminished synthesis of clotting factors. A radioimmunoassay for human thrombin has also been used to measure the generation of thrombin *in vivo*.

Other haemostatic defects in liver disease

Thrombocytopenia seen in hepatic dysfunction may be explained by congestive splenomegaly, folate deficiency, alcoholism or non-specific marrow suppression. Defective hepatic clearance mechanisms may lead to the persistence of fibrin split products and plasminogen activators in the circulation. Qualitative platelet defects, as evidenced by a prolonged bleeding time, have been noted in many patients with liver disease.

Principles of treatment

The treatment of the bleeding patient with hepatic disease and abnormal coagulation parameters is controversial. Generally, the treatment of choice is the replacement of deficient clotting factors. Plasma is the ideal replacement as it contains all the vitamin K factors as well as factors V, VIII:C, fibrinogen and ATIII. Plasma volume considerations, which may limit the usefulness of plasma tranfusion, can sometimes be overcome by plasmapheresis. Platelet concentrates should also be administered as indicated.

Prothrombin-complex concentrates have been used in patients with liver disease to replace the vitamin K-dependent factors. Some concentrates contain more factor VII coagulant activity than others, but they do not contain factor V or ATIII. These preparations have resulted in thromboembolic complications, especially in liver disease.

Malignancy and acquired coagulation defects

Disseminated malignancy may produce changes in the coagulation mechanism by either reducing factor levels or by increasing the levels of factors that cause thrombotic tendencies. The commonest manifestation is DIC caused by: (1) direct activation of the coagulation pathway by tumour 'products' via release of thromboplastins, (2) damage to endothelial cells or circulating cells that trigger or inhibit coagulation reactions (e.g. promyelocytic leukaemias); and (3) association with malignant paraproteinaemia (myeloma, Waldenström's macroglobulinaemia, cryoglobulinaemia, cryofibrinogenaemia, hyperviscosity syndromes).

In the presence of a paraprotein abnormal bleeding may occur due to:

1. Thrombocytopenia.
2. Qualitative platelet defects (coating of platelet membrane).
3. Disturbed fibrinogen–fibrin reactions.
4. Inhibition of coagulation factors (reversible inhibition).
5. Increased fibrinolysis.

Macroglobulinaemia with its paraprotein (molecular weight $>10^6$ daltons) shows similar bleeding tendencies to those in myeloma. Cryoglobulinaemia, due to abnormal globulins which precipitate at temperatures below 37°C, has an associated thrombocytopenia and decreased platelet adhesiveness. The disturbances found in cryofibrinogenaemia are related to the abnormal fibrinogen precipitation causing fibrinolysis and defibrination. The hyperviscosity syndrome with its high plasma paraprotein results in abnormalities of platelet function, thrombosis and tissue hypoxia.

Pregnancy

Pregnancy may be associated with bleeding or thrombotic complications such as:

1. Low-grade DIC with acute or chronic phases.
2. Acute DIC or 'defibrination syndrome' following abortion, abruptio placenta, placenta praevia and other obstetric complications.

Renal disease

In both acute and chronic renal disease there is a tendency towards either thrombosis or bleeding. Common findings are:

1. Prolonged bleeding times with normal platelet count.
2. Decreased adhesion and aggregation of platelets.
3. Increased levels of factor VIII:C, fibrinogen and plasminogen activators.
4. Increased fibrinogen turnover.
5. Decreased fibrinolytic potential (decreased urokinase), together with increased plasminogen activators.
6. High molecular weight FDPs (X and Y) in both plasma and urine.
7. Abnormal prostaglandin metabolism (PGI_2).
8. Decreased ATIII.

Coagulation problems in the new-born

In addition to the hereditary defects in coagulation or platelet function which may be manifest at birth, neonates – particularly the premature infant – have physiological abnormalities of blood coagulation and platelet function and are susceptible to DIC.

Coagulation mechanism
The activity of the coagulation pathway progressively increases from the tenth week of gestation but even in the full-term normal infant activity has not reached the level of the adult. The main abnormality concerns the vitamin K-dependent factors (II, VII, IX and X) which can be only 20–40% of adult levels. Levels of factors V and VIII:C are normal but low levels of XII and XI have been demonstrated. Although the fibrinogen level is normal, a fetal form of fibrinogen is present and is associated with a prolonged plasma thrombin time.

Primary haemorrhagic disease of the new-born
This usually occurs within the first 3 days of life and is an exaggeration of the physiological deficiency of the vitamin K-dependent factors. It is rarely observed when the infant is fed cows' milk as opposed to human milk and is due to the higher vitamin K content of cows' milk. Vitamin K supplementation will correct the defect.

Hepatic immaturity or liver disease
This presents with similar findings to vitamin K deficiency but is not infrequently complicated by the presence of DIC.

DIC
DIC may be triggered by infection, hypoxia or respiratory distress syndrome and there is usually a consumptive element in neonatal liver disease.

Platelet function
This is abnormal in the neonate despite a normal platelet count and is due to abnormal responses to aggregating agents, abnormal platelet factor 3 and nucleotide release, and reduced levels of 5-hydroxytryptamine.

Diagnostic approach
Problems associated with the collection of blood samples from the neonate, including the high PCV and proportion of plasma to citrate anticoagulant, can affect many investigations. Nevertheless, successful identification of haemorrhagic disorders is possible though some investigations may not be possible, e.g. platelet studies, because of the small sample volumes. Investigations should include: family history, full blood count and film examination, prothrombin and APTT, fibrinogen and FDP screen and factor V and VIII assays; all these tests may be performed on capillary blood samples.

Pathological inhibitors of blood coagulation

Pathological inhibitors are by definition not normally found in plasma. Their presence may be associated with a haemorrhagic diathesis. They act as circulating anticoagulants, and can act against single factors (e.g. VIII:C, IX) or against stages of the coagulation cascade (e.g. interference by a paraprotein). In some cases they are produced in response to therapy, e.g. inhibitors to factor VIII:C in haemophilia A, or may occur spontaneously (acquired vWD). Where a single factor is compromised life-threatening bleeding can occur, whereas when a series of reactions are inhibited, bleeding is unusual but thrombosis may occur.

Inhibitors of specific factors

Factor I
Acquired inhibitors of fibrinogen have been reported which interfere with fibrin polymerization[33], fibrinopeptide A[34] and antibodies against fibrinogen following transfusion of patients with congenital afibrinogenaemia.

Factor II
Inhibitors to prothrombin are very rare[35].

Factor V
Inhibitors of factor V have been reported[36]; they have occurred spontaneously but have been noted after treatment with streptomycin and in association with myeloproliferative disorders.

Factor VII
Specific inhibitors of factor VII have not been described.

Factor VIII:C
Inhibitors of VIII:C are the most frequent inhibitor directed against a single factor of the coagulation cascade. They are found in 5–10% of *severe haemophiliacs* (*see* page 594) and occasionally in *mild haemophilia* following treatment. They may occur spontaneously in *non-haemophiliac* patients: in older people with no other associated illness, in association with pregnancy, in drug allergy, collagenous

vascular disease (especially SLE and rheumatoid arthritis), exfoliative skin disease, inflammatory bowel disease, neoplasms and in association with paraproteins. Most non-haemophiliacs with spontaneous factor VIII antibodies are *low responders*, and the antibody appears to be directed against the patient's own factor VIII molecule and not infused material.

vWf[37–39]
The precipitating IgG antibodies that occur in patients with severe homozygous vWD are directed at vWf:Ag, with the indirect loss of VIII:C. Many examples of *acquired* vWD have been described, particularly in association with autoimmune disease, monoclonal immunoglobulins and lymphoproliferative disorders and are due to inhibitors which may be IgG or IgM. The specificity of the inhibitor is directed to the high molecular weight factor VIII component causing molecular dissociation with loss of functional activity in respect of vWf:RiCoF and VIII:C. Although activity against VIII:C is not demonstrable the secondary incremental rise of VIII:C after infusion of plasma or concentrates may not occur.

Factor IX
Spontaneous factor IX inhibitors in non-haemophilia B patients have been described but their occurrence is considerably less frequent than the spontaneous factor VIII antibodies arising in non-haemophilia A subjects.

Factor X
A family with a congential deficiency caused by an 'inactivator' of factor Xa and a 'non-factor X deficient' patient with an inhibitor to factor X have been described.

Factors XI and XII
Factors XI and XII deficiencies are uncommon disorders and inhibitors against these factors have only rarely been described. Examples of inhibitors arising in previously undiagnosed factor XI deficiency following transfusion are well documented[40]. Inhibitor arising in a congenital XI deficient patient, not transfused but with carcinoma of prostate, has been reported[41].

Cases of SLE associated with circulating inhibitors have been described. These patients had normal PT and prolonged APTT and appeared to have a specific factor XI inhibitor. Another patient had an inhibitor that lowered the activity of both factors XI and XII.

Factor XIII
Factor XIII inhibitors have appeared in patients without congenital factor XIII deficiency[42]. In several patients a definite relationship exists between the development of the inhibitor and antibiotic therapy. These inhibitors interfere with fibrin cross-linking in the presence of activated factor XIII.

Tissue thromboplastin
An inhibitor to tissue thromboplastin resulting in a prolonged prothrombin time has been reported[43].

Surgical bleeding

Surgical procedures may result in excessive or prolonged bleeding problems. It is not uncommon for previously undiagnosed mild inherited haemorrhagic disorders to become manifest as a result of surgery. Dental extraction, tonsillectomy and other procedures which depend on normal haemostasis to prevent prolonged bleeding are particularly prone to reveal pre-existing abnormalities.

Haemostatic abnormalities induced by surgical procedures may be due to replacement by transfusion of over 80% of blood volume with stored blood or crystalloid solutions and should be corrected by infusion of FFP and platelets. Colloids such as dextrans, gelatin solutions or human albumin preparations will produce a dilutional effect as well as affecting haemostasis by interfering with the coagulation mechanism or by inhibiting platelet function. Infusion of large volumes of stored blood may induce DIC due to the breakdown of cells and the presence of partially activated procoagulants.

Extracorporeal circulation in cardiopulmonary surgery can result in platelet depletion, coagulation factor deficiencies and DIC. Inadequate heparin neutralization following bypass surgery may result in postoperative bleeding. Primary fibrinolysis following prostatectomy is recognized but is an unusual complication. Excessive bleeding may be found in patients treated with non-steroidal anti-inflammatory preparations and other drugs which inhibit platelet function.

The possibility of inadequate surgical haemostasis must be considered, however reluctantly by the surgeons, when laboratory investigation reveals no abnormality!

Drug-induced coagulation disorders

Clearly, patients being treated with oral anticoagulants, heparin or thrombolytic agents will have an induced coagulation disorder. Over-anticoagulation, inadequate monitoring, synergistic action of other drugs or changes in prescribing may result in spontaneous bleeding or symptoms following minor trauma.

An acquired inhibition of the γ-carboxylation of the glutamic acid residue of the vitamin K-dependent factors is associated with a number of antibiotics of the cephalosporin group. These drugs contain an N-methyl-thio-tetrazole side chain which results in an effect similar to that of the coumarin anticoagulants[44].

Vascular bleeding disorders (non-thrombocytopenic)

Because of its central role in the maintenance of a normal haemostatic mechanism, an alteration to the vessel wall structure or function may lead to disordered 'vascular' haemostasis with a *normal platelet count*. This can be the result of the vessel wall having increased permeability, failure to react and contract following injury or structural abnormalities causing vessel wall weakness.

It is useful to classify vascular disorders as primary or secondary, as follows:

1. Primary, e.g. senile purpura, simple bruising (increased skin fragility), hereditary haemorrhagic telangiectasia (HHT), hereditary connective tissue disorders, e.g. Ehlers–Danlos syndrome, and homocysteinuria.
2. Secondary, e.g. Henoch–Schönlein purpura, dysproteinaemias, drug-induced vasculitis, infection and 'metabolic' purpura.

Primary disorders

Senile purpura

A benign disease affecting elderly patients with characteristic purpuric spots covering forearms and hands. It is believed to be caused by atrophy of the collagen supporting small vessels.

Simple 'easy' bruising
This condition results in many referrals to coagulation clinics and is characterized by purpuric lesions on the arms, buttocks and legs. Laboratory tests often fail to reveal any underlying cause for the purpura which is often benign.

Hereditary haemorrhagic telangectasia (HHT)
HHT is the most common of the hereditary vascular disorders and is transmitted as an autosomal dominant. The vascular abnormalities or lesions appear on the skin or mucosa. Haemostatic abnormalities are associated with the vascular abnormality and include fibrinolysis, abnormal platelet function and low-grade DIC.

Ehlers–Danlos syndrome (EDS)
EDS is characterized by hyperextendable skin, fragile tissues and a tendency to bleed. Many forms of the disorder exist and it is believed to be due to a disorder of connective tissue. It can be transmitted as an autosomal dominant or recessive or as an X-linked recessive trait.

Homocysteinuria
A rare inherited disorder of sulphur metabolism which can be transmitted as an autosomal recessive trait. There are increased levels of plasma homocysteine which can affect intramolecular cross-links required for stabilizing collagen molecules.

Secondary disorders
Henoch–Schönlein purpura
This type of purpura covers a variety of conditions characterized by allergic vasculitis. Common laboratory findings are normal platelet count, high ESR or plasma viscosity and total fibrinogen and normal coagulation screen.

Dysproteinaemias
These disorders include: (1) myeloma, (2) macroglobulinaemia, and (3) cryoglobulinaemia, and may be accompanied by haemostatic abnormalities including thrombocytopenia, abnormal fibrinolysis, circulating anticoagulants or inhibitors, qualitative platelet disorders, low levels of coagulation factor and abnormal fibrin polymerization. Most of these abnormalities are caused by the paraproteins interacting with functional molecules.

Purpura associated with drugs and infection
Drugs can affect the vessel wall by causing changes in permeability or producing immune complexes. Infection, e.g. septicaemia or bacteraemia, may cause direct damage to the vessel wall by circulating toxins.

Metabolic purpuras
This large group includes diabetes, uraemia, scurvy and hypothyroidism.

Platelet disorders

Platelets are essential for the maintenance of a normal haemostatic mechanism (*see* Chapter 2), and alterations to their numbers (*quantitative*) or function (*qualitative*) will affect the dynamic balance of the system. Platelet diseases may be classified according to: (1) decreased platelet numbers (thrombocytopenia); (2) normal platelet numbers (defective function); (3) increased platelet numbers (thrombocythaemia or thrombocytosis); but this is an over-simplification because abnormal function frequently accompanies thrombocytopenia, and thrombocythaemia can be associated with a bleeding tendency which is platelet related. Furthermore, although much discussion centres around platelet deficiencies and the mechanisms responsible for abnormal bleeding, recent research has been oriented towards defining the role the platelet plays in atherosclerosis and the hypercoagulable state. The results of such studies may provide the basis of defining 'new' platelet disorders in the future.

Quantitative disorders of the platelet

The number of circulating platelets is under strict physiological control, with the following characteristics:

1. A survival time in the circulation of 8–10 days.
2. A mean platelet volume of 9.5 ± 1.3 fl.
3. A concentration of between 150 and 400×10^9/l.

The peripheral pool (two-thirds) and splenic pool (one-third) account for most of the platelets in circulation. Marrow-pool kinetics show the following parameters:

1. Marrow megakaryocytes mature in 7–10 days.
2. They each produce between 1000 and 1500 platelets.
3. Most of the megakaryocyte cytoplasm efficiently releases platelets (effective platelet production).
4. Defective platelet production is characterized by abnormal platelet morphology despite normal megakaryocyte appearance.

Thrombocytopenia

The mechanisms responsible for thrombocytopenia are decreased platelet production or increased destruction, utilization, or splenic sequestration.

Decreased platelet production will usually be associated with a decreased number of megakaryocytes in the bone marrow, though ineffective thrombopoiesis can occur analogous to ineffective erythropoiesis. Increased destruction, sequestration or utilization is associated with plentiful megakaryocytes. The concept that effective platelet production is associated with megakaryocyte 'budding' can be shown to be an artefact of platelet aggregation as the appearance is not seen when marrow is collected into EDTA.

Initial investigations will include:

1. Case history and clinical examination.
2. A full blood count (reliance must not be placed on instrument platelet counts).
3. Blood-film examination concentrating on platelet appearances, i.e. morphology, size, shape, and red-cell and leucocyte appearances.
4. A 'template bleeding time' to assess overall platelet function.

Further investigations include:

1. Studies of platelet function including detection of platelet antibodies.
2. Studies of platelet survival.
3. Coagulation screening.

Table 16.10 Causes of thrombocytopenia

Cause	*Examples*
Decreased production	Marrow aplasia Marrow infiltration Myelodysplasia Megaloblastosis Hereditary thrombocytopenias Virus infections Drugs
Decreased survival	Immune mediated: allo- or auto-antibodies AIDS Virus infections Drug-induced
Excessive consumption	Disseminated intravascular coagulation 'Local' intravascular coagulation Microangiopathies Prosthetic heart valves Extracorporeal circulation Structural platelet defects
Sequestration	Splenomegaly

Causes of thrombocytopenia, with some examples, are shown in *Table 16.10*.

A cause of severe (about 20×10^9/l) thrombocytopenia not uncommon to the clinical laboratory is idiopathic thrombocytopenia purpura (ITP). Two forms are encountered: acute and chronic.

Acute ITP

Generally affects children following a febrile (virus) infection. The disorder undergoes spontaneous remission in 80–90% of cases. Transient thrombocytopenia in the neonate occurs when: (1) the mother has ITP, the autoantibody crossing the placenta; and (2) in an analogous situation to haemolytic disease of the new-born, where the mother has been 'immunized' by previous pregnancies but in this case with the formation of antiplatelet antibodies.

Chronic ITP

This type of ITP usually affects adults and has an insidious onset. Petechiae and echymoses are presenting signs. Thrombocytopenia is often in the range 20–80 $\times 10^9$/l while other laboratory tests are usually normal. Platelet survival is short, ranging from hours to a few days and the marrow shows only increased megakaryocytes. It appears to be an autoimmune disorder and has been reviewed extensively[45]. Auto-antibodies may be directed against the GPIb–IX complex.

Thrombocytosis

Thrombocytosis is characterized by a platelet count greater than 400×10^9/l and results from increased and effective production of platelets. However, in some myeloproliferative disorders platelets may be *functionally* defective.

Thrombocytosis is most frequently associated with or secondary to:

1. Malignancy.
2. Inflammatory processes.
3. Iron deficiency.
4. Splenectomy.
5. Drugs.

Thrombocytosis (*see* Chapter 13) is a feature of the clonal proliferation in:

1. Thrombocythaemia (primary thrombocythaemia (PT)).
2. Primary proliferative polycythaemia (PPP).
3. Chronic granulocytic leukaemia.

Qualitative disorders of platelet function

Improved understanding of platelet physiology, ultrastructure and biochemistry has resulted in reappraisal of hereditary and acquired abnormalities of platelet function. Qualitative platelet disorders are either (1) inherited (rare single-gene defects), or (2) acquired (common and of clinical importance). Abnormal mechanisms associated with qualitative disorders include:

1. Failure to adhere to vascular connective tissue.
2. Abnormal aggregation profile.
3. Defective biochemical pathways, e.g. thromboxane synthesis.
4. Abnormal 'secretion' involving intracellular granules.
5. Abnormal contribution to the coagulation pathway (e.g. phospholipid, PF3).
6. Failure to react with circulating plasma proteins (fibrinogen, vWf).

Qualitative inherited platelet disorders

Bernard–Soulier syndrome [46]
This is a rare disorder characterized by:

1. Autosomal recessive inheritance.
2. Moderate to severe thrombocytopenia.
3. Giant platelets.
4. Prolonged bleeding time.
5. Normal aggregation to physiological aggregating agents but a failure to aggregate with ristocetin and bovine fibrinogen.
6. Absence of the platelet membrane glycoprotein heterodimer GPIb–IX.
7. Reduced capacity to adhere to subendothelium.

Bleeding problems may be severe indicating the physiological importance of platelet adhesion in primary haemostasis. The structure of the Bernard–Soulier platelets emphasizes the important interaction between the glycoprotein I complex, vWf and adhesion of platelets to vessel walls.

Laboratory findings in the Bernard–Soulier abnormality are:

1. Normal findings: normal aggregation (with thrombin, ADP, collagen, arachidonate), normal prostaglandin metabolism, and normal release reaction with ADP, collagen and arachidonate.

2. Abnormal findings: bleeding time prolonged, thrombocytopenia, giant platelets, abnormal aggregation (ristocetin, bovine fibrinogen), decreased surface change, decreased sialic acid content, decreased receptor binding, decreased subendothelial adhesion, decreased life span, and absent GPIb–IX.

Bernard–Soulier-like disorders with giant platelets may develop in myeloproliferative disorders, probably as a clonal abnormality. Auto-antibodies blocking the GPIb–IX complex are not associated with changes in platelet morphology.

Glanzmann's thrombasthenia[47, 48]
A rare disorder characterized by:

1. Autosomal recessive inheritance.
2. Normal platelet count and morphology.
3. Prolonged bleeding time.
4. Absent clot retraction (type I).
5. Subnormal clot retraction (type II).
6. Absent aggregation to virtually all physiological aggregating agents.
7. Normal platelet adherence to the subendothelium.
8. Deficiencies in membrane glycoproteins IIb–IIIa.
9. Low (type I) or subnormal (type II) platelet fibrinogen.

It may be the most frequent hereditary qualitative platelet defect. Variation from the characteristic findings suggests heterogeneity in this disorder and includes variation in clot retraction, platelet fibrinogen concentration, amount of GPIIb–IIIa and slight aggregation with ADP and thrombin. Some of these variants may represent asymptomatic heterozygote carriers who may only have a slightly prolonged bleeding time, or molecular variants of GPIIb–IIIa. Quantitative determination of the platelet antigen PL^{A1} or platelet proteins by quantitative gel electrophoresis or using monoclonal antibodies and flow cytometry may be the best way of recognizing heterogeneity and carrier status. The features of Glanzmann's thrombasthenia are as follows:

1. Normal findings: normal platelet count and morphology, normal *shape change* (thrombin, ADP, arachidonate, collagen), aggregation with ristocetin, normal receptor binding (ADP, thrombin), adherence to subendothelium and normal life span.
2. Abnormal findings: long bleeding time; no aggregation with ADP, adrenaline collagen, thrombin or arachidonate; decreased clot retraction; abnormal GPIIb–IIIa; decreased GPIIb–IIIa; decreased PL^{A1} antigen; decreased release reaction with ADP, collagen; and decreased platelet fibrinogen.

'Acquired' Glanzmann's thrombasthenia may account for platelet dysfunction in myeloproliferative disorders and myeloma paraproteins interfere with fibrinogen binding. Auto-antibodies directed against GPIIb–IIIa have been described.

Platelet secretion and storage pool disorders[49]
Until platelet aggregometry was introduced into clinical laboratory practice this group of disorders often went undiagnosed[50]. The findings of variable bleeding tendencies (from mild to moderate severity), inhibition of ADP release, defective collagen-induced platelet responses and absent secondary aggregation in response to ADP or adrenaline are the important diagnostic features of these disorders.

They are functions of defective mechanisms of granular secretion (defective release), defective storage by platelet secreting granules (storage pool defects), or both. Differential diagnosis between the two groups is aided by platelet morphology, estimation of storage granules, measurement of intraplatelet contents and of secreted stored substances, e.g. platelet factor 4, β-thromboglobulin from the α granules, and adenine nucelotides and serotonin from dense granules. Platelet storage and release defects may be inherited or acquired.

Techniques for the measurement of β-thromboglobulin, platelet factor 4 (α granules), adenine nucleotides (ATP, ADP and AMP), 5-HT (dense granules) have supported the findings of abnormal responses with ADP, collagen, thrombin, adrenaline and sodium arachidonate and has resulted in improved classification of a wide variety of hereditary or acquired qualitative disorders which is shown in *Table 16.11*.

Grey platelet syndrome This rare disorder is inherited as an autosomal dominant and refers to the agranular appearance of the platelets in the stained blood film. The defect is due to an absence of α granules and consequently of the associated

Table 16.11 Clinical disorders and laboratory findings in inherited disorders of platelet storage and secretion

Type of defect	*Clinical disorder*	*Laboratory findings*
A. *Storage organelles*:		
Alpha granules (α-SPD)	'Grey platelet' syndrome	1. Deficient in granules and contents (PF4, β-TG) 2. Hypogranular platelets 3. Mild/moderate thrombocytopenia 4. Increased bleeding time 5. Abnormal aggregation with ADP, collagen, adrenaline and thrombin
Dense bodies (δ-SPD)	Hermansky–Pudlak, Chediak–Higashi and Wiskott–Aldrich syndromes. Storage pool disease	1. Prolonged bleeding time 2. Deficiency in dense granules 3. No second-phase aggregation with ADP and adrenaline, no response to collagen, and normal response to arachidonate.
Combined alpha/dense granules (α δ-SPD)		1. Features of both types.
B. *Secretory mechanisms*:		
Thomboxane synthesis	Cyclo-oxygenase deficiency	1. Absent second-phase aggregation, no response to collagen, no response to arachidonate
	Thromboxane synthetase	1. As above
Defective response to weak agonists		1. Poor response to TXA_2 and calcium ionophores 2. Defective formation of arachidonate 3. Defective response to adrenaline 4. Defective response to platelet activating factor (PAF)

SPD = storage pool defect; PF4 = platelet factor 4; β-TG = β-thromboglobulin platelet constituents (alpha-storage pool disease, α-SPD). There is usually a mild thrombocytopenia. Slight abnormalities of aggregation in response to ADP, collagen, adrenaline and, particularly, thrombin are found. The bleeding tendency is generally mild.

Hermansky–Pudlak syndrome This autosomal recessive disorder is characterized by albinism, ceroid-like pigment in macrophages and a bleeding tendency. The platelet count and morphology are normal. The aggregation pattern is characteristic of dense body deficiency (delta-storage pool disease, δ-SPD), i.e. no second-phase aggregation with ADP or adrenaline, no response to collagen and normal response to arachidonic acid. The bleeding disorder may be mild to severe.

Chediak–Higashi syndrome An autosomal recessive disorder characterized by large lysosomal structures in granulocytes in the stained blood film. Thrombocytopenia is usual. The platelet aggregation pattern is typical of dense body deficiency as decribed for Hermansky–Pudlak syndrome above.

Wiskott–Aldrich syndrome This disorder is characterized by thrombocytopenia and microthrombocytes. The mean platelet volume as measured by platelet counting and sizing instruments is 3–4 fl. The disorder is inherited as an X-linked recessive and is also associated with eczema and immunodeficiency. There is a deficiency of dense bodies together with other platelet defects and the aggregation pattern shows poor responses to ADP, adrenaline and collagen. The bleeding manifestations are mainly attributable to the thrombocytopenia.

Defective thromboxane synthesis Whether due to cyclo-oxygenase or thromboxane synthetase deficiency, this disorder is characterized by failure of platelet aggregation in response to arachidonic acid, absent second-phase aggregation to ADP and no response to collagen. An important aspect of diagnosis is to exclude the possibility of cyclo-oxygenase inhibiting drugs.

Defective response to weak agonists This heterogenous group of bleeding disorders encompasses a variety of defects showing abnormalities in platelet aggregation responses to weak agonists and are sometimes associated with macrothrombocytes and thrombocytopenia. The term 'congenital thrombocytopenic thrombopathy' probably includes patients with minor defects demonstrable by aggregation studies.

Acquired qualitative platelet defects [51]

Advances in technology have improved the recognition of acquired qualitative platelet defects as being common causes of clinical bleeding or even thrombotic tendency. As in hereditary storage pool or release disorders the acquired conditions are heterogeneous in nature. *Table 16.12* lists the major clinical disorders associated with the acquired defects.

Drugs and platelet function
The interference of drugs with platelet function is of major importance to any laboratory carrying out platelet function studies. Drugs are the commonest cause of platelet dysfunction by reducing or increasing platelet reactivity. A careful history of prescribed or proprietary drug therapy must be taken before investigating

Table 16.12 Clinical disorders with associated acquired storage pool, platelet function or release defects

Clinical details	*Clinical and laboratory findings*
SLE	Impaired platelet function, normal platelet count
Chronic idiopathic thrombocytopenia	Impaired platelet function when platelet counts are normal
Cyanotic heart disease	Defective response to adrenaline, abnormal 5-HT release
Cardiopulmonary bypass	ADP levels reduced, platelet injury, reduced platelet adhesiveness
Renal disease with uraemia	Bleeding tendency, reduced adhesiveness and retention, defective phospholipid release
Liver disease	Abnormal platelet aggregation, decreased glycoprotein Ib (acquired Bernard–Soulier syndrome)
Dysproteinaemia	Paraproteins interfere with platelet functions
Myeloproliferative disorders:	Associated with bleeding or thrombotic tendencies
Primary thrombocythaemia	Spontaneous platelet aggregation, abnormal platelet function
Primary proliferative polycythaemia	Abnormal platelet function
Chronic granulocytic leukaemia	Abnormal platelet function with ADP, acquired storage pool defect

SLE = Systemic lupus erythematosus

platelet function. Alcohol impairs platelet function and it is not uncommon to investigate patients with bleeding tendencies such as bleeding after dental extraction, bruising, menorrhagia, etc. from whom a history of moderate (70 ml/day) alcohol intake can be elicited. Second-wave platelet aggregation with ADP and adrenaline is reduced. Alcohol withdrawal may be associated with 'rebound' hyperaggregability and may predispose to venous thrombosis and pulmonary embolus [52]. Drugs that affect platelet function are listed in *Table 16.13*.

Figure 16.4 illustrates patterns of platelet aggregation responses with normal platelets and those obtained in various platelet disorders.

Table 16.13 Some common drugs that interfere with platelet function*

Drugs	*Action on platelets*
Platelet cyclo-oxygenase inhibitors:† aspirin, phenylbutazone, indomethacin, sulphinpyrazone	Inhibit endoperoxide production, i.e. thromboxane (TXA_2), prostacyclin (PGI_2)
Prostaglandins: prostacyclin (PGI_2, PGE_1, PGD_2)	Raise cyclic AMP
Membrane drugs: antibiotics, anaesthetics, propranolol	Alter platelet membrane structure and function
Other drugs: heparin, dextran, vinca alkaloids, clofibrate, vitamin E, diuretics, oestrogens, those absorbed in cigarette smoking	Direct effects unknown, although most have been researched

* This list is by no means complete.
† This group, aspirin in particular, have been the subject of intensive research and reviews, because of their effect on platelet prostaglandin synthesis (via their inhibitory effect on cyclo-oxygenase and the production of thromboxane A_2).

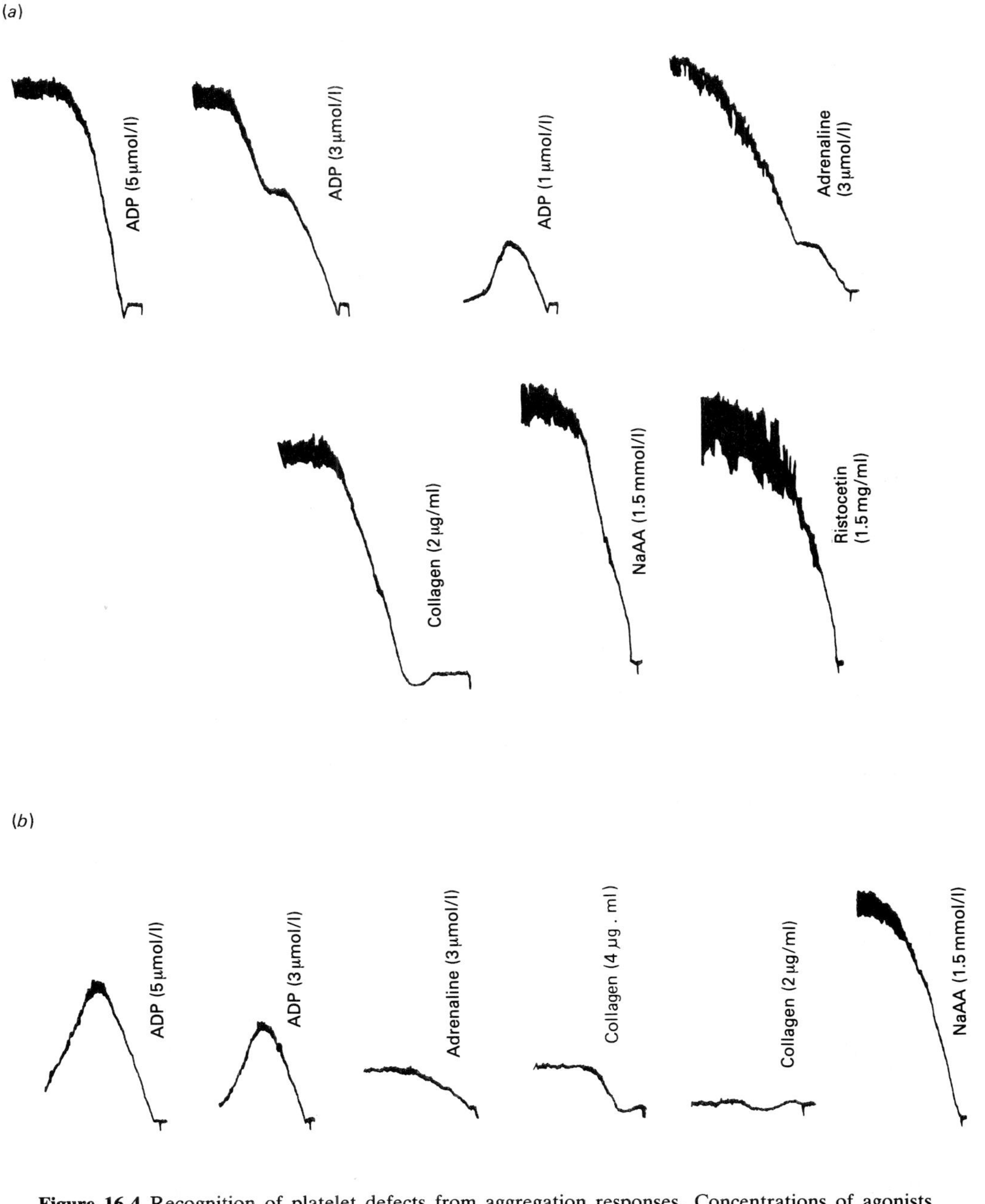

Figure 16.4 Recognition of platelet defects from aggregation responses. Concentrations of agonists represent *final* concentrations. (*a*) Normal responses. (*b*) Storage pool defect: absence or deficiency of dense granules; considerable reduction in releasable ADP; absence of secondary phase of ADP and adrenaline-induced aggregation; defective collagen response; normal response to sodium arachidonate (NaAA); aggregation defects can be corrected by mixing with 'normal' aspirinated platelets. Phospholipase deficiency would give similar responses.

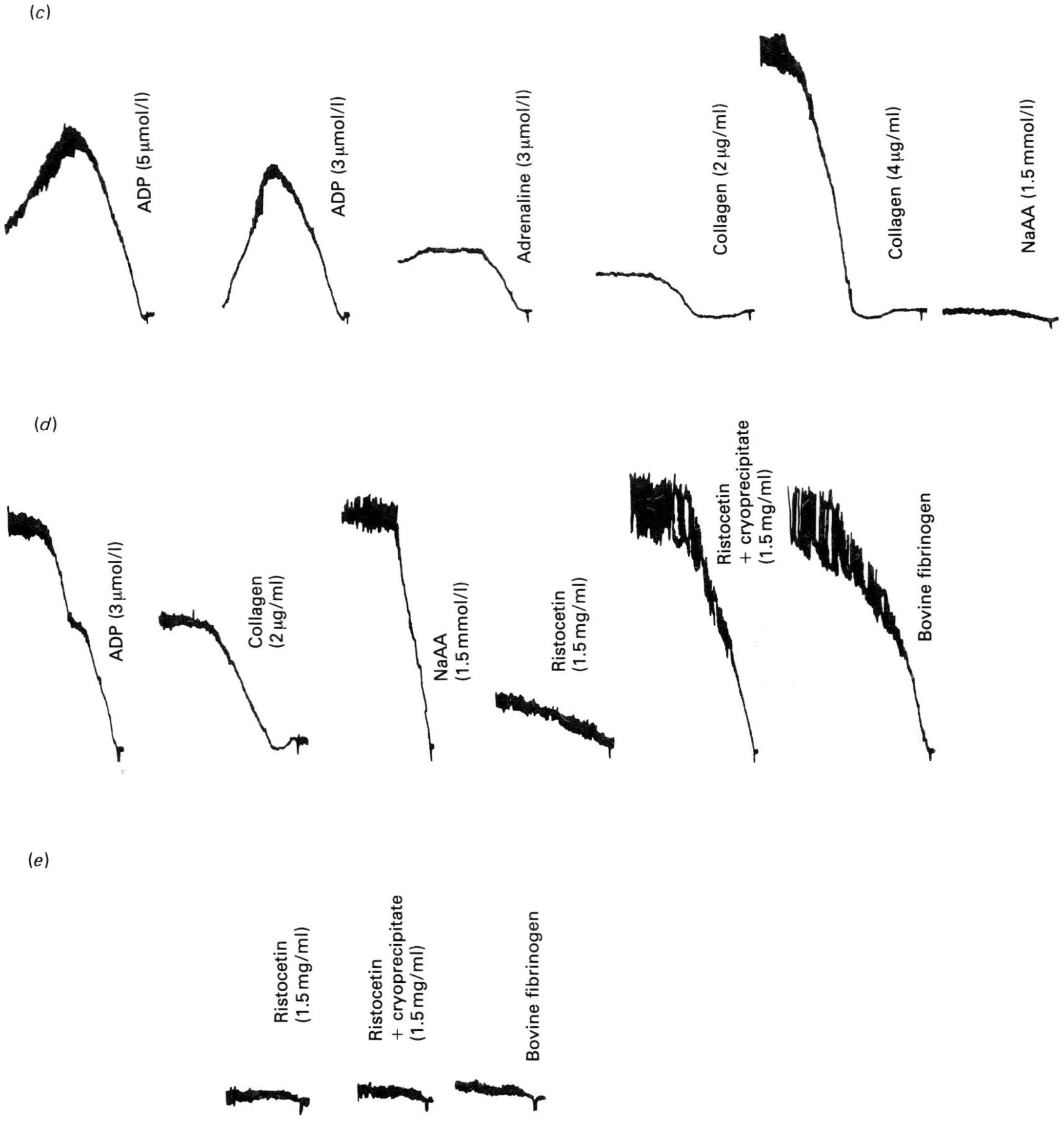

Figure 16.4 (continued) (*c*) Cyclo-oxygenase defect/aspirin defect: lack of secondary phase with ADP and adrenaline; defective response to low-dose collagen (may be corrected by using higher concentrations); no response to NaAA. Similar responses may be seen in congenital thromboxane (TBX) synthetase deficiency. Drugs that inhibit TBX synthetase may give results different from those shown. (*d*) von Willebrand's disease: absent or reduced response to ristocetin (may be corrected by adding cryoprecipitate of normal plasma); normal response to bovine fibrinogen (which is contaminated with vWf:RiCOF); occasionally defective response to collagen. (*e*) Bernard–Soulier syndrome: abnormal response to ristocetin which is not corrected with plasma or cryoprecipitate; no response to bovine fibrinogen.

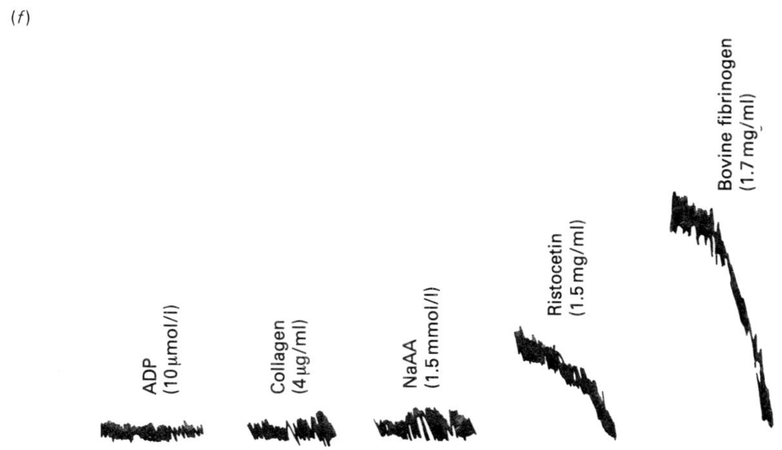

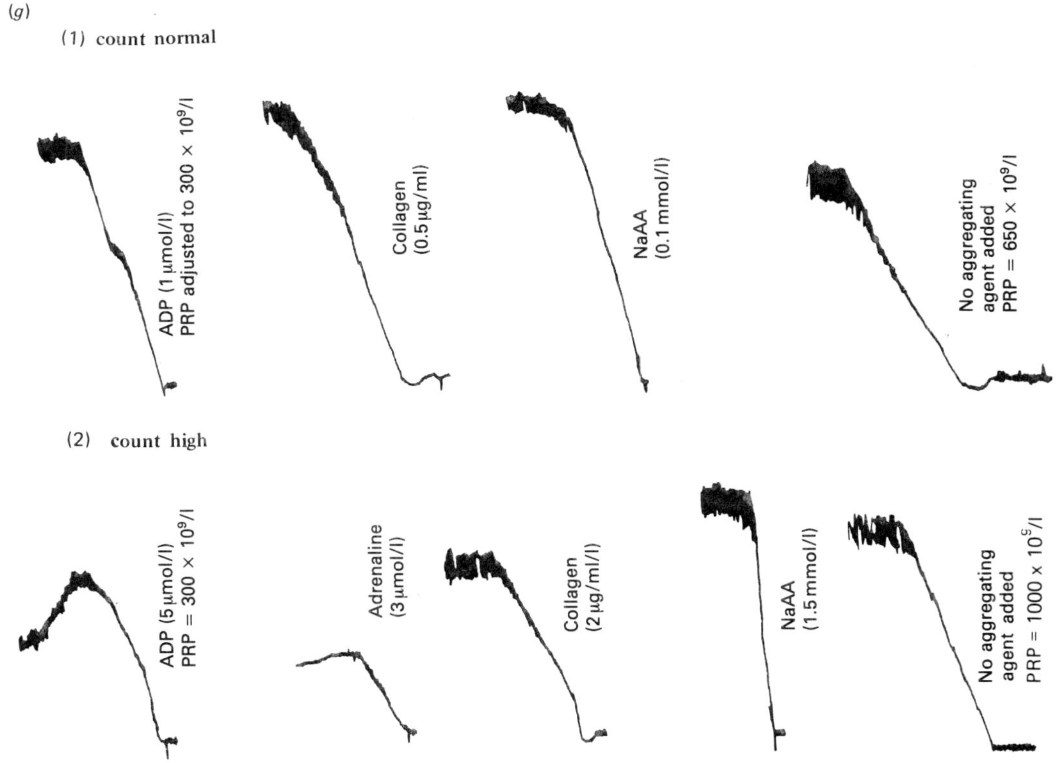

Figure 16.4 (continued) (*f*) Glanzmann's thrombasthenia; no response to ADP, collagen, thrombin, adrenaline or NaAA; some response to ristocetin and bovine fibrinogen. (*g*) Hypersensitive platelets. Example (1): platelet count not excessively high; platelets aggregate spontaneously; increased sensitivity to all aggregating agents. Example (2): very high platelet count causes spontaneous aggregation; at an adjusted platelet count there is evidence of storage-pool type defect (this may be seen in some patients with essential thrombocythaemia and other myeloproliferative disorders); platelets have undergone activation and release in circulation. Spontaneous aggregation is relatively uncommon and these examples illustrate extreme states of hypersensitivity

Investigation of bleeding disorders

Bleeding is a common occurrence. The problem lies in determining whether the bleeding is due to a localized lesion, e.g. gastrointestinal, vascular abnormality of the nasal mucous membranes or due to trauma, or whether the patient has a systemic haemostatic defect. Investigation of bleeding should normally take the form of:

1. Patient's history.
2. Family history.
3. The pattern of bleeding.
4. Physical examination.
5. Laboratory investigation.

Patient's history

Questioning should be directed towards:

1. Establishing whether there is a history of *prolonged* haemorrhage.
2. Establishing whether the prolonged bleeding occurred from more than one site.
3. The form of haemorrhage, e.g. petechiae, purpura, ecchymoses, haematomata, haemarthroses, haematuria, gastrointestinal bleeding, menorrhagia.
4. Establishing whether bleeding occurred spontaneously or after trauma (either accidental or surgical), and in particular direct questioning should determine whether prolonged bleeding (longer than 24 hours) occurred after dental extraction, tonsillectomy, circumcision or umbilical cord separation; dental extraction and tonsillectomy are particularly sensitive indicators of haemostatic efficiency.
5. Drug history: particular attention should be given to analgesic, anti-inflammatory and antihistamine preparations. Many patients do not regard proprietary, unprescribed preparations as drugs and indirect questioning regarding frequency of headaches, muscular or joint pains, dysmenorrhoea, antacids, etc. can be useful in eliciting a history of aspirin ingestion.

It should be remembered that in infants or children a *single* episode of abnormal bleeding may be the first evidence of a hereditary defect and similarly an episode of prolonged bleeding may be the first symptom of an acquired abnormality. Very mild hereditary defects may not be manifest until adult life when trauma or surgery may be complicated by prolonged bleeding.

Family history

A *complete* family tree should be constructed to determine the possibility of an inherited disorder which may be sex-linked recessive, autosomal recessive or autosomal dominant. Careful questioning should include reference to:

1. Siblings, antecedents and descendants who have died, and the cause of death.
2. The possibility of consanguinity.
3. The question of step-parents.
4. The not uncommon and sometimes difficult questions of true parentage and adoption.

A negative family history does not exclude an inherited disorder as the patient may:

1. Have a 'new' mutation.
2. Have distant or unknown affected relatives.
3. Be the only member of the family in which a recessive trait is manifest.

Pattern of bleeding

Bleeding due to vascular/platelet disorders, coagulation defects or consumption of platelets or coagulation factors (with or without fibrinolysis) presents in different ways and is summarized in *Table 16.14*. The pattern of bleeding is important in directing laboratory investigation along particular lines, particularly if the bleeding is acute or severe, e.g. associated with pregnancy, postoperative haemorrhage, or septicaemia.

Table 16.14 The pattern of bleeding in different haemostatic disorders

Vascular/platelet defects	*Coagulation defects*	*Consumption/fibrinolysis*
Usually limited to skin and mucous membranes	Not limited to skin and mucous membranes	No limitation to site of bleeding
Petechiae, purpura, ecchymoses	Bruising common. Subcutaneous or muscular haemorrhages. Haemarthroses	Bleeding from more than one site simultaneously
Immediate bleeding from site of trauma	Bleeding sometimes delayed following trauma	Usually an obvious precipitating cause
Not usually recurrent	Often recurrent from same site or injury	
Bleeding after dental extraction often controlled by local haemostatic measures		

Haematuria and uterine bleeding may be found in each type of defect.

Physical examination

Physical examination is carried out by medical personnel and will include, in addition to current bleeding problems, an assessment of past episodes and in particular the effect of haemarthroses. Close attention is given to the possibility of other disorders that may present with bleeding, e.g. leukaemias, liver disease.

Laboratory investigation

Complex techniques have been introduced for the diagnosis of bleeding disorders, yet it remains possible to recognize most haemostatic abnormalities and make a provisional diagnosis using a minimum number of relatively simple tests, though the final diagnosis and assessment of severity may require more complex procedures.

It is paradoxical that *severe* haemostatic disorders may be demonstrated and identified with a minimum of laboratory tests, whereas patients with *mild* disorders or with doubtful histories often require extensive laboratory investigation using the most sensitive methods available. It is a fact that the great majority of patients referred for investigation do not have a history suggesting a haemostatic defect and it is arguable that they should not be investigated further, particularly by the use of a series of screening tests that are limited in scope and, by their design, are relatively insensitive. Nevertheless, screening for haemostatic defects is often demanded as part of a preoperative 'work-up' and most laboratories have a battery of screening tests in an attempt to cover likely or even unlikely possibilities. Even when the pattern of bleeding in a patient with a definite history of haemostatic defect may indicate which aspect of the haemostatic process is defective, the use of screening tests is still a common approach in many laboratories.

An approach to laboratory investigation

Because of the complexity of the haemostatic mechanism and the range of investigations available, different laboratories may adopt different procedures to satisfy the requirements for:

1. Demonstration of a defect.
2. Identification of the defect (or defects).
3. Assessment of severity.
4. Consequential studies, e.g. recognition of carriers.
5. Monitoring treatment.

Collection of blood samples

Successful laboratory investigation depends upon satisfactory blood samples and these should be taken by staff with a knowledge of the variables that can affect the laboratory results. Important aspects include:

1. Minimum of circulatory stasis.
2. Clean venepuncture to avoid activation.
3. Absence of heparin contamination of blood collected via in-dwelling catheters.
4. Choice of anticoagulant or buffered anticoagulant.
5. Proportion of blood to anticoagulant.
6. The effect of PCV on the proportion of *plasma* to anticoagulant.
7. Handling and separation of plasma to avoid activation and to ensure that time- and temperature-dependent procedures are performed quickly.
8. Recognition of interference by drugs in the haemostatic processes.
9. The effect of stress, emotion and physical activity of the patient on certain parameters.

Screening procedures

Having obtained satisfactory samples a preliminary screening procedure can be performed as shown in *Table 16.15*.

Completion of the above procedures should allow recognition of the great majority of moderate and severe abnormalities. Mild or very uncommon disorders may not be demonstrated. The results may also allow clear recognition that a defect involves either the coagulation, platelet, vascular, or fibrinolytic mechanisms or a combination. A defect in the coagulation pathway may be identified as involving

Table 16.15 Preliminary screening procedure

Test	*Rationale for inclusion*
Haemoglobin, leucocyte count and blood film	Underlying blood disorder (?), platelet morphology
Platelet count	Quantitative values
Template bleeding time	Functional platelet defect (?), capillary abnormality (?)
One-stage prothrombin time	Screen of extrinsic coagulation (factors VII, X, V, II, I, inhibitors)
Activated partial thromboplastin time	Screen of intrinsic coagulation (factors XII, XI, other contact factors, IX, VIII, X, V, II, I, inhibitors)
Thrombin time	Conversion of fibrinogen to fibrin, inhibitors (heparin, FDPs), dysfibrinogen
Clot lysis or euglobulin clot lysis	Screen for fibrinolysis
Solubility of fibrin in urea	Factor XIII availability

FDPs = Fibrin degradation products

phase one (formation of factor Xa), phase two (conversion of prothrombin to thrombin) or phase three (conversion of fibrinogen to fibrin and fibrin stabilization). It is not possible at this stage to differentiate between deficiency and inhibition. *Figures 16.5* and *16.6* show schematic approaches to the interpretation, possible causes and further investigation of abnormalities of the coagulation pathways and platelet disorders, respectively.

An alternative approach is by tabulating the results obtained from screening tests. *Table 16.16* shows the pattern of results with different coagulation factor deficiencies and the further tests that can be used for precise identification. It should always be remembered that combined or multiple deficiencies may be encountered, particularly of the liver-dependent factors and in consumptive coagulopathies. *Table 16.17* shows a similar approach applied to certain platelet disorders.

Table 16.16 Use of prothrombin time (PT), activated partial thromboplastin time (APTT), and plasma thrombin clotting time (TCT) to identify coagulation factor deficiencies

PT	*APTT*	*TCT*	*Deficient factor(s)*	*Further tests*
Abnormal	Abnormal	Abnormal	I	Assay
Abnormal	Abnormal	Normal	II, V, X	Correction studies. Assays
Abnormal	Normal	Normal	VII	Correction study. RVV time. Assay
Normal	Abnormal	Normal	VIII, IX, XI, XII, other contact factors	Correction studies. Assays
Normal	Normal	Normal	XIII	Urea solubility. Correction study. Assay

The possible presence of inhibitors should be revealed by the correction studies.
RVV = Russell's viper venom.

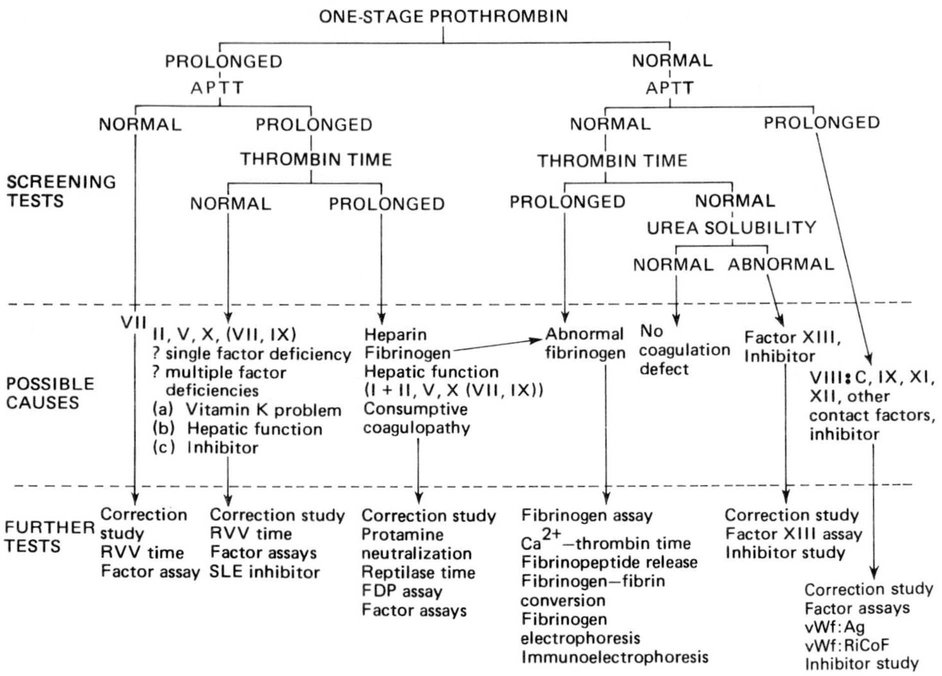

Figure 16.5 A schematic approach to the investigation of coagulation disorders. FDP = fibrin degradation products; RVV = Russell's viper venom; APTT = activated partial thromboplastin time

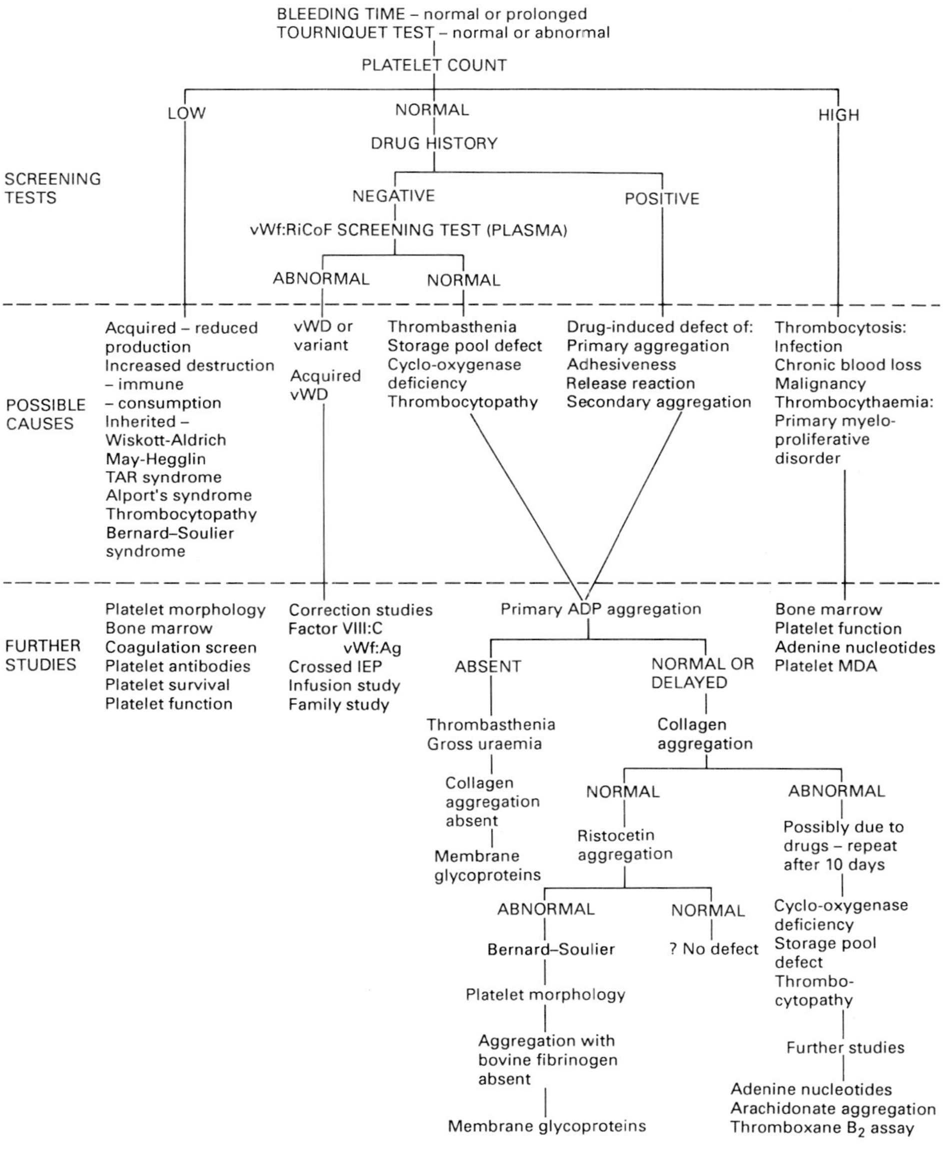

Figure 16.6 A schematic approach to the investigation of platelet abnormalities. IEP = Immunoelectrophoresis; MDA = malondialdehyde

Use of correction studies

The principle of correction studies is to add to the test plasma separate small proportions of normal plasma, adsorbed plasma and aged serum (*Table 16.18*). This approach may be regarded as a 'positive' approach in which *correction* is the significant finding. Absence of correction by the addition of normal plasma indicates the presence of an inhibitor but as the action of an inhibitor may be

Table 16.17 Use of platelet aggregation responses in differentiating certain disorders of platelet function

Aggregation studies				*ADP release*	*Probable disorder*	*Further studies*
Primary aggregation (1st phase)	*Secondary aggregation (2nd phase)*	*Ristocetin*	*Bovine fibrinogen*			
Normal	Normal	Reduced	Normal	Normal	vWD	Correction study
Normal	Normal	Enhanced	Normal	Normal	vWD (IIB)	Assay of VIII:C, vWf:Ag, vWf: RiCoF, 2DCIE
Normal	Normal	Reduced	Reduced	Normal	Bernard–Soulier syndrome	Membrane glycoproteins
Absent	Absent	Normal	Normal	Normal	Thrombasthenia	Membrane glycoproteins
Normal	Reduced	Normal	Normal	Reduced	Aspirin-induced. Storage pool defect. Cyclo-oxgenase deficiency	Thromboxane B_2. Aggregation by arachidonate

2DCIE = two-dimensional crossed immunoelectrophoresis

Table 16.18 Reagents used for correction studies

Reagent	*Factor content*
Normal plasma	All plasma coagulation factors
$Al(OH)_3$ adsorbed plasma	I, V, VIII, XI, XII
Aged serum	VII, X, XI, XII, IX
'24-hour-37°C' oxalated plasma	All except V

immediate (e.g. with factor IX inhibitor) or progressive (e.g. with factor VIII inhibitor), testing soon after addition of the normal plasma and again after 1 or 2 hours' incubation can be informative.

An alternative approach is by demonstrating the absence of, or 'negative', correction by the addition of a series of plasmas with known single-factor deficiency obtained either from subjects with proved deficiency or by preparation in the laboratory by adsorption and by the lability of certain factors in stored or anticoagulated plasma. Plasma may be also depleted of single factors by immune-absorption or antibody neutralization. Failure to correct the defect of the test plasma by the addition of known deficient plasma indicates identical deficiency.

The results of correction studies of a prolonged prothrombin time are shown in *Table 16.19* and of the APTT in *Table 16.20*.

Correction procedures are useful but are qualitative, and in mild deficiency states with only slightly prolonged prothrombin or APTT times a significant pattern of correction may not be obtainable.

Table 16.19 Correction studies applied to a prolonged prothrombin time

Addition of one-fifth volume of				*Factors (s) deficient*	*Further tests*
Normal plasma	*Adsorbed normal plasma*	*Aged serum*	*Oxalated plasma*		
C	C	NC	C	I	Fibrinogen assay
C	NC	NC	C	II	Factor assay
C	C	NC	NC	V	Factor assay
C	NC	C	C	VII, X	RVV time Factor assay
NC	NC	NC	NC	Inhibitor	Protamine neutralization Reptilase time

C = correction; NC = not corrected; RVV = Russell's viper venom

Table 16.20 Correction studies applied to a prolonged activated partial thromboplastin time with normal prothrombin time

Addition of one-fifth volume of			*Factor(s) deficient*	*Further tests*
Normal plasma	*Aged serum*	*Adsorbed plasma*		
C	C	C	XII, XI	Correction with specific deficient plasmas. Factor assay
C	C	NC	IX	Factor assay
C	NC	C	VIII	Factor assay
NC	NC	NC	Inhibitor ? heparin ? specific inhibitor	TCT, protamine neutralization, inhibitor assay

C = corrected; NC = not corrected; TCT = plasma thrombin clotting time

Investigation of increased fibrinolytic activity

Increased fibrinolytic activity is usually secondary to intravascular coagulation and is not uncommon, whereas significant primary fibrinolysis, i.e. without a consumptive coagulopathy, is a rare occurrence.

The recognition of increased fibrinolysis may be by demonstrating the presence of plasminogen activators, monitoring plasminogen levels and the production of free plasmin, or indirectly by the consequences of the action of plasmin on fibrin, fibrinogen and perhaps other substrates.

Tests of increased plasmin production include dilute whole-blood clot lysis, euglobulin lysis time, the use of fibrin plates, plasminogen assay and plasma fibrinogen titre (with and without the addition of protamine sulphate and ε amino-caproic acid (EACA)). The consequences of hyperplasminaemia can be demonstrated by fibrinogen assay, measurement of serum FDP levels and the presence of fibrin monomer. Fibrinolysis secondary to a consumptive coagulopathy may be accompanied by reduced levels of factors VIII:C, V, XIII, ATIII,

Table 16.21 A comparison of certain laboratory investigations in primary and secondary fibrinolysis

	Platelets	*Fibrinogen*	*FDPs*	*Factor II*	*Factor V*	*Factor VIII:C*
Primary fibrinolysis	Normal	Reduced	Increased	Normal	Normal	Normal
Secondary fibrinolysis	Reduced	Reduced	Increased	Reduced	Reduced	Reduced

FDPs = Fibrin(ogen) degradation products.

fibrinogen and platelets, whereas primary fibrinolysis is not associated with the multiple consumption of coagulation factors and platelets. A comparison of the laboratory findings in primary and secondary fibrinolysis is shown in *Table 16.21*.

Quantitative methods

The majority of tests of haemostatic function are qualitative or semi-quantitative and there is usually no simple relationship between the time for the end-point of the reaction or technique and the activity of the factor, or factors, under investigation.

The quantitation or assay of coagulation and other factors of the haemostatic process is necessary for:

1. Confirmation of a suspected defect.
2. Assessment of severity.
3. Monitoring the course of a haemostatic defect.
4. Monitoring therapy.
5. Assay of the activity of plasma fractions or concentrates used for treatment.

Assay procedures can be based on techniques using:

1. Rate of fibrin formation (coagulation factors).
2. Amount of fibrin formed (fibrinogen).
3. Specific antibodies (any factor or component that is antigenic and against which an antibody may be raised).
4. Chromogenic or fluorogenic substrates (components with protease activity).
5. Rate or amount of platelet aggregation (platelet co-factors).
6. Physicochemical methods (fibrinogen, fibrin monomer).
7. Other methods, e.g. luminescence (nucleotides), incorporation of radioactive labels (factor XIII).

With the exception of fibrinogen (measured in g/l), haemostatic factors are measured in mg/l, μg/l or even ng/l, values which usually defy assessment of concentration other than by immunological methods or in certain instances biochemical measurement. Recourse is often made therefore to 'bioassay' methods and comparison with 'normal' activity. A limiting factor in bioassay procedures was a lack of reference preparations. The present availability of reference preparations has allowed comparison of assay methods and the associated variables. The recognition and control of these variables is an important aspect of the day-to-day work of coagulation laboratories.

Assay of coagulation factors is commonly based on the rate and amount of thrombin formation using fibrin formation as the end-point of the reaction. Methods are commonly based on the prothrombin time and activated partial thromboplastin time techniques (one-stage assays) and the thromboplastin generation test (two-stage assays). In all such assay procedures the principle is to provide in excess all the factors necessary for normal thrombin generation and fibrin formation other than the factor to be assayed. Ideally the test system is *totally* devoid of activity of the factor under assay. The corrective effect of the addition of dilutions of the test plasma is compared with the corrective effect of 'standard', 'reference' or 'normal-pool' plasma, the rate of fibrin formation being proportional to the activity of the factor assayed. *Table 16.22* lists assay techniques commonly used for coagulation factors.

Table 16.22 Coagulation factor assays based on a fibrin end-point

Factor	*Technique*
I	Thrombin clotting time of diluted plasma, plasma fibrinogen titre, clot weight, clot opacity
II	One-stage PT, one-stage Taipan snake venom method, two-stage PT
V	One-stage PT
VII	One-stage PT
VIII:C	One-stage APTT, two-stage thromboplastin generation test
IX	One-stage APTT, two-stage thromboplastin generation test
X	One-stage PT, one-stage RVV/cephalin method
XI	One-stage APTT
XII	One-stage APTT
XIII	Weight of stable fibrin

PT = Prothrombin time; APTT = activated partial thromboplastin time; RVV = Russell's viper venom.

The choice of assay technique for the majority of factors is not controversial but the one-stage and two-stage assay of VIII:C is an exception. In general, the performance of each assay is comparable when plasma is assayed against a plasma standard, or concentrate is assayed against a concentrate standard; however, when plasma is assayed against a concentrate or vice versa, the one-stage assay tends to give higher values. Advantages claimed for the two-stage technique are:

1. It is less influenced by activated intermediate products.
2. It is less influenced by changes in the levels of natural inhibitors.
3. It is less influenced by the presence of 'non-specific' inhibitors such as that found in SLE.
4. It does not require a source of plasma totally devoid of VIII:C activity.
5. The low molecular weight coagulant activity is not influenced by the amount of high molecular weight factor VIII present in the substrate plasma used in the one-stage assay.

On the other hand, the difference between one-stage and two-stage values may be in part due to the aluminium hydroxide adsorption procedure of the two-stage assay. The choice between assays may therefore be dictated by the type of material to be assayed and by personal preference. Certainly for routine diagnostic work and for monitoring treatment the one-stage assay can give perfectly satisfactory results. Any assay procedure should fulfil the requirements of specificity, sensitivity, discrimination, and parallelism of standard and test dose response graphs (*see* page 548).

Assays using chromogenic substrates [53]

Chromogenic substrates are short synthetic peptides usually consisting of three amino acids with a chromophore, *p*-nitroaniline (*p*NA), coupled at the C terminal to either arginine or lysine. Enzymatic hydrolysis of the substrates releases free *p*NA which is yellow with a maximum absorption at 405 nm which is quite distinct from the absorption spectrum of peptide-linked *p*NA.

The specificity of the various chromogenic substrates to different serine proteases of the coagulation and fibrinolytic system is determined by the peptide sequence and varies from being virtually specific e.g. S 2222 for Xa and S 2251 for plasmin, to relatively low specificity, e.g. Chr PL is cleaved in varying degree by plasmin, urokinase, thrombin, kallikrein, and other enzymes, though specificity can be improved by the use of selective inhibitors.

Assay procedures are based either on the measurement of the initial reaction rate (kinetic assay) under controlled conditions in the presence of an excess of substrate, or by an end-point technique in which the reaction proceeds for a fixed time and is stopped by the addition of an organic acid. The kinetic assay is more precise but the end-point method is most suitable for large numbers of samples.

The major contribution of chromogenic substrates at present is in providing sensitive and specific assay procedures for factors that were previously difficult to measure, e.g. plasmin, plasminogen and plasminogen activators, the kallikrein system, functional ATIII and low levels of heparin.

Immunological assays

Immunological assays of coagulation factors are particularly useful in distinguishing between absence of functional molecules and the presence of dysfunctional forms and are also routinely used for the measurement of:

1. vWf:Ag (quantitative immunoelectrophoresis, ELISA, 2DCIE).
2. Fibrinogen (radial immunodiffusion (RID), passive agglutination, quantitative immunoelectrophoresis).
3. Fibrin(ogen) degradation products (passive agglutination).
4. Factor XIII (quantitative immunoelectrophoresis).
5. α_1-antitrypsin.
6. α_2-macroglobulin.
7. ATIII.
8. Factor II, VII, IX and X antigens.

Radioimmune assays based on competitive protein binding and immunoradiometric assays (IRMA) can also be used.

Measurement of functional vWf

Assessment of functional vWf activity can be made indirectly by measuring the bleeding time, platelet adhesion (retention in glass bead columns) and by ristocetin aggregation of the patients' platelets. Measurement of ristocetin-induced platelet aggregation is an *in vitro* procedure and does not necessarily completely reflect vWf activity. Nevertheless, the phenomenon is used in assay systems for measuring vWf activity in plasma (RiCoF) using washed normal platelets. There are many reports of monoclonal antibodies which inhibit various aspects of vWf activity and therefore appear to be directed at different epitopes of vWf[54]. Some antibodies result in total inhibition of ristocetin-induced aggregation and can be used in immunological methods as an alternative to RiCoF assay.

Ristocetin co-factor assay (RiCoF)

Principle

The ability of test plasma to aggregate washed platelets in the presence of ristocetin is compared with a reference plasma using a dose-response curve. Various techniques have been used to measure the end-point of the reaction, e.g. optical aggregometry[55], platelet counting using an electronic counter[56,57] and macroscopic aggregation in microtitre plates or in tubes[58,59]. Fixed washed platelets are superior overall to fresh washed platelets and are more convenient.

Preparation of fixed washed platelets

Reagents

1. Acid citrate dextrose (ACD): 0.085 M disodium citrate; 0.064 M citric acid; 0.11 M dextrose. Adjust to pH 4.5 with 0.1 M HCl or 0.1 M NaOH. Sterilize by autoclaving. Store at 4°C.
2. Citrate-saline: 0.15 M (8.76 g/l) NaCl; 0.006 M (1.76 g/l) trisodium citrate. Adjust to pH 7.1 with 0.1 M HCl. Sterilize by autoclaving. Store at 4°C.
3. 4% paraformaldehyde: 18.8 g NaH_2PO_4 $2H_2O$ and 40.0 g trioxymethylene (paraformaldehyde) in 1 litre distilled water. Leave at 56°C overnight to dissolve the trioxymethylene. Cool and adjust to pH 7.3 with 50% NaOH (usually 4–4.5 ml).
4. 0.135 M (21.06 g/l) NaH_2PO_4 $2H_2O$.
5. 1.8% paraformaldehyde. Mix equal volumes of 4% paraformaldehyde and 0.135 M sodium dihydrogen phosphate; to nine parts of the mixture add one part of ACD solution.
6. Storage buffer. 0.05 M (3.4 g/l) imidazole; 0.11 M (6.42 g/l) NaCl; 0.2 g/l sodium azide. Adjust pH to 6.4 with concentrated HCl. Store at 4°C.

N.B. Use reagent bottles with piercable caps to allow sampling without contamination after sterilization.

Procedure A minimum of 50 ml platelet-rich citrated plasma (PRP) is required. Platelets obtained from 500 ml of blood obtained by therapeutic venesection of suitable patients will provide a better yield or, ideally, outdated platelet concentrates. The procedure described is for handling platelet concentrates.

1. Select platelet units free from red-cell contamination if possible. Suspend bags overnight and discard any bag with excess red cells.
2. *Decant* each bag into a sterile 30 ml plastic container. Centrifuge at 170 *g* for 10 minutes to remove contaminating red cells. Decant supernatant PRP into a further 30 ml container.
3. Centrifuge at 1200 *g* for 10 minutes to sediment the platelets (a few remaining red cells may be ignored). Remove supernatant plasma and add 5 ml citrate-saline and resuspend the platelets using a plastic pipette *avoiding bubbles*. Pool the resuspended platelets into a further 30 ml container.
4. Centrifuge at 1200 *g* for 10 minutes and remove supernatant which should be almost clear, and resuspend as above in 5 ml citrate-saline. Make up to 25 ml with citrate-saline and repeat the washing process twice more.

5. Fixation. Remove the supernatant after the final wash and add 5 ml of 1.8% paraformaldehyde to each platelet button. Resuspend the platelets using a plastic pipette, again *avoid bubbles* as much as possible. Leave for a minimum of 2 hours or overnight at room temperature.
6. Washing the fixed platelets. *Add 5 ml of storage* buffer to the platelets in paraformaldehyde. This is an *IMPORTANT* step to dilute the fixative and allow further centrifugation without the formation of aggregates. Resuspend the platelets.
7. Centrifuge at 1200 *g* to sediment the fixed platelets. Remove the supernatant, add 5 ml of *storage* buffer and resuspend. Gentle vortexing is permissible at this stage. Make the volume up to 25 ml with storage buffer and repeat the washing process three times.
8. After the last wash resuspend in 5 ml of *storage* buffer and pool into one container if volumes are appropriate.
9. Count the number of platelets and adjust to 800×10^9/l with storage buffer. Ten units of platelet concentrates will yield up to 200 ml of working, fixed platelet suspension.
10. Store at 4°C. Suitable for use for 4–5 months.

Assay

Reagents

1. Reference plasma.
2. Fixed washed platelets.
3. Ristocetin. The concentration of ristocetin is adjusted to give 3+ aggregation in approximately 15 seconds with a 1 in 3 dilution of normal plasma; this is usually in the range of 4–6 mg/ml which gives a *final* concentration in the test of 1–1.5 mg/ml.
4. Citrated test plasma.

Method Using imidazole buffer pH 7.3 containing 40 mg/ml bovine albumin, prepare dilutions of reference and test plasmas as follows: reference plasma 1 in 3, 5, 10 and 20; test plasma 1 in 3 and 1 in 5. Each dilution is tested at 37°C as follows: in a 75 × 10 mm glass tube, mix 0.2 ml fixed platelets, 0.1 ml diluted plasma and 0.1 ml ristocetin. On additon of the ristocetin start a stop watch and tilt the tube gently over a dark background or a concave mirror and record the time for 3+ aggregation to occur. Each dilution is tested in duplicate and in triplicate if the difference between duplicates is more than 2 seconds. Plot the aggregation times for the dilutions of reference and test plasma on 2 cycle log/log paper. The graphs should be straight parallel lines. Concentration of RiCoF in the test plasma is read from the reference graph and corrected for dilution. RiCoF activity can be expressed in units/ml or as '% normal activity'.
Reference range 60–160% or 0.6–1.6 units/ml.

Notes

1. Though the end-point of the aggregation is to some extent subjective, good precision can be achieved.
2. The addition of bovine albumin to the imidazole buffer for diluting plasmas maintains protein content and reduces the sensitivity of ristocetin aggregation to changes in protein content of the plasma.

Immunoassays of 'functional' vWf

Immunoradiometric assays (IRMA)

Both one-site (fluid phase) and two-site (solid phase) assays have been described for the assay of vWf activity using monoclonal antibodies [60]. Using one-site fluid phase IRMA, the radiolabelled antibody is reacted with antigen (plasma) in fluid and the labelled antibody bound to antigen is separated by selective precipitation using ammonium sulphate and is proportional to the concentration of antigen. Two-site solid phase IRMA is achieved by coating plastic tubes with unlabelled antibody followed by antigen (plasma) and then a second radiolabelled antibody. The radioactivity bound in the second stage is proportional to the concentration of antigen in plasma. Two-site IRMA is generally more sensitive than one-site methods and has been widely applied in the assay of trace proteins. The general procedure is outlined below; the major variables are in determining the optimum dilutions of unlabelled antibody, plasma and labelled antibody.

General procedure for two-site IRMA

Coating Unlabelled antibody is suitably diluted in bicarbonate buffer pH 9.6 and 0.5 ml is added to a series of plastic tubes and placed at 4°C overnight. The tubes are washed once with 3–5 ml of barbitone buffer and once with 4–5 ml distilled water.

Antigen incubation Plasma is suitably diluted in barbitone buffer containing 4% bovine albumin. A standard graph is prepared using dilutions of a reference plasma. All dilutions are assayed in duplicate. 0.2 ml of each dilution is added to coated tubes and incubated at 37°C overnight. Suitable antigen and antibody blank tubes are included. The tubes are drained, washed once with barbitone buffer and again drained.

Incubation with labelled antibody The labelled antibody is suitably diluted and should have an activity of 10–20 000 c.p.m. 0.2 ml is added to each tube and incubated overnight at 37°C. The tubes are placed at 4°C for 24 hours, drained, washed twice with distilled water, drained and the radioactivity measured. Background count is subtracted and the mean value of the duplicate tubes calculated. The bound radioactivity is expressed as a percentage of the total radioactivity added to each tube. The percentage bound radioactivity is plotted against the logarithm of antigen concentration on semilog graph paper.

Enzyme-linked immunoabsorbent assay (ELISA)

Monoclonal antibodies that react with epitopes of vWf:Ag reflect vWf function and can be used in IRMA techniques and should also be suitable for use in ELISA methods. As with IRMA methods the general principles of ELISA methods can be applied to a range of assays. The procedures for ELISA are described in the method given for the assay of vWf:Ag (*see* page 648).

Assay of vWf:Ag by electroimmunoassay (Laurell technique)

Principle

Antigen is placed in a well in an agarose gel containing an appropriate concentration of antibody. On electrophoresis the antigen moves out of the well into the antibody-containing gel. The antigen complexes with the antibody when in optimum concentration and forms a 'rocket' of immunoprecipitate, the height of which is proportional to the concentration of the antigen.

Materials and reagents

1. Electrophoresis equipment incorporating a water-cooled platform (16°C).
2. Water bath at 56°C.
3. Levelling table for pouring the gels.
4. Glass plates, 8 × 8 cm.
5. Agarose.
6. Barbitone-acetate buffer, pH 8.6 (Oxoid, UK), 0.07 I.
7. Anti-vWf:Ag antibody, used at a dilution determined by experiment.
8. Reference plasma.
9. Citrated test plasma.
10. Coomassie Blue staining solution: Coomassie Blue 2 g in 400 ml methanol, 600 ml distilled water and 100 ml glacial acetic acid. Dissolve the stain in methanol using a magnetic stirrer before adding other solutions. Filter before use.
11. De-staining solution: 400 ml methanol, 600 ml distilled water, 100 ml glacial acetic acid. Discard after use.

Method

1. Dissolve 0.15 g agarose in 15 ml distilled water by boiling in a sterile glass container; when dissolved maintain at 56°C in a water bath. Prepare a 15 ml volume for each plate.
2. Prepare barbitone-acetate buffer by dissolving 11.5 g in 1 litre distilled water. Set aside 200 ml for preparation of plates and dilution of samples. The remaining 800 ml is diluted with an equal volume of distilled water (0.035 I) for use in the electrophoresis reservoirs.
3. Clean glass plates thoroughly, finishing with alcohol, and place on the levelling table. Each 8 × 8 cm plate requires 10 ml 1 g/dl agarose solution. Measure 5 ml of 0.07 I barbitone-acetate buffer in a glass container and warm to 56°C. Add 5 ml of the 2 g/dl agarose solution and mix gently avoiding bubbles. To 10 ml of the agarose buffer add 15 μl of anti-vWf:Ag suitably diluted, mix gently and carefully pour on to the levelled glass plate. Allow to cool and solidify. Prepared plates may be stored in a 'wet-box' at 4°C until required.
4. Prepare the electrophoresis equipment using the 0.035 I buffer in the tanks.
5. Cut a row of 3 mm diameter wells in the agarose gel, 2 cm from one edge of the plate.
6. Prepare strips of Whatmann No. 3MM paper to use as wicks.
7. Prepare dilutions of the reference and test plasmas in 0.07 I buffer. For the reference plasma 1 in 2, 1 in 5 and 1 in 10 dilutions are made. Test samples are diluted 1 in 2 and 1 in 5. If low levels of vWf:Ag are expected use neat and 1 in 2 test plasma; if high levels are suspected dilute 1 in 5 and 1 in 10.
8. Place the plate on the cooled platform of the electrophoresis tank with the wells to the cathode side. Place the wicks carefully on each side of the plate ensuring they have been thoroughly soaked in buffer and are making good contact with gel.
9. Pipette 10 μl of each of the reference and test dilutions into the appropriate wells, with the 1 in 2 reference dilution at each side of the plate.

10. Cover the tank and run for 45 minutes at 300 V ensuring that the water cooling is operating. After 45 minutes reduce to 110 V and run for 17–18 hours.
11. After completion of the electrophoresis remove the plates and store in a wet-box for 1 day at 4°C, and then wash the plates in a large volume of normal saline for 1–2 hours.
12. Remove plates from the saline and place on a layer of paper tissues on a level surface. Prepare a double layer of Whatmann 3MM paper of sufficient size to cover the plate and carefully layer over the gel avoiding bubble formation. Cover with several layers of paper tissue and apply an even weight of approximately 2 kg for 20–30 minutes.
13. Carefully remove the paper and dry the gel thoroughly at 37°C or by using a hair dryer.
14. Stain the gel in Coomassie Blue for 20–25 minutes and then differentiate in the de-staining solution until the precipitation peaks are clearly visible, and allow to dry.

Calculation of results

Measure the peak heights in mm from the centre of the wells to the tip of the peak and plot the heights of the peaks against dilution of reference plasma (1 in 2 = 100%, 1 in 5 = 40%, 1 in 10 = 20%) on log/log graph paper and draw a line of best fit through the points. Read off the peak heights of the test plasma from the reference graph; the 1 in 2 dilution is read directly, the 1 in 5 dilution is multiplied by 2.5 and the 1 in 10 multiplied by 5; if neat plasma has been used divide the value by 2. Average the values and correct if necessary for the calibrated value of the reference plasma. Express results in units/ml (100% = 1 unit/ml).

Technical notes

1. Agarose may be stored in suitable volumes in sterile glass containers at 4°C. Boil to redissolve.
2. Barbitone-acetate is relatively insoluble and magnetic stirring is recommended.
3. 10 × 10 cm plates can be used and require 15 ml 1 g/dl agarose and 22.5 μl of antiserum; 12 wells can be cut in these larger plates.

Two-dimensional crossed immunoelectrophoresis (2DCIE) [61]

Principle

Plasma is electrophoresed in one dimension in agarose without antibody. The distance of protein (antigen) migration in the first dimension is estimated by electrophoresis in a second dimension into agarose containing specific antibody.

Reagents and materials

These are identical to those required for the Laurell technique described above.

Method

First dimension 0.15 g agarose is dissolved in 15 ml of buffer by heating. Cool to 56°C and pour onto glass plate or other support medium on a level surface. Cool and store at 4°C for 2 hours in a moist chamber. Wells are cut into the agarose 2 cm from one end of the plate and the plasma sample(s) applied. Electrophorese at a constant 200 V for about 4 hours with cooling. A strip of agarose containing the separated proteins is transferred to a second plate, or alternatively the unwanted agarose is removed leaving the required strip.

Second dimension Agarose containing anti-vWf:Ag is prepared as described for the Laurell method. The molten agarose-antibody is poured carefully on to the plate containing the agarose strip from the first dimension and electrophoresis is repeated at right angles to the original separation. The second electrophoresis is performed at 110 V for 18 hours. Staining and differentiation is carried out as for the Laurell method.

Interpretation
Comparisons are made between normal and test plasma samples of the appearances of the precipitin arcs and the distance migrated by the vWf antigens with particular attention to the position of the precipitin peaks and the shapes of the arcs. Attempts have been made to quantify the 'migration ratios' of the test:normal [62] but this approach is difficult to reproduce.

Enzyme-linked immunosorbent assay (ELISA) of vWf antigen (vWf:Ag) [63]

Principle
Microtitre plates are coated with antibody to vWf:Ag and incubated with diluted plasma; the vWf:Ag in the plasma is bound to the coating antibody. A second, peroxidase-conjugated antibody is added which reacts with the bound vWf. The amount of bound peroxidase-conjugate antibody is determined by colour development of added peroxidase substrate. The colour developed is therefore proportional to the amount of vWf:Ag present in the plasma.

Reagents
1. 0.05 mol/l carbonate buffer pH 9.6 (1.59 g Na_2CO_3, 2.93 g $NaHCO_3$, 0.2 g NaN_3 in 1 litre distilled water).
2. 0.01 mol/l phosphate buffered saline (PBS) pH 7.2 (0.345 g NaH_2PO_4 H_2O, 2.68 g Na_2HPO_4 $12H_2O$, 8.474 g NaCl in 1 litre distilled water).
3. 0.1 mol/l citrate phosphate buffer pH 5.0 (7.3 g $C_3H_4OH(COOH)_3$, 23.87 g Na_2HPO_4 $12H_2O$ in 1 litre distilled water).
4. Enzyme substrate: 80 mg 1,2-ortho-phenylenediamine dihydrochloride in 15 ml citrate phosphate buffer; add 10 µl 20 volumes H_2O_2 immediately before use.
5. vWf:Ag reference plasma.
6. Citrated platelet-poor test plasma.
7. IgG fraction of anti-vWf:Ag antiserum.
8. IgG fraction of anti-vWf:Ag conjugated with peroxidase.
9. 1 mol/l sulphuric acid.
10. Tween 20.

Method
100 µl of anti-vWf:Ag diluted in carbonate buffer is added to each well of a microtitre plate. Incubate for 1 hour at room temperature in a moist chamber. Wash three times with PBS containing 0.5 ml/l Tween, invert and tap to drain. Prepare doubling dilutions of reference and test plasmas from 1 in 10 to 1 in 80 in PBS containing 1 ml/l Tween. Place 100 µl of each dilution and buffer blanks in wells and stand at room temperature for 1 hour. Repeat the washing procedure.

100 µl of peroxidase-conjugated antibody diluted in PBS containing 1 ml/l Tween is added to each well and left for 1 hour at room temperature. Wash the plate twice in PBS containing 0.5 ml/l Tween and once in citrate-phosphate buffer pH 5.0. Add

100 μl of substrate to each well and stand at room temperature for 20 minutes. Stop the reaction by adding 150 μl sulphuric acid to each well.

Read optical densities at 492 nm using a microtitre plate reader and plot optical density against dilutions on log-linear graph paper. vWf:Ag values are obtained by extrapolation from the reference plot.

Reference range: 0.5–1.5 units/ml (50–150% normal activity).

Notes

1. Polystyrene microtitre plates are generally satisfactory but should show uniformity of antibody binding between batches.
2. The optimal dilutions of first and conjugated antibodies are determined by 'chequer-board' titration.
3. Over-coating by using high concentrations of antibody results in reduced assay sensitivity.
4. Coated plates may be stored following washing.
5. Adequate washing is essential between each step of the procedure.
6. Linear graphs can be obtained up to dilutions of 1 in 100 indicating a sensitivity of 0.01 units/ml or less.
7. The activity and amount of hydrogen peroxide is critical for optimum colour development.
8. In vWD variants, non-parallelism between control and test dose-response curves may be found.

Multimeric analysis of vWf

The structure of vWf can be further studied by electrophoresis in polyacrylamide gels (PAGE) containing agarose and sodium dodecyl sulphate (SDS). The SDS disperses molecular aggregates and imparts a uniform electrical charge on the subunits. Polyacrylamide gels have a much smaller pore size than agarose gels, thus impeding the movement of high molecular weight proteins while permitting low molecular weight proteins to migrate more rapidly. Separation is therefore based principally on molecular size rather than electrical charge[64]. The separated protein components can be visualized by a variety of techniques including autoradiography using labelled antibody, electroblotting with immunoenzyme staining, and by luminescence enzyme immunoassay.

Normal vWf shows a range of high, intermediate and low molecular weight multimeric components, each composed of a 'triplet' of bands. To obtain maximum information regarding multimeric structure both 'low resolution' gels (low agarose concentration) to differentiate vWf type I from type II, and 'high resolution' gels to permit further resolution of type II subtypes, should be used. A multicentre comparison of sizing techniques[65] demonstrated the importance of variations in the conditions of electrophoresis.

Detection of inhibitors

Method A: Detection of inhibitors using the kaolin–cephalin time or the one-stage prothrombin time

Principle

Varied proportions of test and normal plasmas are mixed and incubated at 37°C and aliquots of the mixtures tested by the KCCT and/or one-stage PT to demonstrate: (1) the failure of normal plasma to correct a prolonged time; and (2) the ability of test plasma to prolong the clotting time of normal plasma.

Method
Normal and test plasma are mixed in the proportions shown in *Table 16.23*. Prepare each mixture at 2 minute intervals to permit testing at fixed times after mixing normal and test plasmas. After 5 minutes incubation at 37°C, 0.1 ml aliquots of each mixture are tested by the KCCT or one-stage PT as appropriate. The procedure is repeated after 15, 30 and 120 minutes incubation even if the first test clearly shows inhibition. High-titre progressive inhibitors may show prolongation of clotting times after 5 minutes which may be misinterpreted as having immediate inhibition kinetics unless further, progressive inhibition is demonstrated.

Table 16.23 Proportions of normal and test plasma

	Tube				
Plasma	*1*	*2*	*3*	*4*	*5*
Normal	10	8	5	2	0
Test	0	2	5	8	10

Interpretation
Tube 1 will show the baseline time of normal plasma and tube 5 the initial prolonged time. Any extension of the time for tube 2 beyond 1 or 2 seconds in the PT or 5 seconds in the KCCT must be considered as evidence of inhibition by the presence of the test plasma. Failure of tube 4 to show significant correction of the time for tube 5 is evidence of inhibition. The results of tube 3 may be equivocal depending upon the activity of the inhibitor. The effect of inhibitors that react immediately, e.g. heparin, inhibitors of factors V and IX, anti-phospholipid antibody (lupus inhibitor, SLE inhibitor) can be expected to be apparent after 5 minutes' incubation; progressive inhibitors, e.g. against factor VIII:C, show a progressive effect over a period of incubation.

Method B: Kasper technique [66]

This method is particularly suitable for detection of low levels of progressive inhibitor, particularly against VIII:C.

Principle
Based on the APTT, a high ratio of test:normal plasma is used and a 'delta control' is incorporated.

Reagents
Citrated test plasma (TP).
Normal plasma pool or reference plasma used for VIII:C assay (NP).
Kaolin-cephalin (KC) reagent.

Method
In 75 × 12 mm glass tubes, set up the test as shown in *Figure 16.7*. The difference between the clotting time of the test and normal plasma mixtures incubated together and separately is determined.

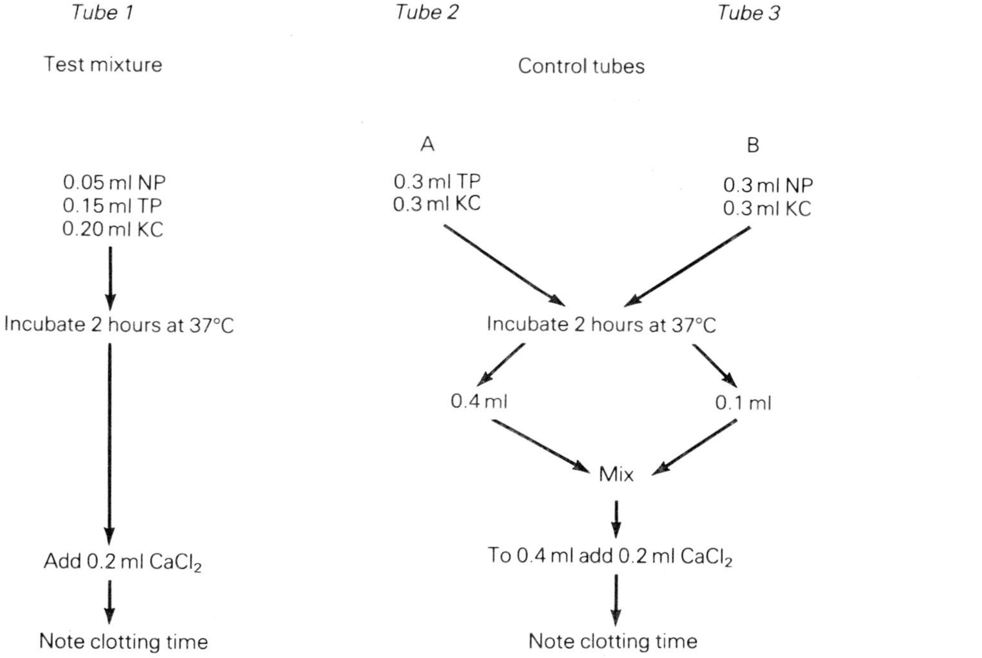

Figure 16.7 Kasper method for detection of inhibitors. NP = normal plasma; TP = test plasma; KC = kaolin-cephalin reagent

Interpretation
The KCCTs of the test mixture and the test/normal plasmas incubated separately are similar if no inhibitor is present. The difference (delta) will exceed 10–12 seconds in the presence of inhibitor.

Notes
1. Delta values exceed 12 seconds in the presence of high or low titre inhibitor.
2. Positive results in this screening test may not be confirmed by inhibitor assay but will result in reduced *in vivo* half-life of infused factor VIII:C.
3. Kaolin is superior to ellagic acid as an activator in the APTT in this method.
4. High titre inhibitors may result in prolonged KCCTs whether incubated together or separately but the delta value always exceeds 12 seconds.

Assay of factor VIII:C inhibitors

Factor VIII inhibitors are classified according to the kinetics of their reaction with factor VIII. Two categories are recognized:

1. Those with simple reaction kinetics by which the antibody can be completely neutralized provided that sufficient VIII:C is present. If further VIII:C is added it is not neutralized and the antigen–antibody complex does not dissociate or possess residual VIII:C activity. They are usually found in patients with classic haemophilia.
2. Those with complex reaction kinetics. On adding VIII:C to the antibody an immediate fast inactivation of the VIII:C occurs. If the reaction reaches equilibrium and more VIII:C is added it may also be inactivated at a similar rate to the first reaction. The antigen–antibody complex may dissociate and may show VIII:C procoagulant activity *in vivo* and in *in vitro* reactions.

Measurement of VIII:C inhibitor can be made by the methods shown in *Table 16.24*.

Table 16.24 Measurements of factor VIII: C inhibitor activity

Technique	*VIII:C source*	*Starting VIII:C level*	*Incubation time* (hours)	*Defintion of one unit of inhibitor*
'Old' Oxford 1-hour technique	Concentrate	100%	1	Destroys 75% of the added VIII:C over 1 hour at 37°C
'New' Oxford 4-hour technique	Concentrate	50–100%	4	Destroys 50% of VIII:C over 4 hours at 37°C
Bethesda	Normal plasma	50%	2	Destroys 50% of the added VIII:C over 2 hours at 37°C

Factor VIII:C inhibitor assay (Bethesda method) [66]

Principle

The Bethesda assay is the method of choice for measuring inhibitors of factor VIII:C. It is based on measuring the residual VIII:C activity remaining after test plasma is mixed with a standard plasma containing VIII:C and incubated for 2 hours at 37°C alongside a control of standard plasma mixed with citrate-saline. The residual VIII:C activity is expressed as a percentage of the residual activity of the control mixture and any inhibitor activity converted to units of inhibitor per ml plasma by the use of a reference graph. One Bethesda unit is defined as that activity that will inactivate 50% of added VIII:C after 2 hours at 37°C.

Reagents

1. Imidazole buffer, pH 7.3.
2. Imidazole buffer, 0.05 M, pH 7.3 containing 0.585 g NaCl/dl.
3. Standard plasma: the source of VIII:C (should contain 1.0 units/ml VIII:C).
4. Test plasma.
5. Plasma containing VIII:C inhibitor previously assayed as an internal control.
6. Reagents for VIII:C assay (*see* page 555).

Method

Mix one volume of standard plasma and one volume of undiluted test plasma and incubate at 37°C. It is recommended that a range of dilutions of test plasma are tested to allow inhibitor levels greater than 1 unit/ml to be assayed. The standard plasma is mixed with an equal volume of buffer and incubated alongside the test mixture. After 2 hours' incubation the test and control mixtures are assayed for VIII:C activity. A reference graph is constructed on log-linear graph paper using the definition that one unit of inhibitor inactivates 50% of added VIII:C as shown in *Figure 16.8*.

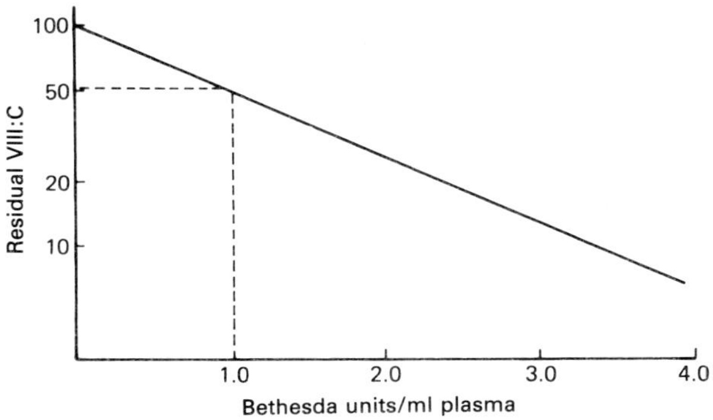

Figure 16.8 Factor VIII:C inhibitor assay: conversion of residual factor VIII:C value to Bethesda units.

A dilution of test plasma with residual VIII:C activity between 25 and 75% may be converted to inhibitor units by reading from the graph and multiplied by the reciprocal of the dilution to give units/ml. Inhibitors with complex reaction kinetics may appear to contain increasing amounts of inhibitor as dilution increases. A dilution which gives a residual VIII:C closest to 50% should be used to calculate the inhibitor level rather than calculating a mean value of dilutions with residual VIII:C between 25 and 75%.

Notes

1. The method can be used to assay inhibitors of factor IX with the incubation time shortened to 30 minutes due to the kinetics of the inhibitor.
2. The Bethesda method uses *plasma* as the source of added VIII:C.
3. It may be difficult to assay levels of inhibitor less than 0.05 units/ml, although the screening test is positive.
4. Inhibitors to porcine VIII:C should be assayed using a standard porcine VIII:C preparation.

Investigation of platelet function

Laboratory tests are used to measure platelet adhesion, aggregation, secretion, prostaglandin production, membrane structure, relationship with the coagulation cascade and response to drugs.

The aim of the laboratory investigation of platelet function is to assess the reactivity of the platelets under well-controlled laboratory conditions and both qualitative and quantitative disorders can be detected in this way (*Figure 16.9* and *see Figure 16.6*).

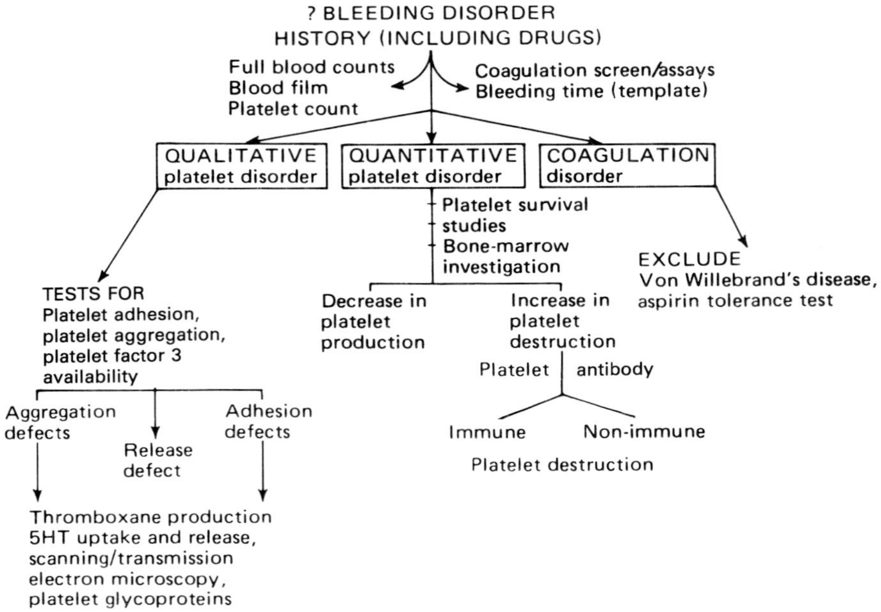

Figure 16.9 The use of platelet function studies in the investigation of a bleeding disorder

Laboratory investigation [67–69]

1. Personal history, including drugs such as aspirin.
2. Full blood count: total count and appearance of platelets.
3. Template bleeding time.
4. Collection of blood, processing and testing within 90 minutes. (N.B. Avoid glass contact during preparation).
5. Platelet adhesiveness;
   (a) Test for physical adhesion, e.g. on glass tubes coated with collagen.
   (b) Test for adhesion-aggregation: platelet retention tests using glass-bead columns.
6. Platelet release reaction:
   (a) Platelet factor 4.
   (b) β-thromboglobulin.
   (c) [^{14}C]5-hydroxytryptamine uptake and release.
7. Platelet aggregation studies by addition of aggregating agents and analysis of aggregation responses.
8. Platelet survival studies.
9. Platelet metabolism, e.g. thromboxane assays.

Thromboxane B_2 assay

Principle

Thromboxane B_2 (TXB_2) is the stable metabolite of thromboxane A_2, the main product of the platelet prostaglandin pathway. This test is now used for the investigation of bleeding and thrombotic disorders.

PRP is stimulated with either collagen or arachidonic acid. After 4 minutes the reaction is stopped by the addition of an equal volume of absolute ethanol. After spinning down the precipitate the supernatant is assayed for TXB_2 by radioimmunoassay.

In addition serum or washed platelets stimulated by thrombin may be used.

Normal range
Arachidonate stimulation, 90–150 pmol/10^7 platelets; collagen stimulation, 5–20 pmol/10^7 platelets.

Interpretation
In cases where an abnormality of the prostaglandin pathway is suspected, this assay may help to determine where the defect lies. For example, if no TXB_2 is produced in response to any aggregation agent, this could be due to cyclo-oxygenase deficiency, thromboxane synthetase deficiency or more commonly aspirin. Aspirin ingestion can sometimes be confirmed by the presence of salicylate in the plasma, but the aspirin effect on platelets persists long after the salicylate is undetectable.

Some patients produce normal amounts of TXB_2 in reponse to arachidonic acid but not to collagen. This indicates that the defect occurs in a step before cyclo-oxygenase. TXB_2 production in Glanzmann's disease is normal.

High levels of TXB_2 have been found in patients with a thrombotic tendency. Some patients with peripheral vascular disease, diabetes and nephrotic syndrome produce higher than normal TXB_2 results although it is a point of debate whether diabetics as a group produce more TXB_2 than normal subjects.

This test is also used to assess the effects of treatment and in platelet survival determinations.

Preparation of samples
1. Stir PRP or washed platelet suspension in an aggregometer with a stimulator of thromboxane production, e.g. collagen, sodium arachidonate (NaAA) or thrombin. After 4 minutes, remove 200 µl and add to 200 µl absolute ethanol in an Eppendorf centrifuge tube. Mix. Store at −80°C until assayed.
2. Serum. Blood in a glass tube is allowed to clot at 37°C for 30 minutes. Centrifuge, remove serum and store at −80°C.

Analysis of platelet nucleotides

Principle
The dense granules or storage pool of the platelet contains ADP but very little ATP, whereas the rest of the cell contains both ATP and ADP. Therefore, in storage pool disorders, both acquired and congenital, there will be a specific lack of ADP (from the dense granules) but no significant reduction of ATP and the ATP:ADP ratio will be raised.

Platelet adenine nucleotides are extracted with perchloric acid and after neutralization are assayed by high-pressure liquid chromatography (HPLC).

Sample preparation for HPLC
Prepare PRP *avoiding contamination with red cells*. Perform a platelet count on the PRP. Take 3 ml PRP with a platelet count of 300 × 10^9/l or equivalent, e.g. 1.5 ml

at a count of 600 × 10^9/l. Place in a 4 ml plastic tube and add dipotassium EDTA according to the following formula:

$$\frac{\text{Platelet count of PRP } (10^9/\text{l})}{300\ (10^9/\text{l})} \times 40 \times \text{volume PRP (ml)} = \mu\text{l EDTA (10 g/dl)}$$

Mix well and centrifuge at 1200 *g* for 20 minutes at 4°C. Decant off the supernatant and discard. Free the platelet button by vortex mixing; this is very important – the platelet button must be well dispersed otherwise nucleotide extraction will be incomplete. Store at −80°C to prevent degradation of nucleotides.

ATP release: luciferin-luciferase method [67]

Principle
When a platelet aggregating agent is added to platelet-rich plasma in the presence of luciferin-luciferase, the ATP released during platelet aggregation will react with the luciferin in a light-emitting reaction:

$$\text{ATP} + \text{luciferin} \xrightarrow[\text{luciferase}]{Mg^{2+}} \text{adenyl luciferin}$$

The light released is measured and recorded by the lumiaggregometer.

Reagents
Luciferin-luciferase 40 mg/ml (Sigma)
ATP standard 100 µM (Sigma)
Arachidonic acid, sodium salt 15 µM (BioData)
Collagen 40 µg/ml (Hormon-Chemie, Munich)

Method
1. Take 18 ml blood into 2 ml 0.19 M sodium citrate in a plastic container, using a 19 G needle and minimum stasis.
2. Prepare platelet-rich plasma (PRP) as for platelet aggregation studies.
3. Prepare platelet-poor plasma (PPP) by centrifuging the remainder of the sample for 10 minutes at 2000 *g*.
4. Adjust platelet rich plasma count to 200 × 10^9/l with PPP.
5. Using 500 µl PPP and 450 µl PRP, add the appropriate amount of freshly prepared luciferin-luciferase (25 µl for collagen, 50 µl for arachidonate) to the PRP in a cuvette in the aggregometer and warm for 1 minute.
6. Add 50 µl of the appropriate agonist.
7. Observe the aggregation and record the luminescence in terms of peak height.
8. When the aggregation is complete add 20 µl (2 nmol) of ATP standard and record the peak height. Then further add 30 µl (3 nmol) of the ATP standard and again record the peak height. Ideally the luminescence peak height should fall between that of the two standards, so if the luminescence peak is low use less standard, such as 10 µl and 15 µl.
9. Plot the standard concentrations as nmoles against peak heights and read off the release peak obtained with each agonist.

Calculation
ATP release is expressed in terms of nmol/10^8 platelets.

$$\text{ATP release} = \frac{\text{nmoles ATP released}}{\text{No of platelets} \times 10^8 \times 0.45}$$

(0.45 is the volume of PRP in the cuvette in ml).

Interpretation
Laboratories should establish their own normal ranges. Reduced ATP release indicates a platelet release defect.

[^{14}C]5-Hydroxytryptamine uptake and release (imipramine method)

Principle
PRP is incubated with [^{14}C]5-hydroxytryptamine (5-HT) and at 30, 60 and 90 minutes aliquots are taken and the amount of 5-HT uptake is expressed as a percentage of the total uptake at 90 minutes, at which time uptake is at a maximum. Imipramine is then added to prevent any further uptake which might produce misleading results when leakage and release are to be studied. A further aliquot is taken 30 minutes after the addition of imipramine to determine the amount of 5-HT which has leaked from the platelets, i.e. that which had entered the platelets but had not been taken into the dense granules. Aliquots of the remaining PRP are then stirred in an aggregometer with either added collagen or incubated with thrombin to measure induced 5-HT release.

Reagents
Imipramine hydrochloride, 31.5 mg in 5 ml distilled water.
Thrombin, 500 units/ml.
Collagen, 40 μg/ml.
Stock [^{14}C]5-HT, 0.01 mmol/l (about 0.4 μCi), stored in 0.5 ml amounts at −20°C.
Streptokinase, 25 000 units/ml, store at −70°C when reconstituted.
PRP, 300×10^9/l.

Method
Prepare 14 counting vials each containing 2 ml scintillation fluid. Add 0.5 ml of 5-HT to 4.5 ml PRP, mix gently and place at 37°C and start a timer. Immediately remove 100 μl into each of two counting vials; the activity represents 100% activity. At 30, 60 and 90 minutes remove 0.5 ml and centrifuge at 1200 *g* for 10 minutes and remove duplicate 100 μl volumes for counting; the loss of activity represents *uptake*. At 90 minutes add 3 μl imipramine (final concentration = 2×10^{-5} mol/l). Leave for 30 minutes at 37°C and remove 0.5 ml, centrifuge, and count 100 μl supernatant in duplicate; any increase in activity represents *leakage*. Remove 1 ml and add 10 μl thrombin and 10 μl streptokinase. Leave on a rotary mixer for 10 minutes, centrifuge, and count 100 μl volumes of supernatant in duplicate to measure *release by thrombin*. Remove duplicate 300 μl volumes of the incubation mixture and place in aggregation cuvettes and add 30 μl of 40 μg/ml collagen (final concentration 4 μg/ml). Stir for 5 minutes, centrifuge, and count duplicate 100 μl volumes to measure *release by collagen*. All samples are added to scintillant and counted in a liquid scintillation counter.

Calculation
Take the average of the duplicate counts.

$$1.\ \%\ \text{uptake} = \frac{\text{Total count} - \text{uptake count}}{\text{total count}} \times 100$$

Calculate uptake at T30, T60 and T90 minutes.

$$2.\ \%\ \text{leakage} = \frac{\text{leakage count} - \text{T90 uptake count}}{\text{total count} - \text{T90 uptake count}} \times 100$$

$$3.\ \%\ \text{release} = \frac{\text{release count} - \text{leakage count}}{\text{total count} - \text{leakage count}} \times 100$$

Interpretation
Platelets are one of the main storage sites for 5-HT which is actively accumulated from the plasma by energy-dependent processes. The association of 5-HT with other storage constituents such as adenine nucleotides in the dense bodies make it a suitable parameter for assessing disorders such as storage pool defects. In this heterogeneous group of disorders lack of dense granules leads to:

1. Impaired uptake.
2. Defective release of labelled amines following collagen stimulation.
3. Rapid reflux from the platelet, which is reflected by 'significant leakage values'.

Defective uptake and release can be found if:

1. The metabolic processes are impaired.
2. There are defects in the prostaglandin pathway leading to abnormal release with collagen despite normal 5-HT uptake.

Preparation of platelets for electron microscopy

Reagent
Freshly prepared glutaraldehyde, 1.2 ml 25% glutaraldehyde and 8.8 ml sodium dacodylate buffer, pH 7.4. Use dust-free plastic ware for all manipulations.

Method
Prepare sufficient PRP to provide a reasonable sized 'platelet-button' after centrifugation. Add 2 ml PRP to 20 ml glutaraldehyde and fix at room temperature for 1 hour. Centrifuge at 1200 *g* for 5 minutes at *room temperature* (cooling to 4°C damages the tubular system of the platelets). Discard the supernatant and re-suspend the platelet button in a minimal amount of buffer.

Measurement of platelet survival using ^{51}Cr labelling

Principle
The platelets from a 500 ml donation of blood are labelled with [^{51}Cr]sodium chromate and reinfused. Post-infusion samples are collected at intervals for 5 days and from the remaining radioactivity a survival curve is plotted.

Collection of blood
A plastic donation pack containing ACD anticoagulant and with two satellite transfer packs is used to collect 500 ml of blood.

Preparation of platelet concentrate

The blood is centrifuged at 16°C and 200 *g* for 30 minutes to obtain PRP, which is separated into a satellite pack. Recentrifuge the PRP at 1200 *g* for 15 minutes and transfer the PPP supernatant to the second transfer pack leaving 15 ml of plasma to re-suspend the platelet concentrate.

Introduce 800 μCi [^{51}Cr]sodium chromate to the re-suspended platelets, mix well and leave at room temperature for 20 minutes. To wash the labelled platelets re-introduce the PPP to the labelled platelets but retaining 30 ml of the PPP in a syringe. Centrifuge the re-suspended platelets at 1200 *g* for 15 minutes and express *all* the contaminated PPP back to the second transfer pack for proper disposal. Introduce the 30 ml of PPP to the deposited, labelled, washed platelets and after re-suspension take up 20–30 ml in a syringe for infusion, without filtration, to the patient. Only approximately 15% of the added ^{51}Cr will have been taken up by the platelets. The red-cell concentrate may be reinfused to the donor (or patient).

Sampling

Duplicate samples (A + B) of blood (13 ml) are taken into 0.4 ml 5 g/l EDTA at 2 minutes and at 1, 3, 8, 24, 36, 60, 72, 96 and 120 hours after reinfusion of the labelled platelets.

Preparation of samples for counting

There are two approaches to the counting of the remaining activity of the labelled platelets. The platelets can be separated from the whole blood by preparing PRP, re-suspending the red cells in saline and again taking the 'platelet-rich' supernatant saline which is pooled with the PRP. Alternatively the activity of the whole-blood samples is counted and the total counts corrected for any red-cell labelling that may have occurred and for any activity in PPP. The latter approach is described below.

Although blood may be stored it is preferable to process the samples as they are collected. Tube A is centrifuged at 1200 *g* for 15 minutes to deposit all the blood cells. The PPP is carefully transferred to a further tube 'C' taking care not to disturb the buffy layer and leaving a small volume of plasma. Sample tube 'B' is centrifuged at 200 *g* for 15 minutes to sediment the red cells, the supernatant plasma is taken off and discarded and the sedimented red cells washed three times with 0.154 mol/l NaCl. The washed red cells are re-suspended in 5 ml 0.154 mol/l NaCl and the PCV determined. Tube A contains all the blood cells with a small volume of plasma, tube B contains washed red cells and tube C contains plasma without cells. The amount of plasma remaining in tube A is considered to be one-tenth of that in tube C.

Calculation

Radioactivity of platelets is calculated from the following formula:

$$\text{Remaining platelet radioactivity} = \mathrm{A} - \left(\frac{C \times 1}{10}\right) - B_{\mathrm{corr}}$$

where A = radioactivity of platelets plus red cells plus a small volume of plasma,

$$B_{\mathrm{corr}} = \mathrm{cpm}\ B \times \frac{\mathrm{PCV\ of}\ A}{\mathrm{PCV\ of}\ B}$$

C = radioactivity of PPP.

The radioactivity of the remaining platelets is plotted against time of sampling or as percentage of the 2-minute sample. Plots should be made on linear and semi-log paper to obtain information regarding loss of platelets from the circulation, i.e. as a function of time or as a random function.

Interpretation
Mean platelet life span is normally 8–11 days with a half-life of 3.2–5.5 days, i.e. a non-linear function.

Notes
1. The measurement of platelet life span may be combined with determining the sites of platelet sequestration by surface scintillation counting.
2. Time zero (T_0) is considered to be when half the platelets have been infused.
3. In the investigation of thrombocytopenic patients, blood-group compatible normal platelets may be used.

Aspirin-platelet regeneration time

Principle
Aspirin irreversibly acetylates platelet cyclo-oxygenase; 600 mg aspirin is sufficient to block the enzyme activity completely and therefore abolish TXB_2 production. Since platelets cannot synthesize protein (cyclo-oxygenase), thromboxane production will be zero for the whole life span of the aspirin-treated platelets. Daily TXB_2 assays after a dose of aspirin will then show a steady rise, to return to pre-aspirin levels due to TXB_2 production by new platelets entering the circulation. When all the 'old aspirin-treated platelets' have been replaced thromboxane generation should equal pre-aspirin values. The time taken for this to occur is the platelet regeneration time which in normal subjects is 8–10 days, i.e. equivalent to the normal platelet life span. Thromboxane levels may be measured in PRP or in serum.

Samples
1. 5 ml citrated blood for preparing PRP. Determine the platelet count.
2. 5 ml clotted blood incubation at 37°C for 30 minutes; platelet count is determined on an EDTA sample.

PRP method
Reagents
40 μl/ml collagen (giving a final concentration of 4 μg/ml in PRP).
30 mmol/l arachidonic acid (giving a final concentration of 1.5 mmol/l in PRP).

Method
In *triplicate* add 30 μl collagen to 300 μl PRP and stir in an aggregometer at 900 rpm at 37°C for 4 minutes. Remove 200 μl from the cuvette and add 200 μl absolute ethanol in a microtube, mix and store at −20°C until assayed. Repeat the procedure but adding 15 μl arachidonic acid.

Serum method
Centrifuge the clotted sample, separate the serum and store at −20°C with a record of the whole-blood platelet count.

Timetable

Prior to aspirin ingestion take two baseline samples. Give 600 mg soluble aspirin, and take blood samples 2 hours later. Further samples are taken daily for 8 days, noting the precise times of sampling.

Assay

TXB_2 in PRP is expressed as pmoles per 10^9 platelets.

TXB_2 in serum can be expressed as pmoles per ml serum provided that the platelet count remains reasonably constant throughout the test; otherwise levels should be expressed in relation to platelet count.

Analysis

Plot TXB_2 levels against time of sampling; the platelet regeneration time is the time taken for TXB_2 levels to return to the pre-aspirin level. In a steady state (production = destruction) the platelet regeneration time is considered to be equal to the platelet life span.

Notes

1. In patients with platelet counts below 50×10^9/l the test loses accuracy and precision.
2. Measurement of TXB_2 is preferred to measurement of platelet malondialdehyde (MDA).

References

1. Hoyer, L. W. and Breckenridge, R. T. (1968) Immunologic studies of antihemophilic factor (AHF, factor VIII): cross reacting material in a genetic variant of hemophilia A. *Blood*, **32**, 962–71
2. Giddings, J. C. (1988) The nature of procoagulant proteins. In *Molecular Genetics and Immunoanalysis in Blood Coagulation*, pp. 93–100. Chichester: Ellis Horwood
3. Tuddenham, E. G. D. (1989) Factor VIII and haemophilia A. *Clin. Haematol.*, **2**, 849–77
4. Zimmerman, T. S., Ratnoff, O. D. and Littell, A. S. (1971) Detection of carriers of classic haemophilia using an immunologic assay for antihaemophilic factor (factor VIII). *J. Clin. Invest.*, **50**, 255–8
5. World Health Organization (1977) Methods for the detection of haemophilia carriers: a memorandum. *Bull. World Hlth Org.*, **55**, 675–702
6. Allain, J.-P., Gaillandre, A. and Lee, H. (1981) Immunochemical characterisation of antibodies to factor VIII in hemophilic and non-hemophilic plasmas. *J. Lab. Clin. Med.*, **79**, 791–800
7. Howard, M. A. and Firkin, B. G. (1971) Ristocetin – a new tool in the investigation of platelet aggregation. *Thromb. Diath. Haematol.*, **26**, 361–9
8. Giddings, J. C. (1988) The nature of procoagulant proteins. In *Molecular Genetics and Immunoanalysis in Blood Coagulation*, pp. 100–19. Chichester: Ellis Horwood
9. Ruggeri, Z. M. (1987) Classification of von Willebrand's disease. In *Thrombosis and Haemostasis* (eds. M. Verstraete, J. Vermylen, R. Lijnen and J. Arnout), pp. 419–45. Leuven: Leuven University Press
10. Ruggeri, Z. M. and Zimmerman, T. S. (1987) von Willebrand factor and von Willebrand disease. *Blood*, **70**, 895–904
11. Manucci, P. M. Ruggeri, Z. M., Ciaverella, N. *et al.* (1981) Precipitating antibodies to factor VIII/von Willebrand factor in von Willebrand's disease: effect of replacement therapy. *Blood*, **57**, 25–31
12. Giddings, J. C. (1988) The nature of procoagulant proteins. In *Molecular Genetics and Immunoanalysis in Blood Coagulation*, pp. 51–71. Chichester: Ellis Horwood
13. Gianelli, F. (1989) Factor IX. *Clin. Haematol.*, **2**, 821–48

14. Kasper, C. K., Osterud, B., Minami, J. Y. *et al.* (1977) Haemophilia B: characterisation of genetic variants and detection of carriers. *Blood*, **50**, 351–66
15. Denson, K. W. E., Lurie, A., De Cataldo, F. and Manucci, P. M. (1970) The factor X defect: recognition of abnormal forms of factor X. *Br. J. Haematol.*, **18**, 317–27
16. Fair, D. S. and Edgington, T. S. (1985) Heterogeneity of hereditary and acquired factor X deficiencies by combined immunochemical and functional analyses. *Br. J. Haematol.*, **59** 235–48
17. Bhavani, M. and Evans, D. I. K. (1984) Carriers of factor VII deficiency are not always asymptomatic. *Clin. Lab. Haematol.*, **6**, 363–8
18. Girolami, A., de Marco, L, dal bo Zanon, R. *et al.* (1985) Rarer quantitative and qualitative abnormalities of coagulation. *Clin. Haematol.*, **14**, 385–411
19. Mariani, G., Hermans, J., Orlando, M. *et al.* (1985) Carrier detection in factor VII congenital deficiency. *Br. J. Haematol.*, **60**, 687–94
20. Giddings, J. C. (1988) The nature of procoagulant proteins. In *Molecular Genetics and Immunoanalysis in Blood Coagulation*, pp. 40–3. Chichester: Ellis Horwood
21. Lane, D. A. and Southan, G. (1987) Inherited abnormalities of fibrinogen synthesis and structure. In *Haemostasis and Thrombosis*, 2nd edn (eds. A. L. Bloom and D. P. Thomas), pp. 442–51. Edinburgh: Churchill Livingstone
22. Miloszewski, K. J. A. and Losowsky, M. S. (1988) Fibrin stabilisation and factor XIII deficiency. In *Fibrinogen, Fibrin Stabilisation and Fibrinolysis* (ed. J. L. Francis), pp. 175–202. Chichester: Ellis Horwood
23. Soff, G. A. and Levin, J. (1981) Familial multiple coagulation factor deficiencies. *Semin. Thromb. Hemost.*, **7**, 112–48
24. Fischer, R. R., Giddings, J. C. and Rosenberg, I. (1988) Hereditary combined deficiency of clotting factors V and VIII with involvement of von Willebrand factor. *Clin. Lab. Haematol.*, **10**, 53–62
25. Lewis, J. H., Iammarino, R. M., Spero, J. A. and Hasiba, U. (1978) Antithrombin Pittsburgh: an α_1-antitrypsin variant causing hemorrhagic disease. *Blood*, **51**, 129–37
26. Owen, M. C., Brennan, S. O., Lewis, J. H. and Carrell, R. W. (1983) Mutation of antitrypsin to antithrombin. α_1-Antitrypsin Pittsburgh (358 met $\rightarrow$ arg), a fatal bleeding disorder. *N. Engl. J. Med.*, **309**, 694–8
27. Kettle, P. and Mayne, E. E. (1985) A bleeding disorder due to deficiency of α_2-antiplasmin. *J. Clin. Pathol.*, **38**, 428–9
28. Kluft, C., Niewenhuis, H. K., Rijken, D. C. *et al.* (1987) α_2-Antiplasmin Enschede: dysfunctional α_2-antiplasmin molecule associated with an autosomal recessive hemorrhagic disorder. *J. Clin. Invest.*, **80**, 1391–400
29. Hilgartner, M. W., Knatterud, G. L. and the FEIBA Study Group (1983) The use of factor eight inhibitor by-passing activity (FEIBA Immuno) product for treatment of bleeding episodes in hemophilias with inhibitors. *Blood*, **61**, 36–40
30. Hedner, U. and Kisiel, W. (1983) Use of human factor VIIa in the treatment of two hemophilia A patients with high-titer antibodies. *J. Clin. Invest.*, **71**, 1836–41
31. Rao, L. V. M. and Rapaport, S. I. (1990) Factor VIIa-catalysed activation of factor X independent of tissue factor: its possible significance for control of hemophilic bleeding by infused factor VIIa. *Blood*, **75**, 1069–73
32. Francis, J. L. (1988) Acquired dysfibrinogenaemia. In *Fibrinogen, Fibrin Stabilisation and Fibrinolysis* (ed. J. L. Francis), pp. 128–56. Chichester: Ellis Horwood
33. Ghosh, S., McEvoy, P. and McVerry, B. A. (1983) Idiopathic autoantibody that inhibits fibrin monomer polymerisation. *Br. J. Haematol.*, **53**, 65–72
34. Marciniak, E. and Greenwood, M. F. (1979) Acquired coagulation inhibitor delaying fibrinopeptide release. *Blood*, **53**, 81–91
35. Scully, M. F., Ellis, V., Kakkar, V. V. *et al.* (1982) An acquired coagulation inhibitor to factor II. *Br. J. Haematol.*, **50**, 655–64
36. Lai-Lu, C. and Yuk-Cheumg, W. (1985) A case of factor V inhibitor. *Am. J. Hematol.*, **19**, 395–9
37. Ingram, G. I. C., Kingston, P. J., Leslie, J. and Bowie, E. J. W. (1971) Four cases of acquired von Willebrand's syndrome. *Br. J. Haematol.*, **21**, 189–99

38. McGrath, K. M., Johnson, C. A. and Stuart, J. J. (1979) Acquired von Willebrand's disease associated with an inhibitor to factor VIII antigen and gastrointestinal telangiectasia. *Am. J. Med.*, **67**, 693–6
39. Sampson, B. M., Greaves, M., Malia, R. G., and Preston, F. E. (1983) Acquired von Willebrand's disease: demonstration of a circulating inhibitor to the factor VIII complex in four cases. *Br. J. Haematol.*, **54**, 233–44
40. Musclow, C. E., Amato, D., Ofosu, F. *et al.* (1988) Transfusion-induced specific anti-factor XI inhibitor in a patient with previously unrecognised factor XI deficiency. *Am. J. Clin. Pathol.*, **89**, 418–22
41. Chediak, J., Madej-Zevin, P., Ratnoff, O. D. *et al.* (1986) Studies on a circulating anticoagulant inhibiting factor XI in a patient with congenital deficiency and carcinoma of prostate. *Br. J. Haematol.*, **63**, 123–33
42. Fear, J. D., Miloszewski, K. J. A. and Losowsky, M. S. (1983) An acquired inhibitor of factor XIII with a qualitative abnormality of fibrin cross-linking. *Acta Haematol.*, **71**, 304–9
43. Tinegate, H. N., McArdle, B. and Qureshi, M. (1984) Falsely prolonged prothrombin time due to an inhibitor of human thromboplastin. *Br. J. Haematol.*, **58**, 347–52
44. Lipsky, J. J. (1983) *N*-methyl-thio-tetrazole inhibition of the gamma-carboxylation of glutamic acid: possible mechanism for antibiotic-associated hypoprothrombinaemia. *Lancet*, **ii**, 192–3
45. Bellucci, S. (1989) Autoimmune thrombocytopenias. *Clin. Haematol.*, **2**, 695–718
46. Berndt, M. C., Fournier, D. J. and Castaldi, P. A. (1989) Bernard–Soulier syndrome. *Clin. Haematol.*, **2**, 585–607
47. Caen, J. P. (1989) Glanzmann's thrombasthenia. *Clin. Haematol.*, **2**, 609–25
48. George, J. N., Caen, J. P. and Nurden, A. T. (1990) Glanzmann's thrombasthenia: the spectrum of clinical disease. *Blood*, **75**, 1383–95
49. Hardisty, R. M. (1989) Disorders of platelet secretion. *Clin. Haematol.*, **2**, 673–94
50. Niewenhuis, H. K., Akkerman, J.-W. N. and Sixma, J. J. (1987) Patients with a prolonged bleeding time and normal aggregation tests may have storage pool deficiency: studies on 106 patients. *Blood*, **70**, 620–3
51. Vermylen, J. and Blockmans, D. (1989) Acquired disorders of platelet function. *Clin. Haematol.*, **2**, 729–48
52. Fink, R. and Hutton, R. A. (1983) Changes in the blood platelets of alcoholics during alcohol withdrawal. *J. Clin. Pathol.*, **36**, 337–40
53. Scully, M. F. and Kakkar, V. V. (eds) (1979) *Chromogenic Peptide Substrates. Chemistry and Clinical Usage*. Edinburgh: Churchill Livingstone
54. Goodall, A. H. and Meyer, D. (1985) Registry of monoclonal antibodies to factor VIII and von Willebrand factor. *Thromb. Haemost.*, **54**, 878–91
55. Weiss, H. J., Hoyer, L. W., Rickles, F. R. *et al.* (1973) Quantitative assay of a plasma factor deficient in von Willebrand's disease that is necessary for platelet aggregation: relationship to factor VIII procoagulant activity and antigen content. *J. Clin. Invest.*, **52**, 2708–10
56. Evans, R. J. and Austen, D. E. G. (1977) Assay of ristocetin cofactor using fixed platelets and a platelet counting technique. *Br. J. Haematol.*, **37**, 289–94
57. Hall, R. and Malia, R. G. (1984) *Medical Laboratory Haematology*, pp. 620–1. London: Butterworths
58. Olson, J. D., Brockway, W. J., Fass, D. N. *et al.* (1975) Evaluation of ristocetin-von Willebrand factor assay and ristocetin-induced platelet aggregation. *Am. J. Clin. Pathol.*, **63**, 210–18
59. Hoyer, L. W. (1982) The assessment of von Willebrand's disease. In *Methods in Haematology, Volume 5. The Haemophilias* (ed. A. L. Bloom), pp.106–21. Edinburgh: Churchill Livingstone
60. Goodall, A. H., Jarvis, J., Chand, S. *et al.* (1985) An immunoradiometric assay for human factor VIII/von Willebrand factor (VIII/vWf) using a monoclonal antibody that defines a functional epitope. *Br. J. Haematol.*, **59**, 565–77
61. Giddings, J. C. (1988) Laboratory methods for immunoanalysis of proteins. In *Molecular Genetics and Immunoanalysis in Blood Coagulation*, pp. 190–1. Chichester: Ellis Horwood
62. Enayat, M. S. and Hill, F. G. H. (1982) Qualitative factor VIIIR:Ag function screening of multiple samples by two-dimensional crossed immunoelectrophoretic technique. *Med. Lab. Sci.*, **39**, 357–62

63. Short, P. E., Williams, C. E., Picken, A. M. and Hill, F. G. H. (1982) Factor VIII related antigen: an improved enzyme immunoassay. *Med. Lab. Sci.*, **39**, 351–5
64. Enayat, M. S. and Hill, F. G. H. (1983) Analysis of the complexity of the multimeric structure of factor VIII-related antigen/von Willebrand protein using a modified electrophoretic technique. *J. Clin. Pathol.*, **36**, 915–19
65. Manucci, P. M., Abildgaard, C. F., Gralnick, H. R. *et al.* (1985) Multicenter comparison of von Willebrand factor multimer sizing techniques. *Thromb. Haemost.*, **54**, 873–7
66. Kasper, C. K. and Ewing, N. P. (1982) Measurement of inhibitor to factor VIIC (and IXC). In *Methods in Haematology, Volume 5. The Haemophilias* (ed. A. L. Bloom), pp.39–50. Edinburgh: Churchill Livingstone
67. British Society for Haematology (1988) Guidelines on platelet function testing. *J. Clin. Pathol.*, **41**, 1322–30
68. Harker, L. A. and Zimmerman, T. S. (eds) (1983) *Methods in Haematology, Volume 8. Measurements of Platelet Function*. Edinburgh: Churchill Livingstone
69. Williams, C. E., Entwhistle, M. B. P. and Short, P. E. (1985) Platelet function tests: a critical review. *Med. Lab. Sci.*, **42**, 262–74

Chapter 17

Thrombosis and hypercoagulable states

In general hospital practice, disordered haemostasis resulting in vascular occlusion due to thrombus formation is more common and results in higher morbidity and mortality than disordered haemostasis resulting in bleeding. Thrombosis can involve the larger vessels of both the venous and arterial circulation. Multiple thrombi in the microcirculation can also occur.

Venous thrombosis results from local generation of thrombin in areas of retarded blood flow. The presence of activated coagulation factors and/or tissue factor probably initiate thrombin formation while impaired defence mechanisms probably lower the threshold at which thrombosis develops[1]. There is no convincing evidence that vascular endothelial damage is a primary mechanism.

In contrast to venous thrombosis, arterial thrombosis is usually the result of vessel wall damage resulting in platelet adherence, aggregation and secretion leading to fibrin formation[2]. Coagulation may also be initiated by tissue factor from disordered endothelial cells.

Platelet thrombi in the microcirculation can result from vessel damage, be due to bacterial toxins, 'thromboplastin-like' substances or associated with treatment with certain cytotoxic drugs[3].

Hypercoagulable states may be classified into inherited and acquired types[4] or as primary and secondary[5]. The terms 'prethrombotic' and 'prothrombotic' state have been used interchangeably with 'hypercoagulability' to describe conditions with an increased risk of thrombosis.

Acquired hypercoagulable states

Acquired hypercoagulability leading to thrombosis is common. Many disorders and 'risk factors' have been identified and major causes are summarized in *Table 17.1*.

Pregnancy

Thromboembolic complications occur during the later stages of pregnancy and particularly in the post-partum period. Progressive changes in coagulation factors are found, notably in the third trimester, with a marked increase in fibrinogen level and also increases of factors VII, VIII:C, IX, X, XII and of vWf:Ag. Significantly, ATIII and protein S levels decrease and there is depression of fibrinolytic activity. The risk of thrombosis is increased in those women confined to bed during pregnancy and who require surgical intervention.

Table 17.1 Acquired hypercoagulable states

1. Abnormalities of coagulation and fibrinolysis:
   - Pregnancy
   - Malignancy
   - Oestrogen therapy and the use of oral contraceptives
   - Nephrotic syndrome
2. Abnormalities of platelets:
   - Myeloproliferative disorders
   - Paroxysmal nocturnal haemoglobinuria
   - Diabetes mellitus
   - Heparin-induced thrombocytopenia
3. Anti-phospholipid antibody syndrome (lupus anticoagulant)
4. Abnormal vasculature and rheology:
   - Venous stasis (obesity, immobilization, postoperatively, advancing age)
   - Chronic vascular disease
   - Hyperviscosity (increased PCV, increased plasma viscosity, gross leucocytosis, sickle cell disease)
   - Thrombotic thrombocytopenic purpura, haemolytic uraemic syndrome
5. Liver disease

Malignancy

The association between malignancy and thrombosis (Trousseau's syndrome)[6] has long been recognized. The overall incidence is 5–15% but with some tumours it may be as high as 50%. Thrombosis may precede the diagnosis of malignancy. In addition to the association between malignancy and venous thrombosis, mucin-secreting adenocarcinomas can result in intravascular coagulation with the typical findings of microangiopathic haemolytic anaemia and thrombocytopenia. Thromboembolism is a common cause of death in patients with solid tumours.

Oestrogens and oral contraceptives

There is a clear association between oestrogens and increased risk of deep-vein thrombosis and pulmonary embolus. Alterations to coagulation factors are found similar to those in pregnancy, though changes in blood flow, rheology and increased distensibility of leg veins resulting in stasis may be more relevant[7].

Nephrotic syndrome

Renal vein thrombosis and systemic thromboembolic complications are associated with nephrotic syndrome. Acquired ATIII deficiency has been suggested as being the cause but has not been substantiated. Other changes in nephrotic syndrome include reduced fibrinolysis and platelet hyperactivity.

Myeloproliferative disorders and paroxysmal haemoglobinuria

Both venous and arterial thrombosis are seen in this group of disorders. In addition to the common types of occlusion, unusual sites of thrombosis can occur, notably in the splenic, portal and mesenteric vessels. Microvascular thrombi causing peripheral ischaemia is another unusual complication. There is no clear relationship between the level of thrombocytosis and the incidence of thrombosis. The most likely mechanism is qualitative abnormality of the platelets.

Diabetes mellitus

The occurrence of platelet micro-aggregates and the demonstration of platelet hyper-reactivity indicates that platelets have a central role, together with changes in the vessel wall, in the thrombotic complications of diabetes mellitus [8].

Heparin-induced thrombocytopenia [9]

Both venous and arterial thrombosis may be associated with this disorder and patients who develop thromboembolism during treatment with heparin should be suspected of having heparin-induced thrombocytopenia. Heparin-dependent antibodies are formed against platelet antigens and cause *in vivo* platelet aggregation and formation of platelet thrombi, and severe thrombocytopenia. These changes usually develop within 10 days of starting heparin therapy.

Lupus anticoagulant; anti-phospholipid antibody syndrome [10]

First described in 1952, the lupus anticoagulant (LA) results in prolongation of coagulation tests dependent on the presence of phospholipid (APTT, KCCT) and occasionally the one-stage prothrombin time, without specifically inactivating any individual coagulation factor. Originally thought to be only associated with systemic lupus erythematosus (SLE), hence the derivation of the term, it is now recognized to be associated with a range of autoimmune disorders, with infections, after treatment with certain drugs and in subjects without obvious immune disorders. The inhibitor has been shown to have anti-phospholipid specificity and may be of IgG or IgM type. Paradoxically, although coagulation tests are prolonged there is rarely a bleeding tendency but there is a high incidence of thrombosis. The presence of LA is associated with the finding of anti-cardiolipin (a negatively charged phospholipid) antibodies (ACL). There is a strong association between the presence of LA and recurrent abortion. The anti-phospholipid antibody syndrome consists of thrombosis, recurrent abortion and the presence of LA and ACL antibodies in the absence of the typical features of SLE.

Abnormal vasculature and rheology

Damage to the vessel wall such as occurs in the various forms of vasculitis may be expected to influence the release or availability of activators and/or inhibitors of the fibrinolytic system. Immobilization with associated venous stasis is a well recognized risk factor. This is particularly true after abdominal or lower limb surgery. No consistent systemic changes in haemostasis testing have been demonstrated.

Hyperviscosity, whether due to elevated PCV, increased numbers of leucocytes, decreased red-cell deformability or increased plasma viscosity can be directly implicated in the development of thrombosis. The thrombotic complications of primary proliferative polycythaemia and sickle cell disease are well recognized.

Liver disease

Reductions of the vitamin K-dependent factors, protein C and protein S, together with antithrombin III (ATIII) are well documented in liver disease and might therefore be expected to result in hypercoagulability. However, concomitant reduction of the vitamin K-dependent procoagulant factors, together with a reduction in the other coagulation factors dependent on hepatic synthesis, usually results in haemorrhagic symptoms rather than thrombotic complications. Nevertheless, low-grade intravascular coagulation can be demonstrated in liver failure and may be due to delayed clearance of activated coagulation products or reduced plasminogen levels.

Inherited hypercoagulable states

The currently recognized inherited hypercoagulable states involve defects in the proteins of the coagulation or fibrinolytic systems; platelet abnormalities have not been identified. Inherited hypercoagulable states are at risk of developing venous thrombosis and, more rarely, arterial thromboembolism.

Although the defects are constant, clinical thrombotic events are episodic and some patients are asymptomatic. The isolated thrombotic events are probably precipitated by clinical or subclinical events which tip the balance of impaired antithrombotic mechanisms. Additional risk factors such as pregnancy, surgery, oral contraception, immobilization, etc. may trigger a thrombotic episode in previously asymptomatic patients. The recognized inherited defects leading to hypercoagulability are shown in *Table 17.2*[11].

Table 17.2 Inherited disorders associated with thrombosis

1. Impaired anticoagulant activity:
   - Protein C deficiency
   - Protein S deficiency
   - Antithrombin III deficiency
   - Heparin co-factor II deficiency?
2. Impaired fibrinolysis:
   - Plasminogen deficiency
   - Dysfibrinogenaemia
   - Plasminogen activator deficiency?
   - Plasminogen activator inhibitor increased
   - Histidine-rich glycoprotein?

Note: The term 'deficiency' includes both quantitative and qualitative defects

Impaired anticoagulant activity

Protein C deficiency

There is a strong association between inherited protein C deficiency and recurrent venous thrombosis. The majority of patients present with levels of 50 units/dl or less of protein C antigen and a comparative reduction in functional activity (type I). Type II protein C deficiency shows normal antigen levels but reduced functional activity, i.e. a molecular variant. The prevalence of protein C deficiency in patients less than 40 years of age with unexplained venous thrombosis is 5–8%. In the general population of The Netherlands the incidence of heterozygotes is reported as one in 16000, though a study of normal blood donors in the USA indicated a prevalence of one in 300 in the absence of thrombotic disease![12] A clinical sign peculiar to heterozygous protein C deficiency is the occurrence of skin necrosis shortly after starting coumarin therapy and is probably due to the very rapid decrease in protein C activity before the slower decrease of the other vitamin K-dependent factors. Homozygous protein C deficiency results in extensive thrombosis of visceral veins or purpura fulminans soon after birth, often leading to death if not treated[13].

Protein S deficiency

The incidence of protein S deficiency is probably similar or more frequent than protein C deficiency. Because protein S is found in two forms in plasma, 40% as free protein and 60% in complex with C4b binding protein, and because protein S activity may differ from total protein S, the classification of protein S deficiency into sub-types is difficult. A proposed classification[14] is shown in *Table 17.3*.

Table 17.3 Proposed classification of hereditary protein S deficiency based on total protein S levels

	Free protein S	*Protein S activity*	*Total protein S*
Type I	Low	Low	Low
Type IIa	Low	Low	Normal
Type IIb*	Normal	Low	Normal

*No cases reported to date

Approximately 70% of cases fall into type I with the remainder in type IIa. Type IIb cases may be expected when dysfunctional protein S is identified.

Antithrombin III deficiency

ATIII deficiency was the first plasma defect to be reported in patients with recurrent venous thrombosis. The prevalence in the general population is one in 30 000–40 000, accounting for 2–3% of venous thrombosis in patients less than 45 years of age. As with protein C and protein S deficiencies the defect is inherited as an autosomal dominant. Not all individuals with ATIII deficiency develop thrombosis but by the age of 50 about two-thirds become symptomatic. Dysfunctional ATIIIs are recognized; type I cases have a parallel reduction in concentration and activity while the much smaller numbers with normal concentration and reduced function are designated as type II. Further subclassification can be made by differentiating function into progressive antithrombin activity and heparin co-factor activity; type III have normal antigen and progressive antithrombin activity with decreased heparin co-factor activity[15].

Heparin co-factor II deficiency

Heparin co-factor II activity is directed solely against thrombin and like ATIII is greatly potentiated by heparin and by dermatan sulphate. Only two families have been described in which reduced levels of heparin co-factor II were associated with venous or arterial thrombosis, but the majority of deficient kindred had no thrombotic symptoms. It is generally accepted that a causal relationship between heparin co-factor II deficiency and thrombosis has not been proved[15].

Impaired fibrinolytic activity

Plasminogen deficiency

Inherited plasminogen defects are reported to account for 2–3% of unexplained venous thrombosis in patients under the age of 45 years. The defect is transmitted as an autosomal dominant; in the heterozygote, plasminogen is about 50% of normal activity and in the only reported homozygote the level was 10%. As in the other inherited thrombotic disorders, type I and type II defects are recognized on the basis of functional activity and concentration [16].

Dysfibrinogenaemias [17]

Rare types of congenital dysfibrinogenaemia develop venous and/or arterial thrombosis below the age of 45 years. A number of mechanisms implicating the abnormal fibrinogen have been suggested:

(a) reduced capacity to bind plasminogen or plasminogen activator resulting in impaired plasmin formation and delayed fibrinolysis;
(b) reduced capacity to bind thrombin, the free thrombin being available to activate platelets;
(c) the functionally abnormal fibrinogen forming rigid fibrin with resistance to plasmin degradation.

Plasminogen activator and inhibitor

At least three families with kindred showing apparent defective release of tissue plasminogen activator (t-PA) associated with venous thrombosis were subsequently shown to have high levels of plasminogen activator inhibitor (t-PAI) [18]. True cases of defective release of t-PA have not been identified.

Histidine-rich glycoprotein

Histidine-rich glycoprotein (HRG) reduces plasminogen binding to fibrin by blocking the lysine binding sites of plasminogen. High levels of HRG might inhibit fibrinolysis by decreasing the transformation of plasminogen to plasmin. Two kindreds showing recurrent thrombosis have been described but did not clearly correlate with high levels of HRG.

Laboratory detection of thrombosis

The diagnosis of venous thrombosis using clinical criteria is insensitive and imprecise. Probably up to two-thirds of venous thrombi are not detected clinically and thrombi are present on only half the occasions when signs and symptoms suggest their presence [18]. Definitive diagnosis depends on techniques such as radiographic venography, radioisotopic scanning, ultrasound or thermography or a combination of these, with specificity and sensitivity over 90%. In occlusive arterial diseases, evidence of a thrombotic component is often lacking.

Despite intensive studies, no single test provides conclusive evidence of the presence of thrombosis. Using an array of methods, supportive evidence can be obtained for clinical or sub-clinical thrombosis. The methods can be separated into three groups:

1. Evidence of the activation of coagulation and thrombin formation by the detection in plasma of:
   (a) fibrinopeptide A released from fibrinogen by the action of thrombin;
   (b) prothrombin fragments F1 and F2 formed by the action of thrombin on fragment 1.2 released by the action of Xa on factor II;
   (c) thrombin–antithrombin complexes formed by the binding of thrombin and antithrombin III;
   (d) protein C activation peptide released by the action of thrombin on protein C.
2. Evidence of platelet activation by the demonstration of:
   (a) formation of circulating platelet aggregates;
   (b) release of platelet factor 4;
   (c) release of β-thromboglobulin;
   (d) formation and release of thromboxane B_2.
3. Evidence of secondary activation of fibrinolysis by:
   (a) euglobulin lysis time;
   (b) presence of cross-linked fibrin fragments;
   (c) presence of fragment Bβ 15–42;
   (d) fibrin complexes.

Note. Methods providing evidence of the activation of coagulation and/or platelets require rigorous attention to specimen collection, anticoagulant used and technical detail and are difficult to ensure in general hospital practice.

Investigation of prethrombotic states

Clinical evidence of a prethrombotic state

The following categories of patients should be investigated:

1. Recurrent thrombosis without precipitating factors.
2. Thrombosis before the age of 45 years (juvenile thrombosis).
3. Family history of thrombosis.
4. Recurrent abortions.
5. Thrombosis at unusual anatomical sites.
6. Arterial thrombosis in the absence of arterial disease.
7. Resistance to conventional antithrombotic treatment.

Strategies for laboratory investigation

The multifactorial causes of thrombosis make it difficult to devise a simple scheme for the laboratory investigation of a prethrombotic state. No single test has been devised which will differentiate between normal haemostasis and the prethrombotic states. A number of strategies have been suggested for the diagnosis of inherited hypercoagulable states.

Manucci and Tripodi[11] propose a two-step procedure. The first step specifies assays (preferably functional) of ATIII, protein C, protein S, plasminogen and fibrinogen. If no abnormality is demonstrated, the second stage is directed at detecting the less common causes of inherited thrombophilia – deficiency of heparin co-factor II, defective release of t-PA and elevated plasma levels of t-PAI.

Rodgers and Schuman[19] proposed a scheme using the relatively simple assessment of the plasma thrombin time and euglobulin lysis time as the first stage, and testing for specific deficiency or abnormality of ATIII, protein C, protein S and heparin co-factor II.

An approach to impaired fibrinolysis has been suggested [20] by the investigation of fibrinolytic potential due to t-PA or PAI defects. The scheme is based on measuring PAI-1 in plasma after 10 minutes venous occlusion. If PAI activity is no longer measurable (due to excess release of t-PA), the patient is considered to have a normal fibrinolytic response. If PAI levels are over 1 unit/ml, further testing of PAI activity and antigen and t-PA levels before and after stasis will distinguish between high PAI levels and poor release of t-PA. The potential value of fibrinolytic tests has been recently reviewed [21].

The approaches described above are primarily designed to identify inherited defects. It has become increasingly apparent that the most frequent cause of thrombosis, *identifiable by laboratory testing*, is probably the lupus anticoagulant (anti-phospholipid antibody). A strategy for the laboratory identification of lupus anticoagulant is described in the 'Methods' section of this chapter.

One of the problems in investigating patients with predisposition to thrombosis is that many are taking oral anticoagulants which depress the activity of protein C and protein S in addition to the activity of the other vitamin K-dependent factors. In this situation comparisons must be made between the levels of coagulant and procoagulant factors in an attempt to establish an underlying defect. In addition, prolongation of the APTT due to anticoagulation may mask the possibility of the lupus anticoagulant. It may not be appropriate to discontinue treatment in order to determine pre-treatment levels of activity.

Antithrombotic therapy

Antithrombotic therapy has been used in the treatment of thromboembolism for over 40 years. The main aims of therapy are the prevention of thrombus formation or the prevention of the extension of existing thrombus by *anticoagulant agents*, and the dissolution of formed thrombus by *thrombolytic agents*.

Anticoagulant therapy

The objectives of anticoagulant therapy are to reduce the potential of the haemostatic mechanism to form thrombus while retaining adequate haemostatic function to prevent haemorrhage. To achieve this balance an understanding is required of the mechanisms involved and of the appropriate techniques for laboratory control. Anticoagulants and their mode of action are shown in *Table 17.4*. The choice of anticoagulant is determined by clinical circumstance.

Oral anticoagulants [22]

The oral administration of 4-hydroxycoumarin derivatives – of which warfarin is a widely used, long-acting form – results in the inhibition of the synthesis of factors II, VII, IX and X, each factor disappearing from the plasma at a rate corresponding to its physiological half-life, with the concurrent appearance and increasing level of inactive precursors termed PIVKA proteins (proteins induced by vitamin K absence or antagonism).

Table 17.4 Anticoagulants and their effect on the haemostatic mechanism

Type	*Effect*
Oral anticoagulants (e.g. coumarins)	Antagonists of vitamin K_1. Inhibition of the synthesis of the functional, vitamin K-dependent clotting factors
Heparin	Interacts with antithrombin III, the primary inhibitor of activated serine proteases of the coagulation cascade
Snake venoms	Act directly on fibrinogen to reduce the level of plasma fibrinogen
Anti-platelet drugs	Inhibit platelet responsiveness to intra- or extracellular stimuli thus reducing the potential for platelet adhesion and aggregation

Mechanism of the action of vitamin K

Vitamin K is fat soluble and is absorbed from the intestine and concentrated in the liver. The daily requirement is about 1 μg/kg. All vitamin K-dependent factors exist as precursor forms in the microsomes of the liver hepatocytes and are identical with the functional plasma proteins except for (1) the ability to bind calcium; (2) low biological activity; and (3) adsorption to barium salts.

Vitamin K is involved in the conversion of glutamic acid residues (glu) on the terminal amino calcium binding part of the precursor protein into γ carboxy-glutamic acid (gla) residues, thus completing the functional protein with normal, calcium-binding, gla domain, polypeptide binding sites. The gla residues enable the vitamin K-dependent proteins to bind to phospholipids and thus form efficient factor Xa and IIa complexes.

When vitamin K is given to patients deficient in the vitamin there is a rise in functional clotting activity within 0.5–2 hours, indicating the 'completion' of existing intracellular proteins rather than *de novo* synthesis.

Mechanism of the action of coumarins

Between 60 and 100% of coumarin adminstered by mouth is passively absorbed by the gut with a peak between 30 minutes and 5 hours. More than 95% of coumarin is protein bound (mainly to albumin) and only the unbound fraction has significant 'anticoagulant capability'. It has a long half-life of 36–44 hours because the protein binding protects it from filtration by the renal glomeruli. Following absorption, coumarin in its free form is bound to the hepatocyte microsomes which regulate protein synthesis, and inhibits the action of vitamin K_1, resulting in an accumulation of intracellular vitamin K-2,3-epoxide which is a product of vitamin K_1 metabolism and is ineffective in the conversion of the PIVKA proteins to functional forms. Three separate menadione (vitamin K) reductases are present in liver, one of which, DT-diaphorase, is completely inhibited by coumarin at a concentration of 5×10^{-8} mol/l.

The induction of coumarin anticoagulation

The aim is to achieve a prothrombin ratio accepted as the optimum therapeutic range (*see* page 677). In general, patients on 10 mg coumarin daily reach the therapeutic range in 5 days, those on 15 mg daily take 3 days and with a dose of

1.5 mg/kg a therapeutic ratio can be achieved in 1 day due to the fall in the level of factor VII (half-life = 4 hours). The usual induction dose for adults is 10 mg on each of the first 2 days. A larger dose is not recommended and should be reduced in certain clinical situations such as abnormal liver function tests, congestive cardiac failure, less than average body weight, age over 80 years and parenteral feeding. The daily maintenance dose should be given at a fixed time, preferably in the evening, with a prothrombin test performed during the day of treatment and the dose adjusted accordingly. By the end of 7 days factors II, VII, IX and X have reached equally low levels and therefore the one-stage prothrombin time and the derived ratio is valid for adjusting dosage. Since the *in vivo* antithrombotic effect of coumarin may not occur until all the dependent factors are equally reduced, a patient may not be considered to be fully anticoagulated until 5–7 days have elapsed. The maximal effect of a dose of warfarin is found 36 hours later and therefore the dose should be given at the same time each day; its effect will be evident 36–40 hours later. The maintenance dose is usually between 3 and 9 mg daily though the response varies widely.

The inevitable delay before coumarin drugs have effect can be covered by the use of heparin which has an immediate anticoagulant effect and which can be withdrawn when the coumarin therapy has had an adequate effect. Because the half-life of protein C is similar to that of factor VII (4 hours) and shorter than the other procoagulant factors, patients with inherited protein C deficiency may be at risk of tissue necrosis or rethrombosis during the induction of warfarin therapy. This is a further reason for the use of heparin during the induction phase.

The concurrent administration of warfarin and of heparin by continuous infusion does not preclude control of warfarin therapy. If heparin treatment is controlled by the APTT (*see* page 682) and maintained at 2–2.5 times the midpoint of the reference range for the APTT, there is little effect on the prothrombin time. If the APTT ratio is >2.5, heparin can be withheld for 4 hours before repeating the prothrombin time.

Laboratory control of oral anticoagulant therapy

With the introduction of coumarin therapy it was recognized that regular laboratory testing by Quick's one-stage prothrombin time test was necessary to prevent disastrous haemorrhagic complications. At that time the only factors recognized to be involved in the test were prothrombin, fibrinogen and calcium and laboratories using the prothrombin time had to prepare their own source of 'thromboplastin'. The availability of Russell's viper venom (RVV) as a powerful coagulant for topical use and its demonstrable thromboplastin activity led to its use as an alternative to brain thromboplastin in the prothrombin time test, and when used to control the clinical effect of coumarin drugs it resulted in haemorrhagic episodes in apparently adequately controlled patients.

The 'discovery' of factor VII (proconvertin) and of its vital role in the effect of coumarins, coupled with the knowledge that RVV is totally insensitive to factor VII activity, resulted in the abandonment of the RVV-activated prothrombin time test for the control of anticoagulant therapy.

Results using the standard Quick's prothrombin time were not entirely satisfactory and the 'prothrombin-proconvertin' or 'P and P' method using diluted plasma was recommended as more suitable for controlling treatment. The identification of factor X, its key role in the coagulation cascade, and its depression by coumarin, together with knowledge that factor IX is also depressed by oral anticoagulants, led to the development of the 'Thrombotest'. The Thrombotest uses bovine brain with added bovine plasma as a source of factor V, in combination with a partial thromboplastin to detect factor IX activity, the components being adjusted to achieve a balance between the factors of the extrinsic and intrinsic pathways.

The problems using the one-stage prothrombin time are known to be mainly due to the source of brain thromboplastin. Not only is there considerable variation in the sensitivity of thromboplastins from different species but different batches of thromboplastin from the same species can also have different sensitivity to reduced levels of the coumarin-sensitive factors.

A further difficulty in achieving standardization was the differing methods of reporting results of the one-stage prothrombin time (PT) – in seconds with comparison to a 'control' time; as a 'percentage index' of test/control × 100; as 'percentage activity' by converting tests in seconds to percentage activity by reference to a graph prepared by testing varying concentrations of plasma diluted in adsorbed plasma to maintain constant levels of factor V and fibrinogen or, less satisfactorily, diluted in saline.

The first attempt to establish a uniform system of testing was introduced in the UK by the widespread distribution of a standardized, phenolized human brain extract, eventually designated as the Manchester Comparative Reagent (MCR). Progress towards uniform representation of reporting was achieved by adoption of the Biggs–Denson model[23]. This model is based on the observation that the PT ratios (derived by dividing the result of the test plasma by the average PT of normal plasma) obtained from two different thromboplastins have a linear relationship. The slope of the plot for any thromboplastin tested against the British Comparative Thromboplastin (formerly the MCR) allowed correction of test ratios and reporting as 'British Comparative Ratio' (BCR). This concept was adopted by the World Health Organization (WHO) in the standardization of thromboplastin against the 1st International Reference Preparation (IRP) IRP 67/40. This preparation was one of five candidate reference preparations of human, rabbit and bovine origin, either 'plain' or 'combined' (a combined reagent contains added factor V and fibrinogen, typified by the Thrombotest reagent). IRP 67/40 was a combined reagent prepared from human brain. Each thromboplastin calibrated against IRP 67/40 was assigned an International Calibration Constant (ICC), the ICC of 67/40 being defined as 1.0.

A number of limitations of the WHO scheme were identified, notably the use of a combined reagent, the requirement that the calibration line should pass through the origin, the fact that the relationship between dissimilar thromboplastins is often non-linear, and problems with statistical analysis[24].

In 1983 the WHO published recommendations[25] which addressed the question of reference thromboplastins, introduced a revised statistical model for the calibration of thromboplastins from which is derived the International Sensitivity Index (ISI), and reporting of results as International Normalized Ratio (INR). These recommendations have been adopted by the ICSH/ICTH[26].

Reference thromboplastins The first reference thromboplastin was the WHO/IRP 67/40 human combined reagent. A second primary IRP was prepared, IRP BCT/253 human plain reagent. The secondary reference preparations, 70/178 rabbit plain and 68/434 bovine combined, have been replaced with IRP RBT/79 rabbit plain, OBT/79 bovine combined, each calibrated directly with 67/40, and BCT/099 human plain. These reference preparations are held on behalf of the

WHO by the Central Laboratory of the Netherlands Red Cross, Amsterdam. Certified reference materials (CRM) based on RBT/79, OBT/79 and BCT/099 are designated CRM 149, 148 and 147 respectively and held by the Bureau of Reference of the European Communities (BCR) (not to be confused with BCR = British Comparative Ratio!) [27]. It is clearly recommended that for the calibration of a working thromboplastin the most similar IRP should be selected, i.e. rabbit against RBT/79, combined against OBT/79 and human brain or placental thromboplastin against BCT/099 [28]. The calibration procedure has been precisely detailed [24,29]. The use of human brain thromboplastin in 1985 was mainly confined to the UK and those countries with historical associations. The withdrawal of human brain thromboplastin from general use, mainly due to possible risks of infection to operatives during manufacture, has therefore made IRPs of human brain unnecessary except for calibrating human placental thromboplastin preparations.

International Sensitivity Index (ISI) The ISI of a commercial or in-house thromboplastin is obtained by comparison with an IRP thromboplastin. When the logarithms of prothrombin times obtained using fresh plasmas of patients on long-term oral anticoagulants and fresh normal plasmas using the reference thromboplastin and the thromboplastin to be calibrated are plotted on the vertical and horizontal axis respectively, an almost linear line is obtained following the equation:

$$\log(\text{prothrombin time}_v) = c \times \log(\text{prothrombin time}_h) + d$$

where c is the slope, d is the intercept and v and h signify the ordinate and abscissa respectively. In principle a primary IRP is used but in practice a secondary RP is usually used. The line is derived using orthogonal regression in which the sum of squared deviations perpendicular to the regression line is minimized and when the variances of the log PT_v and log PT_h are equal. The ISI of the thromboplastin is obtained as the product of the slope c and the ISI of the IRP against which it is calibrated. For example, when a thromboplastin calibrated against RBT/79 (ISI 1.4) has a slope c of 0.9, the ISI of the 'new' thromboplastin is $0.9 \times 1.4 = 1.26$ [30].

The main differences from the Biggs–Denson model are: prothrombin times are used, not ratios; plotting on logarithmic axes; plotting the IRP on the ordinate; the use of orthogonal regression equation. The calibration procedure specifies the use of at least 20 fresh plasmas from healthy subjects and at least 60 plasmas who are stabilized on oral anticoagulants for at least 6 weeks. The collection and handling of the samples is strictly defined.

Detailed description of the ISI calibration procedure is described elsewhere [24].

International Normalized Ratio (INR) INR is the ratio of the patient's prothrombin time to the mean normal prothrombin time when using the primary IRP. In practice, the INR of a patient's plasma is:

$$\text{INR} = \text{prothrombin ratio}^{\text{ISI}}$$

$$\text{or INR} = \text{antilog}(\text{ISI} \times \log \text{ratio}).$$

For ease of determination, tables are usually prepared to convert prothrombin times to INR values for a given mean normal prothrombin time (MNPT).

The potential reliability of the INR depends upon: correct collection, anticoagulation and handling of samples; accurate estimate of the ISI of the thromboplastin; identical technique for determining the prothrombin time as used to determine the ISI; mean normal prothrombin time used to determine the prothrombin ratio.

Clearly, manufacturers of thromboplastins should describe the technique used to determine the ISI. Although ISI should be determined using a standardized manual technique, surveys have shown this is not always the case. If an instrument has been used the type of instrument should be specified. On the other hand, over 50% of laboratories use coagulometers for prothrombin times in the control of oral anticoagulation. This further emphasizes the importance of local determination of the MNPT.

Mean normal prothrombin time [31] The INR depends on the prothrombin ratio which in turn depends on the method of determining the MNPT. Experience indicates that the MNPT in individual laboratories varies from that stated by the manufacturer. It is recommended that each laboratory should determine its own MNPT for a given batch of thromboplastin. The MNPT should be derived from testing at least 20 fresh plasmas from healthy subjects over a period of 5 days. Prothrombin times should be recorded to, at the most, the nearest 0.5 seconds and the mean calculated. Strictly the geometric mean is preferable, though in practice an arithmetic mean gives a value of only 0.1–0.3 seconds difference.

The MNPT must remain constant for any given batch of thromboplastin. Lyophilized or frozen plasma pools may be used for confirming the MNPT only if it has been shown that the mean value of replicate prothrombin times of the reconstituted or thawed plasma is identical to that of the fresh plasma samples.

Clinical aspects of oral anticoagulant therapy [22]

Therapeutic ranges Improved standardization of thromboplastins and overall performance in external quality assessment has permitted the use of higher therapeutic INR ranges than were previously considered desirable and these are detailed in *Table 17.5*.

Table 17.5 Suggested INR ranges in various conditions

INR	*Clinical state*
2.0–2.5	Prophylaxis of deep vein thrombosis (DVT) including surgery on high-risk patients (2.0–3.0 for hip or lower limb surgery)
2.0–3.0	Treatment of DVT; pulmonary embolus (PE); systemic embolism, prevention of venous thromboembolism; in myocardial infarction; mitral stenosis with embolism, transient ischaemic attacks; atrial fibrillation
3.0–4.5	Recurrent DVT and PE, arterial disease including myocardial infarction; mechanical prosthetic heart valves

Surgical procedures during anticoagulant therapy may be associated with an increased risk of bleeding, though the risk is low if the INR is less than 2.0 at the time of surgery.

Resistance to warfarin therapy Failure to achieve adequate anticoagulation, other than because of inadequate dosage or patient non-compliance, may rarely be a hereditary resistance due to reduced activity of vitamin K coenzymes, acquired resistance to coumarin drugs, or bizarre dietary habit. More commonly responsible is interaction with antagonistic drugs. Although the majority of drugs which interact with oral anticoagulants potentiate the action of warfarin, barbiturates, antihistamines and preparations containing vitamin K are frequent causes of resistance.

Bleeding associated with an INR beyond the upper therapeutic range Overdosage, increased sensitivity of the patient due to intercurrent illness and change in drug prescribing, either the introduction of a potentiator or withdrawal of an antagonist, are the commonest causes.

The list of potentiating drugs is considerable with antibiotics, tranquillizers, hypnotics and anti-inflammatory agents being commonly implicated in 'over-anticoagulation', together with dietary influences including alcohol.

Restoration of haemostasis can be achieved by withholding further treatment or intravenous infusion of vitamin K or, if the haemorrhage is life-threatening, by the infusion of fresh frozen plasma or 'prothrombin complex' concentrates, particularly those with a high level of factor VII.

Heparin

Chemistry and pharmacokinetics [32, 33]

Standard, unfractionated heparin from beef lung or porcine mucosa is a heterogeneous polysaccharide with a mean molecular weight of 15 kd and a range of 2–40 kd. Heparin may be divided into two classes on the basis of its affinity to ATIII, class 1 molecules having low affinity and class 2 high affinity. Class 2 molecules can be subdivided into 2A having a molecular weight <5 kd and anti-Xa activity, and 2B with a molecular weight >5 kd and both anti-Xa and IIa activities.

In the last decade much interest has centred on low molecular weight heparins (LMWH) with a mean molecular weight between 4 and 6 kd consisting of both class 1 (75%) and class 2 (25%) molecules, the latter being mainly of 2A type. LMWH have high anti-Xa activity, tighter binding to ATIII and a longer *in vivo* half-life than standard heparin. It is therefore possible that LMWH may be more useful than standard heparin in the prophylaxis and treatment of thrombosis. The hope that LMWH may result in a lower incidence of haemorrhagic complications than standard heparin has not been shown convincingly.

Figure 17.1 summarizes the features of standard and low molecular weight heparins. The mean *in vivo* half-life of standard heparin is 1.5 hours but is dose-dependent with an increase in half-life as the dose increases relative to body weight. Heparin is cleared by the reticuloendothelial system, especially the liver, and excreted in urine. A lower heparin dose may be indicated in patients with hepatic or renal impairment.

Mechanism of action of heparin

Antithrombin III (ATIII) is a very weak serine protease inhibitor. The formation of an equimolar complex between class 2 heparin molecules and ATIII is accompanied by a conformational change in the ATIII molecule which fully activates the arginine reactive site. The inhibition kinetics of the ATIII–heparin complex towards serine proteases is enhanced approximately 1000-fold. *Figure 17.2*

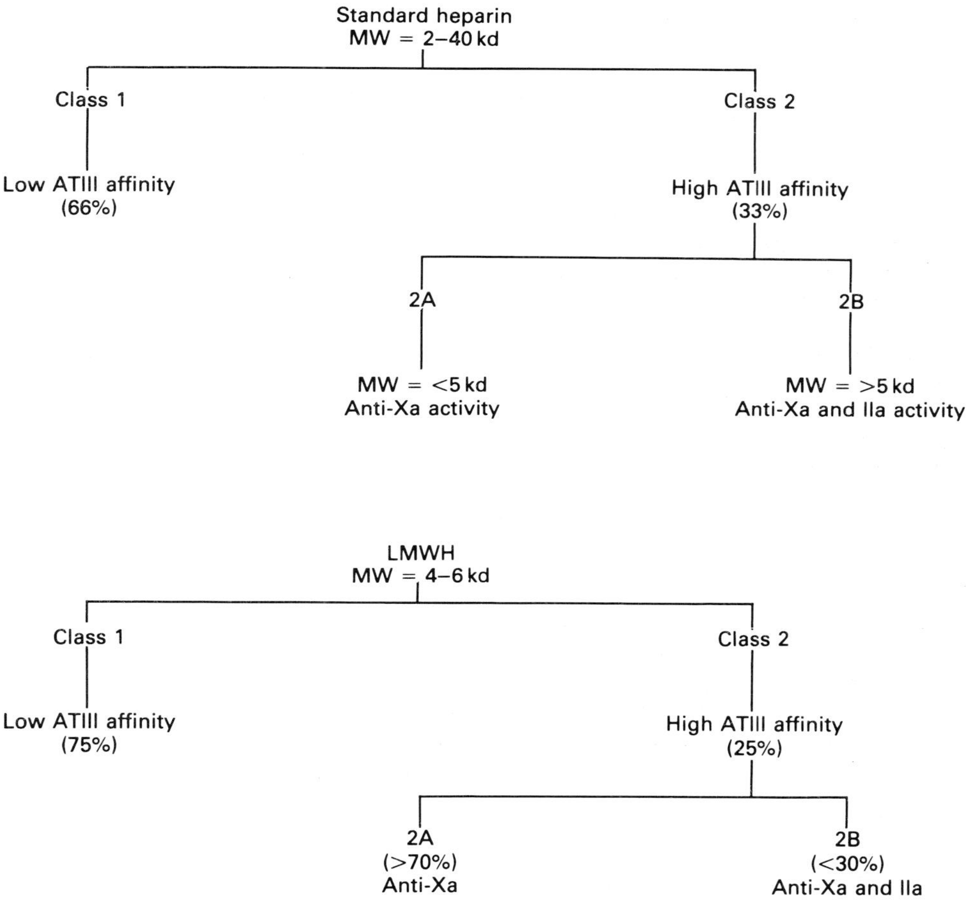

Figure 17.1 Composition and activities of standard and low molecular weight heparins (LMWH)

illustrates the slow action of native ATIII compared with enhanced activity in the presence of heparin, against thrombin, though it is emphasised that the ATIII–heparin complex has activity against all serine proteases with the probable exception of VIIa.

Effect of heparin on platelet function The effects of heparin on platelet function are complex but it is considered that heparin enhances primary aggregation by stimulating the release reaction. This response may also make the platelets refractory to *in vitro* aggregation by agents such as adrenaline and ADP. This heparin effect may be mediated *in vivo* by free fatty acids, as heparin is known to induce the release of lipoprotein lipase and free fatty acid, which are known to be capable of inducing platelet aggregation via the prostaglandin pathway. From a practical point of view it is important to recognize that 'minidose' subcutaneous heparin does not prolong the bleeding time but that large doses (>20 000 units) do so.

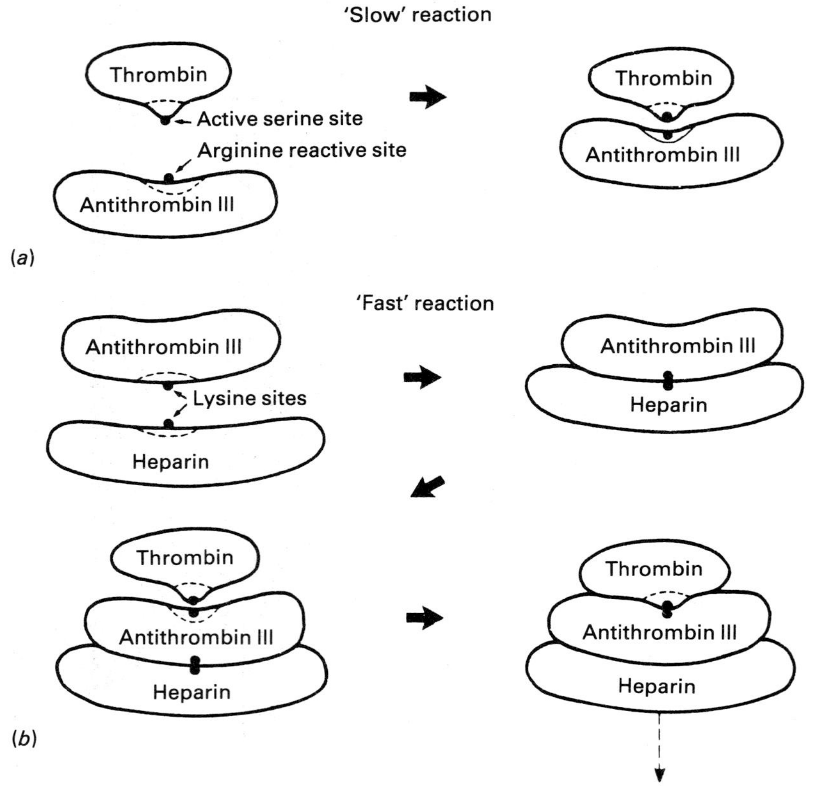

Figure 17.2 Antithrombin III (ATIII) inhibition of thrombin in the presence of heparin

Platelet factor 4 (PF4) Platelet factor 4 is a highly cationic protein capable of combining with strongly acidic substances such as heparin and appears to function by combining with heparin (both endogenous and exogenous) to prevent heparin inhibition of the coagulation system within, and in the vicinity of, platelet aggregates. Although PF4 appears to neutralize heparin, this neutralization does not appear to reactivate thrombin which has already been neutralized by ATIII–heparin. PF4 is released in relatively large amounts whenever platelets are damaged.

Clinical use of heparin

Prophylaxis in the prevention of thromboembolism When there is an increased risk of thromboembolism, e.g. orthopaedic surgery of the lower limbs, heparin is often used in a 'low-dose' regimen to inhibit possible activation of the coagulation cascade and prevent a hypercoagulable state in which Xa generation overwhelms anti-Xa, thrombin formation is enhanced and fibrin formed with a resulting clot. Trace amounts of heparin (low-dose) enhance the anti-Xa activity of ATIII, provided that it is given before thrombin is formed. Low-dose heparin therapy is also of value in preventing the thromboembolic complications of pregnancy.

Use in established thromboembolism Heparin is widely used in the treatment of thrombotic or embolic episodes such as deep-vein thrombosis (DVT) and pulmonary embolus (PE). Its main advantage is that its anticoagulant effect is immediate, particularly in the prevention of the thrombin–fibrinogen–fibrin sequence thus reducing the potential to form and lay down fibrin. It is often used in combination with oral anticoagulants (*see* page 674) to give protection until coumarin drugs produce a significant effect.

Method of heparin infusion Four alternative routes or regimens are used for heparin therapy: (1) 'minidose' subcutaneous; (2) 'full-dose' subcutaneous; (3) intermittent intravenous; and (4) 'continuous infusion' intravenous. The effect of full-dose subcutaneous heparin is somewhat unpredictable and it is not commonly used in hospitalized patients, but when long-term, outpatient heparinization is necessary full-dose subcutaneous treatment may be considered appropriate.

Clinical trials comparing 'intermittent' versus 'continuous' infusion show the incidence of bleeding to be seven times more frequent in patients treated by intermittent therapy and that continuous infusion is equally effective in preventing subsequent thromboembolism. The main advantage of intermittent therapy is that it allows greater patient mobility and does not require significant volumes of intravenous fluids to be administered as is required by continuous infusion.

Dosage of heparin The correct dose of heparin is that amount that inhibits clot formation but does not result in bleeding and it varies considerably from patient to patient. In patients with *thomboembolic disease* a single intravenous infusion of 70 units heparin/kg body weight may produce an APTT between 40 and 120 seconds (baseline 40 seconds) and a plasma heparin level of 0.2–1.0 units/ml. The half-life of heparin in plasma can vary from 0.5 to 6 hours.

Clearly a 'standard dose' regimen cannot be adopted, but an initial dose of 10 000–15 000 units for 'low-risk' patients is recommended, the dose being adjusted for 'high-risk' patients of average weight. Within 30–60 minutes of administration an APTT should be performed to ensure that the required effect has been attained. If the APTT has not reached 2–2.5 times the midpoint of the reference range, further heparin should be given *immediately*; there should not be a delay of 4–6 hours, as is sometimes practised. When the APTT is 2–2.5 times 'normal' the frequency of dosage can be determined by laboratory monitoring. In general the average daily dose required is 20 000–30 000 units by continuous infusion and 5000–10 000 units every 6 hours if therapy is given intermittently.

It should be remembered that PF4 levels are often high following a thromboembolic episode and that the levels will fall within several hours or days, assuming further thomboembolism does not occur. Consequently a patient who initially requires large amounts of heparin to attain the desired therapeutic effect may gradually or suddenly become 'sensitive' and dosage may need to be reduced. On the other hand ATIII levels may fall significantly following thrombotic events, and as the main anticoagulant effect of heparin is mediated by ATIII a patient may appear 'resistant' to heparin but the balance could be restored by infusions of ATIII.

Duration of therapy The risk of continued thromboembolism may remain until endothelialization of the thrombus has occurred which generally takes 7–10 days. Since it requires about 5–7 days for the coumarin effect to be fully established, heparin should be continued for a minimum of 10 days. For recurrent thromboses, heparin should be continued longer as the general view is that heparin is superior to coumarin as an anticoagulant.

Monitoring heparin therapy External quality assessment surveys in the UK show that over 95% of laboratories use the APTT to monitor and control heparin therapy, i.e. assess the overall effect of heparin on coagulability rather than use the plasma thrombin time or measure plasma heparin levels. Although the plasma thrombin clotting time is sensitive to low concentrations of heparin, there is very limited linear relationship between clotting times and heparin level and the test only involves the heparin inactivation of IIa. The APTT fulfils the requirements of being rapid, capable of precision and accuracy, can be readily standardized and controlled, and has a possible sensitivity to 0.1 units heparin/ml plasma. It cannot be overemphasized, however, that different platelet substitute reagents (phospholipid, cephalin) for use in the APTT have greatly varying sensitivity to heparin, some being relatively insensitive. There is evidence from studies in animals that control of LMWH is best achieved by chromogenic assays of anti-Xa and IIa activity[34].

Maintenance of the APTT at 2–2.5 times the midpoint of the reference range is based on clinical trials and is a compromise between the possibility of thrombosis and the risk of haemorrhage.

Notes on factors affecting the effect of heparin

1. Samples should be collected carefully to avoid release of PF4 and tested within 30 minutes.
2. ATIII levels are reduced in pregnancy, liver disease, DIC, continuous heparin infusion and congenital ATIII deficiency. Patients with low levels of ATIII show 'resistance' to heparin therapy.
3. The half-life of heparin is dose-dependent. There is an increase in half-life as the dose increases and it is reduced in massive pulmonary embolism, possibly due to PF4 release.

Side-effects of heparin therapy

Bleeding The most common and important side-effect of heparin therapy is bleeding which occurs in 5–20% of patients receiving full-dose intravenous therapy. Bleeding can take any form but melaena, haematuria, haematoma, ecchymoses and bleeding from the injection or infusion site are the most common. Although controversy exists over the prevention of bleeding by laboratory monitoring, many studies support the view that it is less likely to occur if the APTT time does not exceed 2.5 times the baseline value. Certain groups of patients are more likely to have haemorrhagic complications – associated quantitative or qualitative platelet defects, underlying coagulopathy, hepatic and renal disease, septicaemia and any patient with an anatomical lesion which is likely to bleed, e.g. gastric ulceration, malignant lesion.

Before commencing heparin therapy it is wise to perform a platelet count, APTT, TCT and PT, and if any test is abnormal or prolonged, care should be exercised. Following the start of therapy the PCV and platelet count should be monitored daily in addition to the APTT.

Since the half-life of heparin is short, stopping the drug permits the rapid disappearance of the heparin effect and neutralization by protamine sulphate is not usually necessary. In certain circumstances such as massive haemorrhage and severe liver disease, neutralization may be required with protamine sulphate and 1 mg protamine will usually neutralize 100 units of heparin. Heparins of differing molecular weight may react differently to protamine sulphate neutralization [35]. Excess infusion of protamine should be avoided since protamine itself has an anticoagulant effect (inhibition of the reaction between factors, X, V, calcium and phospholipid). Following protamine neutralization the APTT and TCT should be performed and should be corrected, though the TCT may be shorter than normal since protamine enhances fibrin polymerization. Following heparin neutralization a heparin 'rebound' may occur some hours later which is thought to be due to dissociation of heparin–protamine complexes.

Although unusual, heparin-induced thrombocytopenia may occur and is characterized by progressive thrombocytopenia after a few days' treatment. It is due to a heparin-dependent platelet antibody. Paradoxically, heparin-induced thrombocytopenia may be associated with thrombotic complications. Platelet counts should be performed regularly on patients receiving heparin.

Defibrination therapy

In addition to the neurotoxic or haemolytic effects of some snake venoms, others affect haemostatic mechanisms. Purified fractions of venoms can be used therapeutically as anticoagulants by reducing the level of plasma fibrinogen. Ancrod (Arvin) is purified from *Agkistrodon rhodostoma* venom (Malayan pit viper) and has the following properties:

1. Converts fibrinogen to soluble fibrin by removing fibrinopeptide A.
2. The fibrin monomer produced polymerizes in an end-to-end form which is not cross-linked by factor XIIIa.
3. The reaction is not Ca^{2+}-dependent and is not inhibited by heparin.
4. The clot is readily lysed by plasmin.
5. Does not cause platelet aggregation or release of nucleotides.
6. It can be neutralized by α_2-macroglobulin.
7. One unit of Ancrod is that activity which will clot human fibrinogen in the same time as 1 unit of thrombin.

The therapeutic effect is:

1. Degradation of fibrinogen with clearance of the soluble fibrin from the circulation.
2. Reduction in plasma fibrinogen.
3. Conversion of plasminogen to plasmin but no increase in systemic fibrinolytic activity.
4. Production of FDPs.
5. The blood is relatively hypocoagulable.
6. Reduction in blood and plasma viscosity.

Laboratory control of defibrination therapy

The objective is to reduce plasma fibrinogen levels yet avoid haemorrhagic complications and levels ranging from 0.5 to 1.5 g/l should be maintained depending on the clinical situation. Estimation or measurement of plasma fibrinogen is the only monitoring necessary and the plasma fibrinogen titre (1 in 4 ≡ 0.5 g/l) or fibrinogen quantitation can be used. Simple observation of a blood sample to ensure that a small clot is formed can be used to prevent overdosage. Stored plasma samples should contain added antivenom to prevent *in vitro* fibrinogen loss.

Bleeding complications can be arrested by (1) withdrawing the drug; (2) administration of fibrinogen concentrate; and (3) injection of antivenom.

Anti-platelet therapy [36, 37]

Platelets have an essential role in haemostatic function, particularly by their interaction with vessel walls and their contribution to fibrin formation. This has resulted in the use of drugs known to suppress platelet function in attempts to modify thromboembolic processes.

Of the many drugs or compounds known to alter platelet function acetylsalicylic acid (aspirin), sulphinpyrazone and dipyrimadole, either singly or in combination, have been the most widely used. More recent approaches to the modification of platelet function by drugs have been directed at membrane receptors/binding sites and the stimulation of prostacyclin (epoprostenol) by vascular endothelium. It must be remembered that different forms of thromboembolism almost certainly have differing aetiologies and that it is therefore not possible to make generalizations regarding their efficacy.

Aspirin

The effects of aspirin include (1) inhibition of the platelet release reaction; (2) inhibition of ADP-induced platelet aggregation; and (3) inhibition of adherence to collagen.

The important mechanism is the inhibitory effect of aspirin on the conversion of arachidonate to cyclic endoperoxides, thus blocking thromboxane A_2 synthesis by irreversible acetylation of platelet cyclo-oxygenase.

The inhibitory effect of 300 mg (one tablet) aspirin lasts for the life of the platelet (10–14 days) with a prolongation of the bleeding time for up to 1 week in some cases. Aspirin will not prolong the bleeding time in all subjects and it is difficult to identify those who will have a prolonged time. Aspirin in higher doses also blocks vessel wall cyclo-oxygenase and, hence, prostacyclin production. This effect is, however, short-lived and is regained in a matter of hours in contrast to the effect on platelets throughout their lifespan.

Sulphinpyrazone

The main effect appears to involve the release reaction by competitive inhibition of cyclo-oxygenase but, in contrast to aspirin, the effect is reversible and is dependent on plasma concentration.

Dipyrimadole

The effects of dipyrimadole are also multiple and include (1) the inhibition of *primary* and *secondary* aggregation induced by ADP, collagen and adrenaline; and (2) decreased platelet *adhesion*, by inhibition of platelet phosphodiesterase activity which is responsible for the degradation of cyclic AMP. Since cyclic AMP inhibits many platelet reactions the consequent build-up of cyclic AMP may be responsible for most of the anti-platelet effects of dipyrimadole.

Ticlopidine
Ticlopidine hydrochloride has a unique mechanism of action by modifying the Gp IIb/IIIa complex. This results in inhibition of aggregation by ADP, adrenaline and collagen. The inhibition of function lasts for the lifespan of the platelet.

Laboratory monitoring of anti-platelet therapy
There is no easy approach to ensuring that anti-platelet therapy is effective, and as haemorrhagic complications are not a problem laboratory monitoring is unnecessary.

Thrombolytic therapy

Anticoagulant therapy (oral anticoagulants, heparin, defibrinating agents) and anti-platelet drugs are directed at preventing thrombotic episodes or the extension of existing thrombus. Thrombolytic therapy attempts to induce dissolution of existing thrombus and is used particularly in the presence of extensive venous thrombosis, massive pulmonary embolus, and more recently in myocardial infarction. The principle is to enhance the potential of the physiological fibrinolytic system to produce plasmin by the use of plasminogen activators.

Mechanisms of in vivo thrombolysis

Plasmin has a limited substrate specificity and its controlled production should enhance thrombolysis. The mechanisms of the action and regulation of thrombolysis are:

1. The Sherry hypothesis:
   (a) Thrombus is formed with sufficient absorbed plasminogen to ensure its subsequent lysis.
   (b) Plasminogen activator diffuses into the clot, activates bound plasminogen and the plasmin formed is protected from circulating inactivators and can initiate clot lysis.
   (c) Plasminogen has two phases – (i) a plasma (soluble) phase, from which any formed plasmin is readily neutralized with minimal clot lysis; and (ii) a thrombus (gel) phase from which formed plasmin is in close spatial relationship to the fibrin, is not affected by inhibitors and readily causes clot dissolution.
2. Sharp, Chesterman, Allington hypothesis. This considers that plasminogen activator in the circulation is adsorbed to fibrin/thrombus and that circulating plasminogen is converted to plasmin within the thrombus. This differs from the Sherry hypothesis in that it proposes that the activator is fixed within the thrombus and plasminogen circulates through it.
3. Recent advances in understanding *in vivo* thrombolysis. The relationship between t-PA and the fast-acting PAI has led to the following concept:
   (a) Plasmin is generated in a thrombus and acts on single-chain t-PA which is more reactive with plasminogen and accelerates the formation of plasmin *within* the thrombus;
   (b) External to the thombus, the two-chain forms of t-PA formed by the action of plasmin on single-chain t-PA is rapidly neutralized by fast-acting PAI;
   (c) PAI is less active against single-chain t-PA;

(d) The result is fibrin-specific fibrinolysis limited to thrombus and induces less systemic fibrinolysis.

Factors affecting the rate of thrombolysis

1. The level of fibrinolytic activation.
2. The internal and external structure of the thrombus.
3. Physical changes in the thrombus, i.e. growth, infiltration by fibroblasts and collagen fibres, making the thrombus inaccessible to fibrinolysis.
4. Whether the thrombus has completely occluded the vessel.
5. The type of thrombus:
   (a) Arterial thrombus with densely packed platelets, fibrin strands and leucocytes, which are more resistant to lysis.
   (b) Venous thrombus consisting mainly of red cells and fibrin with few platelets and more susceptible to lysis.
   (c) The extent of fibrin cross-linking by factor XIII which makes the clot more resistant to the action of plasmin.

Thrombolytic agents

Streptokinase (SK)
Streptokinase is produced by β-haemolytic streptococci and has the following properties:

1. It does not activate plasminogen directly but forms a stoichiometric complex with plasminogen (SK–plasminogen).
2. This complex results in conformational changes in the plasminogen molecule and the development of an 'active' site.
3. The active complex then acts inter- or intramolecularly in the conversion of plasminogen to plasmin.
4. In the course of plasmin production, SK is proteolytically reduced to low molecular weight fragments.
5. SK is potent and effective but has the following disadvantages:
   (a) It is antigenic.
   (b) It does not activate fibrin-bound plasminogen in preference to circulating plasminogen.

Urokinase (UK)
Urokinase is a β-globulin excreted in normal human urine from which it can be extracted, or it can be obtained from culture of fetal kidney cells. Unlike SK it directly activates plasminogen to form plasmin and has the following advantages over SK:

1. It has an affinity for fibrin-bound plasminogen (i.e. within a thrombus) in preference to plasma (circulating) plasminogen.
2. It is not antigenic in humans.

In addition to the 'first generation' thrombolytic agents, streptokinase and urokinase, the relatively recent introduction of acylated plasminogen–streptokinase activator complex (APSAC), recombinant t-PA (rt-PA) and single-chain urokinase (scu-PA) has widened the application of fibrinolytic therapy.

Before starting thrombolytic therapy the patient's haemostatic status should be assessed as most will have been treated with oral anticoagulants or heparin. A potential problem in the use of SK is that many patients have antistreptolysin (ASO) antibodies which will inactivate SK, and initial testing to determine the loading dose of SK is sometimes practised.

Although recommendations for laboratory control may differ, the plasma thrombin time with its sensitivity to the degree of hyperplasminaemia, fibrinogen level and the FDPs generated is often the only test performed. Chromogenic assay of plasminogen and the relative ease of obtaining a result may make control of thrombolytic therapy more reliable.

Techniques for the investigation of thrombotic disorders

Evidence of platelet activation

Platelet aggregation ratio (PAR)

Principle
Circulating platelet aggregates are demonstrated by collecting blood into anticoagulant with and without fixative; aggregates will disperse in the sample without fixative and remain in the fixed sample. The ratio of the platelet counts on each sample is determined.

Reagents
Solution A: Trisodium citrate dihydrate 0.475 g, 36% formalin 2.7 ml, 10 ml 1 mol/l phosphate-buffered saline, made up to 100 ml with distilled water. Store at 4°C.
Solution B: As for solution A but without the formalin.

Blood sampling and method
Bring solutions A and B to room temperature. Take four 5 ml syringes and label two syringes as 'A' and two syringes as 'B'. Take up exactly 4 ml solution A into each of the 'A' syringes and 4 ml solution B into each of the 'B' syringes. Exclude any air bubbles to make measurement as accurate as possible.

Apply minimum stasis and by venepuncture using a 21G butterfly set, allow blood to run down the line on to a wad of cotton wool and then take exactly 1 ml blood into each of the four syringes. Mix well within the syringes and dispense into four plastic tubes. Leave the samples at room temperature for 15 minutes to allow fixation of the platelet aggregates and centrifuge at 200 *g* for 8 minutes. Perform duplicate platelet counts on each supernatant and average the duplicate results. Calculate the ratio by:

$$\frac{(A1/B1) + (A2/B2) - (A1/B2) + (A2/B1)}{4}$$

Interpretation
Normal ratio: 0.75–1.20. A ratio of less than 0.75 indicates the presence of circulating platelet aggregates.
Note. If the two values for 'A' or the values for 'B' do not agree the test is invalid.

Platelet β-thromboglobulin in plasma

Principle
β-thromboblogulin (BTG) is a platelet-specific protein released by platelet activation. Increased plasma β-thromboglobulin levels can therefore be interpreted as evidence of *in vivo* platelet activation if liberation of β-thromboglobulin during sample collection can be kept to an absolute minimum.

Sample collection
Blood samples *must* be taken without stasis using a 21G butterfly set, if possible discarding the first 1 ml of blood. Use a 5 ml syringe to collect 2.5 ml of blood and immediately transfer to a tube containing anticoagulant solution. Invert three times and place immediately into melting ice to reduce the temperature rapidly. Because of the critical conditions for sampling and specimen handling it is wise to collect a sample from a normal subject using exactly the same procedure as for the test sample.

Method
Measurement of BTG is by a competitive-binding radioimmune assay technique which is available in kit form (Amersham International, UK).

Platelet factor 4 in plasma

Principle
Platelet factor 4 (PF4) is a low molecular weight protein that is secreted from the α granules of platelets during the release reaction. This occurs when platelets are activated by contact with subendothelial tissues and by a variety of physiological agents such as thrombin, ADP and adrenaline.

Method
Quantitation is by radioimmune assay. Kits are available from commercial sources.

Interpretation
Measurement of PF4 is used to detect the activation of the coagulation system as occurs in myocardial infarction, coronary artery disease and arterial thrombosis. Elevated PF4 levels are also found in subjects with prosthetic heart valves, pulmonary embolus, DIC and venous thrombosis.

Detection and identification of lupus anticoagulants

The possible presence of lupus anticoagulant (LA) may be suggested by one or more of the following: (1) unexplained prolongation of the APTT; (2) fetal loss; and (3) unexplained thrombotic tendency.

The Working Party on Acquired Inhibitors of Coagulation of the ICSH proposed criteria for the diagnosis of LA[38] based on the APTT and one-stage and two-stage factor assays. The criteria were not widely accepted due to the reliance on the APTT as the sole screening test by which a significant number of LA would not be identified.

Detection of LA by the APTT depends on the phospholipid content and composition of the partial thromboplastin, particularly phosphatidyl serine, which ideally should be low in content [39]. Further reagent variables include the choice of activator, i.e. kaolin, ellagic acid, etc., and the buffering capacity of the reagent.

Minimal criteria have been proposed [40] that incorporate the concept of the phospholipid specificity of LA:

1. Abnormality of phospholipid-dependent coagulation test (in most cases an unexplained abnormal APTT).
2. Demonstration that the abnormality is due to an inhibitor.
3. Proof that the inhibitor is directed at phospholipid and not specific plasma coagulation factors.

Approach to laboratory investigation

1. Tests to identify alternative abnormalities:
   (a) one-stage prothrombin time – to exclude deficiencies of factors II, V, VII or X and oral anticoagulant therapy;
   (b) thrombin time/reptilase time – to exclude heparin and the possibility of dysfibrinogenaemia.
2. Screening tests for possible LA:
   (a) APTT – a sensitive reagent must be used;
   (b) kaolin clotting time (KCT) of platelet-poor plasma – possibly the most sensitive test in pregnancy;
   (c) dilute Russell's viper venom time (DRVVT) – possibly the most sensitive test and significantly associated with thrombotic events;
   (d) one-stage assays of factors XII, XI, IX or VIII may show non-parallelism.
   Note. A sensitive APTT test system, which includes a well established normal reference range, can perform as well as other test systems but *no single test system will identify all patients with LA* [41].
3. Identification of inhibitor activity:
   Mixing studies – APTT of test and normal plasma, 1:1 and 4:1 mixtures.
   Notes. Failure to correct the APTT of 1:1 mixture establishes the presence of inhibitor, but correction may occur with low levels of LA. A 4:1 mixture is more sensitive and the 1:1 mixture alone is not recommended. Although LA are generally considered to have an 'immediate' inhibitory effect, a time-dependent pattern has been shown to be found in 10–40% of LA [41,42]. The Kaspar inhibitor screening method (page 650) is entirely suitable.
   When the APTT screening test is only slightly above the upper limit of the reference range, mixing studies may be inconclusive and studies using plasma-agarose gel can be helpful [41,43]. Mixing studies may show a *prolongation* of the APTT or other screening tests; this is more often seen when a 4:1 mixture is used. The unidentified factor in normal plasma responsible for this effect has been termed 'lupus co-factor' [44].
4. Conformation of phospholipid specificity:
   (a) Platelet neutralization procedure (PNP) with the DRVVT – significantly corrects or bypasses inhibitor activity.
   (b) KCT of various mixtures of normal and test plasma (Exner test).
   (c) Thromboplastin dilution test – enhancement of inhibitory effect of LA by decreasing the amount of phospholipid; sensitive but not specific.
   Note. A neutralization procedure using hexagonal phospholipid [45] has been described which appears to distinguish accurately between LA and specific factor inhibitors or deficiencies.

A number of decision algorithms can be constructed for the diagnosis of LA. The starting point can be either the investigation of an unexpected, prolonged APTT, or, in cases of recurrent abortion or a thrombotic tendency, a systematic study starting with the sensitive DRVVT. *Figure 17.3* shows a scheme starting with a prolonged APTT in the presence of a normal one-stage PT.

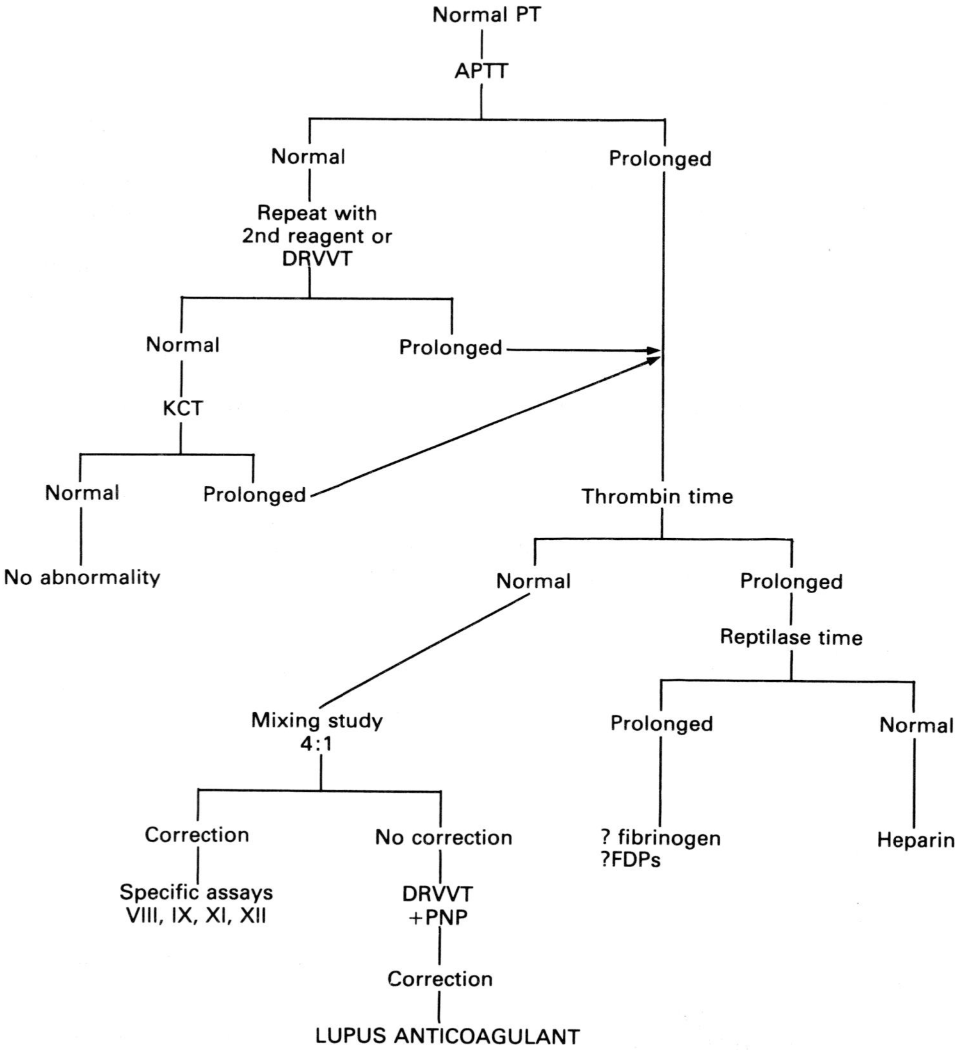

Figure 17.3 Detection and identification of lupus anticoagulant

Pre-analytical variables

Careful blood collection, handling, plasma preparation and storage are essential for the reliable demonstration of LA.

Blood collection

A plastic syringe and 19G needle is used to collect blood into standard citrate solution, with minimal stasis to avoid platelet activation. Evacuated collection systems should be avoided. Samples should be processed as soon as possible and tested within 1 hour of collection. If this is not possible, platelet-free plasma should be stored at −70°C. A control normal plasma should be prepared at the same time.

Preparation of platelet-poor plasma (PPP)

1. Double-spin method
   The citrated blood is centrifuged at 2000 *g* for 10 minutes. The plasma is transferred to a plastic container avoiding the plasma–red cell interface, and recentrifuged at 2500 *g* for a further 10 minutes. The plasma is transferred to a further container and the platelet count which must be $<10 \times 10^9$/l checked.
2. Filtration method
   Filtration of plasma through a 0.22 μm cellulose acetate filter is particularly recommended for use with the KCT and when plasma samples are to be frozen.

Control plasmas

For LA studies control plasmas must be treated as for test plasmas. Commercial, lyophilized plasmas are unlikely to be free of platelets or platelet fragments.

Methods

Methods for PT, APTT/KCCT, Reptilase time and plasma thrombin time are described in Chapter 15 and are standard procedures.

Kaolin clotting time

Principle Following activation by kaolin, PPP is recalcified; the clotting time is influenced by traces of platelet phospholipid, hence the sensitivity to platelet fragments.

Reagents

1. Kaolin: 20 mg/ml in Owren's buffer.
2. Calcium chloride: 0.025M.
3. Filtered or double-spun test and control plasmas.

Method

1. In 75 × 12 mm polystyrene tubes, 0.2 ml of plasma is added to 0.1 ml kaolin suspension.
2. Mix gently and leave at 37°C for 3 minutes.
3. Add 0.2 ml calcium chloride and start stopwatch. Mix gently and leave for 30 seconds before continuous tilting to determine clot formation.
4. Perform test in duplicate.

Kaolin clotting time of mixtures of test and normal plasma – Exner test [46]

Principle Decreasing amounts of normal plasma are mixed with increasing amounts of test plasma and a kaolin clotting time performed on each mixture.

Clotting times are plotted against increasing concentrations of test plasma on arithmetic graph paper. The test is sensitive to the presence of LA and allows recognition of the lupus co-factor effect, and can identify the coexistence of a factor deficiency.

Reagents
1. Kaolin: 20 mg/ml in Owren's buffer.
2. Plasmas and calcium chloride as for the KCT above.
3. Polystyrene 75 × 12 mm tubes.

Method
Test plasma (TP) and normal plasma (NP) are mixed in the proportions of NP:TP 5/0, 4/1, 1/1, 1/4 and 0/5. To 0.2 ml of each mixture add 0.1 ml kaolin and incubate for 3 minutes at 37°C, add 0.2 ml of prewarmed $CaCl_2$ and determine the clotting time.

Plot the clotting times against plasma mixture on arithmetic graph paper.

Interpretation Four patterns are recognized and are illustrated in *Figure 17.4.*

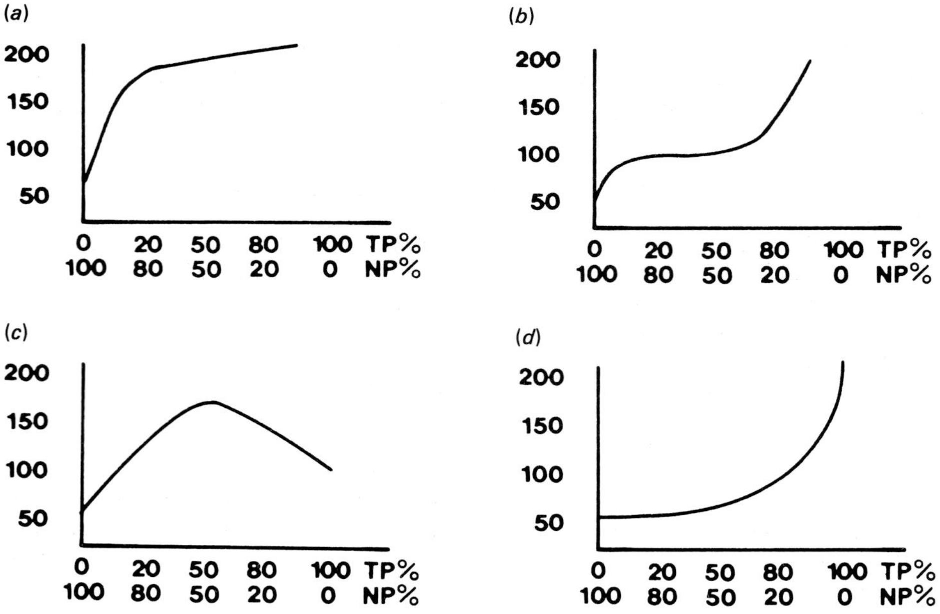

Figure 17.4 Representative graphs obtained by the Exner kaolin clotting time procedure: (*a*) type 1, classical lupus anticoagulant; (*b*) type II, classical lupus anticoagulant and factor deficiency; (*c*) type III, lupus anticoagulant present, no lupus co-factor present; (*d*) no lupus type inhibition present

Dilute Russell's viper venom time (DRVVT)
Principle RVV selectively activates factor X to Xa with consequent conversion of II to IIa. Enhancement of LA inhibition is achieved by decreasing the amount of phospholipid.

Reagents
1. Calcium chloride: 0.025M.
2. Imidazole buffer 0.05M, pH 7.3: 3.4 g imidazole; 5.5 g NaCl. Dissolve in 900 ml distilled water; adjust to pH 7.3 with HCl and make up to 1 litre.
3. Russell's viper venom (Diagnostic Reagents, Thame, Oxon, UK): add 2 ml distilled water to prepare a stock solution of 0.1 mg/ml; store in 20 µl amounts at –20°C. For use dilute 1 in 1000 by adding 10 µl to 490 µl of buffer and further dilute 1 in 20 in buffer (alternatively add 10 µl to 10 ml buffer). The concentration is adjusted to give an RVV clotting time of between 30 and 40 seconds with normal plasma in the reaction mixture.
4. Phospholipid: Bell and Alton platelet substitute (Diagen Reagents, Thame, Oxon, UK). Reconstitute with 5 ml of distilled water for a stock solution and store frozen in 100 µl amounts. For use, thaw and dilute 1 in 8 by adding 700 µl of buffer. Alternative RVV and phospholipid reagents may require different dilutions.
5. Test and control plasmas: PPP prepared as described.

Method To 0.1 ml plasma in a 75 × 10 mm glass tube add 0.1 ml phospholipid, mix and incubate for 30 seconds; add 0.1 ml dilute RVV. Incubate for 30 seconds at 37°C and add 0.1 ml calcium chloride. Record the clotting time.

Interpretation Prolongation of the DRVVT may be due to LA. Some workers recommend calculation of the ratio of clotting time of test:clotting time of normal plasma with a DRVVT ratio greater than 1.1 suggesting the possibility of LA.

Notes
1. The DRVVT is sensitive and relatively specific for LA when the optimum dilution of phospholipid is used.
2. It is not affected by levels of factors XII, XI, IX, VIII, HMWK or PK. Factors V, X, II and I will prolong the DRVVT when levels are below 0.3 units/ml but will be corrected by the addition of normal plasma.
3. Antibodies to factor V will prolong the DRVVT.
4. Ratios greater than 1.1 should be retested using the platelet neutralization procedure; a significant reduction in ratio indicates specificity for phospholipid.

DRVVT and platelet neutralization procedure (PNP)
Principle The prolonged DRVVT due to LA will be corrected by substituting washed, activated platelets for the phospholipid reagent. The phospholipid of platelets is insensitive to the action of LA possibly because of steric hindrance due to the higher affinity of 'prothrombinase complex' than LA for phospholipid binding sites.

Reagents Washed, freeze-thawed platelets: centrifuge citrated blood at 200 *g* for 10 minutes. Remove the supernatant platelet-rich plasma and centrifuge at 2000 *g* for 10 minutes to deposit the platelets which are washed three times with Tris-buffered saline (TBS), (0.15M NaCl (8.766 g/l); 0.05M Tris (6.055 g/l)). Resuspend in TBS and adjust the platelet count to 200–300 × 10^9/l with TBS. Divide into 1 ml aliquots and freeze at –20°C. For use, thaw rapidly and mix well. Commercial platelet preparations are available but freeze-thawed platelets are reported to be more reliable [41].

Method Repeat the DRVVT technique replacing the phospholipid with the platelet preparation.

Interpretation In the presence of LA a significant shortening of the DRVVT is seen in the great majority of LA and the PNP is probably the most specific evidence for anti-phospholipid activity. What represents a significant reduction in the ratio has not been defined, though a 10% reduction has been suggested.

Note Very potent LA may be difficult to correct with washed platelets; a preparation prepared from a higher concentration of platelets may be necessary to shorten the DRVVT time.

Tissue thromboplastin inhibition test (TTI)
Principle Test and control plasmas are tested using the one-stage prothrombin time using increasing dilutions of brain thromboplastin. The test is positive if the results of test and normal plasma diverge with increasing dilution of thromboplastin.

Reagents
1. Rabbit brain thromboplastin.
2. Saline.
3. Calcium chloride 0.025м.
4. Test and control plasmas.

Method Prepare 1/10, 1/100 and 1/1000 dilutions of thromboplastin in saline. Using the diluted thromboplastin perform a one-stage prothrombin time with control and test plasma with each dilution of brain. For each dilution divide the mean time of test plasma by the mean time of the control plasma to give a ratio.

Interpretation The test is positive if the ratios show increasing divergence with increasing dilutions of thromboplastin to eventually give a ratio greater than 1.3.

Notes Although widely used, the TTI test is not specific for LA. False positive results may be seen with specific factor inhibitors and factor deficiencies of both extrinsic and intrinsic systems. One study suggested that 40% of normal subjects will have an abnormal TTI test.

Measurement of the natural inhibitors of coagulation

Understanding and assessment of the coagulant and platelet aspects of haemostasis developed from the use of tests of functional activity, supported later by measurement of the concentration of the protein factors by immunological methods. Paradoxically, the measurement of the natural inhibitors of coagulation developed by the use of immunological methods and more recently by techniques for assessing functional activity. Abnormalities of function due to molecular variants in which normal amounts of protein are associated with abnormal function (type II defects) have switched the emphasis from immunological to functional assays for first phase investigation.

Functional assays are based on clot end-points and/or the use of chromogenic substrates. Total protein of any factor can be quantitated if a suitable specific antibody is available and can be incorporated into a sufficiently sensitive immunological test system. Electroimmunoassay (EIA, Laurell method) and enzyme immunosorbent assay (ELISA) are widely used, and immunoradiometric (IRMA), radioimmune (RIA) and radial immunodiffusion (RID) assays have also been applied.

The general procedure for performing chromogenic assays are all similar and specificity is achieved by the type of chromogenic substrate and the possible addition of natural substrates, co-factors and activators. Similarly, the basic procedures for EIA and ELISA are well established and it would be repetitious to detail methods for factor assays when the only difference is the specificity of the antibody.

The basic principles and procedures are therefore described and any variations necessary for the measurement of specific factors are detailed separately.

Chromogenic assays

Prior to the introduction of chromogenic substrates, the only visible step in the assessment of coagulation was fibrin formation or, in the study of fibrinolysis, the dissolution of fibrin. These end-points are the final stages of a series of enzymatic reactions in one-stage, two-stage or multi-step laboratory procedures. Information regarding the protease activity of an intermediate stage or factor in the coagulation and fibrinolytic pathways is indirectly obtained by ensuring that all other factors of the pathway have normal activity.

The substitution of simple synthetic molecules for the natural substrates allows efficient, accurate and specific assessment of enzyme activity by release of a coloured compound (chromophore). Spectrophotometric measurement of the amount or rate of release of the chromophore allows sensitive quantitation of enzymatic activity.

Characteristics of a chromogenic substrate

The basic structure is a short peptide chain which mimics a natural substrate, linked by an amide bond (hence the alternative use of 'amidolytic assay') to a molecule which becomes coloured when cleaved from the substrate, that is, a chromophore.

A large number of substrate structures specific for different enzymes have been synthesized[47] which determine the specificity, enzyme affinity and catalytic reaction. Enzyme kinetics are determined by the pH, ionic strength and substrate concentration of the reaction system. The chromophore is often *para*-nitroaniline (*p*NA) which has maximum absorption at 405 nm. A satisfactory substrate must also be stable, not show spontaneous hydrolysis and have high solubility in water.

Advantages of chromogenic substrates are high affinity, sensitivity and specificity. Only microlitre quantities of plasma are required and techniques can be performed using microtitre plates and are therefore readily adapted to automation. They can eliminate the need for specific, factor-deficient, plasmas or preparations.

An important disadvantage is that results may not reflect biological activity, may not identify dysfunctional proteins and do not reflect the inhibitory or enhancing effect of co-factors. Interference by plasma pigments, notably bilirubin, with the absorption maximum of the chromophore may be overcome only by considerable plasma dilution.

Chromogenic assay kits are available from a number of commercial sources and provide standardization of methodology and are cost effective unless large numbers of assays are performed. Purchase of the chromogenic substrate and in-house preparation of other reagents may then be more economical.

General ELISA procedure [48]

A double antibody sandwich ELISA on microtitre plates is usually used.

Reagents

1. Coating buffer pH 7.2.
   $NaH_2PO_4 2H_2O$ 0.0025M, 0.345 g; $Na_2HPO_4 12H_2O$ 0.0075M, 2.68 g; NaCl 0.145M, 8.474 g.
   Distilled water to 1 litre, check pH, store at 4°C, stable for 2 months.
   Coating with this buffer is comparable to the widely used carbonate buffer pH 8.9.
2. Washing and dilution buffer pH 7.2.
   To 1 litre of coating buffer add 1 ml Tween 20 and 20.75 g (0.5M) NaCl. Store at 4°C, stable for 2 months.
3. Citric acid-phosphate buffer pH 5.0.
   Citric acid H_2O 0.0347M, 7.3 g; $Na_2HPO_4 12H_2O$ 0.0667M, 23.87 g.
   Distilled water to 1 litre; check pH, store at 4°C, stable 2 months.
4. Colour reagent.
   1.2-phenylenediamine dihydrochloride 8 mg. Citrate-phosphate buffer 12 ml. Mix and add 5 μl 30% v/v H_2O_2.
   Prepare shortly before use. Leave for 5 minutes and check that the reagent remains colourless. Any enzyme contamination will turn the reagent yellow. Use within 1 hour.
5. Sulphuric acid 1 M.
   55.5 ml concentrated (18 M) H_2SO_4 is added *slowly* to about 900 ml distilled water. Make up to 1 litre.

Procedure

1. Coating of wells with antibody.
   To each well of a suitable flat-bottomed polystyrene microtitre plate is added 100 μl of antibody diluted in coating buffer. Cover the plate with plastic film and stand at 4°C overnight. Immunoglobulin fraction of the antiserum must be used, not whole serum. The protein content of diluted antibody should be about 10 μg/ml. Coating overnight is preferable to 1 hour and increases sensitivity and precision. Pre-coated plates may be stored at 4°C for several months if 0.1 ml thiomersal is added to the diluted antibody and the plates wrapped in plastic film.
2. Washing the plate.
   Empty the plate by inversion, tap over layers of tissue to remove residual liquid. Wash the plate by immersion in washing/diluting buffer, leave for 3 minutes, empty and repeat twice more. The presence of Tween 20 in the washing buffer reduces the eventual background colour. An automated plate washer is useful.

3. Incubation with test samples.
   Add 100 µl of test serum and standards diluted in washing/diluting buffer. Cover and stand at room temperature for 2 hours. Sera are generally diluted at least one in two to reduce non-specific reactions. Using the stated volumes the detection limit is about 1–5 ng of antigen/ml. Sensitivity might be improved by adding 30 g/l polyethylene glycol MW 6000 (PEG) to the buffer. Sensitivity may be further improved by leaving the plate overnight at 4°C covered in plastic film.
4. Wash as described in (2) above.
5. Incubation with peroxidase-conjugated antibody.
   100 µl of peroxidase-conjugated antibody diluted in washing/dilution buffer is added to each well. Cover and stand at room temperature for 1 hour. Again, sensitivity may be improved by the addition of PEG or prolonging the reaction time to 2 hours. The dilution of conjugated antibody is adjusted to produce a suitable range of optical densities, usually 1 in 500 to 1 in 2000.
6. Wash as described in (2) above.
7. Colour development.
   Add 100 µl of colour reagent to each well. Cover the plate and stand for 15 minutes or until satisfactory colour has developed. Protect from light during colour development.
8. Stopping the enzymatic reaction.
   Add 150 µl of sulphuric acid to each well. It is important that each well has been reacted with the colour reagent for exactly the same time.
9. Reading results.
   Read in a spectrophotometer using microcuvettes requiring no more than 250 µl, or alternatively using a bottom-reading microtitre plate photometer (ELISA reader).
10. Plot the standard curve on semi-logarithmic graph paper with absorption on the ordinate and $\log_{10}$ concentration of standard as the abscissa.

Primary and conjugated antibody with recommended dilutions for use by ELISA are available commercially.

Electroimmuno assay (Laurell)

The EIA assay of vWf:Ag is described in detail on page 645 and describes the special electrophoretic conditions required for the migration of extremely large molecules. The procedures for EIA of smaller molecules follow the same principles.

Antibodies must be of precipitating type and are available from commercial sources. A 1% agarose is the standard concentration for preparation of the gel. A number of migration buffers are recommended, Tris-barbitone or Tris-barbitone-glycine are often specified and excellent results are obtained with Tris-tricine buffer pH 8.6 (Tris, 38.2 g; tricine, 17.2 g; distilled water to 4 litres). For the quantitation of vitamin K-dependent factor proteins there is the special requirement of the addition of EDTA to the buffer. Electrophoresis with cooling at 1 mA/cm gel width for 18 hours is standard procedure. The dilution of antibody incorporated into the gel and the dilutions of serum are adjusted to give a length of precipitate (25–30 mm) which gives a standard graph with a steep slope. The precipitation peaks may be difficult to define when stained with Coomassie Blue. Enhancement of the rocket by immersing the plate in diluted enzyme conjugate antibody and subsequent colour development is reported to enhance the sensitivity of methods for some antigens [49].

Generally EIA is capable of quantitating levels of antigen as low as 10% of normal concentration. The precipitation peaks below this level may be difficult to define and ELISA is the preferred alternative.

Measurement of antithrombin III

Functional assays

Assays which measure the capacity of a plasma sample to inhibit thrombin over a short period of time in the presence of heparin will overestimate the concentration of ATIII to a small degree due to the presence and action of heparin co-factor II (HCII) [50]. Progressive antithrombin activity in the absence of heparin gives an indication of ATIII activity but is influenced by α_1-antitrypsin and α_2-macroglobulin.

The most appropriate assay for measuring functional activity is a two-stage chromogenic assay:

Stage 1: plasma + heparin → ATIII–heparin complex
Stage 2: ATIII–heparin complex + thrombin → ATIII–heparin–thrombin complex + residual thrombin

chromogenic substrate–*p*NA → substrate + pNA

The change in colour development is therefore inversely proportional to ATIII concentration.

Assays should be designed with a relatively low concentration of heparin to minimize thrombin inhibition by HCII [51]. Other modifications to improve the specificity are the use of bovine thrombin which reacts well with ATIII but poorly with HCII, and factor Xa rather than thrombin since HCII does not react with Xa.

Functional ATIII activity can be determined by clotting assay against either thrombin or Xa. The methods require removal of fibrinogen from the test plasma which results in loss of ATIII activity. The available methods have been fully reviewed [52].

Antigen assays

A variety of immunological techniques have been described, though EIA is the most widely used. The presence of heparin in the test sample influences the migration of ATIII in the gel, making quantitation inaccurate. The conformational change of the ATIII–heparin complex can, however, be useful in identifying abnormal molecular variants. The technique of two-dimensional crossed immunoelectrophoresis (2DCIE) described in Chapter 16 (page 647) does not usually identify molecular variants of ATIII, but if heparin is added to the first-dimension gel, a clear separation between normal molecules with the ability to bind heparin and abnormal molecules with defective heparin binding is obtained [53].

Normal levels

The mean antigen concentration in adults is 150 ng/ml. The range of activity is 84–116% of normal; a similar range of antigen levels is found. Full-term infants have antigen concentrations between 40 and 90% of normal, increasing to adult levels at 3 months of age.

Levels in disease states
Levels are decreased during continuous heparin infusion to between 40 and 80% of normal. L-asparaginase therapy results in marked reduction of values. Liver disease and disseminated intravascular coagulation (DIC) can result in a wide variation of levels with mean values around 60–70%. Proteinuria in nephrotic syndrome results in lowered ATIII levels, 32–100% with a mean level of 62%, and has been implicated in the occurrence of thrombosis in patients with this disorder.

Hereditary ATIII deficiency
Results of progressive and heparin co-factor activities, antigen levels and 2DCIE identify three sub-types (*Table 17.6*).

Table 17.6 Classification of hereditary ATIII deficiency

	Progressive activity	*Heparin co-factor activity*	*Antigen levels*	*2DCIE with heparin*
Type 1	Reduced	Reduced	Reduced	Normal
Type 2	Reduced	Reduced	Normal	Variable
Type 3	Normal	Reduced	Normal	Abnormal

Measurement of heparin co-factor II (HCII)

Functional assay

HCII is most conveniently assayed in plasma by substituting dermatan sulphate for heparin in the standard chromogenic assay (dermatan sulphate has no effect on the rate of thrombin inhibition by ATIII)[51,54].

Antigen assay

Measured by EIA or ELISA.

Normal levels
The concentration of HCII in normal adults is 1.2 ± 0.4 μM.

Levels in disease states
Marked decreases are found in some patients with liver disease, DIC and obstetric complications and are usually associated with parallel decrease in ATIII[51].

Hereditary HCII deficiency
In a few patients described with HCII deficiency the levels have been 40–60% of normal. Inheritance is autosomal dominant and some affected family members have a history of thromboembolism. However, about 1% of apparently healthy subjects have been reported to have HCII levels below 60%.

Measurement of protein C

Functional assays

Clotting methods

Protein C (PC) can be activated by the addition of thrombin [55], thrombin–thrombomodulin complex [56] or the venom of the copperhead snake *Agkistrodon contortrix* (Protac®, Ortho). Activated protein C (APC) inactivates factors V and VIII resulting in prolongation of the APTT proportional to the amount of APC. Apart from being laborious, the clotting methods are difficult to standardize. There is extreme sensitivity to variation in technique as the graphs are very shallow and therefore a small difference in APTT makes a considerable difference to the result. The methods are very sensitive to heparin and are influenced by the levels of factors V and VIII. PC deficient substrate plasma is also expensive.

Chromogenic assay

The incorporation of venom activation into a chromogenic assay [57] has significantly improved the availability and quality of functional assays. Test plasma is activated by venom and APC directly cleaves the chromogenic substrate S2366 (Kabi) or its equivalent. The method is available in kit form from a number of commercial sources.

Note. Discrepancy is found between clotting and amidolytic methods especially in patients treated with oral anticoagulants [58]. The expected difference between activity and antigen levels in patients on oral anticoagulants is not found using the amidolytic assay. This may be due to the fact that the active serine site is located on the heavy chain and the vitamin K-dependent carboxylated glutamic acid residue required for clotting activity is on the light chain.

Antigen assay

PC antigen can be readily measured by EIA or ELISA using polyclonal or monoclonal antibody. With polyclonal antibody EIA detects PC, APC and APC complexed with its inhibitor, APC–APCI. EIA assays are generally higher than the values obtained by ELISA using monoclonal antibody which emphasizes the importance of determining reference ranges for each technique.

Assays of plasma of patients not treated with oral anticoagulants present few problems. Plasma from anticoagulated patients must be electrophoresed in gels containing EDTA, 1.8 g/l of buffer. The calcium chelating effect of the EDTA reduces the differences in mobility between the carboxylated and non-carboxylated (PIVKA) forms of PC antigen. This variation in method applies to EIA of any of the vitamin K-dependent proteins and particularly, in this context, to protein C, protein S and factors II, IX and X (*see* below). Most workers incorporate EDTA in the buffer system as a routine procedure.

Normal levels

International standards for PC allows functional activity to be reported in units/ml. Normal range is 70–140 units/dl. PC antigen levels show a similar range of values with a mean of 4.0 mg/l. Values rise slightly with increasing age. Full-term infants have low levels ranging from 27–40 units/dl as is found with the other vitamin K-dependent factors.

Levels in disease
PC levels appear to be lower in a variety of disorders[59] and any reduction of protein synthesis may be expected to result in reduced levels. Of particular relevance are disturbances of vitamin K metabolism and liver disease. The short half-life of PC (6–7 hours) can be expected to result in rapid changes of activity if the rates of synthesis or consumption are altered.

Hereditary PC deficiency
The prevalence of heterozygous PC deficiency is difficult to establish. Approximately 8% of cases of thrombosis at an early age have PC levels of 50 units/dl or lower. As is found in other coagulation defects, molecular variants are found and the same classification is used – type 1 defects have low activity and antigen levels while type 2 abnormality shows low functional activity with normal antigen levels. A type 3 PC defect has been described with low activity in clotting methods, normal amidolytic activity and normal antigen level.

Interpretation of values in patients on oral anticoagulants

Laboratory investigation of thrombosis is frequently requested on patients who are already on oral anticoagulants. Because PC is a vitamin K-dependent factor, both the functional and antigenic levels are reduced together with those of the procoagulant factors II, VII, IX and X. Functional activities are reduced to a greater extent than antigen levels. Discontinuation of treatment to allow activity and antigen levels to return to normal may not be clinically acceptable.

PC status can be assessed by determining the antigen level in relation to those of the vitamin K-dependent procoagulants. This approach requires a stable level of anticoagulation and, because of the differing half-life of PC and that of most of the procoagulant factors, should not be attempted until the INR has been stable for at least 2 weeks. In 'normal' individuals taking oral anticoagulants PC *activity* correlates well with factor II *activity* and there is similar agreement between the antigen level of PC and those of factors II, IX and X[60,61]. Comparison with factor VII antigen levels would be a logical choice because of the similar half-life to PC, but a precipitating antibody to VII antigen for use by EIA is not available.

Although there is some difference between the antigen levels of factors II, IX and X and that of PC at different levels of anticoagulation[61], the availability of antibody to factor II is a satisfactory compromise. Levels of factor II and PC antigens are determined by EIA and expressed as the ratio of PC antigen: II antigen as follows:

No deficiency	=	>0.6
Doubtful	=	0.5–0.6
Probable deficiency	=	<0.5

Measurement of protein S

Protein S (PS) is present in normal plasma in two forms, complexed with C4b binding protein (60%) and in a free state (40%). As the free PS is functionally active and the bound form is not, assays have been devised to measure both total and free PS.

Functional assays

The role of PS as co-factor to APC has been used in methods based on prolongation of a one-stage Xa clotting time[62] or the APTT[63]. Functional assays require PS-deficient plasma which is not readily available, and the activation of PC. Commercial kits are not currently available for the assay of functional PS which must reflect the problems involved.

Antigen assays[64]

Crossed immunoelectrophoresis provides a means of determining the relative proportions of free and complexed forms. Electrophoresis at 4°C in the first dimension minimizes the dissociation of the C4b–PS complex and the free PS migrates more rapidly to the anode than the complex. Second dimension electrophoresis at 25°C into gel containing IgG anti-PS and subsequent staining shows the proportions of free and complexed forms.

Standard EIA may reveal double peaks due to the different mobilities of the two forms of PS though results may correlate well with alternative methods of measurement. Extended electrophoresis at room temperature encourages dissociation of the complex allowing measurement of total PS. Clearly, assay of free PS is not possible by EIA of whole plasma.

RIA using high plasma dilution and prolonged incubation prior to assay encourages dissociation and measures total PS.

ELISA can be used to measure total PS if interference by C4b can be excluded. The semi-quantitative assessment by 2DCIE and the inability of EIA, RIA and ELISA to measure the functionally active free PS has resulted in the development of a method in which C4b and C4b–PS complex can be removed from plasma leaving the free PS available for immunological assay in addition to the measurement of total PS[65].

Polyethylene glycol (PEG) precipitation of plasma to separate free PS

Reagent

An 18.75% solution of PEG 8000 is prepared in distilled water and stored at 4°C in a tightly closed container. This concentration is critical and can be checked by freeze drying 1 ml amounts and weighing the residue. *If too much PEG is added to plasma some of the free PS will precipitate. Conversely, if too little is added there will be incomplete precipitation of the C4b–PS complex.*

Method

200 µl of test plasma is warmed to 37°C for 5 minutes and 50 µl prewarmed PEG added (final PEG concentration 3.75%). Cap the tube and mix twice for *5 seconds* using a vortex mixer and leave for 30 minutes in melting ice. Centrifuge for 10 minutes at 2500 *g*. Carefully remove the supernatant and test immediately or store at –40°C. A standard plasma is treated in the same manner.

Assay

Whole plasma and PEG-precipitated supernatant are assayed by the method of choice against standard plasma and PEG-treated standard plasma respectively.

Expression of results
Values for PEG-treated plasma are corrected for dilution by multiplying by 1.25. Free PS can be expressed as % or units/dl of the total PS of the standard plasma, or as % or units/dl compared with the free PS (PEG-treated) standard plasma.

Reference ranges
Using an ELISA technique, reference ranges[66] were:

Normal adults, from standard plasma graph: total PS: 74–112 units/dl (mean 92.9)
free PS: 27–63 units/dl (mean 60.3)
Normal adults, from free PS standard graph: free PS: 75–123 units/dl (mean 94.8)
Full-term infants, free and total PS: 20–35% of normal adult values.

Acquired changes in PS levels
Simultaneous reductions of free and total PS are found in pregnancy (40–80% of normal), oral contraceptives (70–90% of normal) and liver disease (20–100% of normal). Elevated levels of C4b binding protein are found in acute inflammation resulting in a shift of PS from the free to the bound form.

Hereditary PS deficiency [64]
Approximately 70% of deficient subjects have 50% normal total PS with comparable reduction in free PS (type I). The remaining 30% have total PS in the normal range but most is complexed and is therefore accompanied by low free PS (type II). Patients with dysfunctional PS have not yet been described but would be expected to have free and total PS in the normal range with low functional activity.

Assessment of PS values in patients on oral anticoagulants
In non-deficient patients PS *activity* correlates best with factor IX activity but less well with antigen levels[60]. In reported cases[62] of both type I and type II all but one of the activity levels were less than 35 units/dl. Free PS antigen is generally above 65 units/dl.

Comparison of PS and factor II antigen ratios of non-deficient and deficient patients probably requires different interpretation from those found in PC-deficient subjects on oral anticoagulants.

Assessment of fibrinolytic status [67]

Collection of samples

The quality of results depends on patient preparation and the techniques of blood collection, handling and storage. Activation of coagulation, platelets and fibrinolysis must be avoided. Preparation of the patient should include a 12-hour overnight fast including the avoidance of alcohol and refraining from smoking on the morning of sampling. The patient is rested for 20 minutes and samples taken with a 21G needle with minimal stasis and free blood flow. Samples are transferred into pre-cooled plastic tubes containing 0.109M sodium citrate without HEPES buffer and placed in melting ice.

Collection of samples after venous occlusion

Inflate the blood pressure cuff to mid systolic/diastolic pressure and maintain for exactly 10 minutes. Maintaining the pressure, collect samples into pre-cooled plastic tubes containing sodium citrate and place in melting ice.

Sample processing

Within 20 minutes of collection centrifuge at 2000 *g* for 10 minutes at 4°C. Separate the plasma into pre-cooled plastic tubes, place in melting ice and commence the euglobulin lysis test 30 minutes after sample collection. Other assays are started with the remaining plasma or freeze and store at –20°C or lower temperature.

Euglobulin clot lysis time (ECLT)

Tests such as whole blood and dilute whole blood clot lysis can be used to assess fibrinolytic activity and are mainly applied to the investigation of clinically significant hyperfibrinolysis resulting in haemorrhagic states. In the context of the investigation of hypercoagulable states, the ECLT is used to demonstrate hypofibrinolysis by prolongation of the lysis time.

The euglobulin fraction of plasma contains fibrinogen, plasminogen, plasminogen activators (PA), most of the fast-acting plasminogen activator inhibitor (PAI-1) and C1-inactivator. Inhibitors of fibrinolysis, α_2-antiplasmin, α_2-macroglobulin and α_1-antitrypsin, are not present in the euglobulin fraction.

Until 1983 the ECLT was considered to be an indication of reduced PA activity. It is now recognized that PAI-1 is present in the euglobulin fraction and that an extended ECLT may be due to either a decrease in PA, inhibition by PAI or a plasminogen defect. Reports of patients and families with reduced plasma PA or defective release of PA prior to 1983 must be considered with caution.

Method variables [68]

The initial dilution of plasma, pH at which euglobulins are precipitated, method of acidification, the possible addition of compounds to enhance precipitation, the buffer for dissolving of the precipitate, fibrinogen concentration, the method of clotting the euglobulin extract and the monitoring of clot lysis, will all affect the result. Whatever protocol is determined, it must be strictly adhered to and a reference range determined by each laboratory.

The technique described on page 568 is quite satisfactory, though dissolving the precipitate in 0.1M Tris-HCl containing 0.1% Tween 80 and clotting the euglobulin solution by the addition of 1 unit of thrombin in 0.025M calcium chloride are suggested changes in the method. An additional possible modification is dissolving the euglobulin in half the original plasma volume with the addition of flufenamate (15 mM final concentration) to block C1-inactivator inhibitor activity [69].

The ECLT of pre-occlusion plasma is in the order of 100–300 minutes and post-venous occlusion ECLT 30–60 minutes, depending on the method used.

Measurement of tissue plasminogen activator (t-PA)

t-PA is an active enzyme which complexes with PAI unless fibrin is present. Levels show a diurnal variation of 25% and therefore samples should be collected at a fixed time, preferably in the morning while fasting and at rest as previously described.

Functional assays

Sampling into standard sodium citrate results in *in vitro* inactivation of t-PA by PAI-1. The protocols of certain assays require immediate acidification of the sample to pH 4.0 by the addition of acetate buffer to block the inactivation. An alternative is to collect the sample into 0.5M citric acid/sodium citrate pH 4.0[70] which is more convenient when samples are collected away from the laboratory.

Functional activity is measured by chromogenic assay. Two types of assay are available in kit form from at least six commercial sources:

1. Fibrin is immobilized in microtitre wells, test plasma is added and the t-PA adsorbed to the fibrin. After washing to remove inhibitors, plasminogen is added in excess and the plasmin generated is quantitated by reaction with the chromogenic substrate S2251 (Kabi) or an equivalent.
2. Test plasma is mixed with plasminogen in the presence of fibrinogen fragments (prepared by cyanogen bromide treatment of fibrinogen) to enhance the conversion of plasminogen to plasmin which is measured by its action on substrate S2251.

Notes

1. Standardization can be achieved by using the International Standard of t-PA prepared from human melanoma cells.
2. Reference ranges depend on sample preparation and the assay procedure.
3. The acidification procedure increases plasma t-PA levels several fold.
4. Euglobulin fraction may be substituted for plasma.
5. t-PA activity in pre-occlusion plasma is very low and measurements are usually only of value in post-occlusion samples.

Antigen assay

ELISA using anti-tPA monoclonal antibody is useful when samples cannot be processed promptly. Antigen is stable at room temperature for 8 hours, for 48 hours at 4°C and 1 year at –20°C. PAI does not interfere with the assay.

Note

t-PA antigen can be detected in small amounts in pre-occlusion samples but is of limited value in routine investigation[71]. Values rise four-fold in post-occlusion samples from normal individuals.

Measurement of plasminogen activator inhibitor (PAI)

Over 95% of PAI activity in plasma is due to the fast-acting inhibitor PAI-1. One unit of PAI is defined as that activity which neutralizes one unit of t-PA activity.

Functional assay

Chromogenic methods are available in kit form from several commercial sources. t-PA is added in excess to plasma to form t-PA–PAI complex plus residual t-PA;

plasminogen is added together with fibrinogen fragments to generate plasmin which is measured by its amidolytic action on substrate S2251.

Antigen assay

There is reasonable correlation between ELISA assay of PAI-1 and functional activity.

Interpretation
Normal level in plasma is 10 units/ml which can rise to 100 units/ml in the third trimester of pregnancy. PAI-1 levels are increased in many clinical situations associated with thromboembolism and assay of post-occlusion samples, in combination with the ECLT, is extremely valuable in the assessment of fibrinolytic status[71].

Measurement of histidine-rich glycoprotein (HRGP)

HRGP in plasma is readily assayed by EIA. Interest is focused on demonstrating elevated levels above the 60–155% normal range, which may lead to reduced fibrinolysis due to impaired binding of plasminogen to fibrin.

Measurement of plasminogen

Reduced levels or molecular variants of plasminogen result in diminished plasmin formation and hypofibrinolysis. Functional assay should be used for screening for plasminogen deficiency or abnormality.

Functional assay

Early measurements of plasminogen activity were made by adding activated preparations to fibrin plates previously heated to destroy endogenous plasminogen.

The lysis of casein by plasmin generated from the action of streptokinase on plasminogen and measurement of liberated tyrosine using Folin and Ciocalteau's reagent, is a more direct method of quantitation.

Activity is more easily and accurately measured using a chromogenic assay. Streptokinase is added to plasma and the plasmin generated is measured by its activity against substrate S2251 (Kabi).

Antigen assay

Plasminogen can be readily measured by most immunological methods due to its relatively high concentration in plasma. Two-dimensional crossed immunoelectrophoresis can be used to identify abnormal molecular forms of plasminogen.

Heparin assay

The clinical situations requiring the monitoring of heparin therapy and recommended methods are summarized in *Table 17.7*.

Table 17.7 Clinical situations and methods of heparin assay

Clinical situation	*Recommended methods*
Continuous heparin infusion for the prophylaxis or treatment of thrombotic episodes	Standardized APTT test
Low-dose heparin	Standardized APTT test. Amidolytic method with chromogenic substrate
Heparinization in 'bypass' surgery using extracorporeal circulation	Heparin–protamine neutralization test
Heparin therapy in the presence of a consumptive coagulopathy	Heparin–protamine neutralization. Amidolytic method with chromogenic substrate

Heparin–protamine neutralization test

Principle

The lowest amount of protamine sulphate necessary to neutralize the heparin in the test plasma is determined using a thrombin clotting time technique. The result may be expressed as heparin concentration in plasma (units/ml) or as the amount of protamine required to neutralize the total heparin content of the plasma by reference to the PCV and total blood volume.

Reagents

1. Stock solution of protamine sulphate. Dilute an ampoule of 1 g/dl protamine sulphate with imidazole buffer (*see* page 533) to give a 50 mg/dl solution (1 in 20 dilution).
2. Working protamine sulphate solutions. A range of working solutions are prepared from 5–50 mg/dl as shown in *Table 17.8*.

Table 17.8 Working protamine solutions in heparin–protamine neutralization test

	Tube									
Solution	*1*	*2*	*3*	*4*	*5*	*6*	*7*	*8*	*9*	*10*
Stock protamine, 50 mg/dl (ml)	0.1	0.2	0.3	0.4	0.5	0.6	0.7	0.8	0.9	1.0
Buffer (ml)	0.9	0.8	0.7	0.6	0.5	0.4	0.3	0.2	0.1	0
Protamine sulphate (mg/dl)	5	10	15	20	25	30	35	40	45	50

3. Thrombin. Approximately 20 NIH units/ml, adjusted so that 0.1 ml thrombin will clot 0.2 ml normal plasma at 37°C in 10 ± 1 second. Maintain dilute thrombin solution at 4°C in a plastic container.
4. Citrated test PPP.
5. Normal plasma. To control thrombin activity.

Method

To 0.2 ml test plasma is added 20 μl buffer in a 75 × 10 mm tube, warm to 37°C and add 0.1 ml thrombin and note the clotting time. If the clotting time is within 1 second of that of the normal plasma clotting time there is no demonstrable heparin content. A prolonged time indicates the presence of heparin and the test is repeated substituting 20 μl of the protamine sulphate solutions for the volume of buffer to determine the *lowest* concentration of protamine that restores the clotting time to that of the normal plasma. The small volumes of protamine sulphate are best measured and delivered using a 20 μl positive displacement pipette after carefully wiping the exterior of the capillary. Incubate the plasma and protamine mixture for 2 minutes before adding the thrombin. The initial choice of protamine concentration depends on the degree of prolongation of the thrombin time, e.g. over 50 seconds commence with 50 mg/dl and less than 50 seconds commence with 25 mg/dl. If 50 mg/dl fails to correct the thrombin time, 40 μl volumes may be used or higher concentrations of protamine prepared.

Calculations

An example of results and calculations is as follows:

Concentration of added protamine sulphate (mg/dl):	5	10	15	20	25	30	35	40	45	50
Thrombin times:	50	50	40	20	13	10	11	10	11	10

The minimum concentration that corrects the thrombin time is 30 mg/dl.

Plasma heparin level (units/ml)

1 mg heparin is equivalent to 100 units of heparin.
Weight for weight neutralization by protamine is assumed.
If 20 μl 30 mg/dl protamine is sufficient to neutralize the heparin in 0.2 ml of plasma,
then 100 μl of protamine is sufficient to neutralize the heparin in 1 ml plasma;
or 30 μg protamine is sufficient to neutralize the heparin in 1 ml plasma;
or there is 30 μg of heparin in 1 ml plasma.
If 1 mg ≡ 100 units then 30 μg = 3 units/ml.

Total plasma heparin From the above example 30 μg protamine neutralize the heparin in 1 ml plasma. Assuming a total blood volume of 70 ml/kg and, for example, a PCV of 0.400 l/l and a body weight of 80 kg then:

$$\frac{\text{concentration of protamine sulphate } (\mu g) \times \text{blood volume (ml/kg)} \times \text{body weight (kg)} \times (1 - \text{PCV}) \text{ correction to plasma volume}}{1000 \text{ (to convert } \mu g \text{ to mg)}}$$

= amount of protamine sulphate required to neutralize the circulating heparin, or by substitution:

$$\frac{30 \times 70 \times 80 \times (1 - 0.400)}{1000} = \begin{array}{l}100.8 \text{ mg protamine or} \\ 10 \text{ ml } 1 \text{ g/dl protamine sulphate}\end{array}$$

Note

With the range of protamine sulphate solutions suggested above, the limit of sensitivity is 0.5 units heparin/ml.

Assay of plasma heparin using chromogenic substrate

Heparin may be assayed using a chromogenic substrate. Two substrates can be used, S2222 (Kabi) which measures excess factor Xa after neutralization by heparin–ATIII complex, or Chromozym TH (Boerhinger) by measuring excess thrombin activity.

Principle using S-2222

Heparin + ATIII ⟶ heparin/ATIII complex

Heparin/ATIII + Xa (excess) ⟶ heparin/ATIII/Xa + residual Xa

S-2222 $\xrightarrow{\text{residual Xa}}$ peptide + *p*NA (measured at 405 nm)

Principle using Chromozym TH

Heparin + ATIII ⟶ heparin/ATIII complex

Heparin/ATIII + thrombin (excess) ⟶ heparin/ATIII/thrombin + residual thrombin

Chromozym TH $\xrightarrow{\text{residual thrombin}}$ peptide + *p*NA (measured at 405 nm)

Methods

Both methods are available in kit form. Using S-2222 the liberated pNA may be measured by initial rate or end-point techniques, with Chromozym TH an initial rate method is recommended by the manufacturer. Unless normal plasma is added to the reaction the assay of heparin assumes a normal ATIII level.

Note

The advantage of chromogenic assay is that, with the exception of ATIII, the results are not affected by the overall clotting characteristics of the test plasma.

References

1. Thomas D. P. (1988) Overview of venous thrombogenesis. *Semin. Thromb. Hemost.,* **14**, 1–8
2. Buchanan, M. R. (1988) Mechanisms of pathogenesis of arterial thrombosis: practical sites of inhibition by therapeutic compounds. *Semin. Thromb. Hemost.,* **14**, 33–40
3. Byrnes, J. J. and Moake, J. L. (1986) Thrombotic thrombocytopenic purpura and the hemolytic-uremic syndrome: evolving concepts of pathogenesis and therapy. *Clin. Haematol.,* **15**, 413–42
4. Comp, P. C. (1990) Overview of the hypercoagulable states. *Semin. Thromb. Hemostat.,* **16**, 158–61
5. Schafer, A. I. (1985) The hypercoagulable states. *Ann. Intern. Med.,* **102**, 814–28
6. Rickles, F. R. and Edwards, R. L. (1983) Activation of blood coagulation in cancer: Trousseau's syndrome revisited. *Blood,* **62**, 14–31
7. Tooke, J. E. and McNichol, G. P. (1981) Thrombotic disorders associated with pregnancy and the pill. *Clin. Haematol.,* **10**, 613–30
8. Banga, J. D. and Sixma, J. J. (1986) Diabetes mellitus, vascular disease and thrombosis. *Clin. Haematol.,* **15**, 465–92
9. Carreras, L. O. (1980) Thrombosis and thrombocytopenia induced by heparin. *Scand. J. Haematol.*, Suppl., **36**, 64–83

10. Vermylen, J., Blockman, D., Spitz, B. and Deckmyn, H. (1986) Thrombosis and immune disorders. *Clin. Haematol.,* **15**, 393–412
11. Manucci, P. M. and Tripodi, A. (1988) Inherited factors in thrombosis. *Blood Rev.,* **2**, 27–35
12. Miletich, J. P., Sherman, L. and Broze, G. (1987) Absence of thrombosis in subjects with heterozygous protein C deficiency. *N. Engl. J. Med.,* **317,** 991–5
13. Miletich, J. P. (1990) Laboratory diagnosis of protein C deficiency. *Semin. Thromb. Hemost.,* **16,** 169–76
14. Comp, P. S. (1990) Laboratory evaluation of protein S status. *Semin. Thromb. Hemost.,* **16**, 177–81
15. Tollefsen, D. M. (1990) Laboratory diagnosis of antithrombin and heparin cofactor II deficiency. *Semin. Thromb. Hemostat.,* **16**, 162–8
16. Girolami, A., Lazzaro, A. and Simioni, P. (1988) Thrombotic manifestations in plasminogen deficiency and in plasminogen abnormalities. *Thromb. Hemostat.,* **60**, 528
17. McDonagh, J. N. and Carrell, N. (1987) Disorders of fibrinogen structure and function. In *Hemostasis and Thrombosis, Basic Principles and Clinical Practice* (eds R. W. Colman, J. Hirsh, J. Marder and E. W. Salzman), pp. 301–17. Philadelphia: J. B. Lippincott
18. Kernoff, P. B. A. (1989) Thrombosis and antithrombotic therapy. In *Postgraduate Haematology* (eds A. V. Hoffbrand and S. M. Lewis), pp. 672–95. Oxford: Heinemann
19. Rodgers, G. M. and Schuman, M. A. (1986) Congenital thrombotic disorders. *Am. J. Hematol.,* **21**, 419–30
20. Nguyen, G., Horellou, M. H., Kruithof, E. K. O. *et al.* (1988) Residual plasminogen activator inhibitor activity after venous stasis as a criterion for hypofibrinolysis: a study in 83 patients with confirmed deep vein thrombosis. *Blood,* **72**, 601–5
21. Davidson, J. F. and Walker, I. (1987) Assessment of the fibrinolytic system. In *Haemostasis and Thrombosis* (eds A. L. Bloom and D. P. Thomas), pp. 953–66. New York: Churchill Livingstone
22. British Society for Haematology (1990) Guidelines on oral anticoagulation: second edition. *J. Clin. Pathol.,* **43**, 177–83
23. Biggs, R. and Denson, K. W. E. (1967) Standardisation of the one-stage prothrombin time for the control of anticoagulant therapy. *Br. Med. J.,* **i**, 84–8
24. Kirkwood, T. B. L. (1983) Calibration of reference thromboplastins and standardisation of the prothrombin time ratio. *Thromb. Haemost. (Stutt.),* **49**, 238–44
25. WHO Expert Committee on Biological Standardisation (1983) *Thirty-third Report.* WHO Technical Report Series, 687, 81–105
26. Loeliger, E. A. (1985) ICSH/ICTH recommendation for reporting prothrombin time in oral anticoagulant control. *Thromb. Haemost.,* **53**, 155–6
27. Lewis, S. M. (1987) Thromboplastin and oral anticoagulant control. *Br. J. Haematol.,* **66**, 1–4
28. WHO Expert Committee on Biological Standardisation (1977) *Twenty-eighth report.* WHO Technical Report Series 610, 14
29. WHO (1986) *Recommended Methodology for Using WHO Reference Preparations for Thromboplastin.* Geneva
30. Loeliger, E. A., Poller, L., Samama, M. *et al.* (1985) Questions and answers on prothrombin time standardisation in oral anticoagulant control. *Thromb. Haemost.,* **54**, 515–17
31. IMLS Haematology Scientific Advisory Committee (1986) Recommendations for the laboratory determination of the International Normalised Ratio. *IMLS Gazette*, November, 603–5
32. Thomas, D. P. (1981) Heparin. *Clin. Haematol.,* **10**, 443–58
33. Choay, J. (1989) Structure and activity of heparin and its fragments: an overview. *Semin. Thromb. Hemost.,* **15**, 359–64
34. Doutremepuich, C., Lalanne, M. C., Guyot, M. *et al.* (1989) Laboratory control of heparin and heparin fragment treatment: an experimental study. *Semin. Thromb. Hemost.,* **15**, 373–7
35. Racanelli, A., Hoppensteadt, D. A. and Fareed, J. (1989) *In vitro* protamine neutralisation profiles of heparins differing in source and molecular weight. *Semin. Thromb. Hemost.,* **15**, 386–9
36. Turpie, A. G. G. (1981) Antiplatelet therapy. *Clin. Haematol.,* **10,** 497–500
37. Turpie, A. G. G. (1988) Clinical studies: evidence for intervention with specific antiplatelet drugs in arterial thromboembolism. *Semin. Thromb. Hemost.,* **14**, 41–9
38. Green, D., Hougie, C., Kazmer, F. J. *et al.* (1983) Report of the working party on acquired inhibitor of coagulation: studies of the lupus anticoagulant. *Thromb. Haemost.,* **49**, 144–6

39. Kelsey, P. R., Stevenson, K. J. and Poller, L. (1984) The diagnosis of lupus anticoagulants by the activated partial thromboplastin time – the central role of phosphatidyl serine. *Thromb. Haemost.*, **52**, 172–5
40. Triplett, D. A. and Brandt, J. T. (1988) Lupus anticoagulant: misnomer, paradox, riddle epiphenomenon. *Hematol. Pathol.*, **2**, 121–43
41. Triplett, D. A. (1990) Laboratory diagnosis of lupus anticoagulants. *Semin. Thromb. Hemost.*, **16**, 182–92
42. Clyme, L. P. and White, P. F. (1988) Time dependency of lupus-like anticoagulants. *Arch. Intern. Med.*, **148**, 1060–3
43. Cassidy, P. G., Triplett, D. A. and LaDuca, F. M. (1985) Use of the agarose gel method to identify and quantitate factor VIII:C inhibitors. *Am. J. Clin. Pathol.*, **83**, 697–706
44. Lo, S. C. L., Oldmeadow, M. J., Howard, M. A. and Firkin, B. G. (1989) Comparison of laboratory tests used for identification of the lupus anticoagulant. *Am. J. Hematol.*, **30**, 213–20
45. Rauch, J. and Janoff, A. S. (1989) Distinguishing plasma lupus anticoagulants from antifactor antibodies using hexagonal phase phospholipids. 53rd Annual Meeting of American College of Rheumatology, Cincinatti, Ohio, June 12–17
46. Exner, T., Richard, K. A. and Kronenberg, H. (1978) A sensitive test demonstrating lupus anticoagulant and its behavioural patterns. *Br. J. Haematol.*, **40**, 143–51
47. Friberger, P. (1983) Synthetic peptide substrate assays in coagulation and fibrinolysis and their application on automates. *Semin. Thromb. Hemost.*, **9**, 281–300
48. Technical Data. General procedure for ELISA. Dakopatts a/s, Glostrup, Denmark
49. Han, P. and Nathan, I. V. (1987) Enzyme enhancement for the measurement of protein C. *Clin. Lab. Haematol.*, **9**, 409–13
50. Tran, T. H. and Duckert, F. (1985) Influence of heparin cofactor II (HCII) on the determination of antithrombin III (AT). *Thromb. Res.*, **40**, 571–6
51. Tollefsen, D. M. (1990) Laboratory diagnosis of antithrombin and heparin cofactor II deficiency. *Semin. Thromb. Hemost.*, **16**, 162–8
52. George, A. J. (1988) The laboratory investigation of thrombotic disorders. In *Critical Factors in Haemostasis* (eds C. E. Williams, P. E. Short, A. J. George and M. B. P. Entwhistle), pp. 120–2. Chichester: Ellis Horwood
53. Fischer, A. M., Beguin, S., Strenberg, C. and Dautzenberg, M. D. (1987) Comparative effect of heparin and heparan sulphate on two abnormal antithrombin type 3 variants. *Br. J. Haematol.*, **66**, 213–7
54. Tollefsen, D. M. and Pestka, C. A. (1985) Heparin cofactor II activity in patients with disseminated intravascular coagulation and hepatic failure. *Blood*, **66**, 769–74
55. Francis, R. B. Jr and Patch, M. J. (1983) A functional assay for protein C in plasma. *Thromb. Res.*, **32**, 605–13
56. Francis, R. B. Jr (1986) A simplified PTT-based protein C assay using the thrombin–thrombomodulin complex. *Thromb. Res.*, **41**, 337–44
57. Francis, R. B. Jr and Seyfert, U. (1987) Rapid amidolytic assay of protein C in whole plasma using an activator from the venom of *Agkistrodon contortrix*. *Am. J. Clin. Pathol.*, **87**, 619–25
58. D'Angelo, S. V., Comp, P. C., Esmon, C. T. and D'Angelo, A. (1986) Relationship between protein C antigen and anticoagulant activity during oral anticoagulation and in selected disease states. *J. Clin. Invest.*, **77**, 416–25
59. Miletich, J. P. (1990) Laboratory diagnosis of protein C deficiency. *Semin. Thromb. Hemost.*, **16**, 169–76
60. D'Angelo, A., Gilardoni, F., Seveso, M. P. *et al.* (1987) Anticoagulant and antigenic levels of protein C and protein S in patients on stabilized oral anticoagulant treatment (Abstract). *Thromb. Hemost.*, **58**, 406
61. George, A. J. (1988) The laboratory investigation of thrombotic disorders. In *Critical Factors in Haemostasis* (eds C. E. Williams, P. E. Short, A. J. George and M. B. P. Entwhistle), pp. 144–6. Chichester: Ellis Horwood
62. Comp, P. C. and Esmon, C. T. (1984) Recurrent venous thromboembolism in patients with a partial deficiency of protein S. *N. Engl. J. Med.*, **311**, 1525–8

63. Kamiya, T., Sugihara, T., Ogata, K. *et al.* (1986) Inherited deficiency of protein S in a Japanese family with recurrent venous thrombosis: a study of three generations. *Blood,* **67**, 406–10
64. Comp. P. C. (1990) Laboratory evaluation of protein S status. *Semin. Thromb. Hemost.,* **16**, 177–81
65. Comp, P. C., Doray, D., Patton, D. and Esmon, C. T. (1986) An abnormal plasma distribution of protein S occurs in functional protein S deficiency. *Blood,* **67**, 504–8
66. Woodhams, B. J. (1988) The simultaneous measurement of total and free protein S by ELISA. *Thromb. Res.,* **50**, 213–20
67. Davidson, J. F. and Walker, I. D. (1987) Assessment of the fibrinolytic system. In *Haemostasis and Thrombosis* (eds A. L. Bloom and D. P. Thomas), pp. 953–66. New York: Churchill Livingstone
68. George, A. J. (1988) The laboratory investigation of thrombotic disorders. In *Critical Factors in Haemostasis* (eds C. E. Williams, P. E. Short, A. J. George and M. B. P. Entwhistle), pp. 158–61. Chichester: Ellis Horwood
69. Kluft, C. and Brakman, P. (1975) Effect of flufenamate on euglobulin fibrinolysis: involvement of C1 inactivator. In *Progress in Chemical Fibrinolysis and Thrombolysis* (eds J. F. Davidson, M. Samama and P. C. Desnoyers), pp. 375–81. New York: Raven Press
70. Ranby, M., Sundell, I. B. and Nilsson, T. K. (1989) Blood collection in strong acidic citrate anticoagulant used in a study of dietary influence on basal t-PA activity. *Thromb. Haemost.,* **62**, 917–22
71. Bachmann, F. (1990) Laboratory diagnosis of impairment of fibrinolysis in patients with thromboembolic disease. *Semin. Thromb. Hemost.,* **16**, 193–7

Index